Textbook of Rural Medicine

Textbook of Rural Medicine

EDITORS

John P. Geyman, MD

Professor Emeritus
Department of Family Medicine
University of Washington
Seattle, Washington

Thomas E. Norris, MD, CPE

Associate Dean, University of Washington School of Medicine
Executive Director and Medical Executive
UW Physicians Network
Professor of Family Medicine
Adjunct Professor of Medicine and Biomedical Informatics
University of Washington
Seattle, Washington

L. Gary Hart, PhD

Research Professor
Director, WWAMI Rural Research Center
Department of Family Medicine
University of Washington
Seattle, Washington

McGRAW-HILL
Medical Publishing Division

New York   St. Louis   San Francisco   Auckland   Bogotá   Caracas
Lisbon   London   Madrid   Mexico City   Milan   Montreal
New Delhi   San Juan   Singapore   Sydney   Tokyo   Toronto

McGraw-Hill

A Division of The **McGraw·Hill** Companies

TEXTBOOK OF RURAL MEDICINE

1234567890 FGRFGR 09876543210

ISBN 0-07-134540-X

This book was set in Palatino by The PRD Group Inc.
The editors were Martin Wonsiewicz, Susan R. Noujaim, and Muza Navrozov.
The production supervisor was Richard Ruzycka.
The text was designed by Joan O'Connor.
Quebecor Printing/Fairfield Graphics Inc. was printer and binder.

The book is printed on recycled, acid-free paper.

Library of Congress Cataloging-in-Publication Data

Textbook of Rural Medicine/editors, John P. Geyman, Thomas E. Norris, L. Gary Hart.
    p. ; cm.
  Includes bibliographical references and index.
  ISBN 0-07-134540-X
  1. Rural health services. I. Geyman, John P., 1931-II. Norris, Thomas E. III. Hart, L.
Gary.
  [DNLM: 1. Rural Health Services.   2. Rural Health. WA 390 T3548 2000]
RA771.T49 2000
362.1'04257--dc21
                                                              99-088756

Contents

Contributors

Note: Numbers in brackets following the contributor's name refer to chapters written or cowritten by the contributor.

DAVID A. ACOSTA, MD [8, 9]
Associate Director, Tacoma
Family Medicine
Clinical Associate Professor
Department of Family Medicine
University of Washington
Seattle, Washington

JAMES R. BLACKMAN, MD [22]
Assistant Dean, Regional Affairs
  and Rural Health
University of Washington
Seattle, Washington

NANCY CAMPBELL-HEIDER, PhD, RN [4]
Associate Professor
School of Nursing
Project Director, Family Nurse Practitioner Program
State University of New York at Buffalo
Buffalo, New York

KATHERINE HILL CHAVIGNY, PhD,
  FACE [29]
Consultant, China Medical Board
Portland, Oregon

JOHN B. COOMBS, MD [20]
Associate Vice President
Medical Affairs for Clinical Systems and Networks
University of Washington
Seattle, Washington

IAN D. COUPER, MBBCh, BA [28]
Department of Family Medicine
Medical University of South Africa
Durban, South Africa

JENNIFER DEAVILLE, PhD [27]
Institute of Rural Health
Newtown, Powys
Wales, United Kingdom

JOHN DEWAR, MD [12]
Clinical Assistant Professor
Department of Family Medicine
Canton, New York

SHERRILYNNE S. FULLER, PhD [15]
Associate Professor and Head
Division of Biomedical Informatics
Department of Medical Education
University of Washington
Seattle, Washington

JOHN P. GEYMAN, MD [23]
Professor Emeritus
Department of Family Medicine
University of Washington
Seattle, Washington

PAUL GORMAN, MD [15]
Assistant Professor
Division of Medical Informatics
  and Outcomes Research
Oregon Health Sciences University
Portland, Oregon

L. GARY HART, PhD [3, 6]
Research Professor
Director, WWAMI Rural Research Center
Department of Family Medicine
University of Washington
Seattle, Washington

RICHARD B. HAYS, MBBS, PhD, FRACGP [26]
Professor of General Practice and Rural Health
Chair of General Practice and Rural Health
James Cook University
School of Medicine
Townsville, Queensland, Australia

PETER J. HOUSE, MHA [21]
Director, Programs for Healthy Communities
Clinical Assistant Professor
Department of Family Medicine
University of Washington
Seattle, Washington

JEFFREY HUMMEL, MD, MPH [5]
Clinical Instructor
Division of General Internal Medicine
University of Washington
Seattle, Washington
Clinic Chief
University of Washington Physicians Network
Seattle, Washington

CHRISTINA A. KUENNETH, MPH [14]
Research Analyst
UC Davis Health System
Office of Rural and Regional Alliances
  and Telehealth
Sacramento, California

JOHN WYNN-JONES, FRCGP [27]
Institute of Rural Health
Newtown, Powys
Wales, United Kingdom

WALTER L. LARIMORE, MD [19]
Associate Clinical Professor
Department of Family Medicine
University of South Florida
Kissimmee, Florida

ERIC H. LARSON, PhD [3]
Associate Director for Research
WWAMI Rural Health Center
Department of Family Medicine
University of Washington
Seattle, Washington

DONALD A. B. LINDBERG, MD [15]
Director, National Library of Medicine
National Institutes of Health
Bethesda, Maryland

DANA CHRISTIAN LYNGE, MD [10]
Assistant Professor
Department of Surgery
University of Washington
Seattle, Washington
Staff Surgeon
Division of General Surgery
VA Puget Sound Health Care System
Seattle, Washington

DAVID MASUDA, MD, MS [15]
Acting Instructor
Division of Biomedical Informatics
Department of Medical Education
University of Washington
Seattle, Washington

IAN R. McWHINNEY, MD, FRCGP,
  FCFP, FRCP [11]
Professor Emeritus
The University of Western Ontario
Department of Family Medicine
Center for Studies in Family Medicine
London, Ontario, Canada

PETER M. MILGROM, DDS [13]
Professor and Director
Dental Fears Research Clinic
Department of Dental Public Health Sciences
University of Washington
Seattle, Washington

IRA MOSCOVICE, PhD [17]
Rural Health Research Center
Division of Health Services Research and Policy
University of Minnesota
Minneapolis, Minnesota

IAIN J. MUNGALL, FRCGP [27]
Institute of Rural Health
Greynog
Newtown, Powys
Wales, United Kingdom

THOMAS S. NESBITT, MD, MPH [14]
Medical Director
UC Davis Health System
Offices of Rural and Regional Alliances
  and Telehealth
Sacramento, California

Contributors

VANESSA NOBLE, BA [28]
Department of History
University of Natal
Durban, South Africa

THOMAS E. NORRIS, MD, CPE [16]
Associate Dean, University of Washington
School of Medicine
Executive Director and Medical Executive
UW Physicans Network
Professor of Family Medicine
Adjunct Professor of Medicine
  and Biomedical Informatics
University of Washington
Seattle, Washington

SUSAN REHM, MBA [19]
Manager of Practice Development
American Academy of Family Physicians
Leawood, Kansas

THOMAS C. ROSENTHAL, MD [4]
Professor and Chair
Department of Family Medicine
State University of New York at Buffalo
Buffalo, New York

STEPHEN J. REID, BSc, MBChB [28]
Centre for Health and Social Studies
University of Natal
Durban, South Africa

HUIMAN REN, MD [29]
President and Professor
Xi' Medical University
People's Republic of China

THOMAS C. RICKETTS, PhD [2]
Deputy Director
Cecil G. Sheps Center for Health Services Research
Associate Professor of Health Policy and Administration
School of Public Health
The University of North Carolina at Chapel Hill
Chapel Hill, North Carolina

ROGER A. ROSENBLATT, MD, MPH [1]
Professor and Vice Chair
Department of Family Medicine
University of Washington
School of Medicine
Seattle, Washington

THOMAS C. ROSENTHAL, MD [4]
Professor and Chair
Department of Family Medicine
State University of New York at Buffalo
Buffalo, New York

JAMES T. B. ROURKE, MD, MCISc,
  CCFP(EM) [25]
Associate Professor
Department of Family Medicine
The University of Western Ontario
Director, Southwestern Ontario Rural Medicine
Education, Research and Development Unit
Goderich, Ontario, Canada

M. ROY SCHWARZ, MD [29]
President, China Medical Board
China Medical Board
New York, New York

JEFFREY A. STEARNS, MD [24]
Associate Professor of Family and Community Medicine
Director, Rural Medical Education Program
University of Illinois College of Medicine-Rockford
Rockford, Illinois

PATRICIA TAYLOR, PhD [6]
Washington, DC

DAVID TISHENDORF, BJ [13]
Martin & Tishendorf
Seattle, Washington

FRASER TUDIVER, MD [12]
Sunnybrook Health Science Center
North York, Ontario, Canada

ANTHONY WELLEVER, MPA [17]
Rural Health Research Center
Division of Health Services Research and Policy
University of Minnesota
Minneapolis, Minnesota

ROBERT L. WILLIAMS, MD, MPH [21]
Department of Family and Community Medicine
University of New Mexico
Albuquerque, New Mexico

HAROLD A. WILLIAMSON, Jr., MD, MSPH [7]
Professor and Chair
Department of Family and Community Medicine
University of Missouri-Columbia School of Medicine
Columbia, Missouri

Contributors

L. THOMAS WOLFF, MD [12]
Department of Family Medicine
State University of New York
Syracuse, New York

GEORGE E. WRIGHT, PhD [18]
Associate Professor
WWAMI Rural Health Research Center
University of Washington
Seattle, Washington

JOHN WYNN-JONES, FRCGP [27]
General Practitioner and CME Tutor
Director of the Institute of Rural Health
Wales, United Kingdom

ZHOADA ZHANG, MD [29]
President and Professor
West China University of Medical Sciences
People's Republic of China

Foreword

*T*he birth of a new century is not unlike the birth of a child. It is cause for celebration, a time for forgetting the nausea and backaches of pregnancy and the pains of childbirth, a time for planning an environment that will support the healthy development of the new infant. This book, launched at the turn of the twenty-first century, is an attempt to look ahead in reassessing the critical issues in *rural* health and *rural* health care. While there is careful thought given to what has led us to this point in history—and it is essential to get our facts right about this—the goal is to lay out directions that can address the important challenges that lie ahead.

Rurality, as complex and varied as it is around the globe, has much to do with scarcity—the scarcity of resources (people, money, technical support) and the scarcity of alternatives or options. Past solutions have tended to emphasize various ways to *access* services, a critical need in the future as well as in the past. But as this book indicates, access may be the least of the important issues that need to be addressed. The significant risks to good health relate more closely to socioeconomic, behavioral, genetic, and environmental issues than to the availability of health care services. This is equally true for rural and urban sites, and for both settings too little has been done to address these adequately.

Another fundamental concern is the need for integrated community development. Health is not an island. One cannot separate good health from decent education, viable jobs, a sustainable environment, government that works for the needs of people, and the emotional/spiritual well-being, which comes from having a sense of control over the vagaries of life. How these things play out in rural settings, and how aggressive the attempts are to address each of them in turn, has much to do with rural health status.

Much has been made in the past of the possibility that *rural* solutions to today's problems might become a model for urban and global solutions to modern life. Indeed, the relatively small scale and limited scope of rural challenges might lead to manageable approaches that could not be tackled in more complex and densely populated regions. Issues of individual rights versus the broader public good offer a particular promise in this light. Much of the progress in rural health during recent years has explored such an agenda. Examples are in the development of improved transportation, communication, and precare programs, rather than expansion of specialty health services to rural communities. Therein lie many of the policy issues and agendas that need to be addressed as we progress into the new century.

Those who are interested in rural health should swim the widest river and climb the highest mountain for this book! No prior publication has attempted to address such a comprehensive list of issues, addressed to so many audiences. One will find here information that is relevant and current on clinical care, education and training for physicians and other rural practitioners, health system organization and management, and rural health policy in America and other parts of the world. The editors have chosen authors for the individual chapters who have devoted a professional lifetime to exploring some of the most critical issues in rural health and rural health care. In so doing, each chapter stands out as part of a larger tour de force on one of the last century's most perplexing and important challenges and one of our greatest future opportunities.

Thomas Allen Bruce, M.D.,
  D.Sc. (hon), F.A.C.P., F.A.C.C.
Professor Emeritus and former Dean
  of the College of Medicine
University of Arkansas
  for Medical Sciences, Little Rock
Program Consultant and Adviser, W. K. Kellogg Foundation
Battle Creek, Michigan.

Preface

Why a book on rural health care? Many reasons, not the least of which is that there has been so little published work on this often neglected but important part of the nation's health care system. In the United States, about 20 percent of Americans live in rural areas (over 50 million people), while only 9 percent of the nation's physicians practice there. The challenges of rural health care are formidable and often quite different in both kind and scale to health care in metropolitan areas. Health care providers in rural settings must be generalists, often facing difficult situations with few resources, and must do the best they can to provide the best possible quality of care. There has been a tendency for many years for health professionals to settle preferentially in metropolitan areas, so that federal and state governments have had a need to develop varied strategies in an effort to promote the choice of rural practice, as well as retention there, for health professionals.

Rural America is in transition, and many of the old stereotypes of rural life and health care are no longer valid. In some areas, rural populations have stopped declining and are growing. Farming and some of the extractive industries have been in decline, but manufacturing and other more technological occupations are on the increase in many rural areas. Rural America has become more diverse than ever before, and the needs for improvements in rural health care have never been more important.

This book is the first of its kind to explore and update what is now known about the content, needs, and special problems of rural health care. Our goal is to then move beyond that knowledge base to profile strategies that have been found useful by various rural health professionals in developing improved quality of care for rural communities and their residents. Our target audience includes clinicians representing varied disciplines practicing in rural areas, as well as clinician-teachers, residents in training, medical students with rural health interests, and other health professionals interested in rural health care. This book should also be of value for health services researchers and others interested in health policy and the special problems of rural health care.

As editors, all three of us have had extensive experience and a long-standing interest in rural health care. Two of us (JPG and TEN) have together practiced over 30 years in rural settings, with more than 20 years' experience teaching in family practice residency programs particularly oriented to the training of rural family physicians. The third editor (LGH) has spent over 20 years in policy-oriented research of rural health care and heads the Rural Health Research Center at the University of Washington School of Medicine.

Initial attention is focused on an overview of rural health care, including the patients, providers, communities, population-based care, and research directions. Next we examine special clinical problems and approaches in rural health care, including emergency and obstetric care, surgery, mental health, dental care, and home care. We then direct our attention to organization and management of rural health care, including rural hospitals, regional networks, economics and practice management, telehealth, medical informatics, and approaches to quality improvement and community-oriented primary care. Finally, we focus on education for rural practice and lessons which can be learned from five different countries elsewhere in the world also dealing with the challenges of serving the health care needs of rural citizens.

To the extent that this book leads to greater interest and understanding of rural health needs and promotes more active strategies to improve the quality of care for rural people, this book will have been a success.

John P. Geyman, MD
Thomas E. Norris, MD, CPE
L. Gary Hart, PhD
Seattle, Washington

PART ONE

Overview of Rural Health Care

*T*he purpose of Part I is to provide an overview of the rural health care milieu, from the changing economic, demographic, and social populations who live in rural places through the providers who practice there to the issues and processes that result in the federal policies that heavily influence the rural health care delivery system. Having an understanding of the larger rural situation is essential for sound judgment when one is making decisions about individual care, local public health, or federal policy changes.

Chapter 1 provides a broad overview of the rural environment and its health needs, presented in broad and integrative brush-strokes, with an emphasis on the overlap between the physical environment, national health care delivery trends, the rural population, and the health care needs of rural residents. Chapter 2 is devoted to describing the nation's rural population in terms of its demography, socioeconomic status, health insurance coverage, health status, and access to and use of the health care delivery system. The distribution of rural physicians and issues associated with it as well as the importance of teamwork between them and different types of providers in effective rural health care delivery are described in Chaps. 3 and 4. Chapter 5 describes how practice in rural communities lends itself to evidence-based medical practice and public health interventions. It provides the framework and tools for this difficult but often health-promoting practice orientation. Finally, Chap. 6 provides an overview of some of the issues and processes associated with federal policies regarding rural health care delivery during the past two decades and into the future.

In some cases, issues that might have been placed within Part I are found in following parts of this text, especially in Part III, "Organization and Management of Rural Health Care," and Part IV, "Education for Rural Practice." Portions of many chapters provide the substance that fills in much of the detail briefly touched upon in this broad overview of the rural health care setting. For instance, Part III includes a series of chapters on the organization and management of rural health care that address specific issues such as hospitals, telehealth, and economics that are covered here in Part I.

The chapters of Part I provide an overview that allows the reader to better understand how the chapters of Parts II through V fit into the complicated rural health care mosaic. In addition, they spotlight those aspects of rural health care delivery that are markedly different from their urban counterparts.

L. Gary Hart

The Health of Rural People and the Communities and Environments in Which They Live

ROGER A. ROSENBLATT

*T*he elderly Native American woman visited the Indian Health Service doctor in Nespelem, a small market town on the Colville Indian Reservation in eastern Washington, where the Public Health Service clinic is located. She wheezed and clutched her chest, alarming the young doctor and the nurse helping him.

The electrocardiograms and chest x-rays were negative. Further history elicited the fact that the woman lived near Battle Mountain, a remote peak high in the Okanogan highlands, which a multinational corporation was proposing to pulverize with explosives in order to leach out gold with cyanide. The woman had already lived through three federally inspired contractions of the Colville Indian Reservation, each instigated when the dominant white culture found something of value they wished to exploit: gold, timber, water rights, soil. Now they were planning to destroy the mountain where she lived, leaving a million tons of poisoned water where the trout used to run. The Indian Health Service doctor prescribed a bronchodilator, commiserated with the woman, and wondered what he could possibly do in a land riddled with clear-cuts, cyanide-laced tailings, and polluted rivers.[1]

BEGINNING AT THE BEGINNING— DEFINING WHAT WE MEAN BY RURAL

Rural America is as diverse as the people who live in it. From American Indians on western reservations to the glitterati gracing the slopes of Aspen to African-American teenagers in the Mississippi delta, rural America defies simplification. Rural inhabitants are young and old, rich and poor, immigrants and aboriginal descendants, and they come in every hue in the human genetic palette.

What connects them—and what makes it both reasonable and important to write a book about their health care—is the fact that rural communities share certain characteristics that affect both health and health care. Rural areas are characterized by their remoteness from large cities and by their relatively small populations. In a world in which most people live in large metropolitan areas, rural dwellers are those who continue to live in smaller places. And in making this choice, rural dwellers do without ready access to the dense net of services— including health services—that characterizes the urban environment.

Rural America is part of a continuum that begins in isolated Athabascan villages on the Alaskan tundra and extends to relatively large and sophisticated market towns on the U.S. mainland. In parts of the world like South Africa or China, rural townships far from the cities have a high population density, although there may be no recognizable city center and few if any services. For the purposes of this text, we use the convention most common in American demography: rural areas are defined as those places outside of "urbanized areas," where an urbanized area is defined as a "continuously built-up area with a population of 50,000 or more."[2]

But we acknowledge that this definition is in many ways arbitrary. It should be noted that even the Census Bureau's statistical definition of *rural* is controversial and that different components of the federal government use different approaches to the definition of *rural*.[2] As we enter the twenty-first century, the whole concept of spatial isolation becomes more problematic, buffeted as we are by the explosion of communication technologies and increasing globalization in the manufacture and sale of everything, from hair spray to dialysis machines. It is entirely possible that this will be the last century in which it will make sense to write a textbook on rural health. As fiberoptic and satellite networks extend their electronic tendrils to distant corners of the globe, the very notion of isolation and separation will be transformed.

Yet, for the moment, "rural America" comprises identifiable places with common sets of problems and potentials. From the volunteer ambulance corps that brings patients to the door of the rural emergency room to the regional medical center that trains the doctors, rural patients and practitioners grapple with a spectrum of similar issues as they strive to maintain health, prevent disease, and deal with the inevitable illnesses that we all share.

THE INTERSECTION BETWEEN LIVING IN A RURAL AREA AND HEALTH

The Health Status of Rural Populations

After one controls for population characteristics such as age, gender, and race, rural populations are, in general, neither sicker nor healthier than people living in urban areas.[3] But rural people have some unique health care needs that derive from specific rural environments and the nature of the residents of these areas.

Health care status is exquisitely sensitive to sociodemographic factors. Who you are—your age, ethnicity, race, education, gender, marital status, and occupation—has much more to do with your health than your proximity to doctors, hospitals, or other people.[4] Because of the diversity of rural areas, it is both impossible and inaccurate to state that rural populations are more or less healthy than their urban counterparts.

The more relevant observation is that certain rural communities, by virtue of the characteristics of the people that live there, are exposed to greater hazard or carry a disproportionate burden of disease. There are certain industries that are almost entirely rural in nature and are particularly dangerous to the people who pursue them. Forestry is a good example of a dangerous calling, from the people who fell trees to the saw operators who cut them up. Exposure to toxic herbicides and pesticides is a problem endemic to farm workers, particularly those who work on field crops that require periodic spraying.[5]

But the extractive industries related to agriculture and mining no longer employ large portions of the rural population and thus have a statistically negligible effect on the health status of aggregate rural populations. These industries have a tremendous impact on the character of rural environments and thus affect health indirectly, as we shall see later in this chapter. But because the occupational patterns of rural areas are rapidly converging with those in urban areas, the traditional link between rural location, specific occupations, and their health consequences has been broken. It remains critical to investigate the health risks within specific communities, but it is crucial to individualize both the approach and the response to the issues in any specific community.

The more significant impact on health for specific rural populations comes not from occupation but from socioeconomic status. At the risk of oversimplification, there has been an increased widening in the economic fortunes of rural America. Certain rural areas—blessed by climate, geography, and the patina of popularity—have become boom communities, with skyrocketing real estate prices and a broad array of services.[6] These services include sophisticated health care systems and often a full retinue of medical and surgical specialists, lured not only by the quality of life but by a clientele that can afford to pay for the very best.

At the same time, another set of rural communities is literally withering, depopulated by the decline in the fortunes of agriculture and by a change in the way primary agricultural products are produced. Farms have grown steadily larger throughout the century, and mechanization has reduced the number of workers needed to grow soybeans, cut trees, or make paper. In places without the ability to attract tourists or wealthy retirees, children leave for education and jobs and rarely come back. These are the places that face a constant struggle to maintain even their basic services, and complex, capital-intensive services like those needed to produce medical care are often the most vulnerable.

As Ricketts points out in Chap. 2, there are no overall differences in broad patterns of mor-tality and morbidity when one compares urban and rural counties; that in itself is a triumph of modern public health and health care. But if one were to break the rural amalgam down into its many facets, it would be evident that health status is directly tied to income, education, employment, race, and ethnicity. Rural areas with large minority populations, high unemployment, poor education, and meager incomes have impaired health status, stemming from both the increased stress and the risks that go with social disadvantage.[7]

As we examine health and health care in rural areas, it is useful to keep in mind the path-breaking work presented in the book *Why Are Some People Healthy and Others Not? The Determinants of Health of Populations.*[4] As seen in Fig. 1-1, the health of an individual or a group of individuals is both the cause and the consequence of a range of factors, from genetic endowment to environmental threat. The truth of this relationship is even more plain in the rural environment, because there the causal interplay is often evident on the surface, as in the case with which we began this chapter.

This revelation—which has some of the power and potential of biblical truth—carries important implications for those who would

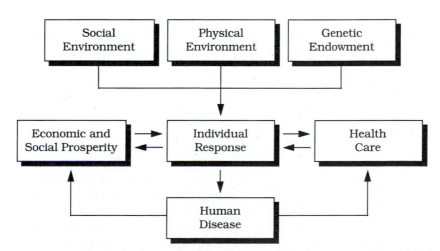

FIGURE 1-1 *The Multifactoral causes of human disease. (Adapted from Evans RG, Barer ML, Marmor TR: Why Are Some People Healthy and Others Not? The Determinants of Health of Populations. New York, Aldine de Gruyter, 1994, p 53.)*

understand and provide rural health care. Although little can be done about the genetic endowment (although even this is not immutable), the physical and social environment are human constructs and therefore every bit as malleable as the spectrum and complexity of the health care system. In the same way, well-being and prosperity are the products of human organization, particularly in the way the fruits of economic activities are distributed among people. As we work to improve the well-being of rural people, we need to devote time to all aspects of the equation.

As we acknowledge the larger truths that proclaim the close ties between social organization, the distribution of wealth, and individual health status, we should not forget the quite distinct subpopulations of rural America. These populations have special health problems that derive from either their occupational status or their cultural identity or some combination of the two. Although America may be seen as a huge cultural Waring blender, the spread of WalMart stores and McDonald's outlets does not eradicate all differences between population groups.[8]

Even with the decline of the resource-based extractive industries—such as agriculture, forestry, and mining—these economic activities are almost exclusively practiced in rural places. Because all of these pursuits wrest goods from the ground, they involve hard work, exposure to potentially toxic chemicals and dangerous natural products, and increased rates of traumatic injury. Special occupational health concerns such as the safety of tractors or the appropriate use of herbicides and pesticides require cooperation between those who study occupational health and those who provide rural health care. In areas where extractive industries remain important, the health care system and the public health system must incorporate these concerns.

Rural Populations with Special Health Needs

Other distinct communities exist within rural America, based on cultural and ethnic factors rather than occupational ones. American Indians were an exclusively rural people at the time of European settlement, and the renaissance of many Indian tribes during the last decade has its base on the rural reservations, to which the Indians were confined 100 years ago. Because Indian peoples generally own land collectively and have deep-seated cultural ties to the land and its use, they have a vested interest in maintaining the physical and functional integrity of the land they manage. With this as a base, tribes have become involved in issues that relate to the sustainability of rural lifestyles and the public health and environmental issues that affect human lives.

At the same time, Indians living in rural areas have relatively high burdens of disease, often due to the total disruption of their traditional lives after European contact. Having survived the genocidal policies of early governments and the settlers they sponsored, the Indians, not surprisingly, have borne a disproportionate burden of infectious disease, alcoholism, and mental illness. The creation of the Indian Health Service soon after World War II began a process of bringing health services to these scattered rural enclaves, and the Indian Health Care Improvement Act (PL 94-437) gave the Indians their first opportunity to provide health services for themselves.[9] Indian health remains a major subarea of rural health care in general and an area where the intersection of two cultures will create opportunities both for creativity and for ongoing conflict.

A second population group with a very high rural representation is that of migrant agricultural workers.[10] Much of American agriculture is based on the availability of cheap labor, both seasonal and permanent. Because American citizens are unwilling to perform the poorly compensated, arduous labor associated with seasonal agricultural work, this work has been done largely by streams of migrants who follow the crops from south to north as they ripen in the spring and summer. As a result, there are millions of people, many living in small rural agricultural areas, whose lives revolve around the crops.

This group is critical to the study of rural health because they, like the Indians, exist outside the dominant cultural system. Although the majority of these workers are Hispanic, they are by no means homogeneous. There are at least three distinct migrant streams in the United States, and each tends to draw its core of workers from clusters of workers in different distant countries, from Mexico and Central America in the West to Puerto Rico in the Northeast. Grafted onto the dominant Hispanic stream are other cultural groups who share much of the misery and dislocation of the Hispanic migrants.

The health consequences of migrant labor are enormous; this topic deserves a book of its own. Poverty exacts its own price, but it is complicated by substandard housing, an itinerant lifestyle, and grueling labor. Migrants, even those who "settle out" and become full-time residents of the communities where they work, tend to live at the fringes of the dominant society. Educational opportunities for children are limited, and both agricultural producers and consumers have a vested interest in maintaining a cheap, mobile, and docile labor force. It is no surprise that these migrant populations experience a disproportionate share of disease.

Just as in the case of the American Indian, the federal government has created a rudimentary health care system for migrant laborers. The migrant health clinics sponsored by the federal government provide some health care for these populations, but the funding is far short of the amount needed to provide ongoing care. The whole issue of migrant health is further complicated by controversies over immigration. Since many of the migrants are undocumented aliens, they are often reluctant to seek care even when it is available. Solutions tend to rely upon local community leaders who are able to craft creative health care programs that meld public and private programs and bridge the tension and hostility that often exist between the private health care system and the health centers created under federal and state sponsorship.

The third and probably largest of the cultural groups with a disproportionate rural presence is African Americans in the rural South.[11] If the problems of the Indian stem from colonialization and the problems of the migrant from economic exploitation, the problems of rural African Americans can be traced directly to slavery. Even today, almost 150 years after the Emancipation Proclamation, there are large rural communities of people who live in segregated poverty, with poor schools, rudimentary health care, and limited opportunities. Although segregation and slavery no longer exist as legal entities, there are literally millions of people whose economic and social horizons are shaped by the legacy of hundreds of years of indenture.

The problem is complicated in rural areas again by the lack of services. Although health care has improved throughout rural America, the health care system in most towns is designed to accommodate the employed middle class. With high unemployment and underemployment rates among rural African Americans, health care opportunities are limited. The Community and Migrant Health Programs of the federal government again sponsor clinics in these rural outposts, but the supply of care only begins to approximate the depths of need.

All three of these rural groups share some central defining characteristics: poverty, isolation, and cultural apartness. Each group has suffered significant discrimination and exploitation and continues to live apart from the dominant culture. Although health care is only one of the social services needed for members of these cultural groups to thrive, it is a critical and important part. The federal government and some state governments have tried to use their scarce resources to build health care programs, but these tend to remain at the fringes of the established systems, without the resources needed to provide even rudimentary care to all who need it.

The challenge for those involved in rural health is to try to weave these groups into the existing health care systems. The growth of managed care networks paradoxically makes the problem more difficult, since distant corporations, particularly those driven by profit, have little incentive to create health care programs for those who cannot afford to pay for care.[12] Responsibility thus shifts increasingly to state governments, where entrenched prejudice and the economic self-interest of developers and agribusiness may prevent any significant disruption of the exploitative status quo. The only practical solution is likely to be adoption of some sort of universal health care entitlement that allows even these disenfranchised groups to buy medical care in the open market, thus giving them the purchasing power that will encourage provider groups to make care available.

HEALTH CARE SYSTEMS IN RURAL AREAS

The interlocking determinants of health summarized by Fig. 1-1 apply to all people, no matter where they live. The genetic endowment of rural populations in the United States does not differ substantially from that of their urban counterparts. As we have discussed above, rural places do differ from urban places in the physical context, although the differences even among rural areas are so great that it is difficult to make meaningful summary comments. Although the vaunted rural independence may persist among some populations in some places, there is certainly no evidence that rural people have personalities that differ from those of people living in cities.

The most dramatic difference between rural and urban areas from the perspective of the determinants of health and disease is in the construction of the local health care system. Health care is one of the most complex, technologically demanding, and capital-intensive activities in which human beings are engaged. Producing the full range of health care is far more complex than building a computer or even a spacecraft and consumes a much larger proportion of the nation's wealth.

Thus it is totally impossible for any rural area, no matter how wealthy or sophisticated, to provide locally all the medical care the local population needs or will consume. Even in the most remote and impoverished U.S. village, substantial care either comes from outside the community or is sought by people traveling to obtain care. We know from our research that although rural populations may use somewhat lower levels of health care services than urban dwellers, the differences are relatively small. The big contrast is in where the care takes place: while urban residents can find most of their medical care close to home, rural residents must often travel for essential services.

The major consequence of this relationship is that rural areas must devise methods to ensure that local patients have access to a full range of services irrespective of the point of delivery.[13] In an ideal system, the rural health care system provides a logical portal to the larger health care system. The ideal system, of course, does not exist. The real world is much less disciplined, and rural people at times go elsewhere for care they could have received at home and go without care because it is unavailable locally. However, the goal is to enable rural people to receive the same spectrum of care as their urban counterparts.

The most difficult decision involves the package of services that should be available locally. At one time, not that distant, this decision was simple. Small towns were served by general practitioners (GPs) working in solo practices. The scope of practice of the GP became the service configuration available to the town. Larger towns might have several GPs, but both specialization and cooperation were rare, and more doctors did not necessarily mean a broader range of services.

Today, the solo general practitioner is an anachronism. The very notion that one individual could have either the knowledge or the fortitude to provide continuous services to any population of people has disappeared from American medicine. Even in those rare cases where individual doctors work alone, they almost invariably share parts of their professional lives, from after-hours call to hospital attending responsibilities to peer review. For roughly the second half of the twentieth century, medical practice in the rural United States has revolved around group practice, usually composed of two to five family physicians or general practitioners at the core. This group would often be complemented by nonphysician practitioners such as physician assistants or nurse practitioners and might include selected specialists such as a general surgeon or obstetrician-gynecologist.

As this book is being written, a second major transition is occurring in the organizational nature of rural practice: the growth of practice networks, a topic covered in detail in Chap. 17.[12] Whereas the rural group practice had its organizational base within the rural community, rural networks often have their headquarters in a large rural referral center or in an urban center that has historically served as a referral center for the rural town. Whether through voluntary amalgamation or by purchase, the rural group practice is slowly but inexorably becoming part of organizations whose governance, values, and objectives rest in the hands of people who no longer live in the local community.

The result of these changes is that decisions about how to provide services to rural communities have moved further away from the communities themselves.[14] When communities were served by solo practitioners, there was an intimate and reciprocal relationship between practitioner and patient. Each depended on the other to a very large extent, payment was in cash or kind, and there were very few intermediaries between the patient and the doctor. As both medicine and society have become more complex, the relationship has become both more complex and more distant. Today, even in the smallest rural community, medical care decisions are the product of the choices not only of the individual patient but also of distant insurance companies, managed care plans, emergency medical service districts, and state and federal regulators.

We should be careful not to overly romanticize the beneficent rural GP in the Norman Rockwell painting, sitting in calm and dignified

repose by the child's bed. The GP is probably sitting so still because he has fallen asleep; after being on call for the last three nights, he is exhausted. In addition, he has little to offer the family except the comfort of his presence while the child's body fights whatever illness afflicts him. Today's rural doctors may work for distant corporations that pay their salaries, but by virtue of being cogs in a much larger wheel, they can tap into a vast array of resources in addressing their patients' problems. It is for these reasons that the medical care rural people receive more and more resembles that of their urban cousins.

This increase in complexity and capability does not come without cost. The problem for the rural community is that critical decisions about local health care reside in other people's hands, and the decisions that are made may be shaped by forces insensitive to—or ignorant of—the needs of rural communities. Rural hospitals may shrink or be closed because they no longer make sense within a larger corporate strategy, although they might have been profitable as independent entities run by nonprofit local governing boards.[15] Physicians may enter or leave a community depending on the personnel strategies of a multisite practice, rather than because of recruitment enticements offered by local groups of concerned citizens. And insurance products may appear and disappear as rapidly as a summer storm, driven by their relative profitability in rural areas rather than by any particular change in the composition or demand of the rural market.

The same forces that are buffeting rural areas exist, with a vengeance, in urban markets as well. The primary difference, and it is a critical one, is that many rural communities are dominated by one major provider of service. Where the urban dweller may be inconvenienced when his or her insurance plan changes coverage, there are always alternatives. This may not be true in a rural area. And where the urban patient can choose among hospitals and doctors, the rural patient can often exercise that choice only by getting in the car and driving to another town. Competition, which is the fundamental tenet of America's approach to health care, may be more of a concept than a reality in many rural areas. And the often convulsive gyrations of large corporations in search of profit may batter small rural communities, much as the rutting of elks endangers smaller organisms unfortunate enough to be in the way.

The major challenge during this next phase of rural health care will be to develop mechanisms that give local people some measure of input into and control of the health care decisions that are being made on their behalf.[16] Short of the establishment of a national health care system—a mirage that fades into the distance every time we step in its direction—this will require new governance structures for old organizational forms. One possibility would be for private health care corporations to allow public representatives to sit on their boards and in so doing speak for their rural constituents. Regulatory controls on health care organizations might also be used to ensure that rural communities have some say in shaping their health care systems. Although rural patients have in many cases benefited from the stability and breadth of care provided by these larger corporate structures, the cost has been a loss of local control. Whether the bargain has been for good or ill, the trend toward greater consolidation is an inexorable consequence of the increasing complexity of the medical endeavor.

THE CHANGING NATURE OF RURAL AMERICA

The nature of rural life is changing rapidly in the United States, and these changes will have pervasive influences on rural health care needs and the anatomy of the rural health care delivery system. The defining demographic characteristic of rural life is low population density. As the population of the United States grows, driven by natural increase and high immigration rates, rural areas also gain population. More and more towns that were previously defined as "rural" using the standard Census Bureau definitions now pass the threshold into demographic urbanity, an acknowledgment that the density of population has created urban conditions through growth. And the majority of other communities still within the rural demographic boundaries have added substantial population.

These trends are widespread but spotty. As mentioned earlier, those agricultural communities without other economic pursuits and that lack recreational amenities are shrinking in many parts of the country. Changes in the economic vitality of different rural areas have created an environment of boom and bust; both situations present significant problems for those who manage and live in rural communities.

Communities that are shrinking in size have the problem of demographic instability complicated by a dwindling economic base. In the health care arena, demographic decline is accompanied by loss of basic services. Since health care is a complex labor- and capital-intensive undertaking, it is extremely sensitive to changes in the structure, wealth, and size of the market population. Hospital closure and physician loss are the two most immediate and potentially catastrophic consequences for these communities, and there are no simple solutions for towns facing this kind of involutional spiral.[17]

But the booming communities have their own problems. Much of the rural economic boom is driven by the recreational community, tourists, retirees, and the explosion of second homes.[6] Rapid population growth can be extremely destabilizing, particularly in rural communities that have traditionally been hostile to any meaningful form of growth regulation or land use planning. Although new residents, both temporary and permanent, bring money into the community, the jobs that are created are usually low-paying service jobs, offering little real opportunity for individual growth. And the ravages of development—sprawl and crassly commercial franchises that metastasize in the rural landscape—destroy the charm and integrity of the towns they afflict.

The end result is developmental polarization: collapsing rural communities at one extreme and metastatic suburban sprawl at the other. These forces, especially in the absence of any meaningful land use planning, often overwhelm more deliberate attempts to plan for basic services, such as health. If we conceptualize health in the broadest sense, we must recognize that rapid population fluxes in either direction are destabilizing.

The only antidote to this disequilibrium exists at the state and national levels. First, population stabilization is critical, not only for the planet but for the communities where people settle. This will require a combination of family planning services and immigration control to harness the continuing population explosion. Although this is not a problem usually appreciated in the rural context, rural communities are not immune to the problems caused by uncontrolled population growth.

Second, state and federal economic policies must mandate rational land use planning if we are to preserve the cultural and physical uniqueness of different rural communities. Although collective action is in some ways antithetical to American capitalism, there must be a meaningful balance between the rights of the individual to develop land and the rights of the community to a peaceful and healthful environment. It is impossible to disentangle the health status of rural people from the health of the communities in which they live.

THE IMPACT OF ENVIRONMENTAL DISRUPTION ON RURAL AMERICA

Environmental change has a disproportionate effect on rural communities because they are by definition closer to and more dependent on the natural environment. The impact on health is clear and direct, both by affecting the economic infrastructure of rural America and by changing the characteristics of the biosphere upon which humans depend for life itself. Although this text concerns itself primarily with the nuts and bolts

of the health care system as it addresses human diseases, the major new threats to health in the coming century are more likely to come from the human environment.

Environmental changes are both local and global in nature. We have alluded to some of the more local changes in discussing some of the economic pursuits that are specific to rural areas, in particular logging, mining, and agriculture. All of these industries have in common their extractive nature: they depend on taking something out of or from the earth. These undertakings are not in and of themselves harmful; humans, like other living organisms, have the capacity to live in equilibrium with the earth. Their pursuits become harmful when they puncture the envelope of equilibrium that protects the earth and the living creatures that depend on it for sustenance. It is at that point that traditional rural pursuits can affect the health of the ecosystem and its inhabitants, including the human community.

Humans are unique among living organisms in their power to transform and degrade the living environment; this is more than a theoretical danger in rural America. The agricultural miracle that has allowed the United States to feed itself and many of its neighbors with a slender 1 or 2 percent of its work force has come at the price of transforming the landscape into a series of industrial monocultures. Huge feeding stations for cattle, coupled with the use of antibiotics to increase productivity, have introduced virulent pathogens such as *Escherichia coli* into the food supply. Pesticides on apples may have estrogen-like effects on those who eat them. Indiscriminate logging creates huge mud slides, stream sedimentation, and loss of biological habitat, with an attendant decline and eradication of many of the interwoven families of species that contribute to the essential biodiversity of the planet. And mines contaminate the landscape with cyanide and toxic metals, as in the example cited at the beginning of this chapter.

Although none of these problems is specific to rural America, many of the practices are fostered by the local economies associated with different rural places. Most rural agricultural workers would argue that they have little choice as to the agricultural practices they use. The ruthless discipline of the market rewards those who are most efficient, and economic "efficiencies" neglect the downstream costs, both concretely and metaphorically, that result from practices that destroy the earth. These practices inevitably harm the health of the people who share that earth, both through causing disease and by creating unhealthy living conditions.

The alternative to creating rural environmental damage is for rural residents to support a set of rules and regulations that protect environmental values while creating a level economic playing field where all can compete using sustainable techniques. It makes no sense to bathe mountainsides in cyanide in order to extract gold, but local rural towns often chase the mining companies because they promise a few temporary jobs. Sustainable forestry techniques actually are more likely to lead to stable employment by helping to eliminate the boom-and-bust cycles that devastate the small community mills. And less dependence on agricultural chemicals saves money both directly and indirectly while increasing the safety and quality of the food supply.

The second source of potential environmental harm is global in nature, with global warming perhaps the most ominous development for many rural areas. Rapidly increasing global temperatures caused by the accumulation of greenhouse gases have devastating effects on agricultural systems and may make certain marginal areas uninhabitable. It has been predicted that rising global temperatures could result in widespread forest death in as much as one-third of the world's forested areas, which would create economic havoc both by further decreasing fiber availability and by changing the attractiveness of areas that are not recreational and retirement magnets.[18] The United States must take a leadership role in advancing global policies to address this threat; rural Americans can play a major role by demonstrating how global warming will affect them personally.

THE DEVELOPMENT OF RURAL HEALTH CARE IN THE TWENTY-FIRST CENTURY

This chapter has attempted to provide a framework through which to understand not only the current anatomy of the rural health care system but also the issues that rural America will face during the next century. While we have typically concentrated on the doctor and the patient, the places where they work, and the ways they get paid, the health issues confronting rural America are much broader. Although it is easier to stay within our safe intellectual domain, it is perilous to do so. Rural America and rural health care are much more embedded in the overall society. The advantages are that the fruits of technology are available to most people most of the time, no matter where they live. The dangers are in the increasing instability of the social and physical structures upon which the health of the earth and its biological populations depends.

We know incontrovertibly that traditional health care—episodic and preventive care directed at the individual—has less impact upon longevity and health status than the health of the society and the environment.[4] If we want to truly improve the health of rural Americans, we must think of health in a multidimensional sense, including all the factors that allow people to lead safe, creative, and fulfilling lives.[19, 20] One of the most exciting practical ways of measuring health has been developed by one of our most rural states: Vermont. In an annual report entitled *The Social Well-Being of Vermonters*, the state of Vermont has developed an index of social well-being that measures not only such traditional aspects of health as infant mortality rates and childhood immunizations but also such other behavioral health issues as cigarette smoking and teen pregnancy rates. To this are added other critical indicators such as poverty, income disparities, violence, and educational status.[21]

This approach has enormous promise for all of rural America because it focuses on the issues that have the most impact on individual and group well-being. Such an index can be fashioned using existing data and can be customized to include the topics of most interest to a community, county, region, or state. Environmental issues such as clear-cutting of forested land or water pollution can be added, measured, and tracked over time. The data can allow communities to decide where to direct their limited resources and how to work collectively across geopolitical boundaries to achieve common goals.

Most of the effort and attention of the past century has gone into ensuring a basic framework for the delivery of traditional services in rural areas. The challenge for the future is to broaden our concept of what constitutes health care, create a structure that provides incentives for those services that have the most impact on populations, and adapt these systems to rural areas. This will involve a philosophical revolution, since it is very difficult for us as individuals or as groups to focus beyond the crises at hand. This crisis-oriented mentality leads to vast investments in curative health services but scant attention to the long-term issues that often create these problems in the first place.

Rural America has the advantage of being composed of social units that the human mind can perceive, understand, appreciate, and change. Although rural communities tend to be conservative and resistant to change, they exist on a manageable scale. To the extent that some communities are able to grapple with the more fundamental problems that affect their well-being, they can develop models that will improve health care and well-being throughout the entire society.

REFERENCES

1. Carrel C: Excavating ecotopia. *High Country News* 30(1):10–13, 1998.
2. Ricketts TC, Johnson-Webb KD, Taylor P: *Definitions of Rural: A Handbook for Health Policy Makers and Researchers.* Bethesda, MD, Federal Office of Rural Health Policy, Health Resources and Services Administration, U.S. Department of Health and Human Services, 1998.
3. Miller MK, Stokes CS, Clifford WB: A comparison of the rural-urban mortality differential for deaths from all causes, cardiovascular disease and cancer. *J Rural Health* 3:23–34, 1987.
4. Evans RG, Barer ML, Marmor TR: *Why Are Some People Healthy and Others Not? The Determinants of Health of Populations.* New York, Aldine de Gruyter, 1994.
5. Pratt DS: Occupational health and the rural worker: agriculture, mining, and logging. *J Rural Health* 6:399–417, 1990.
6. Pooley E: The great escape. *Time* 150:52–61, 1997.
7. Weinert C, Burman ME: Rural health and health-seeking behaviors. *Annu Rev Nurs Res* 12:65–92, 1994.
8. Voss PR, Fuguitt GV: The impact of migration on southern rural areas of chronic depression. *Rural Sociol* 56:660–679, 1991.
9. Indian Health Service: *Trends in Indian Health.* Rockville, MD, Office of Public Health, Indian Health Service, U.S. Department of Health and Human Services, 1997.
10. Dever A: Profile of a population with complex health problems. *Migrant Health Newsline* 8:1–15, 1991.
11. Lyson TA, Falk WW: *Forgotten Places: Uneven Development in Rural Areas.* Lawrence, KS, University Press of Kansas, 1993.
12. Moscovice I: *Rural Health Networks: Forms and Functions.* Minneapolis, MN, University of Minnesota, Rural Health Research Center, 1997.
13. Amundson B, Rosenblatt R: The Rural Hospital Project: conceptual background and current status. *J Rural Health* 4:119–138, 1988.
14. Gold M: Beyond coverage and supply: measuring access to healthcare in today's market. *Health Services Res* 33:223–242, 1998.
15. Maine Rural Health Research Center: Ready or not: rural hospitals are changing. *Rural Health News* 4, 1997.
16. Schlesinger M, Gray B, Carrino G, et al: A broader vision for managed care: Part 2. A typology of community benefits. *Health Affairs* 17:26–49, 1998.
17. Hart LG, Pirani M, Rosenblatt RA: Causes and consequences of rural small hospital closures from the perspectives of mayors. *J Rural Health* 7:222–245, 1991.
18. Flavin C, Dunn S: *Rising Sun, Gathering Winds:*

Policies to Stabilize the Climate and Strengthen Economies. Worldwatch Paper #138. Washington, DC, Worldwatch Institute, 1997.

19. Kindig DA: Purchasing population health: aligning financial incentives to improve health outcomes. *Health Services Res* 33:223–242, 1998.

20. Roos NP, Black CD, Frohlich N, et al: A population-based health information system. *Med Care* 33:DS13–DS20, 1995.

21. Murphy D: *The Social Well-Being of Vermonters 1998.* Waterbury, VT, Agency of Human Services, State of Vermont, 1998.

CHAPTER 2

The Rural Patient

Thomas C. Ricketts

Dr. Ohmart has been having difficulty with a patient, Clara, who is 25 weeks pregnant. There are signs of trouble with the fetus, and he reflects on the advice he was given a few months ago at a CME session for rural physicians: "Ask your OB consultant to step in and review the pregnancy." Ohmart can't visualize one of the already overworked obstetricians from Hays, Kansas, spending three hours driving to and from Oakley, Kansas, to offer his opinion, and there will probably be a problem getting the patient over to Hays— especially if that opinion might be that all was fine, and Ohmart needed to continue with what he was doing. Another suggestion he got was that he alert the "local neonatologist" if he anticipated problems. His neonatologist is also in Hays and he will be leaving soon, meaning that the nearest neonatologist will be in Denver, 250 miles to the west. This is all too familiar to Ohmart as he reflects on his decision to set up practice in Oakley and stick with it.

Clara speaks little English; she came to Oakley 6 months ago with her husband, who works for a meat packing company. He and she had been working the fields between Mexico and the Canadian border in the spring and summer for the previous three years, so she has little knowledge of the health care system she is about to enter. She's apprehensive and shy, but Ohmart has been able to counsel her when the translator from the county social services office was available or the few times her husband could come into the office. There's a new wrinkle in the case now: her mother-in-law has been able to come up from Mexico to help when the baby is delivered, and Ohmart thinks the older woman might be giving Clara some herbal remedy that has caused the irregular heartbeats. The mother-in-law is from a small village in southeastern Mexico and is not good with Spanish herself. She speaks a local language more akin to what the Mayans might have spoken.

The family has a phone out at their trailer 18 miles from town; if there is an emergency, the volunteer EMS group may be able to help quickly, but they still have not been able to get the phone company to set up the 911 system where Clara lives because she's in an exchange owned by a small cooperative company that can't afford the "switch" that links them into the country emergency system. Ohmart is more worried that if something does happen quickly and he needs to get Clara to a hospital with a neonatal ICU, he'll have little time to arrange for the proper triage, and there's always the question of which way to go, Hays or Denver, depending on who is on call or available. He's been working with the small local hospital in trying to set up referral and triage protocols due to the restructuring of the emergency services to meet the new Rural Hospital Flexibility Rules. As one of only three doctors on the staff of the hospital, a lot of the administrative responsibility falls on him. In this case, he's chair of a regional committee that takes him out of town two days and nights each month. Perhaps, he muses, this new medical resident who's coming through for a month-long stay will feel comfortable with obstetrics and maybe know a thing or two about what he's seeing. "He'll have to learn fast," he thought as he finished glancing through the chart. "I just hope Clara comes in today"; getting a ride from the remote corner of the county where they live is not always easy.

Ohmart knows he'll have a hard time with payment for the delivery even if everything goes well. Clara has been able to pay $10 and $20 at some of the visits, but sometimes she's downcast and has to let him know she can't pay anything. Her husband's firm, a large multistate company, offers a "bare bones" insurance policy that has a high co-payment and would cost him $80 a week to put Clara on. His pay of $6.50 per hour doesn't allow them much leeway since they've bought the trailer. "They'll try to pay what they can," he marked on the pink form inside the folder, where his office manager had written the note "Should we carry them?" in big letters.[1]

*T*he issues facing Clara and Dr. Ohmart are typical of what happens in a rural community. Patients are sometimes isolated from medical care and physicians from referral resources by relatively great distances. There are often gulfs in communication between the urban health system and the realities of the rural system. Many rural communities must cope with extremes of cultural diversity, where there are few to provide support for minority patients; moreover, many who work in rural places are poor and often are not able to get health insurance coverage. These specific characteristics apply to many patients in many places, but they are more likely to be encountered in a rural community, especially in the South and Southwest or along the three migrant "streams" that

bring agricultural labor into the heartland and up the East and West Coasts, following crops and opportunities.

Rural places can be very different from each other; they include irrigated agricultural places in western Kansas, like Oakley, but they also can be located in the more prosperous dairy farmlands of the upper Midwest or the timber areas of the Maine backwoods or of the upper Northwest. They can be the sandy tobacco lands of the eastern plans of North and South Carolina and Georgia, or the fishing and resort areas of the Ozarks. The diversity of rural America can be seen in its landscape, which ranges from southern swampland to arctic mountain ranges.

The Economic Research Service of the U.S. Department of Agriculture has developed a rural typology that provides a useful categorization of the communities in which rural patients reside (Table 2-1). This typology, which is applied to counties, summarizes the diversity of rural economic and social conditions among nonmetropolitan counties as seven major overlapping themes or types. Four county types reflect dependence on a particular economic specialization: farming, manufacturing, mining, and government. Three county types—persistent poverty, federal lands, and retirement-destination—reflect other important social themes. These types of communities set a tone for a medical practice, but they need to be considered in the context of the region in which

TABLE 2-1   CLASSIFICATION FOR USDA ERS TYPOLOGY OF PRIMARY ECONOMIC ACTIVITY

Six Economic Activities (number of counties)	Five Policy Areas (number of counties)
1. Farming-dependent (556)	1. Retirement destination (190)
2. Mining-dependent (146)	2. Federal lands (270)
3. Manufacturing-dependent (506)	3. Commuting (381)
4. Government-dependent (244)	4. Persistent poverty (535)
5. Services-dependent (323)	5. Transfers-dependent (381)
6. Nonspecialized (484)	

Key: USDA, U.S. Department of Agriculture; ERS, Economic Research Service.

they occur. A farming-dependent county in the Southeast may have a significant African-American minority, even a majority population, whereas one in the upper Midwest may be almost exclusively white and middle class. A mining-dependent area of the Appalachians may be more reflective of the decline of the coal industry, whereas a newly expanded western mining county based on a new technology may have a very different age and gender structure.

We think of "rural" in different ways, and rural people think of themselves in ways that may affect how they seek medical care and comply with medical advice. The way that rural America is viewed may affect how rural health care systems are treated and rural practitioners are viewed. According to rural sociologists Michael Miller and Al Luloff, popular images of rural America can be distilled into five categories[2]:

1. Positive images—"Rural life is friendly and neighborly."

2. Negative images—"Rural life is monotonous and boring or provincial and narrow-minded."

3. Antiurban sentiment—"Urban living is too fast or impersonal and uncaring."

4. Agrarian values—"Agriculture is natural and the family farm is the backbone of American democracy."

5. Wilderness values—"Open areas are good and healthy places, and solitude contributes to health."

These attitudes may explain some of the specific problems of working with rural people when one is considering their willingness to adhere to recommended therapies or preventive behavior or the incidence of depression and other behavioral conditions. In helping the clinician understand the rural patient, it is useful to look at some of the dominant activities or ecologic characteristics of rural populations and relate those to potential special health care needs. This system (Table 2-2) relates some of

TABLE 2-2   RURAL CHARACTERIZATIONS AND HEALTH SERVICES IMPLICATIONS

Rural Characterization	Health Services Implication
1. Use of the land	Agricultural injuries, recreational injuries: snowmobiles, all-terrain vehicles.
2. Delimited area	The area may relate to a central medical facility, referrals will be possible only to a limited number of specialists.
3. Small population	Occurrence of disease is masked by small numbers; calculation of rates is difficult.
4. Dispersed population	Travel time to care is often very great; transportation can be problematic for poor persons; communications systems may be less than optimal.
5. Identity as countryside	Rural attitudes toward medicine and health care may be inflexible and reflect "country" beliefs in independence and neighborliness. Health care–seeking behavior may be influenced by strong social visibility and belief systems.
6. Isolation from technology	Late innovation, greater travel time to technology or to training, provider isolation.

these fundamental characteristics of rural populations to health services. These fundamental characteristics of rural populations have implications for health services but are more often used to explain observed phenomena than to propose hypotheses to understand rural health. This interpretation of rural characteristics can help us when we examine problems in health services delivery. For example, we can imagine that an issue of access to technology for a rural population would combine problems of distance that have contributed to late adoption of newer treatments and that lack of a sizable, concentrated population would make it difficult to make optimal use of a complex service or provide the means to support its existence in a rural context.

DEMOGRAPHICS

Historically, rural areas have been thought of as having small populations, a dependence on farming, larger family size, and more conservative lifestyles and politics. The populations of rural places remain smaller, but farming is clearly no longer a defining characteristic. Less than 7 percent of the rural population is now engaged in farming, and that proportion will fall to below 5 percent by the beginning of the new century. Rural places may continue to be more conservative and, on balance, include larger families, but this is not consistent enough across all rural places to allow those generalizations to define what is rural. Agriculture, fishing, mining, and forestry, however, are still predominantly rural occupations, and the consequences of those types of employment have strong implications for the structure of the health care needs of rural places.

In 1993, there were 2228 of a total of 3141 counties (or county equivalents) for the nation as a whole, containing 83 percent of the nation's land and 21 percent (51 million) of its people, that were classified as nonmetropolitan. In 1992, nonmetropolitan counties accounted for 18 percent of U.S. jobs and 14 percent of earnings. Rural America is larger in size than all but five of the world's nations and holds a population larger than that of South Africa, Canada, and Australia combined and almost as large as that of France. But the fact that rural America is a minority part of the nation's economy, although a key minority, means that sometimes policies crafted in the urban political centers are less than appropriate or have unanticipated negative effects on rural places.

The term *rural* was first used by the U.S. Bureau of the Census in 1874, when it was defined as a county population of 8000 or more living outside of cities or towns. That population threshold was changed to 2500 in 1910. The Census Bureau now defines *urban* as comprising all territory, population, and housing units in urbanized areas and in places of 2500 or more persons outside urbanized areas. The terms *urban, urbanized area,* and *rural* are specifically defined by the Census Bureau. Other federal agencies, state agencies, local officials, and private groups may use these same terms to identify areas based on different criteria.

SOCIOECONOMIC STATUS AND TYPES

Rural residents have two strikes against them with regard to risk factors for acute illness and trauma: poverty and increased personal risk-taking behaviors. These factors are also highly correlated with educational level. Rural residents who finish high school and go on to college are likely to move to urban areas permanently, leaving lower average education levels in rural areas. The poverty rate for the rural population has remained higher over recent years, at 15.9 percent versus 13.2 percent. Rural minorities are even more often poor, with 35.2 percent of rural blacks falling below the federal policy guideline compared to 26.9 percent of urban blacks.[3] The economic conditions of rural places are not always matched by the social services or economic support systems that can assist needy populations. Traditionally, rural states in the South and West have relatively more restrictive welfare eligibility rules and fewer benefits. Families that stay together are ineligible for the major welfare program, Aid to

Families with Dependent Children (AFDC), in nearly half the states. Those living on family farms often exceed the "assets test" because of the appraised value of farmland or nonproductive property; therefore, despite having very low incomes, they are ineligible for benefits. Rural inhabitants, therefore, are in general more likely than urban inhabitants to have low educational achievement, to experience higher unemployment, and to live in poverty. They are also more likely to be ineligible for welfare benefits and more likely to engage in recreational (snowmobiling, hunting, boating) and occupational (mining, agriculture, timbering) activities that put them at higher than average risk for injury. Many of the rural poor do not receive public assistance, do not live in public housing, do not receive food stamps, are not covered by Medicaid, and do not have access to medical care.[4] This cycle holds the potential to negatively affect the health of rural Americans, particularly poor rural Americans.

The trends affecting the rural portions of the nation ebb and flow. There have been periods of in-migration (1970s), out-migration (1980s), and apparent revival (1990s); but these overall changes cannot be applied to all rural communities or regions. In the last 20 years the proportion of the rural work force employed in farming has decreased from 14.4 percent in 1969 to 7.6 percent in 1992. The largest share of rural jobs and employment growth today comes from the services sector, which employs more than half of all rural workers. Manufacturing is also a big provider of rural jobs, employing 16.9 percent of the rural work force, but this proportion is down from 20.4 percent in 1969.[5] Communications technologies offer new opportunities to rural places. The timeless appeal of pastoral surroundings combined with advanced telecommunications technologies and an increase in "virtual offices" is reversing decades of migration to the cities. Since 1988, job growth in nonmetropolitan areas has outpaced that in urban areas, 2.2 percent compared with 1.3 percent between 1990 and 1994, particularly in communities with a strong technological infrastructure. The population in rural counties has increased overall at a 1 percent annual growth rate, triple the rate of the 1980s. With more people comes more money, and the income for rural residents has grown an average of 5.1 percent annually since 1990, reversing a 20-year trend of negative wage growth. The numbers of telecommuters have grown from 2 million in 1988 to some 11 million in 1998.

HEALTH INSURANCE

Nonmetropolitan residents are slightly less likely than metropolitan residents to be insured for their health care costs, particularly by private insurance. Analysis of the March 1997 Current Population Survey indicates that 16.3 percent of the nonmetropolitan population was uninsured, compared to 15.5 percent of metropolitan persons.[6] Health insurance coverage fell for metropolitan and nonmetropolitan residents between 1987 and 1997, but at a slower rate for the nonmetropolitans. Those who are uninsured in rural America tend to be uninsured longer; for those who lost health insurance during the 28-month period of January 1992 through April 1994, the nonmetropolitan population had the longest spells without health insurance, 7.2 months, compared with 4.9 months for people living in suburbs.[7]

Health insurance coverage for rural residents may be affected by the availability of plans. Rural people are more often employed in smaller firms or on farms and in agriculture-related work that is organized into smaller companies. This employment pattern is consistent with lower rates of coverage.[8,9] The lack of insurance has been found to be associated with the type of care people receive; uninsured persons had 45 percent fewer total hip replacements, 29 percent fewer coronary artery bypass grafts, and 74 percent fewer total knee replacements than insured persons.[10] The uninsured were also more likely to receive no treatment for certain conditions. Among children, the uninsured were 1.8 times more likely to receive no care for a recurring ear infection and 1.7 times more likely to not get care for asthma.[11] Uninsured children were also much less likely to have overall access to ambulatory care, as measured by having a regular physician, having after-hours care available, and having a history of contact with physicians.[12] There have been few studies that simultaneously consider rural residence, use of health care services, and insurance status; however, Mueller et al. found that use of physician services was lower overall for rural persons, but especially for rural minority groups, particularly Latinos and rural Asians or persons of "other" race.[13]

HEALTH STATUS

The patterns of rural land use, occupations, and recreational choices create a picture of health care needs that varies from that of urban places, independent of the age and sex structure of communities. Trauma from use of farm and garden equipment is much more likely in rural areas; chronic diseases related to pesticide and herbicide exposure is more prevalent; and trauma

from crashes of snowmobiles, off-road vehicles, and boats is far more common in rural than in urban places. The severity of automobile crash injuries is clearly much greater in rural places due to higher speeds and poorer road conditions; trauma-related mortality, especially for motor vehicle crashes and related to the use of guns, is disproportionately higher in rural areas.[14]

The mortality and morbidity patterns of rural America, as compared with urban patterns, do not show a distinctive and consistent disadvantage for rural residents.[15] But these general comparisons are plagued by the same classification problems discussed in this chapter—the aggregation of widely divergent populations and communities into large, gross classifications that are meant, primarily, to be consistent across the nation. There are, however, clear regional patterns of rural disadvantage: much higher infant mortality in the rural Southeast, for example, and those conditions are clearly related to the differences in income and education between those rural regions and other parts of the nation.

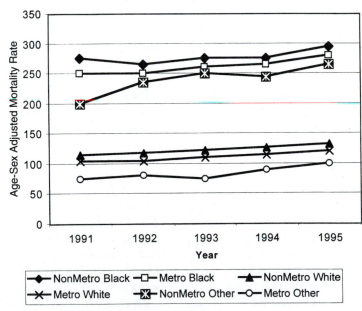

FIGURE 2-1 Diabetes mortality by race and geographic residence, 1991–1995. (From Ricketts TC: In Howard A (ed): Unpublished Analysis of March 1998 Current Population Survey Data. Chapel Hill, NC, University of North Carolina at Chapel Hill, Cecil G. Sheps Center for Health Services Research, 1998.)

Geographic patterns of morbidity and mortality vary by race and ethnicity. Figure 2-1 illustrates the consistent differences in mortality for persons of white, black, and "other" races for diabetes. Nonmetropolitan blacks have the highest mortality rates of all groups, and nonmetropolitan whites have higher rates than metropolitan whites. This pattern of differential mortality by race and rural-urban residence is similar for cardiovascular disease.

It is also clear that there are some difficulties inherent to rural America that make it difficult to clearly understand rural morbidity and mortality patterns. With jurisdictions that have small populations, there is the potential for the masking of disease occurrence, since rates will not be stable and analysts may tend to ignore or not account for the very high fluctuation. Smaller populations also limit the capacity of health service and public health agencies to compile adequate statistics to characterize the health pattern of smaller places.

HEALTH CARE UTILIZATION AND ACCESS

Ensuring equitable access to health care is an important public policy goal for the nation. A significant body of research and policy analysis has focused on documenting access problems for vulnerable populations and suggesting policy options to eliminate access barriers.[16,17] Rural populations have often been viewed as especially vulnerable with respect to access to health care because of poorly developed and fragile health infrastructures, high prevalence rates for chronic illness and disability, socioeconomic hardships, and physical barriers such as distance and availability of transportation, including a lack of public transportation.[4]

Access is measured by a variety of individual sociodemographic characteristics that are known to influence the use of health care.[18,19] Health insurance coverage is important because, controlling for other characteristics, individuals with coverage for health care are more likely to have a usual source of care and to have more physician visits as well as less likely to report problems in obtaining care.[20,21] Data on usual sources of care, sites of care, and travel and waiting times are also important measures of access. A usual source of care—a regular place at which individuals seek medical care when they are sick or need advice about their health—is viewed as an entry point to the health care system and is seen as increasing continuity of care. Because of concern about differences in quality or continuity across sites of care, we report on variation in reported regular care sites. Other dimensions of the usual care site that may be related to access are travel and waiting times: the time associated with making a physician contact may be viewed as one of the resources involved in obtaining care.

Access to health care services in rural versus urban areas has been explored by health services researchers for decades. Rural residents are, on average, poorer, older, and—for those under age 65—less insured than persons living in urban areas.[22-24] Rural Americans also report more chronic conditions and describe themselves as being in poorer health than urban residents. Further, injury-related mortality and the number of days of restricted activity are higher in nonurban areas.

Access to health care in rural areas is complicated by different patterns of employment and insurance coverage among rural residents. Rural residents are more likely to be self-employed; if they are employed by firms, these firms are smaller than those in urban areas. Consequently, employment-related insurance benefits may be less widespread and less generous.[25] State-focused studies have found that urban families have more insurance coverage than their rural counterparts and that rural families pay a higher proportion of their income for insurance premiums.[23,26]

We have seen that insurance coverage differs for metropolitan and nonmetropolitan areas. It has been suggested that residents in rural areas are less likely to have private insurance coverage through their employers because of the industries they work in and the larger share of part-time workers. An examination of the 1996

Medical Expenditure Panel Survey (MEPS) data on health insurance coverage supports these assumptions. Rural residents were less likely to have private health insurance through their employers, unions, or self-owned businesses. Only 54 percent of rural residents had insurance coverage through their employers, as compared with 63 percent for urban residents, using data from the MEPS survey. Some 20 percent of rural respondents were uninsured, compared to 16 percent of urban residents.

The 1994 Access to Care supplement of the National Health Interview Survey included a question on whether there was a time in the year preceding the survey when an individual needed care but was unable to obtain it. Overall, only 3 percent of respondents indicated that they had needed care and could not obtain it. This did not vary by type of geographic area. However, there is a small difference in ability to obtain eyeglasses: 3.2 percent of residents in metro areas and 2.9 percent of individuals in counties that are both adjacent to a metro area and have their own city reported being unable to get eyeglasses compared to more than 4 percent of those in rural areas. Rural residents are more likely than their urban counterparts to delay getting care due to financial barriers. Although only 7.9 percent of urban residents reported delaying care due to cost, 11 percent of residents in rural counties adjacent to metro areas and including a city reported a delay in care, as did 10 percent of those in counties adjacent to a metro area but without a city of more than 10,000. Delays due to cost were reported by 12 percent of respondents in counties not adjacent to a metro area but with a city and 10 percent of residents in the most rural counties (not adjacent to a metro area and no city of more than 10,000).

Most people, approximately 85 percent of both metro and nonmetro residents, report having a usual source of care. However, metro residents more often say that their usual source is a community, school, or county clinic or a health maintenance organization (HMO) or prepaid group. For those who received care in the last year but did not have a usual source of care,

doctors' offices remained the most common site of care for both metro and nonmetro residents, though the latter group were more likely to obtain care at this site. Nonmetro residents were again less likely to receive care in a community clinic or HMO than those in metro areas. More rural people (14 percent) than metro residents (8 percent) reported that they did not have a usual source of care because their provider had moved or closed.

Travel times to doctors' offices are, on average, longer for rural residents than for their urban counterparts. The average travel time for metropolitan residents was 17 minutes as compared to 19 minutes for nonmetropolitan residents (median time, 15 minutes for both groups). Although a greater percentage of urban residents reported traveling more than 1 hour to their usual source of care (2 percent versus 1 percent for rural residents), more rural residents traveled between 30 and 60 minutes to obtain care (17 percent as compared to 14 percent for urban residents). Waiting times for an appointment for routine care are also considered indicators of access; on average, rural residents (mean 3 days; median 1 day) had to wait fewer days for an appointment with their physicians than urban residents (mean 6 days; median 1 day). While 14 percent of both metropolitan and nonmetropolitan residents waited less than a day for an appointment, 14 percent of metropolitan residents, as compared to 8 percent of nonmetro residents, waited more than a week for an appointment.

Approximately three-quarters of the population had at least one doctor's visit in the previous 12 months. Although the proportion with at least one visit is lower for residents of all types of nonmetropolitan counties as compared with residents of metropolitan counties, the difference is small. For persons with at least one visit in the preceding year, the average number of visits is uniform across place of residence (approximately six visits). Overall, rural residents report higher levels of chronic conditions, but they do not visit the doctor more frequently than do urban residents.

Residents in nonmetropolitan counties without a city of 10,000 or greater were more likely to have been hospitalized in the previous year (9 percent for rural counties adjacent to metropolitan areas; 10 percent for rural areas not adjacent to metropolitan counties). This higher rate may reflect any number of factors, including higher accident rates, underlying characteristics such as age or health status, or inadequate ambulatory care.

The mean number of physician visits in the past year reported by urban and rural residents were compared according to selected demographic groupings. For those under age 65, few statistically significant differences were found, although the general trend was for rural people to report fewer doctor visits. Where significant differences exist across the rural-urban continuum, it was often those living in counties not adjacent to metro areas and with a city of 10,000 or more who had fewer visits than those in metro areas. In particular, those who were employed, Hispanic, residing in the Midwest or West, or situated within the middle-income range ($35,000 to $49,999) had fewer visits than their counterparts in metropolitan areas.

Although the elderly have more visits, on average, than the nonelderly, the patterns for this population appear similar. Among those residing in nonmetro counties, individuals in counties not adjacent to metro areas and with cities of 10,000 or more most often were different from those living in metro counties. Of the former group, males, African Americans, those in the Northeast and the West, and those with good health status had fewer visits than those in urban counties.

ENVIRONMENTAL HAZARDS

The rural environment—especially where agriculture, mining, forestry, and fishing are important or dominant parts of the economy—presents extraordinary threats to health. Agriculture brings the use of pesticides and herbicides as well as heavy and potentially dangerous machinery. Mining is a consistently hazardous industry, and persons involved in fishing and forestry are at much higher risks of trauma. A review of the causes for visits to a single rural emergency department (ED) found that work-related injuries accounted for 12.5 percent of over 12,000 injuries. Rural workers who were injured were more often older; the mean age of patients injured on the job was 33.8 years (range 16 to 77 years), compared with a mean age of 27.7 years for all injury visits. The most common mechanisms of work-related injuries were overexertion (20 percent); cut or pierced by sharp implements (16 percent); falls (16 percent); struck by object (13 percent); and transportation-related injuries (5 percent). Sprains and strains were the most common types of injury sustained (27 percent), followed by wounds to upper limbs (18 percent), contusions (12 percent), and fractures (10 percent). Of the 1539 patients coming to the ED with occupational injuries, 12 percent were transported via ambulance. Most (91 percent) were treated and released from the ED, with the remainder hospitalized. The mechanisms of injury that most commonly resulted in hospitalization involved being struck by an object (21 percent) or a vehicle (19 percent), falling (20 percent), being crushed (10 percent), and being hurt by machinery (15 percent). Of workers requiring hospitalization, 97 percent were male, and the average length of hospital stay was 4.4 days.[27]

Exposure to cancer-causing agents is recognized as a hazard of rural life for both farmers and farm workers, and also for persons living near fields that are sprayed with pesticides or where runoff is likely. This results in higher than average rates for farm populations of brain, stomach, lymphatic and hemopoietic, lip, prostate, and skin cancer.[28] There have been a number of programs that have attempted to lower the risks of cancer and agricultural injury; these were sponsored by the National Institute of Occupational Safety and Health,[29] the National Cancer Institute, and the U.S. Department of Agriculture, along with many state agricultural extension services and foundations involved in prevention. The Appalachian Leadership Initiative in Cancer (ALIC) is an example of the combination of local public health agencies, clinicians, and the Agricultural Extension Service network of agents and support units in land-grant universities to address problems specific to rural populations.[30]

SPECIAL RURAL PROBLEMS

The health status of rural residents is, on average, remarkably robust, given the generally lower availability of resources. It is, however, misleading to take the average to represent the specific conditions faced by the substantial number of rural communities having far fewer than the mean number of providers compared to population. In 1997, there were 20.6 million people living in nonmetropolitan areas designated as Health Professional Shortage Areas. There are parts of rural America that are losing population as their economies shrink or are transformed from labor-intensive agriculture to automated agribusiness or range use. There is a large swath of the heartland—279 counties in the states of Wyoming, Montana, North and South Dakota, Kansas, and Nebraska—that is losing population to out-migration and a significant decline in births. In 1995, these counties had less than half of their average annual number of births during the period 1947 through 1956. Birth numbers in these counties are now close to what they were in the worst parts of the Depression. These rural places present the challenge of "downsizing" their health care resources and relying on older physicians and other clinicians working in aging facilities. There are other rural counties in the eastern and western United States that also have been "left behind" by the economic boom of the 1990s. They present special problems of access and disease. Depression among farmers—brought on by economic stress—for example, is an emergent problem in rural America.

There are special rural situations related to the geography and ethnography of places. Alaska, with its vast spaces, presents a real logistic problem for the transportation of patients and access to health care, for as much as one-third of its population lives outside of Anchorage, Fairbanks, and Juneau. The Alaska Native population, like many aboriginal groups in the nation, has dealt with special susceptibilities and a cultural view of health and health care that has often not fit well into the prevailing Anglo–western European health care delivery system. Most Native American communities in the lower 48 states are centered on rural reservations, where the former and current Indian Health Service Systems have struggled to adjust their limited resources to meet the needs of populations that are often unemployed at rates 10 times those of the surrounding areas, where behavioral illness and conditions are endemic due to the social and economic displacement of the groups. These specific population issues must be addressed in the context of distance and, often, isolation from the complex and supportive social and technical structures of cities.

SUMMARY AND POLICY ISSUES

The policies developed by national and state governments often have to consider inclusive populations. "Rural" America is an example, and rural health policy is developed from a perception that there is a general problem with health care access and health status for all rural Americans. This, we know, is not completely true. The most pressing needs are in the portion of the nation we call rural. So far, we have created policies that designate places and populations as underserved or as having professional shortages. Rural places are often designated, but the service options available are often not scaled to meet the needs of the particular community. Comprehensive federally qualified health centers need a sufficiently large population to justify their construction and funding. Even the placement of a physician in a rural community is problematic, since physicians now are very resistant to solo practice. This would make it hard for a small community to support multiple professionals when the population need is calculated to be equal to less than a full-time equivalent. We have also created a financial support system for health services for certain classes of people with low incomes through the Medicaid program. The Medicaid system has depended on the cooperation of social service systems and private providers to determine eligibility and to accept the payments offered. Often, the more rural places have social structures that stigmatize the indigent seeking assistance or a more conservative set of providers who see Medicaid as a handout to the undeserving poor. We have also created a national system of health insurance for the elderly and disabled, but one that discriminates on the basis of geography, paying rural providers less. These initiatives serve many needy people well, but they all suffer from a rigidity in their structure that does not consider many of the special problems attendant to rural life.

These gaps between the structure of health policy and the realities of rural health needs are not restricted to rural communities; they are problems that affect the entire health "system." Dr. Ohmart's experiences with referrals in rural Kansas are repeated in urban areas, but the problems are usually due to gaps in communication and culture rather than great distances and scarce resources. But Dr. Ohmart is in a place where the potential for economic pressures on his practice come from having too little to support his chosen work rather than from a system that has reduced payments to the clinician because someone has decided that too much is being spent in some insurance plans or managed care contracts. American health policy must reconcile the awkward balance of health care as an economic activity, which says that efficiency is the highest good, with its social and cultural imperatives, which say that care is the goal of our society. Although we may see ourselves as one big market, it is the caring impulse that ties us together as humans.

Because of the relationship between our economy and institutions and professions in health care, a great deal of attention is paid to payment policies for hospitals divided by rural and urban distinctions and less attention is given to the specific effects that one's distance from a primary care professional has on one's health. This is not necessarily irrational; it is precisely because health is tied closely to economics that we can make the argument that hospital payment policies affect health care needs and health status. It is not very satisfying to succeed in changing those payment policies when you want to change the very poor health status of the rural poor in a neglected corner of a southeastern state, but it may be that reforming payment policies is the only way to progress toward that goal at that time. Nevertheless, it is imperative that we also recognize when the more direct approach is feasible and effective.

For Dr. Ohmart and his patient Clara, he would probably not be worrying about his ability to get his patients to the right kind of care when they needed it if our payment policies for Medicare and Medicaid did not distinguish between rural and urban providers. The higher income potential might have brought other physicians into the area, and the small hospitals might have been able to structure a referral and transportation system that could have either moved Clara to care when she needed it or brought it to her via telemedicine or on a rotating schedule.

REFERENCES

1. Ohmart C: "I practice in the rural wilderness." *Kansas Med* Spring 1966, pp 11–12.
2. Miller MK, Luloff AE: Who is rural? A typological approach to the examination of rurality. *Rural Sociol* 46:608–625, 1981.
3. Cook PJ: Recent indicators send mixed signals about rural economic performance. *Rural Conditions Trends* 9(2):2–8, 1999.
4. Rowland D, Lyons B: Triple jeopardy: rural, poor and uninsured. *Health Services Res* 23(6):975–1004, 1989.
5. Service ER: *Understanding Rural America.* Washington, DC, US Department of Agriculture, 1995, pp 2, 5.

6. Ricketts TC: In Howard A (ed): *Unpublished Analysis of March 1998 Current Population Survey Data.* Chapel Hill, NC, University of North Carolina at Chapel Hill, Cecil G. Sheps Center for Health Services Research, 1998.

7. US Census Bureau: *Dynamics of Economic Well-Being: Health Insurance. 1992–1993: Who Loses Coverage and For How Long?* Washington, DC: US Department of Commerce, 1996.

8. Hoffman C: *Uninsured in America: A Chart Book.* Washington, DC: Kaiser Commission on Medicaid and the Uninsured, 1998.

9. Custer WH: *Health Insurance Coverage and the Uninsured.* Atlanta, GA, Georgia State University, Center for Risk Management and Insurance Research, 1999.

10. Hadley J, Steinberg E, Feder J: Comparison of uninsured and privately insured hospital patients: condition on admission, resource use and outcomes. *JAMA* 265(3):374–379, 1991.

11. Stoddard JJ, St Peter RF, Newacheck PW: Health insurance status and ambulatory care for children. *N Engl J Med* 330(20):1421–1425, 1994.

12. Newacheck PW et al: Health insurance and access to primary care for children. *N Engl J Med* 338(8): 513–519, 1998.

13. Mueller KJ, Patil K, Boilesen E: The role of uninsurance and race in healthcare utilization by rural minorities. *Health Services Res* 33(3):597–610, 1998.

14. Chen B et al: Geographical variation in mortality rates from motor vehicles. *J Trauma* 38(2):228–232, 1995.

15. Miller MK, Farmer FL, Clarke LL: Rural populations and their health, in Beaulieu JE, Berry DE (eds): *Rural Health Services: A Management Perspective.* Ann Arbor, MI, AUPHA Press / Health Administration Press, 1994, pp 3–26.

16. Aday LA et al: *Evaluating the Healthcare System: Effectiveness, Efficiency, and Equity,* 2d ed. Chicago: AHSR Health Administration Press, 1998.

17. Aday LA: Equity, accessibility, and ethical issues: is the U.S. health care reform debate asking the right questions? In Rosenau PV (ed): *Health Care Reform in the Nineties.* Thousand Oaks, CA, Sage, 1993.

18. Berk ML, Schur CL, Cantor JC: Ability to obtain health care: recent estimates from the Robert Wood Johnson Foundation National Access to Care Study. *Health Affairs* 14:139–146, 1995.

19. Mueller KJ, Patil K, Ullrich F: Lengthening spells of uninsurance and their consequences. *J Rural Health* 13(1):29–37, 1997.

20. Spillman BC: The impact of being uninsured on utilization of basic health care services. *Inquiry* 29(4):457–466, 1992.

21. Weissman JS, Epstein AM: The insurance gap: does it make a difference? *Annu Rev Public Health* 14:243–270, 1993.

22. American College of Physicians: Rural primary care. *Ann Intern Med* 122(5):380–390, 1995.

23. Hartley D, Quam L, Lurie N: Urban and rural differences in health insurance and access to care. *J Rural Health* 10(2):98–108, 1994.

24. Braden J, Beauregard K: *Health Status and Access to Care of Rural and Urban Populations.* Rockville, MD, Agency for Health Care Policy and Research, 1994.

25. Frenzen P: Health insurance coverage in U.S. urban and rural areas. *J Rural Health* 9(3):204–214, 1993.

26. Mueller KJ, Beavers SL: Insurance status among HIV+ Nebraskans. *J Health Soc Policy* 10(1):53–64, 1998.

27. Williams J et al: Work-related injuries in a rural emergency department population. *Acad Emerg Med* 4(4):277–281, 1997.

28. Blair A et al: Cancer among farmers: a review. *Scand J Work Environ Health* 11(6):397–407, 1985.

29. Connally LB et al: Developing the National Institute for Occupational Safety and Health's cancer control demonstration projects for farm populations. *J Rural Health* 12(4):258–264, 1996.

30. Couto RA, Simpson NK, Harris G (eds): *Sowing Seeds in the Mountains: Community-Based Coalitions for Cancer Prevention and Control.* Bethesda, MD: National Cancer Institute, 1994.

CHAPTER 3

The Rural Physician

Eric H. Larson L. Gary Hart

In the 1991 film *Doc Hollywood*, Michael J. Fox portrays a young physician fresh out of residency on his way to a career of tummy tucks, face lifts, and liposuction treatments in Los Angeles. While driving cross country, he is waylaid by the residents of a small town desperate to recruit a new doctor to replace the aging, lovable curmudgeon of a doctor who has tended to the medical needs of the townsfolk for several decades. Eventually, the brash young doctor finds true love, saves the life of the curmudgeon/physician, handles his first breech delivery in the back of a station wagon without assistance, and learns the true meaning of being a healer. And (it hardly needs reporting) he abandons the false and empty life he had planned in Los Angeles for a rich and fulfilling career as a small-town physician.

W hile idealizing rural practice and rural life in the service of romantic comedy, the film described above manages to evoke the moments of harrowing loneliness in rural medicine as well as the deep satisfaction that many rural physicians derive from their multiple roles as community members, community leaders, confessors, and healers. The desperation of the town's residents to recruit and retain a new physician also resonates with a stark rural reality in the United States—the continuing maldistribution of physicians, which creates physician shortages in rural areas during an era when the United States is arguably oversupplied with physicians overall.

This chapter describes the evolution of the rural physician shortage, federal and professional responses to that shortage, and the current practice characteristics, demography, and distribution of rural physicians in the United States. Finally, the short- and long-term issues and trends that may affect the supply of physicians willing and able to serve rural populations in the future are assessed.

THE EVOLUTION OF PHYSICIAN MALDISTRIBUTION

The shortage of physicians willing to practice in rural settings is not a new problem in the United States. In the early years of the twentieth century, America was being transformed from an agrarian rural society into an urban industrial one. At the same time, medicine was transformed both socially and scientifically by forces as broad as the germ theory of disease, the professionalization of medicine, the rise of the hospital in its modern form, the reform of medical training, and the concentration of medical research and training in large urban universities. In the late nineteenth century, Louis Pasteur, Joseph Lister, and Robert Koch had revolutionized the Western understanding of disease as well as infection and its prevention. The power of the germ theory was demonstrated brilliantly in the control of epidemics of bubonic plague in San Francisco in 1900–1909 and later in the movement to assure safe milk supplies in Amer-

27

ican cities, where epidemics of diarrheal diseases sent infant mortality soaring every summer.[1] Interestingly, the power of the germ theory of disease to improve the health of human populations most often found expression in urban settings. Since the time of Hippocrates, health and place were linked in the medical imagination. In *Air, Waters and Places,* Hippocrates wrote of the relative healthfulness of the countryside compared to the city. In the eighteenth century, William Cadogan, in his famous (and in many respects remarkably modern) 1749 essay on the care of infants, observed that foundlings sent to the countryside survived at much higher rates than those who remained in London. More generally, he observed that "In the lower Class of Mankind, especially in the Country, Disease and Mortality are not so frequent, either among the Adult, or their Children."[2]

The "urban penalty" in morbidity and mortality was a well-understood phenomenon for centuries and was used as an argument for social reform in the nineteenth century.[3] Ironically, when the reasons for the penalty were finally understood in terms of the germ theory, the perception of the relative healthfulness of cities compared to the country was transformed. As cure became increasingly possible, the perception of the healthfulness of the countryside gave way to a notion of cities as places where the modern physician—relying on the latest in science, technology, and research—cured patients. Improved public health practice prevented many people from getting sick in the first place. Asepsis and infection control—along with the development of general anesthesia, technology, and the increasing professionalization and specialization of medicine—also transformed and enhanced the role of the large urban hospital.[3] In the nineteenth century, it could be argued that hospitals existed primarily to provide the poor and destitute a place to die and young physicians and anatomists a place to learn anatomy. With the rise of a professionalized medicine invigorated by the germ theory and technological change, hospitals became centers of research, scientific advance and, most important, cure. As the locus of scientific medicine became concentrated in large cities, rural populations, which had generally enjoyed better health than urban ones, suddenly found themselves disadvantaged in their ability to access medical care.

During the same time, rural doctors found themselves disadvantaged within their profession. As Seipp[4] points out, in the years after World War I,

> The steady rise in the proportion of new medical graduates pursuing specialization served not only to reduce the pool of general practitioners from which replacements might be drawn. Specialization, together with the increasing importance of its counterpart, the hospital, magnified both the sense of professional isolation of rural practitioners and the disparity in the kind of care they could render as compared to their urban counterparts.

As early as 1921, Frank Billings, the president of the American Medical Association (AMA), was concerned about a "dearth of medical men to supply the needs of the rural population" and their inability to obtain timely access to the latest in medical knowledge. Billings further lamented that the "country physician lacks modern facilities for diagnosis and for the needed hospital treatment of his patients."[4]

Just as the rural physician shortage is nothing new in the United States, neither is government and private sector involvement in trying to decrease the maldistribution of resources. As the leading professional organization for physicians, the AMA strenuously protected the autonomy of the private physician and effectively helped prevent most government involvement in the direct provision of care in the years before World War II.[5,6] However, several government and private programs have, over the years, attempted to improve the availability of physicians to rural residents. These programs included efforts of the Children's Bureau and the programs associated with the Sheppard-Towner Act, passed in 1921, which improved access to maternal and infant services for isolated rural populations; various public health improvement programs; and medical school loan-forgiveness programs. A fellowship program started by the Commonwealth Fund in the 1930s encouraged physicians to practice in rural areas. Medical cooperatives were started by state farmers' unions, and health insurance was provided by the New Deal–era Farmers Security Administration (FSA).[4–6] At one point in the 1930s, one-quarter of the population of the Dakotas was covered by FSA insurance.[5] Although medical care was sometimes locally effective for a time, the overall shortage of rural practitioners did not decrease. Rural populations continued to be underserved and rural physicians continued to work in difficult circumstances, increasingly isolated from the mainstream of their profession.

In the years after World War II, Hill-Burton rural hospital construction efforts significantly increased the number of hospital beds per capita and helped improve and modernize hospitals all over the country. Employer-based insurance plans (largely among large urban-based companies) began to insure larger numbers of people, and medical practice moved toward a group practice model. None of these developments had much effect on the shortage of physicians in rural areas of the United States. Rather, the relative shortage and disparity with urban areas persisted and, in many instances, worsened. Medical specialization accelerated, decreasing the number of general practitioners available to serve the needs of rural populations.[7] Comprehensive health insurance was generally not available to rural populations (though there were exceptions). Accelerating technological change also made it more and more difficult for doctors and hospitals to keep up with their urban counterparts.[4,8]

THE PRIMARY CARE MOVEMENT

In the 1960s two developments, one legislative and one professional, led to significant changes in the orientation of medical training—changes that, in turn, had far-reaching consequences for rural health care. First, Medicare and Medicaid, established in the mid-1960s, significantly increased the demand for generalist physicians. Medicare dollars also provided a steady income to rural hospitals, though at a lower rate per patient than to urban hospitals.[4,8] Second, a public and professional consensus regarding medical specialization—that it had gone too far—grew. In 1930, there were approximately 80 generalists for every 20 specialists. By the late 1960s, that ratio was reversed.[7] In 1967, James Bryan spoke to the Family Health Foundation of America and said, "What confronts us today is a societal monstrosity; a profession that is standing on its head. Its management function, its generalist coordinator, lies at the bottom of the heap—we must somehow right this pyramid and stand it on its base."[9]

Four different medical education commission reports released in the 1960s insisted on the need to train more of what have come to be called *primary care physicians* oriented toward general practice, continuity of care, preventive health, and care of the individual as a member of a family and community. In 1969, the American Board of Family Practice was established, which promoted a new generalist specialty called *family medicine*. At about the same time, some departments of internal medicine and pediatrics also began developing primary care training programs.[4,7,8] The federal government also promoted primary care training through its Title VII programs.

Although none of these developments occurred with rural physician shortages specifically in mind, they did address one of the most fundamental problems underlying physician shortages in rural America: the shortage of physicians trained as generalists. As the 10th Council on Graduate Medical Education (COGME) report noted, "Nothing affects the location decision of physicians more than specialty. Unfortunately for rural areas, the more specialized the physician, the less likely it is the physician will settle in a rural area."[10]

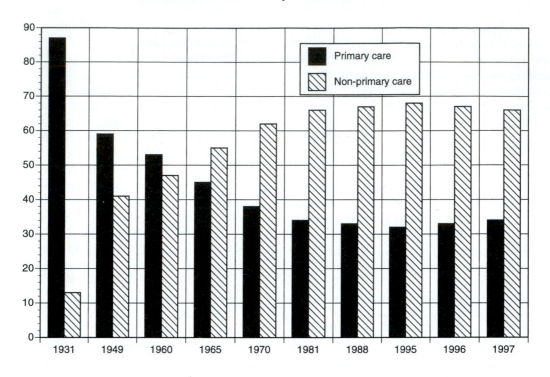

(Source: COGME,1998; ARF, 1999)

FIGURE 3-1 Percentage of primary care and non-primary care physicians, selected years—
1931–1997.

Generalist physicians are the most appropriate kind of physicians for rural areas, given that the population base of small and remote rural areas cannot economically support specialist physicians. The effect of the changes described above (and other developments in the health care market) was to arrest the decline in number of physicians practicing in the primary care disciplines of general practice, family practice, general internal medicine, and general pediatrics. Figure 3-1 shows the decline in the proportion of physicians practicing in primary care since 1931. AMA projections suggest that the proportion of new medical graduates entering primary care will increase over the next decade. In 1997, some 38.2 percent of graduates entered primary care residency programs. The AMA model also suggests that the proportion

entering primary care will stabilize in the year 2007 at about 45 percent,[11] near COGME's goal of 50 percent.[12] However, the results of the 2000 national medical student/residency match are disturbing. Despite decades of primary care rhetoric, the number of family medicine matches has declined for the third consecutive year (by 10 percent overall and by 20 percent for U.S. born and trained medical school seniors).

FEDERAL INVOLVEMENT

In contrast to educational interventions, which addressed the shortage of primary care doctors generally, some federal programs were targeted directly at redressing the geographic maldistribution of physicians. The National Health Service Corps (NHSC) was established in 1970 and deployed physicians and other health professionals to underserved communities throughout the United States. By 1979, the NHSC had a budget of $140 million,[8] including funds for scholarships and loan forgiveness for recent medical graduates willing to serve from 2 to 4 years in underserved communities. The first 12 of many Area Health Education Centers (AHECs) were established in the 1970s, in part for the purpose of reducing the maldistribution of health care providers.

The federal government also sponsors Community Health Centers (CHCs) throughout the country, including clinics for migrant and seasonal farm workers, the homeless, and underserved urbanites. The configurations of these clinics are myriad, involving state and local authorities as well as nonprofit organizations and foundations. Though not uniformly distributed in the underserved areas of the United States, CHCs provide care for about 10 percent of the uninsured population of the United States, or about 4 million people. NHSC providers often staff CHCs. The federal government has also provided 10 percent Medicare bonus payments to providers working in designated Health Professional Shortage Areas (HPSAs) to help induce providers to locate and stay in underserved areas. In addition, the designation of Rural Health Clinic makes it possible to receive cost-based reimbursement for Medicare and Medicaid patients. The federal government also supports research on rural health and telehealth through HRSA's Office of Rural Health Policy, established in 1988,[4,8,10] and Office for the Advancement of Telehealth, established in 1998.

THE RURAL PHYSICIAN POPULATION

Despite the efforts of governments and private organizations, a large part of the rural population of the United States continues to be underserved by physicians. As noted above, the decline of generalism in the physician population is one of the key factors explaining that maldistribution. However, there are intrarural and regional differences in the characteristics and severity of the physician shortage, which are explored below. To begin with, however, it should be noted that in 1997 there were 594,706 physicians providing care to patients in the United States. Although 20 percent of the U.S. population lives in nonmetro counties, only about 9.7 percent (57,645) of those physicians provided care in nonmetro counties. When restricted to primary care generalist specialties only (family practice, general practice, general pediatrics, and general internal medicine), the rural/urban inequity in physician-population ratios is only slightly reduced. Nationally, there are about 78 primary care physicians engaged in patient care for every 100,000 Americans. In metro counties, there are 85 per 100,000 population, compared to 49 in nonmetro counties. Clearly, the rural/urban disparity persists. However, it is important to understand that this disparity is far more severe in some rural locations and less so in others.[13]

In considering the rural physician shortage, it is important to differentiate rural places by region and type of rural county. There are many ways to think about "rurality," as noted in Chaps. 1 and 2. Two important dimensions for rural residents and physicians involved in providing care to rural residents are level of local urbanization and the degree of geographic isolation from large urban centers. The size of the largest town in a nonmetropolitan county is often related to the general level of services available locally. A nonmetro county that includes a city of 25,000 people is likely to have a much more sophisticated hospital and greater access to at least some medical specialists than a nonmetro county where the largest town has only 3000 inhabitants. Isolation from large metropolitan centers where the highest-level services are available is also an important issue. Far from specialists and tertiary hospitals, what is a trivial referral to a specialist in the city becomes a request that a patient leave home and family for treatment, incurring major inconvenience, more stress, and possible loss of income.

A county-level definition of rurality developed by the U.S. Department of Agriculture incorporates these two dimensions into a nine-group taxonomy called the *Urban Influence Codes.*[14] Two types of metropolitan counties and seven types of nonmetro counties are defined based on the size of the largest town in the county and whether or not the county is adjacent to a metropolitan county. The importance of these dimensions for the level of underservice is clearly seen in Fig. 3-2, which shows the generalist physician/population ratios for the nine types of counties. In general, the counties with the smallest towns, whether adjacent or nonadjacent to metro areas, have the lowest number of primary care physicians for their residents. It should be kept in mind that these less populated places are also less likely than larger places to have specialist physicians available. In larger places, some primary care may be performed by other specialists, especially obstetrician/gynecologists.

Rural counties with large towns of more than 10,000 residents have less severe shortages of primary care doctors. The residents of the most isolated counties with the lowest populations are the most disadvantaged in terms of the number of primary care physicians available to care for them (38 primary care physicians per 100,000 residents). Isolated counties have been the last to benefit when physician supply increases. Kindig and Movassaghi noted that, between 1975 and 1985, the number of primary care physicians per 100,000 people grew three times faster in the United States overall than it did in the smallest and most isolated rural counties.[15] Larger rural counties increased the number of generalist physicians at a rate slightly higher than the overall U.S. rate.

There is also a regional dimension to the

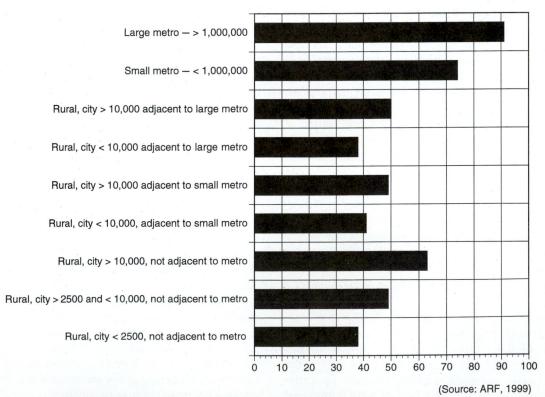

(Source: ARF, 1999)

FIGURE 3-2 Primary care physicians active in patient care per 100,000 population, 1997.

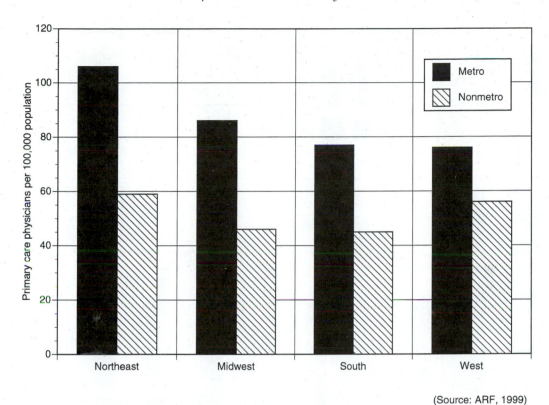

(Source: ARF, 1999)

FIGURE 3-3 *Primary care physicians per 100,000 population by census region and metro vs. nonmetro location, 1997.*

maldistribution of physicians across the rural/urban dimension. As shown in Fig. 3-3, the Northeast has the highest number of primary care physicians per 100,000 population in the country for both its rural and urban populations, but the largest within-region rural/urban gap. The lowest levels of availability of primary care physicians in nonmetro areas are in the South and Midwest, while the Pacific region has a relatively high rural physician/population ratio (56 per 100,000) and the smallest rural/urban gap. Figure 3-3 points out the importance of understanding what is meant by the term *maldistribution*. On the one hand, the greatest maldistribution is in the Northeast region—that is, the Northeast has the largest rural/urban inequity. On the other hand, the Midwest and South have the lowest level of primary care physician availability, albeit in the context of overall lower physician availability (i.e., a smaller rural/urban gap).

When region and the dimensions of rurality measured by the Urban Influence Codes are combined, as they are in Fig. 3-4, other patterns are observed. In general the figure reflects the facts about maldistribution that could be gleaned from Figs. 3-2 and 3-3. However, recall that Fig. 3-2 indicated that the most isolated places with the lowest populations have the lowest generalist physician/population ratios. Figure 3-4 shows that this is not true for the Northeast and not as pronounced in the West. Rather, the problem of very low ratios is concentrated in the Midwest and the South. In general, the Northeast is exceptional for its high physician/population ratios in rural counties. Rural counties of the other three regions of the country, with the occasional exception of

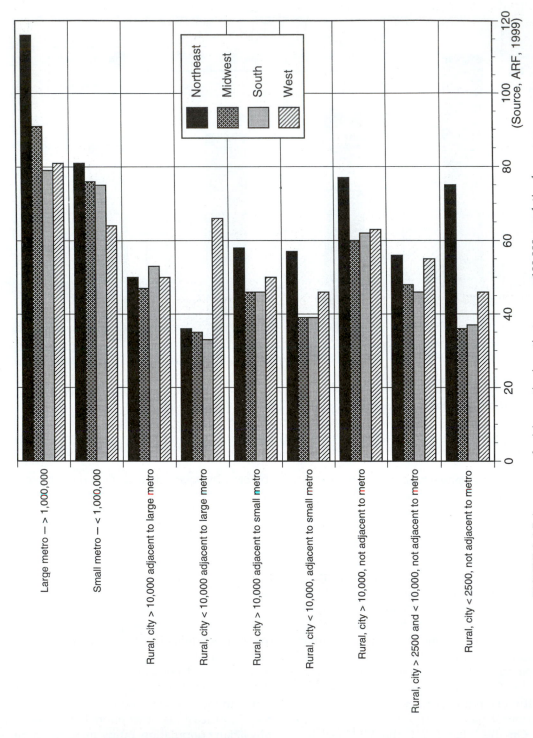

FIGURE 3-4 Primary care physicians active in patient care per 100,000 population by census region, 1997.

the West, have far fewer physicians to meet the needs of their populations than the Northeast.

SPECIALTY DISTRIBUTION

As noted above, the rural physician population is composed mostly of generalist care physicians practicing in the specialties of family practice, general practice, general pediatrics, or general internal medicine. However, the mix of primary care physicians varies substantially depending on the type of rural county. Figure 3-5 shows the physician/population ratios for

several different physician specialties in the seven classes of rural counties identified by the Urban Influence Codes. The figure shows that, even within the generalist care specialties, general pediatricians and general internists tend to concentrate in larger rural counties. Family and general practitioners make up the lion's share of the physicians in smaller and more isolated counties. In addition to the primary care specialties, the figure shows the contribution of two specialties, general surgery and obstetrics/gynecology, that are important to the rural provider mix, especially in larger rural areas. General surgeons and obstetrician/gynecologists are significantly more common in nonmetro

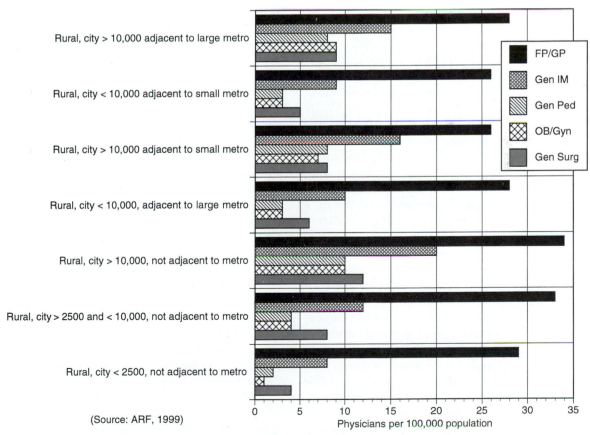

(Source: ARF, 1999)

FIGURE 3-5 Selected patient care physician specialists per 100,000 population in nonmetro counties, 1997.

counties with cities larger than 10,000, where the patient base is large enough to support such specialists.

The scarcity of obstetrician/gynecologists in smaller rural settings can have an effect on the willingness and ability of family practice physicians to provide obstetric care. Obstetricians are often consulted by family physicians, and the ability to refer patients efficiently to obstetricians (and, if necessary, to neonatologists and hospitals with neonatal intensive care units) is particularly important to ensuring good birth outcomes in more isolated rural populations. It is for this reason that the regionalization of perinatal care has been a major research theme in the study of rural health services throughout the 1980s and 1990s. The improvement in birth outcomes among rural residents as a result of the regionalization of perinatal care is one of the most important rural health success stories of the past 20 years.[10,16–21] The availability of obstetricians in regional centers is essential to sustained success in this area.

Figure 3-5 also suggests the declining role of general surgeons in the constellation of locally available care for rural residents. In part this is a function of the increasing specialization of surgical training, which tends to concentrate surgeons in larger urban centers where a sufficient patient base exists to support surgical subspecialization. General surgery is becoming a less common specialty overall, and rural communities have special difficulties in recruiting and retaining general surgeons because there exists little in the way of training programs that prepare general surgical residents for the challenges and special rewards of practice in rural settings.[22–24] Additionally, there is little consensus on the proper scope of surgical service in rural hospitals.[25] Low surgical volume, typical of rural hospitals, has been associated with poor outcomes for some complex procedures, while favorable outcomes for many common procedures do not appear to be associated with surgical volume.[26,27] Many rural hospitals use visiting surgeons from urban or regional centers, and this solution to providing surgical care is apparently becoming more common.[10,28] Questions about quality assurance and continuity of care provided by visiting surgeons have been raised, and it remains to be seen whether this surgical solution is a safe and effective one for rural populations.[28]

GENDER AND RURAL PRACTICE— AN EMERGING ISSUE

The U.S. physician work force is currently in the middle of a profound demographic transformation. Women made up 7.1 percent of the work force in 1970 and 15.3 percent by 1986.[29] In 1997, women made up 23.8 percent of the active physicians in the United States.[13] Currently, medical school enrollments in the United States are approaching 50 percent female, indicating that, as older physician cohorts retire, the proportion of women in the physician work force will continue to increase. AMA data indicate that by the year 2000, some 45 percent of first-year residents will be women.[11] The implications of this transformation for rural health care are large and potentially troubling.

Women are relatively more likely than men to select and practice in generalist specialties like family practice and general pediatrics rather than other specialties. In fact, women made up more than 50 percent of the first-year residents in pediatrics in 1997 and about 43 percent of new family practice residents (U.S. medical school graduates only).[11] Overall, 46.2 percent of female graduates selected primary care specialties, compared with 32.8 percent of male graduates. Women were also relatively more likely than men to select obstetrics/gynecology, a specialty with a significant primary care component. The fact that women are making up an ever-growing part of the physician work force and are more likely than men to enter primary care specialties would seem to bode well for physician supply in rural areas, since the most important underlying cause of the rural physician shortage has been the undersupply of primary care physicians.

However, there is another dimension to the gender transition of the physician work force; women, though they enter primary care specialties more often than men, are far less likely to practice in rural settings. This can be clearly seen in Fig. 3-6. When women do choose rural settings, they are more likely to choose larger rural communities over smaller, more remote ones. The reasons for this particular aspect of maldistribution are not well understood, though Doescher and coworkers suggest a range of factors that could be particularly important in discouraging women from working in rural settings.[29] These include the prevalence of solo and private practice in rural settings, gender bias, and the difficulties in accommodating spousal careers in rural settings. Women, who often face disproportionate demands on their time because of family role expectations, are more likely than men to choose salaried positions that allow for considerable schedule flexibility, as opposed to the inflexible schedule and lifestyle implications of solo or private practice in a small town. A major goal for rural health services research over the next decade is to identify factors that could attract women to rural practice and to learn what can be done to mitigate the factors that make it relatively unattractive to women currently.

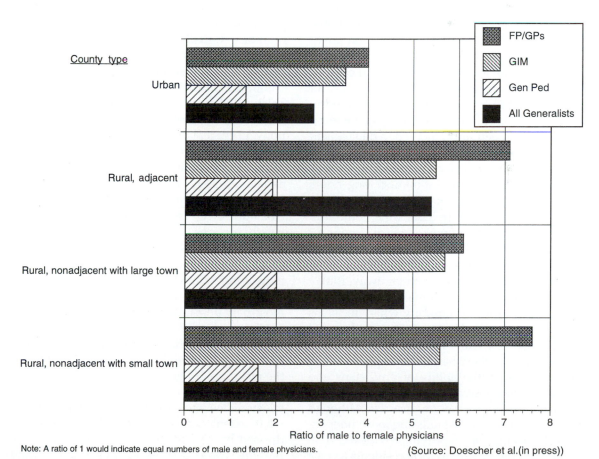

Note: A ratio of 1 would indicate equal numbers of male and female physicians.   (Source: Doescher et al.(in press))

FIGURE 3-6 Ratio of male to female physicians in generalist specialties, by location, 1996.

MANAGED CARE AND TELEHEALTH— INCREASING FINANCIAL VIABILITY, DECREASING ISOLATION?

One of the most important recent changes affecting all of American medicine is the emergence of managed care. (Managed care and networks in rural areas are discussed in detail in Chap. 17.) Beginning as an urban organizational form, it was slow to penetrate rural markets. However, by 1995, some 90 percent of all rural counties were in the service area of at least one health maintenance organization,[10] though the percentage of the population enrolled in managed care remains low in rural areas relative to urban ones, with only about one-third the rate of enrollment compared to urban populations. The appropriateness of the managed care model in rural areas continues to be hotly debated, just as it is throughout the country. In rural areas, however, communities and physicians are confronted with some particularly difficult choices.

Managed care brings with it economies of scale that could not otherwise be generated in small rural communities. By bringing some rationality to on-call and emergency department coverage as well as support for continuing medical education, managed care organizations may mitigate some of the isolation and long hours that have made rural practice unattractive to many physicians.[10] At the same time, communities and physicians may experience significant loss of control over local health care resources. When the hospital is controlled from far away and the physician is paid from far away, it may be very difficult to assert, defend, and maintain the interests of the community when decisions are made about the future of the local hospital or physician practice. Physician independence, often especially cherished by rural providers, is lost. Also lost is the ability of physicians and hospitals in a community to provide an informal safety net for the poor and uninsured. Although community-owned hospitals and local independent physicians may expect to provide a certain amount of charity care to local residents as part of their mission, most managed care organizations are profit-making enterprises with little sense of obligation to uninsured members of the community. Though managed care organizations may take on Medicaid-covered patients, the working poor, who make up a large part of many rural populations, can be left without a health care alternative.

Managed care may address some of the seemingly never-ending problems of maintaining financial viability and ensuring some semblance of a personal life for rural physicians. Telehealth technology may address two other perennial problems of the rural physician: staying current in one's field and consulting with medical specialists. The development of the Internet and the National Network of Libraries of Medicine services such as *Loansome Doc* have put a vast medical literature on the computer screens of physicians in the most isolated of rural communities. E-mail consultation and discussion groups can make significant contributions to ending the professional isolation that has so hampered physicians throughout this century. Telehealth technologies also offer the ability to engage distant specialists in real-time consultation and clinical problem solving (see Chap. 16). Video teleconferencing and "store and forward" technologies can support services such as teleradiology. However, these technologies often create problems even as they solve others. One unresolved issue, for example, is how telehealth services will be reimbursed. Another question involves licensure and malpractice insurance for physicians providing services remotely but across state lines. While these technologies are still in their infancy and for the most part unstandardized, they will undoubtedly play a large role in decreasing the isolation of the rural physician and the rural patient from specialists. Another issue to consider is whether the meaning of "geographic maldistribution of physicians" will be changed in an era where telemedicine technologies are ubiquitous. To what extent can a physician shortage be redressed by physicians who are not physically present? More pointedly, how can telehealth help both overworked rural generalist physicians and the remote and underserved populations they serve?

THE FUTURE OF RURAL PHYSICIANS

Throughout the twentieth century, the ability of rural communities to retain the services of physicians and the willingness and ability of physicians to practice in rural settings have been driven by social and technological changes that affected medical practice in urban and rural areas. The professionalization of medicine and medical education, the germ theory of disease, the modernization of the hospital, and the development of anesthesia had enormous effects on urban as well as rural medicine. Such changes often had vast social and demographic effects as well. Many of those changes found unique expression in rural America in the form of a maldistribution of physicians and a sense that rural places had become unhealthy because they were served by small hospitals and generalist physicians who had been left behind in their profession. It is important to keep in mind, as we consider the future of the rural physician, that it is these larger forces affecting all of American medicine that will affect the future of the rural physician more than anything else. Efforts to redress specific rural problems can help if they are carefully targeted, but technological change, the medical marketplace, and the continuing reassessment of the role of government in ensuring access to care for all its citizens is what matters most. The unique problems of rural physicians and the populations served by them are localized expressions of larger societal choices about ensuring access to health care providers.

REFERENCES

1. Meckel RA: *Save the Babies—American Public Health Reform and the Prevention of Infant Mortality 1850–1929.* Baltimore, Johns Hopkins University Press, 1990.

2. Cadogan W: *An Essay upon Nursing, and the Management of Children, from Their Birth to Three Years of Age.* London, General Committee of the London Foundling Hospital, 1749.

3. Rosenberg CE: *Explaining Epidemics and Other Studies in the History of Medicine.* Cambridge, England, Cambridge University Press, 1992.

4. Seipp C: *Rural Health Care in Historical Perspective.* Chapel Hill, NC, University of North Carolina, Rural Health Research Program, 1990.

5. Starr P. *The Social Transformation of American Medicine.* New York, Basic Books, 1982.

6. Ladd-Taylor M: "My work came out of agony and grief": mothers and the making of the Sheppard-Towner Act, in Koven S, Michel S (eds): *Mothers of a New World: Maternalist Politics and the Origins of the Welfare States.* New York, Routledge, 1993.

7. Geyman JP, Hart LG: *Primary Care at the Crossroads: Progress, Problems and Policy Options.* WAMI Rural Health Research Center working paper #22. Seattle, WA, University of Washington, 1993.

8. Rosenblatt RA, Moscovice IS: *Rural Health Care.* New York, Wiley, 1982.

9. Bryan JE: A summary report on the regional conferences on comprehensive medical care for the American family. *GP* (suppl):17, 1967.

10. Council on Graduate Medical Education: *Physician Distribution and Health Care Challenges in Rural and Inner-City Areas—Tenth Report.* Washington, DC, COGME, 1998.

11. Kletke PR: The projected supply of allopathic physicians, 1997 to 2020. American Medical Association—Physician Marketplace Report. Chicago, AMA, 1999.

12. Council on Graduate Medical Education: *Physician Workforce Policies: Recent Developments and Remaining Challenges in Meeting National Goals—Fourteenth Report,* Washington, DC, COGME, 1999.

13. Area Resource File. Washington, DC, Bureau of Health Professions, Health Resources and Services Administration, February 1999.

14. Ricketts TC, Johnson-Webb KD, et al: *Definitions of Rural: A Handbook for Health Policy Makers and Researchers.* Rockville, MD, Federal Office of Rural Health Policy, Health Resources and Services Administration, 1998.

15. Kindig DA, Movassaghi H: The adequacy of physician supply in small rural counties. *Health Affairs* 8(3):63–76, 1989.

16. Gortmaker S, Sobol A, et al: The survival of very low-birth weight infants by level of hospital of birth: a population study of perinatal systems in four states. *Am J Obstet Gynecol* 152:517–524, 1985.

17. Rosenblatt RA, Reinken J, et al: Is obstetrics safe in small hospitals?—Evidence from New Zealand's regionalised perinatal system. *Lancet* 149:98–102, 1985.

18. Rosenblatt RA, Mayfield JA, et al: Outcomes of regionalized perinatal care in Washington state. *West J Med* 149(1):98–102, 1988.

19. Nesbitt TS, Connell FA, et al: Access to obstetrical care in rural areas: effects on birth outcomes. *Am J Public Health* 80:814–818, 1990.

20. Larson EH, Hart LG, et al: Is non-metropolitan residence a risk factor for poor birth outcome in the U.S.? *Soc Sci Med* 45(2):171–187, 1997.

21. Nesbitt TS, Larson EH, et al: Access to maternity care in rural Washington: its effect on neonatal outcomes and resource use. *Am J Public Health* 87(1):85–90, 1997.

22. Sabo RR: Surgical practices in rural communities: challenges and opportunities. *Bull Am Coll Surg* 79(4):6–10, 1994.

23. Stevick JA, Mullis EN, et al: Perspectives of rural surgical practice in Georgia. *Am Surg* 60(9):703–706, 1994.

24. Saver BG, Bowman R, et al: *Barriers to Residency Training of Physicians in Rural Areas.* WWAMI Rural Health Research Center working paper #46. Seattle, WA, University of Washington, 1998.

25. Williamson HA, Hart LG, et al: Rural hospital inpatient surgical volume: cutting edge or operating on the margin? *J Rural Health* 10(1):16–25, 1994.

26. Luft HS, Bunker JP, et al: Should operations be regionalized? The empirical relation between surgical volume and mortality. *N Engl J Med* 301:1364–1369, 1979.

27. Welch HG, Larson EH, et al: Readmission after surgery in Washington state rural hospitals. *Am J Public Health* 82(3):407–411, 1992.

28. Hanlon CR: Itinerant surgery: outreach or outrage? *Bull Am Coll Surg* 74(10):6–8, 1989.

29. Doescher MP, Ellsbury KE, et al: The distribution of rural female physicians in the United States. *J Rural Health,* in press.

CHAPTER 4

The Rural Health Care Team

THOMAS C. ROSENTHAL   NANCY CAMPBELL-HEIDER

Mrs. M., a 28-year-old mother of two girls under 6 years of age, presented with her third pregnancy to a rural family practice office at 8 weeks gestation. She was a self-employed housekeeper for several families in the community, and her husband was a supervisor in the local salt mine. Together they raised a few beef cattle each year for themselves and for sale. By 16 weeks, her uterine size exceeded expectations and twins were confirmed by ultrasound. She was referred to the local obstetrician and managed jointly. At 38 weeks, with blood pressure rising and fetal movement decreasing, she underwent a cesarean section. At surgery, one member of the family practice group assisted the obstetrician and two other family practice partners took care of a twin apiece as the boys, weighing almost 6 pounds each, were delivered. The mother and newborns went home on the fifth postpartum day. The public health nurse called the office on day 9 concerned that the twins did not seem to be nursing well. Mrs. M. looked careworn when the twins' weight loss was confirmed in the office later that day. Mr. M. was found outside in the pickup with his daughters. He was worried but felt helpless because of his wife's independence. Mrs. M said that her husband was busy enough without having to worry about her. After some in-office discussion, the couple reassigned household jobs. Mr. M. took some delayed vacation time and hired a neighbor to feed the cattle. The public health nurse visited daily and checked in with the office nurse, who organized neighbors to provide casserole dinners for the family. Supplemental bottle feedings were introduced and assigned to Mr. M. and the girls. One week later, the home nurse had coifed Mrs.

M.'s hair and Mr. M. joined his wife in the examination room. She was animated but still looked a bit sleepless. The whole office cheered when, with permission, 7- and 8-ounce gains were announced over the office intercom.

Rural primary care is not simple. The locus of responsibility for organizing health care is the primary care office, where most patients gain entry to medical service. The patient is the recipient of services delivered over time, by the same provider, in a manner more comprehensive than is generally recognized. Receptionists to physicians seem aware of the important role that caregivers, both formal and informal, play in the health care team. A sense of community ownership elaborates a sense of responsibility. This case history illustrates how a team of generalists, specialists, home nurses, office staff, family, and community can work together in patient-specific and nontraditional ways. When a family's usual coping skills and patterns became disorganized, the health care providers were able to recognize a spectrum of needs and assist the family in making adjustments to maximize support. A complicated pregnancy was managed with the community obstetrician, the home health nurse took an interventional approach and became an active team leader, the office nurse engineered task assistance for meals, and the employer adjusted work schedules.

Rural care systems erect fewer barriers to mixing nonprofessionals and professionals into complex teams that address specific needs across vocational boundaries with little attention to hierarchy. Caregivers often have a personal appreciation of community-specific social and environmental impacts on illness. Continuity relationships witness the changing course of chronic problems and multiple interventions. Many overworked rural physicians have discovered that it is the formal and informal caregivers working in a multifaceted team that advance their own career satisfaction and improve patient outcomes.

In this chapter the concept of team care as it exists in rural America is described and the reader will become aware of naturally occurring health care teams. The way teams influence patient care and decision making is explored. The importance of teams to quality care and patient satisfaction is demonstrated and a strategy to implement team management is discussed.

DEFINING TEAMWORK

Russell and Branch described the world champion Boston Celtics of the 1970s as a team of specialists whose performance—like a team of specialists in any field—depended both on individual excellence and on how well they worked together.[1] Senge characterizes teamwork as an "alignment" resulting in a group that functions as a whole with a common direction, synergy, and very little wasted energy.[2] Effective teams mine the resources of all members to enable problem solving in complex situations. Basic to this effort is a high level of trust and interdependence, which enables team members to count on and complement the actions of others. Team dialogue allows the group to explore complex issues from different viewpoints. Conflict resolution depends on the mutual respect shared by participants.

Teams are particularly important among knowledge workers, including those in the increasingly complex health care arena.[3] Like all teams, health care teams are affected by their organizational context, the nature of their work, participants, available recruits, resources, and operative divisions of labor.[4] In traditional hierarchical organizations such as those involved in health care, the physician is usually designated as the team leader regardless of circumstances. There is considerable research, much of it from the nursing literature, substantiating that collaborative decision making improves patient outcomes and that patient participation improves satisfaction.[4,5]

RURAL SYSTEMS

Because rural providers usually live in the communities they serve, they assume a visible and valued community status. Community and patient needs, no matter how trivial, compete with the provider's needs, no matter how great. Being aware that problems not dealt with by the rural primary care office will not be dealt with at all drives the rural doctor to longer hours of more intense work.[6,7] To meet this demand, a successful rural generalist office evolves into a well-organized team where employees have carved out clear roles and articulate a remarkably uniform mission. Each player expresses responsibility for patient outcomes. The word *team* is used often, and job satisfaction is more pervasive than burnout.

Health care organized in terms of teams offers more than the sum of its parts. Some offices are very simple teams that focus on getting patients scheduled and into the rooms where they see the physician. More elaborate practices assign coordinated responsibilities to all individuals who interact with the patient. In these practices, patients are assigned the appropriate amount of time, screened for chief complaint and preventive needs, assessed for satisfaction after care, and followed up after the visit.

Inherently collaborative, primary care is the most common rural model. Several health professionals (minimally a physician and a nurse) work closely together to offer care that is more comprehensive than it would be if they worked in isolation. The sense of a team often matures into a system capable of addressing complexity by seeing both the whole and the parts within it. Inevitably these rural teams transcend the biomedical model of disease, achieving a bio-psychosocial model.[8]

COMPONENTS OF PRIMARY CARE

A primary care medical unit must meet several service parameters. It is the patient's *first contact.* The office is accessible for each new problem or episode of care and for acute as well as chronic care. Patients identify the unit as their regular source of care and use it over a period of time, or *longitudinally.* As a *comprehensive* service, the unit must arrange for all types of health care services, even those not provided within the facility. This includes referrals for consultation, management of specific conditions, or support services like home care. Providers and staff must be prepared to deal with symptoms and signs as well as diagnosable conditions, preventive care, functional complaints, and social problems on the premises or by referral. Primary care teams tolerate ambiguity, aware that many problems will not achieve standard diagnostic nomenclature status. *Coordination* of care is achieved through problem lists tracked from visit to visit. Providers are consistent and medical records well designed.[9]

The rural primary care unit has a geographically defined eligible population, is able to identify the individuals within that population who obtain care from the office, and addresses social issues even while providing minor surgical services in the office. Intuitively, they practice case management. Figure 4-1 illustrates the nature of rural family practice. Individuals are networked into a family system, an office system, and a community. Relationships are perceived to have a past, present, and future that adds connectivity to caregivers, patients, and community in a unique and potentially therapeutic model.

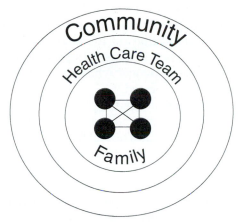

FIGURE 4-1 *Rural primary care practice embeds the family within a system influenced by the health care team and the community.*

DEFINING THE RURAL TEAM

The patient is always a member of the health care team. At its simplest, the doctor and the patient make up a team. Nearly always, a receptionist and office nurse participate. If the patient is referred, a specialist joins the team. Home care, nutritional counseling, social services, and mental health counseling involve other partners. Recently insurance carriers and health maintenance organizations (HMOs) have assumed an ever more active role in the care process. It is useful to explore the multiple teams that assemble and reassemble to provide longitudinal, comprehensive, and coordinated care in a rural practice.

The Physician/Patient Team

The patient and physician assume one of three partnership models within which to structure their relationship. In the *passivity model,* the physician makes the decisions. Up to 50 percent of patients believe their role to be passive. The patient describes symptoms in response to the physician's inquiry and relies on the physician to provide the most appropriate care plan. The patient then follows the care plan. There is relatively little opportunity for the patient to understand the complexities of his or her condition in this model, nor is there an opportunity for the patient to recognize when the plan is not proceeding as expected.[10]

In the *guidance model,* the physician provides more complex instructions that the patient is expected to carry out. Though he or she is somewhat better informed in this case, the patient is offered limited choice and accepts the physician's directions. The physician is still unlikely to become informed of the patient's barriers to wellness or the patient's belief system. The third model, *participation,* scripts the physician as a chief adviser who helps patients to help themselves. Patients are active in decision making, planning, and outcome monitoring.[10]

Getting the patient to actively participate is not always easy. Creating this level of communication can be facilitated by asking the patient to state what fears and feelings are evoked by the problem, what ideas he or she has about the causes of the symptoms, and how the symptoms are affecting the patient's life or functions.[11] Another technique asks patients to visualize themselves in 5 years and relate who is in the vision with them and what they are doing. This technique will often help patients focus on perceptions.

Creating an active participant can be very worthwhile. Patients will expose errors in the provider's assumptions about their abilities, perceptions, and expectations. Active patients report less discomfort, greater improvement in their general health status, and greater satisfaction with their physicians.[12]

The Family

The office workup and examination of Jimmy, an 8-year-old bed wetter, were negative and his parents wanted the problem fixed. During her interview, the family nurse practitioner (FNP) learned that every time Jimmy wet the bed, his older sister, Julie, teased him until he cried. The parents reacted by punishing Julie for hurting her brother's feelings. The FNP and physician were concerned that Jimmy's recalcitrant enuresis problem was partly due to complex family dynamics. From several options presented, the family chose to use positive reinforcement. The parents limited fluids after dinner, took turns getting Jimmy up at night, and on dry days placed a gold star on a calendar in his room. The FNP worked with the older sister to develop understandings that would help Jimmy and called Jimmy's teacher to alert her to contributory school stress. By the third month he was dry.

The family is affected by the disease of any member. In this case the parents needed assistance in recognizing how stress and negative reinforcement were affecting Jimmy. Once this was identified, the parents were guided through a redefinition of communication patterns. The FNP was also able to refocus the family from a limited organic model of disease to a broader understanding of illness. A team reappraisal and recruitment of the teacher effected a pleasingly positive outcome.

During a health crisis, the family routine becomes disorganized until the family adjusts or adapts to the change. Effort and focus are shifted to the illness or to compensating for the individuals affected by the illness. There is a coexistent struggle to recreate family balance. The provider can assist by identifying the peripheral fallout from illness, exploring how family patterns are interrupted, assessing family vulnerabilities and resources for coping, and encouraging the implementation of constructive problem solving.[13] These strategies prevent families from employing illness as a path to secondary gain.

Chronic disease associated with aging has stressed the resourcefulness of some families. Currently 22 million American households have at least one person caring for a relative.[14] Rural residents are spending more time than urban residents in providing care to family members. Farm families are more likely to provide care for a family member in their home than any other group of caregivers. Women, whether rural or urban, bear the greatest burden of caregiving.[15] If there is little outlet for endless demands, the caregiver may experience a cycle of neglect or abuse. An interdisciplinary team is best suited to assess the willingness of an informal caregiver and answer questions such as: What equipment would help? Do they get relief? Do they understand the disease process? Do they have ideas for improved function or concerns about medications?

The Community

Mr. J., a 32-year-old volunteer fireman, presented with nausea and vomiting and a 20-pound weight loss. The workup revealed adenocarcinoma of his left adrenal gland, with metastases. After failure of the first course of chemotherapy, the oncologist confirmed that only experimental regimens could be offered. The gas station where Mr. J. worked offered no health insurance and his bills were soaring. He was dying and leaving his family penniless. Brain metastases caused seizures that alarmed his wife and children, and it was beyond the ability of the home health nurse or the physician, who made daily visits, to reassure them. Mr. J. was admitted to the hospital for intravenous feeds (at his request) and mannitol to relieve brain edema. His depression was overwhelming. The nursing supervisor, the hospital's chief executive officer, and the physician agreed to allow Mr. J.'s poker buddies to visit during the evenings. One Saturday they played all night. Mr. J.'s intermittent confusion did not improve his poker game, but each player donated his winnings to the family anyway. Bystanders contributed to the table; even the parish priest, who visited regularly, did so. "Jack's Day," including pony rides, was organized as a weekend softball tournament at Fireman's Park. Several people from the family practice office and the ambulance crew "abducted" Mr. J. from the hospital so that he might be present at the event. He was the center of attention for 2 hours, and $20,000 was raised. Mr. J. slipped into a coma and died the next afternoon.

This case illustrates how a community can provide additional emotional and financial support for patients and their families. The team consisted of the physician, oncologist, office staff, priest, hospital personnel, friends, family, and volunteer firemen. This highly complex team maximized the patient's quality of life to the end and provided the family with additional resources. The synergism arose out of an open acceptance of nontraditional team participants and created outcomes unattainable through a pure biomedical model.

To outsiders, rural communities tend to be defined geographically and viewed as if they were monothematic. However, they accommodate church groups, ethnic groups, occupational groups, generational cohorts, social cliques, hobbyists, and many other subgroups.[16] Physicians often find themselves associated with several diverse groups. Offers to form new teams or new initiatives for someone in need often start as tentative inquiries to the physician, whom many view as a skilled and unbiased participant. The physician can often facilitate great accomplishments with just a little encouragement.

Another side of community health care is community-oriented primary care (COPC), in which the physician's practice takes a proactive approach to caring for the community by defining and characterizing the community, identifying health problems, developing programs to address problems, and monitoring the effectiveness of interventions.[17]

In many ways rural communities are both better defined and better suited to make great gestures in managing the needs of their own. The primary care office can catalyze these activities by providing effective leadership.

Intradisciplinary Professional Teams

Distance alone dictates that rural patients are referred to specialists somewhat less often than urban patients. Fewer than 5 percent of patients are referred—a rate that is not affected by the number of patients seen per day.[18–20] In a comanagement strategy, specialists provide short-term or one-visit care for patients with continuing assistance to the primary care physician. As a result, the efficiency of care is improved without sacrificing effectiveness.[21] Cancer chemotherapy is one common example where comanagement can be useful. Rural generalists often administer complex chemotherapy regimens to patients in their offices between the patient's visits to the oncologist. As a result, the rural generalist retains significant control in the patient's ongoing care and the specialist is provided with highly instructive feedback that enhances the rural physician's case-based knowledge.

Generalists use a cognitive process that incorporates factors such as probable/improbable, immediate/remote danger, resources/compliance, cost/benefit, baseline condition/potential outcome, patient/physician expectations, and epidemiology/personal experience to arrive at treatment decisions. If an expected response is not achieved in the anticipated time interval, the "tryout" logic circle is entered again. Referrals may be considered during the first cycle or after several. "Tryout" logic results in first-visit definitive care in up to 93 percent of ambulatory encounters but depends on longitudinal relationships[22] (see Fig. 4-2).

In contrast, the specialist regularly deals with situations perceived to be more acute or episodic and is inclined to apply the "rule out" approach by training and experience. Because the patient is considered to be at immediate

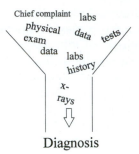

Diagnosis

FIGURE 4-3 *Specialty care is often a limited process whereby data are gathered at presentation, processed according to the conditions present at presentation, and acted on within a limited time. (From Rosenthal TC, Riemenschneider T, Feather J: A generalist-patient-specialist alliance for the nineties. Am J Med 100:338, 1996, with permission.)*

risk, delay could lead to greater morbidity and diagnosis is sought by ordering all relevant tests to rapidly eliminate errant possibilities. The "rule out" logic format requires more immediate use of resources as is appropriate for hospitalized or dangerously ill patients. These logic formats are so ingrained that many generalists begin referral letters to specialists with a request to rule out a list of concerns[22] (see Fig. 4-3).

Ideally a generalist or specialist might choose to apply the "tryout" and "rule out" logic formats according to different patient presentations, and to some extent this happens. However, in practice, physicians develop routine approaches to patients that predictably exemplify one or the other of these two formats, creating management plans that can seem illogical to the other participants in the generalist, specialist, and patient triad.

Informal partner-to-partner referrals are also important. Rural physicians are more likely to practice in single-specialty small groups than are urban physicians.[6] Partners orchestrate close symbiotic relationships. As business partners, they resolve issues of operations management; but as practice partners, they depend on each other for coverage, protected time, quality fol-

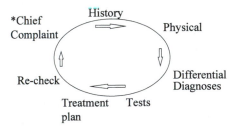

FIGURE 4-2 *primary care is a continuum of care in which each component of the patient-provider interaction is updated at each encounter, building on the findings from the previous encounter. (From Rosenthal TC, Riemenschneider T, Feather J: A generalist-patient-specialist alliance for the nineties. Am J Med 100:338, 1996, with permission.)*

low-up, and mutual responsiveness delivered within a shared philosophy of medical care and patient management. They must know each other's habits, trust each other's judgment, and depend on each other's allegiance to their patients. Charting habits must be uniform enough to facilitate frequent sharing of information. Yet partners must allow professional growth and change. Generally these complex goals are achieved through frequent, often daily, face-to-face or telephone encounters. The patient receives continuity of care from one provider yet has access to second opinions during hospitalizations, urgent visits, or when a given condition requires deliberation or counsel.

Interdisciplinary Professional Relationships

Nurse practitioners and physician assistants bring important skills to a rural office, including expanded clinical capacity, teaching skills, alternate perspectives, and improved patient communication. Counseling individuals, families, and groups is a major part of nurse practitioner practice. Traditional gender-role stereotypes have reinforced hierarchy among health care professionals, particularly between physicians and nurses, but team models reach their potential when they are collaborative and nonhierarchical.[23]

Non-advanced-degree office nurses perform triage and screening for phone calls, walk-in patients, and scheduled patients. They often encounter the patient from a less pressured, less formal perspective than the physician. The office nurse often has a day-to-day perspective on the patients' interactions with the office and guides patients and families in the execution of care plans. The nurse often has two contacts with a patient per visit, before and after the physician has seen the patient. These offer teachable moments during which the nurse can judge the patient's understanding of treatment protocols or instructions. In many rural offices, the nursing staff organizes formal patient-

education programs such as prenatal classes and smoking cessation.

The nurse can be more effective if office protocols or care plans for commonly encountered problems are developed jointly with the physician staff.[24] Thinking ahead about routine approaches to upper respiratory infections, earaches, abdominal pain, or suicide threats can improve the quality of triage and increase patient satisfaction.

Staff members greet patients, make appointments, obtain and record administrative data, carry out the provider's instructions, and deal with insurance companies. Office staff and managers must share the clinical vision to create the operational and financial methods that carry it off. The better informed they are, the more capable they will be of projecting the office mission and making informed decisions when the provider is not immediately available. An informed staff is better able to provide community insight and express continuity principles of primary care.

Some 15 percent of patients have social issues that affect their ability to gain wellness.[16] Social workers can add focus on family issues, housing conditions, employment, and poverty. They provide linkages to other agencies and match programs to family needs. The social worker's perspective enhances the assessment and definition of many complex problems.

Because it can be difficult to gain access to physical and occupational therapy, some rural primary care offices have modified exam rooms to accommodate such therapists. This arrangement encourages joint management and more timely responses to evolving treatment needs such as medication changes or the injection of joints during the rehabilitation process.

The rush to return patients home from the acute care setting has resulted in an increase in the number and acuity of home care patients. Home visits offer insights about the patient's family resources. The visiting nurse often functions as case manager. This team role is acknowledged by encouraging calls to the office.

Because home care is cost-effective only when the family can provide some of the care, the primary care office must coordinate a mixed professional and lay team to achieve success.[14,25]

Mental Health

More than half of all Americans with mental health problems are treated only in the primary medical care setting.[26] These patients represent 10 to 15 percent of the patients seen.[27] Some 20 percent of patients with mental health issues have problems related to material needs, one-third have difficult family relationships, another third have personal adjustment crises, and the remainder suffer significant psychiatric difficulties.[28] There are no rural/urban differences in the rate, type, or quality of outpatient treatment, but while rural residents make significantly fewer mental health specialty care visits, they are more likely to attempt suicide.[29]

Rural-specific barriers to care include fewer mental health providers, inadequate insurance, a stigma associated with mental health needs, and decreased confidentiality. As a result, rural patients often piece together support from friends, family, and pastors.[30] Their intuitive integration of mental health, social health, and physical health makes it most likely that they will seek professional care in the rural primary care office.[31]

Patients who are seen once in specialty treatment and returned to their generalist for continuing care have outcomes at 6 months equivalent to those patients cared for only by the specialty clinic.[21] If travel to a provider was involved, only 50 percent of patients signed up for consultation. However, if they were offered the opportunity to participate in a collaborative mental health approach in the primary medical setting, 91 percent of rural mental health patients were enrolled.[32] Travel does present a barrier to specialty treatment for rural mental health patients.

A typical rural mental health team consists of a family physician, a nurse practitioner, and a clinical psychologist or mental health social worker who collaborate to arrive at a diagnosis and treatment strategy. The family physician assumes the responsibility for medication prescriptions, often in consultation with the therapist. Good outcomes are dependent on good communication between the patient, therapist, and physician.[20,33] Integrating mental health care into the primary care setting affords the physician convenient access to a second point of view on troubling patients, enhancing the work of both providers.[27]

THE STRATEGY: COMMUNICATION IN TEAMS

The implementation of a team strategy within a busy rural office can seem impossible. The authors have studied several offices in rural upstate New York that have implemented weekly office staff meetings to promote the idea of teamwork. The agendas are often surprisingly simple. Everyone in the office—clerical, nursing, and medical staff—is expected to bring a case of a complex patient, frequent user, or problem patient to the meeting. Half of the cases discussed result in shared commiseration only. For the remainder, however, specific strategies are developed to assist the patient or employee. One staff member, often a nurse, is assigned to the case. This individual implements problem-solving strategies arrived at by the group or serves as the focus of contact with the office to improve consistency and responsiveness to the patient and family. The assigned contact person often assumes a very proactive approach by contacting the family to initiate problem solving. The contributions provided by front-office staff are frequently insightful and expand the perceptions of the provider staff. Offices successfully using a meeting often control the time tightly and proceed even if key members of the office are unavailable at the appointed time. Substituting a care plan for the stress felt by staff members actually enhances confidentiality, decreases interruptions, and saves time.

Conceptualizing and then actualizing a team-care approach moves the rural primary care office from a focus on how individuals function to how the whole system functions. When staff members view themselves as important contributors to patient outcomes, coordination occurs at multiple patient contact points and a case becomes actively managed. The patient and the family obtain case-appropriate assistance with the many peripheral problems associated with illness, such as insurance, transportation, and information resources. More problems are effectively handled by informed team members without interrupting the physician. Even moderate case management has resulted in significant cost savings in high-risk prenatal care, asthma, and chronic heart disease—conditions that often lead to high acute care utilization unless they are approached in a holistic fashion.[34]

Communication outside the office can also facilitate a holistic team approach. Making a referral outside the office can be complicated. The office must negotiate insurance coverage, patient denial and delay, missed appointments, payer regulations, and transportation problems. If there is too much workup prior to referral, the physician is accused of mimicking the specialist or wasting time. If there is too little, the problem may be miscategorized for lack of definition and precious patient resources may be wasted.[22] The rural physician can increase the likelihood that a patient will return for follow-up by informing the specialist of the broad range of issues being followed. This results in a better-informed specialist and better bidirectional communication.

Good communication can also overcome covert or overt messages about the "boonies" that may interfere with the teamwork needed if the condition requires shared care over time. The patient will return to the rural provider for routine general health care and will frequently seek supportive advice or reassurance. For example, the child with heart problems continues to see the rural generalist for immunizations, growth and nutrition assessment, school adjustments, and family counseling.

A successful patient-centered care plan between any two providers depends on successful completion of four steps. After judging the patient's needs, desires, premorbid condition, prognosis, and resources, the rural primary care provider must instruct patients about options and expectations. This discussion establishes the purpose of the referral, the patient's responsibility, the primary care provider's continuing role, and the specialist's anticipated actions; this is called *engagement*. The generalist next must *anticipate* the issues raised by the referral and provide the specialist with a clear description of the problem, prereferral workup, interventions, contributing factors, differential diagnoses, and anticipated procedures.[36] Two appointments should be scheduled, one with the specialist and a postreferral visit with the primary provider. During the *feedback* phase, letters document communication, intentions, and information transfer and provide a structure for quality management. In the final phase, *reassessment*, standards of care are judged and shortcomings are dealt with. The postreferral visit allows patients to share fears, express concerns, and explore barriers to implementing treatment.[22]

TEAMS AND QUALITY

Quality management calls for outcome goals with measurable objectives that are communicated to all participants, including the patient. With little effort, a formal team review process can be implemented on a regular basis. Some offices implementing team concepts simply record the patient objectives outlined at their weekly staff meetings and review each case during the first part of each meeting. More sophisticated tracking includes creation of detailed clinical pathways for each patient and outlining of specific objectives along a time line. This adds a time-sensitive dimension to team meetings.[24]

Agencies outside the office can participate in the weekly meeting. For example, one practice convinced the county mental health department and the home health agency to assign a specific caregiver to patients from the practice, and this caregiver attends the weekly staff meetings held over a brown-bag lunch.

Patients cared for by teams report greater opportunity for communication and a fuller sense of their own participation in treatment. As a result, their perception of quality improved, as did verifiable measures such as blood pressure.[36,37]

PROBLEMS WITH TEAM CARE

There are challenges to adopting a team approach to patient care. To be empowered, staff must receive some authority to make decisions. Traditionally, nurses and physicians were socialized to operate in a hierarchical treatment setting. Conversely, social workers and psychologists are socialized to the shared authority model. These differences in professional socialization can affect collaborative practice. Although physicians must assume responsibility for medical care, they are not necessarily the best qualified in all aspects of the care plan. Physicians interested in team care generally respond to instructions or suggestions about patient management issues no matter what their source. Successful teams see their task as exploring patient situations from multiple perspectives in order to intervene in uniquely effective ways. It is this aura of curiosity that facilitates the open communication found in successful team practices.[27]

Allowing multiple members of the team to communicate on substantive issues with patients will invariably lead to discovery of areas of disagreement or complaints. Inevitably performance concerns will be reported to one member of the team about another. Such discoveries need to be addressed as opportunities to improve team performance. Performance reports—informal and formal, positive and negative—need to be handled in a matter-of-fact manner and viewed as contributions to the puzzle that will make the team better. It is particularly important for the physician to accept

criticism, as this will reinforce others in viewing teamwork as the goal.

Just as each office member contributes different perspectives, so will outside consultants. The cardiologist's main focus may be the impact of heart disease on the cardiovascular system. The primary care office may prioritize the impact of illness on the patient's daily activities. These distinctions potentiate mismatches regarding the timing of referrals, utilization of resources, and management. When the office functions effectively as a team, conflicts can be shared from several perspectives, leading to better-informed decisions that are made with greater confidence.

Competition, role definitions, and problem ownership can usually be worked out over time with ample discussion of issues and feelings. These are temperaments not often shared in medical offices. The economics of health care are important, and this needs to be considered like any other issue. Office staff are remarkably sensitive to economic issues from patient and provider points of view.

AN EXAMPLE FROM RURAL PRACTICE

The school nurse practitioner referred a 14-year-old boy to the rural family practice office after discovering a heart murmur during a routine pre-football physical exam. The boy had been well and active but had not seen a health care provider in several years. The office nurse (RN) conducted an intake history with the boy and his mother, which revealed an incomplete immunization history. The RN and the family attend the same church; the RN was therefore able to inform the physician that the parents had separated some months earlier. She was surprised this did not come up during the history screen and sensed the mother to be withdrawn, a bit rattled, and anxious.

The physician confirmed a loud but innocent patterned murmur and described the workup plan to the boy and his mother. Being acutely aware of the mother's withdrawn posture, the physician asked the boy if he had any concerns regarding the murmur. The boy reaffirmed his desire to play football. The same question to the mother met with an anxious inquiry about how much an electrocardiogram (ECG) costs. The physician probed to discover that the family had no health insurance and the father had made no child-support payments during the last two months.

At the weekly staff meeting, the office RN brought up this family as her family of concern for the week. It was decided that the team could get the boy covered by a Medicaid program and could attempt to introduce the mother to a broader support system. The office manager called the county social services department and arranged an urgent appointment for Medicaid enrollment. The nurse called the family and encouraged the boy to return for the ECG, which proved to be normal. The office manager explained the new Child Health Insurance Plan and agreed to wait for payment. A cardiology referral was scheduled to follow approval of the Medicaid application. Immunizations were brought up to date.

The office nurse called the mother the next day to report normal laboratory results. During the conversation, she discovered that the son is often not at home when his mother calls from the restaurant where she cooks evenings, and he would seldom say where he had been. The nurse arranged for her own son to invite the boy over for dinner.

A pediatric cardiologist agreed to accept the Medicaid referral and confirmed an innocent murmur that she felt was loud because the boy is athletically thin. During a follow-up visit, the mother was full of questions about the cardiologist's report but accepted the plan for her son to play football again. The mother was scheduled for a physical examination and the office RN called the school nurse practitioner to verify the sports clearance.

Upon the mother's return for her gynecologic exam, the physician encouraged her to seek counseling from the county mental health department for her situational depression. At the next weekly meeting, the county mental health social workers updated the office and the physician decided to start an antidepressant medication. Football practice motivated the boy to improve his study habits.

He spent his evenings at home and joined his mother for a few sessions with the counselor.

MANAGED CARE'S IMPACT ON RURAL TEAM CARE

Managed care provides an economic basis for a biopsychosocial team approach to health care. The majority of care is initiated in the primary care office and financial barriers to consultations are lessened as patients are encouraged to seek service from the most efficient source.[38] The rationale for managed care comes from studies showing that, even when patient mix is controlled for, generalists use fewer resources than specialists to achieve similar results.[22] By moving generalists beyond coordinating care to controlling resources, managed care introduces new traps into the doctor/patient relationship and specialists become concerned about reduced autonomy.[22] Managed care also challenges an office by periodically seeking patient feedback on the appointment process, waiting time, and staff responsiveness.

This may be less of a change for the rural primary care office than feared. Rural providers have always been concerned about resource utilization in the typically underinsured environment of rural America. Capitation models ensure the rural practice a steady income stream, most likely at rates that are standard across the state and above traditional rural rates. HMOs should be able to provide information about utilization and demographics that the rural practice has not had access to before.[39]

CONCLUSION

Practitioners and patients do not exist in a vacuum. They are not independent entities but belong to complicated, intersecting systems whose relationship to one another is in constant flux. The patient/physician interaction occurs in the context of family, community, and other health care providers.[16] While taking charge of medical care, physicians will enhance their ability to provide healing if the patient's teams communicate effectively. To accomplish this, the physician will need to endorse the team's function and accept new collaborators. The reward will be improved outcomes, improved patient satisfaction, and improved community perception of service quality. When enrolling in the rural primary care office, the patients must feel that they have come to the right place. Patients inherently understand that health care depends on a network of human relationships. They expect understanding and compassion at all contact points. Most of all, they want to be confident that their team competently applies the mysteries of medical science within a holistic model.

REFERENCES

1. Russell W, Branch T: *Second Wind: Memoirs of an Opinionated Man.* New York, Random House, 1979.
2. Senge PM: *The Fifth Discipline: The Art and Practice of the Learning Organization.* New York, Doubleday, 1990.
3. Kelley RE: *How to Be a Star at Work.* New York, Times Business, 1998.
4. Strauss A, Fagerhaugh S, Suczek B, et al: *Social Organization of Medical Work.* Chicago, University of Chicago Press, 1985.
5. Baggs J: The nurse-physician collaboration: the challenge of collaboration, in Suchman A, Botelho RJ, Hinton-Walker P (eds): *Partnerships in Healthcare: Transforming Relational Process.* Rochester, NY, University of Rochester Press, 1998.
6. Rosenthal TC, Rosenthal GL, Lucas C: Factors determining physician practice location: the results of a 1990 survey of New York State residency-trained family physicians. *J Am Board Fam Pract* 5:265, 1992.
7. Farley T: Integrated primary care in rural areas, in Blount A (ed): *Integrated Primary Care: The Future of Medical and Mental Health Collaboration.* London, Norton, 1998.
8. Engel GL: The need for a new medical model: a challenge for biomedicine. *Science* 196:129, 1977.

9. Starfield B: *Primary Care: Concept, Evaluation, and Policy.* New York, Oxford University Press, 1992.
10. Greenfield S, Kaplan SH, Ware JE Jr, et al: Patients' participation in medical care. *J Gen Intern Med* 3:448, 1988.
11. McWhinney I: The need for a transformed clinical method, in Stewart M, Roter D (eds): *Communicating with Medical Patients.* Newbury Park, CA, Sage, 1989.
12. Brody DS, Miller SM, Lerman CE, et al: Patient perception of involvement in medical care: relationship to illness attitudes and outcomes. *J Gen Intern Med* 4:506, 1989.
13. Vaughan-Cole B, Johnson MA, Malone JA, et al: *Family Nursing Practice.* Philadelphia, Saunders, 1998.
14. Braus P: When the helpers need a hand. *Am Demogr* 20:66, 1998.
15. Horwitz ME, Rosenthal TC: The impact of informal caregiving on labor force participation by rural farming and non-farming families. *J Rural Health* 10:266, 1994.
16. Glenn ML: *Collaborative Health Care: A Family-Oriented Model.* New York, Praeger, 1987.
17. Nutting PA: Community-oriented primary care: an integrated model for practice, research, and education. *Am J Prev Med* 2:140, 1986.
18. Christensen B, Sorensen H, Mabeck C: Differences in referral rates from general practice. *Fam Pract* 6:19:1989.
19. Armstrong D, Britten N, Grace J: Measuring general practitioner referrals: patient, workload and list size effects. *J R Coll Gen Pract* 38:494, 1988.
20. Rosenthal TC, Shiffner J, Panebianco S: Physician and psychologists' beliefs about factors influencing successful psychology referrals. *Fam Med* 22:38, 1990.
21. Drummond D, Thom B, Brown C, et al: Specialist versus general practitioner treatment of problem drinkers. *Lancet* 336:915, 1990.
22. Rosenthal TC, Riemenschneider T, Feather J: A generalist-patient-specialist alliance for the nineties. *Am J Med* 100:338, 1996.
23. Campbell-Heider N, Pollock D: Barriers to physician-nurse collegiality: an anthropological perspective. *Soc Sci Med* 25:421, 1987.
24. Bertram DA, Rosenthal TC: Implementation of an in-patient case management program in rural hospitals. *J Rural Health* 12:54, 1996.
25. Anderson K: Is it still home sweet home care? *Business Health* January:42, 1993.

26. Regier DA, Narrow WE, Rae DS, et al: The defacto U.S. mental and addictive disorders service system. *Arch Gen Psychiatry* 50:85, 1993.

27. Blount A: *Integrated Primary Care: The Future of Medical and Mental Health Collaboration.* London, Norton, 1998.

28. Huntington J: *Social Work and General Medical Practice: Collaboration or Conflict?* London, Allen, 1981.

29. Rost K, Zhang M, Fortney J, et al: Rural-urban differences in depression treatment and suicidality. *Med Care* 36:1098, 1998.

30. Fox JC, Merwin E, Blank MB: De facto mental health services in the rural south. *J Health Care Poor Underserved* 6:434, 1995.

31. Hill CE, Fraser GJ: Local knowledge and rural mental health reform. *Commun Mental Health J* 31:553, 1995.

32. Katon W, von Korff M, Lin E, et al: Collaborative management to achieve treatment guidelines: impact on depression in primary care. *JAMA* 273:1026, 1995.

33. Rosenthal TC, Shiffner J, DiMaggio M: Factors involved in successful psychotherapy referral in rural primary care. *Fam Med* 23:527, 1991.

34. Newell M: *Using Nursing Case Management to Improve Health Outcomes.* Gaithersburg, MD, Aspen, 1996.

35. Westerman RF, Hull FM, Bezemer PD, et al: A study of communication between general practitioners and specialists. *Br J Gen Pract* 40:445, 1990.

36. Lerman C, Brody D, Caputo C, et al: Patients' perceived involvement in care scale: relationship to attitudes about illness and medical care. *J Gen Intern Med* 5:29, 1990.

37. Orth J, Stiles W, Scherwitz L, et al: Patient exposition and provider explanation in routine interviews and hypertensive patients' blood pressure control. *Health Psychol* 6:29, 1987.

38. Rosenthal TC, James P, Fox C, et al: Rural docs, rural networks and free market health care in the nineties. *Arch Fam Med* 6:319, 1997.

39. Weiner J: HMOs and managed care: implications for rural manpower planning. *J Rural Health* 7:373, 1991.

CHAPTER 5

Population-Based Medicine: Links to Public Health

JEFFREY HUMMEL

P opulation management represents a convergence of clinical medicine and public health which, in many ways, is part of the tradition of rural medical practice. Primary care physicians practicing in rural settings have always faced a wider scope of practice than their urban counterparts, often resulting in a loss of boundaries between areas of medical specialty. One aspect of this expanded scope of practice is the overlap between acute clinical practice and the many environmental and community factors influencing morbidity and mortality of individual patients. For example, a primary care provider in a Southeast Alaskan Native community may find it difficult to interact with a group of preadolescent boys without pondering the odds each of them faces and the many factors that place them at high risk for depression and suicide as they enter their teen years.[1]

Although rural practice has always carried with it an opportunity for a population-based approach to health care delivery, there is now available to rural providers a conceptual framework and a wide array of new tools that are of major value to practitioners of population management. The goal of this chapter is to review recent developments that are directly applicable to situations faced by clinicians in rural settings as they seek to improve their effectiveness in managing the morbidity and mortality in the populations they serve. Probably the best way to introduce these new tools and to provide a context for the conceptual framework is by beginning this discussion with a case study.

CASE STUDY: STARTING A POPULATION-MANAGEMENT PROGRAM IN A RURAL COMMUNITY

The Decision to Try Something Different

Hamlet is a rural community in a western state; it has a population of about 5000, and is surrounded by another 2500 people in neighboring smaller towns who receive their medical care in Hamlet. With the exception of a small tourism industry, the economy of Hamlet is almost totally dependent on dry-land farming, which relies on seasonal irrigation using both water and hydroelectric power from a nearby major river 50 miles away. There are two clinics in the town as well as a small community hospital; these serve a population that is 40 percent Hispanic and 60 percent Anglo. Most of the Hispanic population receives its care at the larger of the two clinics, called the Hamlet Family Practice Clinic, which is staffed by three physicians, a physician assistant, a public health nurse, three medical assistants, and two licensed practical nurses. The clinic has a computerized billing system, while appointments and medical records are all documented on paper. Approximately half of the Hispanic population resides permanently in the community, while the other half is made up of a migrant population that is present during the 9-month work season and varies significantly in individual composition from year to year. The two medical clinics in Hamlet have a close working relationship; they provide cross-coverage of the hospital, with a history of cosponsoring community service events.

One of the physicians and the public health nurse at the Hamlet Family Practice Clinic have been reading about recent advances in the United Kingdom in providing organized care to populations with chronic illness, and they have been learning about the results of a large study in Britain clarifying the importance of careful management of type II diabetes.[2] This physician and the nurse have become concerned that they do not know how they are doing in managing the diabetics they see in their practice, and they would like to start a population-management program to improve the outcomes for the diabetic patients at their clinic and in their community. The physician recently attended a conference at a major metropolitan center "on the coast" in which some interesting ideas were presented, including a paper outlining a model of chronic disease management.[3] At the conference the physician was introduced to several types of programs for applying this model to diabetes care.[4,5] This physician and nurse are impressed enough with these ideas that they decide to try to do something similar on their own and start a diabetes management program. They discuss their ideas with the other providers in the clinic and, at a planning meeting, they pose the following questions[6]:

1. What are we trying to accomplish?
2. What changes might we make that could result in an improvement?
3. How will we know that a change is an improvement?

After several weeks of discussion, the five providers finally settle on the following answers to their questions:

1. "We are trying to improve the delivery of care to the diabetic patients of the community so that interventions known to be effective are made available to every person with diabetes. We are trying to improve the self-management skills of every person in the community with diabetes."

2. They were able to think of a long list of potential changes they might make. Among the ideas they liked best are the following:

   - "We need a way of defining our entire population of diabetics served by the clinic—i.e., we need a registry."
   - "We need to have a clear set of interventions known to be effective on which to base our clinical management strategy for each diabetic."
   - "We need to set outcome goals for carrying out those interventions among the target populations."
   - "We need a way to monitor our outcomes—i.e., how we are doing in achieving those goals."
   - "We need a way to remind ourselves which tasks need to be done on each diabetic patient every time that patient comes to the clinic."
   - "We need a way to teach patients how to manage their own diabetes better."

3. In order to determine whether any of their changes were making any positive difference, they would need data they currently did not have. A registry containing the names of all diabetics as well as key interventions and dates would give them the necessary data to detect improvement.[7]

In the course of their discussion, which took place in a series of meetings and conversations over several months, they became more precise about whom they were trying to serve. They agreed that their "community" meant the entire population of the town and the surrounding communities, including seasonal migrant workers who are in the region for only several months a year. They understood that their power to have an impact on diabetes outcomes would initially be limited to the patients seen in the clinic and those who could be induced to come to the clinic through outreach activities. They discussed opportunities for collaboration with the other clinic and the hospital as well as a state-run diabetes project that the public health nurse had learned about. They made a list of organizations in the community, including the surrounding towns, with which they might work to overcome such barriers as distance from the clinic, hours of clinic availability, language and culture, migrant workers afraid of legal problems related to immigration status, and inability to pay for services. They came to the conclusion that, although there were probably many diabetics in the greater Hamlet community who were either undiagnosed or receiving suboptimal care, they would have to start small with a pilot project and only expand their efforts once they had learned how such a program worked. For that reason they chose to begin by identifying the diabetics who had come to their clinic during the preceding year. They reasoned that once they had set up a program that was working well, with demonstrable improvements in outcomes, they could expand it by forming linkages with the other clinic in Hamlet to reach a wider population.

Identifying the Population

The five providers began their project by looking for ways to make lists of names of all the diabetics who had come to the Hamlet Family Practice Clinic during the previous 12 months. They came up with four ways of identifying such diabetics:

1. They could use ICD-9 billing codes from the past year pertaining to diabetes.
2. They could ask the single lab that does all their blood work for a list of those patients with test results meeting the criteria for diabetes.
3. They could ask the three local pharmacies for lists of patients who had received prescriptions for medications used only by diabetics.
4. They could review the charts of active patients and make a list by hand.

Despite the fact that they did not have a computerized medical record, the physicians realized that they could use computer searches for three of these four methods. The billing system, when queried for all billings for diagnosis codes 250.0 through 250.9, gave a list of 145 patients with a diabetes-related diagnosis who were seen in the clinic in the prior 12 months. They asked the laboratory, which was 90 miles away, to run a computerized query of all patients from their clinic with a fasting blood glucose equal to or greater than 126 or a random blood glucose equal to or greater than 200. This method yielded a list of 85 names. They asked the pharmacies in the town to search their computerized records and give them a list of all patients who received a prescription for a sulfonylurea, metformin, insulin, and two other diabetes medications that one of the physicians had prescribed. The pharmacy search yielded a list of 179 names. No one had the time to look through all of the medical records.

Registry and Decision Support

It was now clear to everyone that a computer would have to be used to keep track of the list of diabetics and add new people to the registry as new cases were identified. The providers decided to use the clinic's capital budget to purchase a desktop computer equipped with a modem for this project. The physician assistant at the clinic had used a spreadsheet at home, and she offered to set up a registry. Using the lists of diabetic patients from each source, a registry including 215 patients was built. The charts on each of the 215 people identified were pulled; it was then found that six were deceased and seven had left the area. The providers were able to think of three additional patients who were not on this list. This gave them a total of 205 diabetic patients with which the registry could be started.

The modem gave clinic personnel direct access to a web site at the state university's school of medicine on which was posted an evidence-based guideline for diabetes that was very similar to the diabetes guideline they had from the Agency for Health Care Policy and Research but more up to date. Using the guidelines for diabetes management, they proceeded to set up their registry, in which each row pertained to a diabetic patient and each column represented a clinical parameter that the group wished to follow. The spreadsheet, which was structured as shown in Table 5-1, allowed them to track the following variables: patient name; age; gender; smoking status; systolic and diastolic blood pressure; most recent low-density lipoprotein (LDL), high-density lipoprotein (HDL), triglyceride, and total cholesterol; date of most recent LDL, HDL, triglyceride, and total cholesterol; value of most recent HbA1c; date of most recent

HbA1c; result of most recent urine microalbumin; date of most recent urine microalbumin; date of most recent dilated retinal examination; date of most recent monofilament examination for neuropathy; result of most recent monofilament test; and whether the patient was currently on an angiotensin-converting enzyme (ACE) inhibitor, a beta blocker, or aspirin.

They decided that they would add data to the spreadsheet each month. At the beginning of each month, they would copy the data onto a new sheet for the next month and save the

TABLE 5-1   *A PORTION OF THE REGISTRY FOR DIABETES DESIGNED BY THE HAMLET FAMILY PRACTICE CLINIC*

ID	Patient Name	Age	Cigs	BP— Syst	BP— Diast	LDL	LDL Date	HDL	HDL Date	Total Chol	Total Chol Date
1	Gonzales, Jesus	52	Quit	160	70	195	9/18/1998	54	9/18/1998	282	9/18/1998
2	Pfaff, Bud	53	Quit	154	80	139	12/29/1998	42	12/29/1998	247	12/29/1998
3	Dunker, Joe Bob	78	Yes	132	84	189	12/16/1998	61	12/16/1998	274	12/16/1998
4	Ruiz, Maria	79	Yes	130	86						
5	Sanchez, Hector	80	Yes	148	78						
6	Hidalgo, Angelica	44	Yes	112	70	96	12/4/1998	67	12/4/1998	177	12/4/1998
7	Foster, Wanda	52	Yes	180	110	184	12/3/1998	40	12/3/1998	247	12/3/1998
8	Foster, Gus	62	Yes	154	90					224	5/1/1998
9	Ramirez, Leo	31	No	116	70	141	1/7/1999	43	1/7/1999	205	1/7/1999
10	Chavez, Fifi	77		142	68	75	3/22/1999	34	3/22/1999	137	3/22/1999
11	Lawton, Ida	78	Yes	130	70						
12	Person, JT	74	Yes	168	78	72	4/8/1999	62	4/8/1999	151	4/8/1999
13	Thomas, Willard	54		120	72						
14	Castro, Raul	84	Yes	150	88	171	12/24/1997	80	12/24/1997	282	12/24/1997
15	Latourette, Ann	38	Yes	116	80	103	8/20/1998	44	8/20/1998	224	8/20/1998
16	Algodon, Pedro	39	Yes	124	92						
17	Fonseca, Maria	70	Quit	166	74	129	3/17/1999	54	3/17/1999	211	3/17/1999
18	Manring, Burt	70	Quit	138	84	107	3/9/1999	43	3/9/1999	166	3/9/1999
19	Zamora, Cleo	47	Yes	120	88	104	9/28/1998	38	9/28/1998	175	9/28/1998
20	Rockhill, Duke	52		150	100	100	3/31/1999	40	3/31/1999	197	3/31/1999
21	Ochs, Sim	26		100	60	161	8/31/1998	62	8/31/1998	228	8/31/1998
22	Waller, Wendi	30		124	88						
23	Gustavson, Pearl	58	Yes	142	94		3/3/1999	45	3/3/1999	459	3/3/1999
24	Hawthorne, Judd	67		130	64			41	12/22/1998	239	12/22/1998
25	Hayter, Cheri	36	Yes	100	60						
26	Martinez, Juan	52		136	100						
27	Catalan, Octavio	46	No	110	60	121	2/4/1999	42	2/4/1999	213	2/4/1999
28	Gandara, Noemi	42	Yes	130	80	114	1/21/1999	24	1/21/1999	166	1/21/1999
29	Reina, Chester	52	Yes	130	80	130	11/17/1998	44	11/17/1998	237	11/17/1998
30	Felton, Harry	55	Yes	124	80	76	1/5/1999	33	1/5/1999	154	1/5/1999
31	Lopez, Jose Luis	53	Yes	142	92	106	12/18/1997	39	12/18/1997	217	12/18/1997

last month's data sheet so that they could track improvements over time.

Measuring Improvement

While it took the group a month to set up the registry, it gave them a tool to measure improvement as the project developed. The physician assistant bought a book describing ways to do simple descriptive data analysis using the spreadsheet, and she generated a report on outcomes for this population of diabetics. The following information about the management of diabetics at the clinic was discovered. Of the 205 adult diabetics identified, 45.4 percent had received at least one HbA1c during the prior 12 months; of the 93 who had been tested, 38 (40.9 percent) had values above 8.0. A blood pressure had been recorded in the records of 198 (96.6 percent) diabetic patients; of those, 69 (34.8 percent) had a pressure greater than 140/90. Smoking status had been recorded on 153 (74.6 percent) diabetics; of those, 42 (27.5 percent) were currently smoking. A total of 91 (44.4 percent) had had their LDL tested; 53 (58.2 percent) had a value greater than 130 or had triglycerides too high for the LDL to be measurable.

A staff meeting was held to review the data they had gathered. One of them pointed out that their performance was not that bad compared with the national average.[8] Another physician had been sure they were doing better than that and wondered whether the data were correct. The public health nurse pointed out the opportunity for improvement and imagined out loud how it would feel to see the outcomes presented on a graph (Fig. 5-1). They agreed to have a brainstorming session over dinner to review their list of things they could do that might lead to an improvement.

Identifying the Team

At their brainstorming session—attended by the three medical doctors (MDs), the physician assistant (PA), and the public health nurse (PHN)—they discovered that some of their ideas involved delegating work to the licensed practical nurse (LPN), one of the medical assistants, and two of the phone receptionists at the clinic, all of whom were fluent in Spanish. They decided that from then on the core team of the diabetes initiative, as they now referred to their project, should consist of the entire clinic

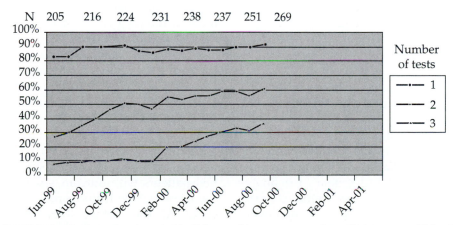

FIGURE 5-1 *Percent of patients with diabetes with one, two, or three HbA1c tests within the prior 12 months. Improvement in process measure of HbA1c testing of diabetics from the Hamlet Family Practice Clinic.*

staff, since most of the efforts to improve outcomes would result in changing the work flow, at least to some degree, for all of the clinic staff.

Point-of-Care Reminders

One idea that they decided to implement immediately was to put a bright orange circle sticker on the front of each chart as a flag to remind the medical assistants and physicians that it was the chart of a diabetic patient. They believed this would reduce the chance that they would realize only after a diabetic had left the clinic that the patient was overdue for an intervention. They also developed a standard paper data entry form that was to be kept at the nursing station in the clinic. It would be the medical assistant's job to put the data entry form in the outside pocket of the chart whenever a patient was seen. This data entry sheet included a place to mark the blood pressure (BP), findings on the foot examination, and a reminder of the intervals for repeating standard monitoring tests for diabetes—including HbA1c, lipid profile, eye examination, and microalbumin screening. The data entry form included a checklist of medications to review on each diabetic patient, including aspirin, beta blockers, and ACE inhibitors. The data entry form would be placed in a basket after the patient visit, and the new data would then be entered into the registry.

Work Redesign

After a month, the group discovered that the job of reviewing the chart in the exam room with the patient added too much work to the short time available for dealing with the patient's chief complaint, which was usually not related to his or her diabetes. Although the providers were trying hard to remember to do everything, all too frequently they found, after the patient had left the clinic, that they had overlooked the need to order a HbA1c or an eye exam. They discovered that the data entry process worked much better if the LPN reviewed all charts on diabetics prior to a visit to see whether there had been an HbA1c result in the previous 6 months, a microalbumin test or an eye exam in the previous year, and a lipid profile in the preceding 2 years. The LPN highlighted each item that appeared to be overdue and then placed the data entry sheet in the front of the chart as a reminder to the busy physician to quickly review the state of a patient's diabetes when he or she was seen for unrelated complaints.

Data Entry

The data entry forms were removed from the chart at the end of each visit and placed in a basket in the nursing station. One of the receptionists was taught by the PA to work with the spreadsheet to a level where she could accurately enter the data collected during an office visit. At the end of each day the data entry forms were picked up by this receptionist, who entered the data.

The group found a way to flag laboratory orders on patients identified as having diabetes; this led the laboratory to write "diabetic patient" automatically in the comments section of the laboratory result slip. One of the medical assistants was assigned to pull lab results for diabetic patients out of the pile of lab slips after the physician had reviewed them and to put them in the data entry basket to be entered in the registry spreadsheet.

The PHN was instructed to review the registry during the first week of each month to identify patients in need of further intervention. She reviewed the charts on all the diabetics to be sure that any tests or interventions performed during the previous month were accurately entered into the new sheet in the registry. During this review of the updated registry, she identified patients with outcomes that were outside the recommended guidelines, who were to be contacted for further intervention. This included patients due for an eye exam, patients whose BP was above 130/80, patients who were smoking, those whose LDL was above 100, patients whose most recent HbA1c was above 8.0, patients who were spilling more than 30 μg/mL of albumin in their urine and were not on ACE inhibitors, and patients with neuropathy who had not been counseled on foot care.

Patient Education

The group decided to send their PHN to the closest regional center to receive training and certification as a diabetes educator. The PHN already had the job of identifying patients via the registry who were due for a test or in need of further intervention. She added to this the job of calling the patients in to have laboratory tests done and medications adjusted, and of counseling interventions focused on assessing patients' readiness and skills needed for behavior change. The PHN followed patients who needed case management for behavior modification or special training for specific aspects of their care, such as smoking cessation, glucose monitoring, weight loss, diet, and exercise. Much of the follow-up of this work after the initial visit was done by telephone.

Monitoring Outcomes

The PA who was adept at using the spreadsheet continued to generate reports every 2 months showing the percent of the clinic's diabetic population meeting the guideline recommendations for each clinical parameter. The outcomes were divided into three categories: (1) metabolic control, (2) coronary artery disease risk factors, and (3) microvascular disease. In each of the three categories, improvements were monitored with both process and outcome measures. These measures for the clinic were organized as shown in Table 5-2. A computer-generated list of patients who were outside the guideline recommendations was routinely printed.

After several months of generating these reports, the group discovered that they were able to see a fairly prompt improvement in process measures, as shown in Fig. 5-1. The outcome measures were much slower to respond, but after a year, a decline could be seen in the number of diabetic patients with HbA1c values above 8.0 and with blood pressures greater than 140/90. There were improvements in the num-

TABLE 5-2   PROCESS AND OUTCOME MEASURES USED IN THE HAMLET DIABETES INITIATIVE

Outcome Category	Process Measure	Outcome Measure
Metabolic control	Percent of patients with 2 or more HbA1c tests in prior 12 months.	Percent of patients with most recent HbA1c value > 8.0.
CAD risk factors	1. Percent of patients with LDL measured in prior 12 months. 2. Percent of patients for whom smoking status is recorded. 3. Percent of patients with BP recorded in prior 6 months.	1. Percent of patients with LDL > 130. 2. Percent of patients currently smoking. 3. Percent of patients with BP > 140/90.
Microvascular disease	1. Percent of patients for whom microalbumin has been measured within the prior 12 months. 2. Percent of patients with documented monofilament exam of feet in prior 12 months. 3. Percent of patients with dilated retinal exam in prior 12 months.	1. Percent of patients with microalbuminuria who are not on ACE inhibitors. 2. Percent of patients who are insensate who have not been trained in care of the diabetic foot.

Key: CAD, coronary artery disease; LDL, low-density lipoprotein; BP, blood pressure; ACE, angiotensin-converting enzyme.

ber of diabetic patients on beta blockers, ACE inhibitors, and aspirin.

Community Linkages

The PHN returned from her diabetes educator training with a list of contacts she had made during the training session. These included several state agencies that were supporting similar projects in urban areas. The clinic began a regular correspondence with the head of the state diabetes project, who helped them to obtain educational materials for diabetics in both English and Spanish and offered to help them look for grant money to support an expansion of the project. The PHN also made contact with the nearest office of the American Diabetes Association, which provided the curriculum for a class on home glucose monitoring.

The LPN contacted the priest in the local Catholic church, who offered to provide an evening meeting place for diabetes classes for the Spanish-speaking community. He agreed to contribute to the cost of pamphlets, in Spanish, to be distributed within the parish, that described the Hamlet Family Practice Clinic program. One of the medical assistants contacted a local minister and community activist who was based at the Presbyterian church but also gave sermons at the Methodist church. Both denominations agreed to inform their congregations about the program, and they encouraged expansion of the diabetes initiative to include the other clinic in town, where many of their congregation received their care.

This effort resulted in a conversation with the physicians at the other clinic about ways to collaborate in the care of diabetes in the entire community. The providers in both clinics agreed to get together, informally at first, to discuss the Hamlet Diabetes Initiative program and to look for ways of expanding it to include the other clinic and the hospital.

POPULATION MANAGEMENT

Population management can be defined as an approach to clinical medicine in which an entire defined population in its community is viewed as the context through which disease-specific individualized patient care is delivered. A major emphasis is placed on identification of factors that put members of the population at increased risk for morbidity and mortality. A population-based approach ensures special attention to reducing barriers to disease-modifying interventions and ways of reaching patients who may be "falling through the cracks."

Historically, physicians in clinical practice have directed their efforts toward helping patients who present to their offices. A population-based approach to clinical medicine differs from usual practice in that it integrates many aspects of public health practice—such as an emphasis on patient education, community linkages, and health promotion/disease prevention—into individualized patient care in a clinical practice setting. Population-based medicine is directed toward common conditions that lend themselves to a systems approach to care. The first step is to identify all the patients in the clinical practice who have the condition. Perhaps the most important difference between population-based medicine and usual care is the emphasis on choosing measurable outcomes that reflect the best evidence-based medical practice. These measurable outcomes are used to assess the impact of changes that are made in the systems used to deliver care, so that the systems can be improved to achieve optimal outcomes.[9]

The case study shows how several motivated providers in a rural clinic might go about approaching diabetes in their community. Another example might be asthma, in which a project would begin by identifying the total population of asthmatic patients within a community.[10] Patient education would be targeted at ensuring that every asthmatic patient had an optimal set of easily accessible medications and understood how to use them properly. Efforts would focus on ensuring that each patient knew how to interact with the medical profession and specifically when to call for help. Patients who were "lost to follow-up" would need to be identified and tracked down to make sure they knew how to monitor their own peak expiratory flow, how to use inhaled steroids correctly, and when to call the clinic for early medical intervention. The goal would be improved outcomes, as measured by functional status, and avoidable emergency room visits or hospital admissions.

POPULATIONS IN RURAL AMERICA: EPIDEMIOLOGIC CONSIDERATIONS

The populations in rural America vary significantly from region to region, but there are some demographic factors that are of importance in any rural community.[11]

Ethnic/Racial Composition

Much of the rural United States includes a major representation of people of ethnic background other than northern European. The rural Southeast has a large percentage of African Americans and, in some places, populations of Caribbean origin. Populations of Hispanic rural workers, traditionally thought of as characteristic of the Southwest, are found throughout the rural United States and are heterogeneous in their lifestyles. Some live permanently in rural communities, some come to the United States from Mexico for several months at a time and then return, while others travel the migrant stream from Texas to Iowa and to Washington State. Native Americans, although found in highest percentages in Alaska and the West, live throughout the United States.[12] Each ethnic group carries specific patterns of risk for specific health conditions. For example, Hispanic, Native American, and African-American communities have a significantly higher prevalence of diabetes and other risk factors for coronary artery disease than is found in many other ethnic groups.[13,14] A population-based approach in each of these geographic areas requires planning to include the ethnic and racial mix of the community.

Socioeconomic Status

In general, rural communities have a greater proportion of people of low socioeconomic status as compared with many urban areas; this is reflected in higher rates of underemployment and lower per capita income. The socioeconomic and ethnic composition of a rural community plays a significant role in types of diseases that are important in the community. Risk-taking behaviors—including tobacco use, alcohol consumption while operating motor vehicles, and unsafe sexual behavior—may be high in many rural communities.[15] A rural health care provider needs to maintain a relationship with multiple socioeconomic strata in the community to understand the dynamics that may be working to increase the disease patterns within the population.

Types of Occupations

Although some rural communities have opportunities for jobs in manufacturing and the information industry, a high percentage of occupations are often related to agriculture or other industries managing natural resources, such as logging, mining, or fishing, or to service industries that support those industries in the community. Occupations involving the management of natural resources have a major effect on the patterns of injury in rural communities. The incidence and severity of injuries in the agricultural, logging,[16] and fishing industries[17] are proportionately greater than is commonly seen in urban settings. The focus of a population-based medical intervention may vary between communities depending on the economic structures that support the population.

Barriers to Receiving Medical Services

Medicine has traditionally depended on patients calling or presenting to a clinic and requesting service as a first step to receiving medical services. In rural communities, barriers to care include distances to a clinic, lack of insurance or resources to pay for services, and cultural and language differences between the health care delivery system and those individuals needing services. This is often reflected in higher rates of undertreatment of conditions such as depression, diabetes, hypertension, and heart disease. Since a population-based approach requires seeking out those individuals who are not coming to a clinic to receive medical care, one of the major issues that must be addressed is identification of those at whom the intervention should be targeted.

A MODEL FOR DISEASE MANAGEMENT

During the 1990s, significant advances, through randomized controlled trials, were made in Europe and the United States in identifying medical interventions that result in improved clinical outcomes.[18] One impetus for this new scrutiny of the effectiveness of medical interventions has been the growing accountability of delivery systems for the management of increasingly scarce health care resources. Due in no small part to competition between provider groups on the basis of price, a major emphasis of efforts to manage resources has shifted to chronic diseases, which account for approximately 75 percent of health care costs and affect nearly 50 percent of Americans.[19] There are demographic reasons to assume that the chronic disease burden of the United States will increase in the future, including aging of the "baby boom" generation. In addition, technological advances in the treatment of such previously fatal illnesses as coronary artery disease, diabetes, cancer, and human immunodeficiency virus (HIV) infections result in increased disease management rather than cure. There is no reason to suppose that rural communities will not have an at least proportional increase in the future prevalence of chronic diseases.

As more of the U.S. population acquires some form of prepaid health insurance, there has been a growing realization that the way to optimally manage both clinical outcomes and costs associated with chronic illnesses is to keep patients healthy and to manage chronic diseases in ways that minimize preventable complications. The growing discipline of chronic disease manage-

ment is important to a population-based perspective in two ways: (1) much of the morbidity and mortality in any population is predictable on the basis of the chronic diseases found in that population and (2) the tools for identifying patients, monitoring progression, and intervening for better outcomes with chronic diseases are of direct utility in any type of clinical effort targeted at a defined population. Much of the work in chronic disease management is directed toward teaching patients ways to better manage their own health. This includes teaching them how to succeed in behavior change (such as quitting smoking or losing weight), how to improve or preserve functional capacity in the face of slowly progressive or chronic illness, and how to interact optimally with the medical profession. The goal is to help patients use health care resources wisely and ensure that important signs and symptoms are reported early.[20]

Lessons from Managed Care

The experience of staff-model capitated managed care organizations in the United States such as the Group Health Cooperative of Puget Sound and Kaiser Permanente has been important in demonstrating that the population of patients for whom a capitated delivery system is responsible includes members who do not come in seeking medical attention.[21] Barriers to care that have the effect of prolonging the time that a chronic condition goes untreated serve to reduce the opportunity that health care providers have to reduce a patient's risk of preventable complications. The basic concept is that a delivery system is at financial risk for the high economic and social cost of chronic illness complications regardless of whether or not the patient is motivated or has been educated to participate in activities that will reduce that risk. In an urban health maintenance organization (HMO), the cost of deteriorating functional status in individuals with chronic illness may be best measured in medical service costs to the delivery system. In a rural community, the lower population density and greater interdependence among community members means that deteriorating functional status of individuals may result in a greater impact on the social fabric of the community.

The management of chronic disease is fundamentally different from treatment of acute or self-limited illness in two important respects: (1) interventions by definition will not result in a cure and (2) the prolonged time course of chronic illness tends to increase the importance of patient self-management as well as change the dynamic of office-based physician-patient interventions. There is evidence to suggest that morbidity and utilization costs associated with chronic illnesses may be lower when patients are helped to engage in specific behaviors that are shown to maintain health and minimize preventable complications (such as quitting smoking or starting to exercise more), improve or preserve functional capacity, and interact optimally with the medical profession.[20]

Chronic illnesses as diverse as diabetes, depression, reactive airway disease, and HIV/AIDS share a number of common characteristics affecting outcomes in the primary care setting. All of these conditions require complex diagnostic and treatment algorithms for optimal management, which may change with medical advances. Many chronic diseases affect patients' psychological and physical energy levels to the point where they may cause depression, lack of exercise, strain on family or friends, and greater dependency on the medical profession.

Essential Tasks for Patients with Chronic Illness

Research has shown that there are four essential tasks that patients with chronic illnesses must accomplish if they hope to maintain a productive life.[22]

1. They must engage in activities to promote health and build physiologic reserve, including those involving exercise, nutrition, social activation, and sleep.
2. They must interact with health care providers

and systems and adhere to recommended treatment protocols.
3. They must monitor their own physical and emotional status and make appropriate management decisions on the basis of symptoms and signs.
4. They must manage the impact of their illness on their ability to function in important roles, on their emotions and self-esteem, and on their relationships with others.

The flow of patients in physicians' offices, however, has historically been structured to support the ability of physicians to interview and examine patients with acute diseases in patient-initiated visits, one at a time, in an interaction built around the process of arriving at a diagnosis and a treatment. Although such advances as the problem-oriented medical record[23] and the application of decision modeling[24] to clinical medicine have led to a highly organized framework for diagnostic and therapeutic decision making, the resulting system does not necessarily lend itself to the tasks of facilitating changes in patient behavior or methodically monitoring multiple metabolic functions at intervals of many months over a period of years. It is useful to think of the work of primary care as occurring in at least two different workload streams, both of which compete for the busy clinician's time and energy and all of which must be carefully managed if patients are to receive the highest quality of care. Those two streams are acute episodic care and chronic care/preventive care. Acute care involves the approximately 60 to 70 percent of primary care in which a patient seeks an office visit, the sooner the better, for assistance with a new or recurrent problem requiring diagnosis and treatment that either resolves or stabilizes over a finite period of time and sometimes results in death. Chronic care pertains to the ongoing management of conditions for which there is no cure, often involving a common final pathway for organ-system malfunction, and for which complications arise over time. Preventive care is the proactive effort to reduce morbidity and mortality outcomes in conditions for which the periodic use of screening, vaccination, education, and behavior change techniques have been shown to be effective. As the physicians at the Hamlet Family Practice Clinic discovered, there is a strong tendency to focus on acute care needs of patients for many reasons, including (1) the expectation that a patient's chief complaint will be addressed, (2) the availability of an array of diagnostic tests and medications available for evaluation and treatment of acute complaints, and (3) a medical culture in which it is usually considered a greater omission to miss ordering a diagnostic test than it is to miss an opportunity to work on changing a patient's behavior to improve functional status.[3] It is common for patients with chronic illness to fit into the acute care–based structure of physicians' offices by presenting with a list of specific acute complaints that may or may not be related to the underlying chronic condition. It is easy for providers to focus on the patient's acute care list, since the acute needs may be more pressing, and often both provider and patient may have come to a tacit agreement that there is little that can be done for the chronic condition. Particularly in settings where providers are very busy and there is pressure to see four to six patients per hour, there may simply not be enough time to address any of the four essential tasks. Consequently, patients with chronic conditions are often on their own to deal with matters that directly affect their health and their health care costs, without medical guidance, as the medical profession continues to focus attention on more acute issues.[25]

Essential Tasks for Providers Treating Patients with Chronic Illness

For organized medicine to manage chronic conditions in a manner that optimally preserves health and avoids preventable, costly complications, it must systematically address three essential functions:

1. It must assure the delivery of those interventions (evaluations and treatments, both medical and psychosocial) that have been shown by rigorous evidence to be effective.
2. It must empower patients to take responsibility for the management of their conditions.
3. It must provide information, support, and resources to assist patients in learning specific self-management tasks.

The management of chronic illness involves more resources and time than are generally available to primary care providers, who are invariably inundated with the never-ending demands of acute episodic care. In many ways, managing chronic diseases in a busy office setting is similar to running a large medical intervention research trial in the middle of a primary care practice. This is a useful analogy. Large medical intervention research studies involve multiple complex tasks (patient selection, intervention, and data collection) that must be carried out systematically for a large population of patients, each of whom usually begins the study at a different time. The only way that such a venture can be carried out is with interdisciplinary teams of health care workers following specific protocols and using large computerized data management systems.[3] By borrowing from the medical research community the tools and techniques for managing large groups of patients with similar conditions, the medical profession can put sufficient energy into the needs of chronic care patients to improve the care they receive while continuing to handle the acute care workload. Fortunately all the tools for this endeavor have recently become widely available in integrated delivery systems. Among the many rapid changes in the health care profession during the 1990s, some of the most important are the computerization of medical record keeping,[26] the rise of evidence-based medicine,[18] and the development of interdisciplinary primary care teams.[27]

Wagner et al., in Seattle, have proposed a conceptual model for understanding the interactions of different facets of chronic disease management that have been shown to be of potential benefit in improving clinical outcomes.

This model is illustrated in Fig. 5-2.[28] Three general categories of organizational support have been shown to be effective in improving outcomes in chronic disease management. These are (1) clinical information systems[29]; (2) decision support, such as point-of-care reminders[30]; and (3) delivery system redesign.[31]

Clinical Information Systems

Numerous types of clinical information systems are in use today, and many aspects of these systems are available in rural settings. At one end of the spectrum, there are now completely electronic medical records in which all clinical data, including laboratory and pharmacy information, is entered both as text in progress notes and into data entry screens. Even without a fully integrated computerized medical record, many organizations have developed computerized results-reporting functions, by which laboratory and pharmacy data are available to the clinician at the point of service. In organizations with computers available only for scheduling or billing functions, some of the more sophisticated spreadsheet and database programs can be used to build registries of patients with chronic diseases. In general, by investing in increasing levels of computer sophistication, an organization can greatly decrease the amount of work needed to retrieve data and increase the ease with which data can be used to generate reports to guide physician behavior.

For optimal results in chronic disease management, electronic medical records are used for three purposes: (1) to identify all patients meeting criteria for inclusion (i.e., to build a registry of all patients with a specific condition); (2) to identify individual patients with a chronic disease for whom an intervention is indicated, according to evidence-based guidelines; and (3) to provide feedback to providers and to the organization regarding areas of disease management in which goals are or are not being met. The clinical information system serves as a powerful tool that an organization can use to track large populations of individuals, so that patients with a chronic conditions stand a minimal risk of falling through the cracks.

In 1996 Balas et al. published a review of 98 randomized clinical trials assessing the clinical value of computerized information services.

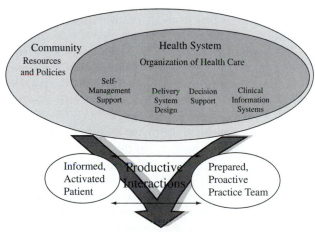

Functional and Clinical Outcomes

FIGURE 5-2 *The chronic illness care model: a conceptual model for disease management. (From Wagner EH: Chronic disease management: what will it take to improve care for chronic illness?* Effect Clin Pract 1(1):2–4, 1998, with permission.)

They found four types of information system interventions that make a significant difference in primary care process-of-care outcomes. These are (1) provider prompt/reminders delivered at the point/time of service, (2) computer-assisted treatment planners, (3) interactive patient education/therapy, and (4) patient prompt/reminders.[32]

A growing number of evidence-based guidelines are available from multiple sources to guide providers in achieving high standards of care and to minimize unnecessary variation in treatments for patients with chronic conditions. Decision-support activities serve to bring those guidelines to providers at the point at which care is delivered and can be used in the absence of a computerized clinical information system. Another way a delivery system can increase decision support to primary care providers is via rapidly available specialty consultation by telephone and e-mail. The opportunity for timeliness of decision support can be greatly enhanced by increased use of computers in clinical practice. One sophisticated example of computerized decision support is the use of patient-specific "pop-up" reminders at the point of service, informing a provider that a patient is overdue for a specific intervention.

In the case study in Hamlet, the providers were not slowed down by the relatively low use of computers in their practice. They used the billing system as a means to search for patients with diabetes and supplemented that search with other sources of information, including the use of computers outside their clinic in the pharmacies and the lab. They built a very functional registry using software that comes preloaded on most home PCs, and they used this in a way that gave them valuable feedback regarding their progress in achieving the goals they had set for themselves.

Delivery System Redesign

Rural providers seeking to set up a population-based program for disease management face many obstacles. One major challenge is to sepa-rate the workload stream of chronic disease management from the flow of acute care well enough to make sure that the chronic disease work gets done without compromising communication between the physician and people performing the work of population-based medicine. One way to accomplish this is to work as an interdisciplinary team using nursing and other ancillary resource people, including pharmacy, physical therapy, or nutrition team members. In a rural setting, the lack of motivated individuals with the necessary skills may be a significant barrier to developing such a team. However, many rural physicians understand intuitively that the nurse working in their office is "on their team"—a lesson that many urban physicians find harder to learn.

There are several ways in which clinical practice can be redesigned to keep acute care demands from crowding out the needs of patients with chronic illness. The physicians at the Hamlet Family Practice Clinic quickly learned to delegate many of the chronic disease tasks to nonphysician team members. Their nurse was put in charge of maintaining the diabetes registry, while the receptionist entered data and the physician assistant generated the reports.

One way to start working as a team is to schedule a patient visit with both the physician and the nurse together. A patient-specific treatment plan can be developed in a joint visit, and the nurse can then follow up on most of the patient education aspects of the plan by telephone or during nursing visits. This leaves the physician free to deal with the demands of acute care. In the United Kingdom, in both urban and rural settings, one successful technique has been to designate a single morning of each week for structured visits by patients with a single disease, such as diabetes or asthma, with both a physician and a nurse.[33] During such a visit, the agenda is limited to the chronic disease, and there is a checklist to assure that all the necessary items are covered. Also during such a visit, another physician and a midlevel provider can cover the acute care demands for the clinic. A pharmacist or dietician can be included, with structured visits to help conduct patient education either one on one or in groups.

In a rural setting, the greatest challenge may be the difficulty in finding qualified people with the skills to do many of the tasks that are required in disease management. The Hamlet Family Practice Clinic was fortunate, but they still needed to train a medical assistant and a phone receptionist to perform certain supervised clinical tasks to improve the performance of the team. Scarcity of motivated team members makes reliance on available community resources all the more essential.

Community Linkages

The risk posed by the social isolation of rural providers and the relatively small size of medical practice groups in most rural towns magnifies the interdependence of the community in a way that may be taken advantage of by physicians in rural practice. There are many organizations in rural communities which may participate in ways that are helpful in promoting the population management of a disease. In many small towns, veterans groups and service organizations such as the Elks and Eagles are stronger than they are in cities. Occupational and employment-based organizations such as a Commercial Fishermen's Association or a Grange may offer activities that are of use in outreach. As the hypothetical experience in Hamlet demonstrates, churches and other faith-based affiliations can serve as powerful allies, both in developing community support and in educational activities. Small-town pharmacies can be a source of data and expertise that can be of value in a disease-specific population-based program.

Many common diseases are represented by national organizations with chapters in nearby regional centers. Organizations such as the American Diabetes Association, the American Heart Association, and the American Lung Association can provide resources and suggest partners for collaboration. Occasionally a state-funded initiative like the Diabetes Control Pro-

gram (which the Hamlet team discovered) may exist as an unused resource to assist in efforts of this kind.

The challenge for rural providers is to weave all of these aspects of community life, modern informatics, and clinical medicine into a program that can produce improvements in the outcomes of diseases that have a major impact on the members of the community. The clinic in Hamlet had providers with the motivation, skills, and resources to make such a program a reality. Their success was due to their hard work and organizational skills—a success that can be duplicated with other diseases in other communities.

LESSONS FROM THE CASE STUDY

1. The hypothetical case study presented above is an example of a population-based approach to management of a chronic disease because it targets an entire population of patients with the disease. The program planners wisely chose to start small, with a subpopulation, while they developed and perfected their processes of population-based care. This allowed them to then build on success as they spread the program to the entire population of diabetics in the community.

2. The Hamlet diabetes initiative was a team effort. Its leaders may not have realized it at the outset, but there was no way that an endeavor this complex could have been carried out by one physician. Not only did one physician not have all the skills necessary, but one physician could never find the time to do all of the tasks that this project entailed. A clinic such as this may or may not be functioning as a team at the outset of such a demanding project. What made them function as a team was not the decision to be a team but rather the performance challenge that they had set for themselves and could not accomplish without teamwork.[34]

3. The Hamlet diabetes initiative was a working example of process improvement methodol-

ogy in action. The key steps in the improvement methodology[35] include asking the following questions:

- *What are we trying to improve*? In this case the improvement was better management of diabetics, defined as better metabolic control, reduced coronary risk factors, and better monitoring of small vessel end-organ disease.
- *What changes might be made that would result in an improvement*? The changes made included most of the components of the chronic illness care model. A readily available technology was used to build a registry, decision support was employed, the work flow was redesigned, activation of patients for better self-management was emphasized, and connections with community resources were made. Each change emerged as a suggestion of one of the people on the team running the project and became a specific part of the overall effort.
- *How will we know that a change is an improvement*? The data the team chose to monitor were selected precisely because they would serve as markers for improvement. The measures of improvement included both process measures (e.g., percent of patients with HbA1c within 6 months) and outcome measures (e.g., percent of patients with HbA1c above 8.0). The reports that were generated provided feedback enabling the team to see whether the changes they had made were resulting in improvements.

4. One of the greatest challenges faced by the community will be how to support such a program financially. Evidence is emerging that improvements in intermediate outcomes may be associated with lower utilization of such high-cost services as emergency department visits, hospitalization, and specialty services.[36] The challenge for these providers will be to fund this program, which provides more intensive services in primary care and therefore increases primary care costs, when the savings resulting from improved outcomes will be accrued by insurance companies, which are at risk for global (specialty and hospital) costs. There are several strategies for doing this, which may work to greater or lesser degrees from community to community depending on state law and payer mix.

- In many states, Medicaid will pay for educational group visits that can be administered primarily by an RN but in which an MD participates.
- More intensive services delivered to diabetic patients by an MD/RN team can often be billed at a higher level under the MD, provided the MD was present during crucial parts of the visit.
- Under capitated plans, many of the interventions resulting in better outcomes can be done through follow-up telephone encounters with an RN certified diabetes educator at a cost that is significantly lower than bringing the patient into the clinic for one-on-one teaching.

CONCLUSION

By combining the tools that have been developed in such diverse fields as improvement methodology, informatics, desktop PC computing, organizational team function, managed care, evidence-based medicine, chronic disease management, and public health, a group of highly motivated primary care physicians working in a rural setting can develop one or more population-based programs targeted at specific diseases in the populations they serve. These programs are energy-intensive, and finding ways to pay for them in a mixed payer system remains a challenge. However, clinical medicine is changing in ways that make clinicians more attentive to previously overlooked clinical issues and to the needs of previously overlooked populations. A rural setting provides an ideal environment for the application of a population-based approach to health.

REFERENCES

1. Gessner BD: Temporal trends and geographic patterns of teen suicide in Alaska, 1979–1993. *Suicide Life Threat Behav* 27(3):264–273, 1997.
2. Treating type 2 diabetes. *BMJ* 317:691–726, 1998.
3. Von Korff M, Gruman J, Schaefer J, et al: Collaborative management of chronic illness. *Ann Intern Med* 127(12):1097–1102, 1997.
4. Friedman NM, Gleeson JM, Kent MJ, et al: Management of diabetes mellitus in the Lovelace Health Systems' Episodes of Care program. *Effect Clin Pract* 1(1):5–11, 1998.
5. Wagner EH: More than a case manager (editorial). *Ann Intern Med* 129(8):654–656, 1998.
6. Berwick DM, Nolan TW: Physicians as leaders in improving health care: a new series in Annals of Internal Medicine. *Ann Intern Med* 128(4):289–292, 1998.
7. Nelson EC, Splaine ME, Batalden PB, Plume SK: Building measurement and data collection into medical practice. *Ann Intern Med* 128(6):460–466, 1998.
8. Kerr CP: Improving outcomes in diabetes: a review of the outpatient care of NIDDM patients. *J Fam Pract* 40(1):63–75, 1995.
9. Rivo ML: It's time to start practicing population-based health care: you don't have to be part of an integrated delivery system to optimize care for populations of patients with common conditions. *Fam Pract Mgt* 5(6):37–46, 1998.
10. O'Connell JM, Howe RS, Sayles SM, et al: Results of a telephone-based asthma management pilot program. *J Clin Outcomes Mgt* 6(4):22–30, 1999.
11. Pearson TA, et al: Rural epidemiology: insights from a rural population laboratory. *Am J Epidemiol* 148(10):949–957, 1998.
12. Manson SM, Callaway DG: Health and aging among American Indians: issues and challenges for the biobehavioral sciences. *Am Indian Alask Native Ment Health Res* 1:160–200, 1988; discussion 201–210.
13. Lee ET, et al: All-cause mortality and cardiovascular disease mortality in three American Indian populations, aged 45–74 years, 1984–1988: the Strong Heart Study. *Am J Epidemiol* 147(11):995–1008, 1998.
14. Fitzgerald JT, Anderson RM, Gruppen LD, et al: The reliability of the diabetes care profile for African Americans. *Eval Health Prof* 21(1):52–65, 1998.
15. Lillie-Blanton M, et al: Race/ethnicity, the social environment and health. *Soc Sci Med* 43(1):83–91, 1996.
16. Holman RG, et al: The epidemiology of logging injuries in the Northwest. *J Trauma* 27(9):1044–1050, 1987.
17. Conway GA, et al: Preventing deaths in Alaska's fishing industry. *Public Health Rep* 110(6):700, 1995.
18. Sackett DL, Richardson WS, Rosenberg W, Haynes RB: *Evidence-Based Medicine: How to Practice and Teach EBM.* New York: Churchill Livingstone, 1997.
19. Hoffman C, Rice D, Hai-Yen S. Persons with chronic conditions: their prevalence and cost. *JAMA* 276(18):1473–1479, 1996.
20. Lasker RD, et al: *Improving the Quality and Cost-Effectiveness of Care by Applying a Population Perspective to Medical Practice. Medicine and Public Health: The Power of Collaboration.* New York, New York Academy of Medicine, 1997, pp 77–89.
21. McCulloch DK, Price MJ, Hindmarsh M, Wagner EH: A population-based approach to diabetes management in a primary care seting: early results and lessons learned. *Effect Clin Pract* 1:12–22, 1998.
22. Wagner EH, Austin BT, Von Korff M: Organizing care for patients with chronic illness. *Milbank Q* 74(4):511–544, 1996.
23. Weed LJ: The problem oriented record as a basic tool in medical education, patient care and clinical research. *Ann Clin Res* 3(3):131–134, 1971.
24. Greene HL, Johnston W, Lemcke D: *Decision Making in Medicine: An Algorithmic Approach,* 2nd ed. St. Louis, Mosby, 1998.
25. Wagner EH, Austin BT, Von Korff M: Improving outcomes in chronic illness. *Managed Care Q Rev* 4(2):12–25, 1996.
26. Garibaldi RA: Computers and the quality of care—a clinician's perspective. *N Engl J Med* 338(4):259–260, 1998.
27. Christianson JB, Taylor RA, Knutson DJ: *Restructuring Chronic Disease Management: Best Practices and Innovations in Team Based Treatment.* San Francisco, Jossey-Bass, 1998.
28. Wagner EH: Chronic disease management: what

will it take to improve care for chronic illness? *Effect Clin Pract* 1(1):2–4, 1998.

29. Marshall PD, Chin HL: The effects of an electronic medical record on patient care: clinician attitudes in a large HMO. *Proc AMIA Symp*, 1998, pp 150–154.

30. Kelly W, Bilous R, Murray G, et al: The clinical value of computerized information systems: a review of 98 randomized clinical trials. *Methods Progr Biomed* 56(2):205–210, 1998.

31. Aubert RE, Herman WH, Waters J, et al: Nurse case management to improve glycemic control in diabetic patients in a health maintenance organization: a randomized, controlled trial. *Ann Intern Med* 129(8):605–612, 1998.

32. Balas EA, Austin SM, Mitchell JA, et al: The clinical value of computerized information systems:

a review of 98 randomized clinical trials. *Arch Fam Med* 5(5):271–278, 1996.

33. Dickinson J, Hutton S, Atkin A, Jones K: Reducing asthma morbidity in the community: the effect of a targeted nurse-run asthma clinic in an English general practice. *Respir Med* 91(10):634–640, 1997.

34. Katzenbach JR, Smith DK: *The Wisdom of Teams: Creating the High Performance Organization.* New York, HarperCollins, 1993.

35. Langley GJ, Nolan KM, Nolan TW, et al: *The Improvement Guide: A Practical Approach to Enhancing Organizational Performance.* San Francisco, Jossey-Bass, 1996.

36. Sheils JF, Rubin R, Stapleton DC: The estimated costs and savings of medical nutrition therapy: the Medicare population. *J Am Diet Assoc* 99(4):428–435, 1999.

The Emergence of Federal Rural Health Policy in the United States

L. GARY HART   PAT TAYLOR

*T*he purpose of this chapter is to briefly describe the emergence of rural health policy at the federal level over the past quarter of a century. The development of the various policy players is briefly described, as is the process by which federal legislation and regulations are developed. Obstacles are discussed that currently prevent rural health care from being more effectively addressed at the federal level. The major rural health issues during the first decade of the twenty-first century are also projected.

This chapter might more aptly be entitled "The Partial Reemergence of Rural Health at the Federal Level." Rural health was a dominant issue at the federal level during the agrarian colonial times. During that period, rural places were generally thought to be more healthy than urban ones, and it was the cities that were seen as dirty and sickness-ridden. Over the following 200 years, a profound demographic transition from an agrarian society to an urban one was accompanied by a shift in the nation's political power structure, its chief concerns, and its population locus. By 1990, approximately three-quarters of the population lived in cities of 50,000 or greater population.[1] During the last three decades of the twentieth century, there was a reemergence of policy issues and sometimes action at the federal level in terms of rural health. This is still only a partial reemergence, however, because no one would argue that these developments have come even close to leveling the political playing field between rural and urban interests.

Although the rural population of the United States is approximately as large as the total rural and urban population of Great Britain (i.e., well over 55 million), relatively little is known about the health care delivery milieu within the rural United States.[2] Between 75 and 80 percent of the U.S. population is located within urban areas. Research resources and attention are concentrated on the populous urban areas and most recently on the managed care revolution. National policy is largely designed to solve urban health care delivery problems, with rural interests left in the backwash to negotiate policy and regulation patches to lessen unintended adverse rural consequences. High technology and specialized medical care interests centered in urban areas lead the public and policymakers to view the rural health care delivery system as a lower-order appendage of the urban system. The consequent view is that the rural population is utterly tied to urban areas for the preponderance of its medical care. If the access of local rural populations to health care is made worse because of policies aimed at reducing urban public expenditures, it is judged as an acceptable trade-off because of the latter's increased use of more sophisticated urban services. This trivialization of the rural health care delivery system is of more than academic interest. It creates the context within which federal and state policy decisions are made. During this time of dynamic health care delivery change, with its emphasis on cost containment, decisions made within this context have the potential to profoundly influence the viability of the rural health care delivery system along with local economic development and, at a personal level, to intrusively degrade personal access to quality care while increasing the personal costs of care. It is imperative that policymakers and others have a realistic view of the rural health care delivery system.

As can be appreciated from the previous five chapters, the rural health care system has strengths and critical needs; it is also extremely varied and vulnerable. Rural environments and residents are diverse, and it is not possible that one cookie-cutter set of congressional policies and administrative regulations will adequately address health care issues in both rural and urban venues. Because of their unique sites, varied histories, cultures, economies, settlement patterns, and health status, rural populations present problems that even extremely complicated administrative regulation systems based on national policies cannot adequately address. In fact, complicated regulations in and of themselves place a disproportionately large burden on rural health care delivery systems when compared to their urban counterparts. As reimbursement administrative burdens increase, lower-volume providers (e.g., smaller, remote rural hospitals, solo practices, and small provider groups) expend a greater proportion of their reimbursement revenue on administrative and accounting overhead than do their larger-volume urban counterparts. They also have a more difficult time procuring fiscal reimbursement and accounting expertise at a price they can afford.

There are other circumstances that make rural health care delivery unique and critical to local rural residents, such as long travel distances, low population densities, diseconomies of scale, high rates of fixed overhead per patient revenue, and unique social environments.[3] The rural population is proportionately older than the urban population, and the ethnic and social character of rural populations varies dramatically from one part of the country to another. These circumstances make it crucial that health services be locally available to rural populations. When local medical care services are not available, the long travel distances, with their concomitant delays in obtaining acute care, increase patient suffering and often result in detrimental outcomes. Locally available medical services reduce the travel time and expenses that local rural residents incur when they obtain care. Federal policymakers who consider the costs and benefits of public medical care programs usually consider only the costs to the government and seldom the costs to rural residents associated with extended travel and care delay, especially for the poor and elderly. And finally, a critical aspect of the health care delivery system in small and remote rural towns is its vulnerability. These local systems, with their small numbers of providers and sparse resources, are tenuously balanced to meet the needs of their residents while providing adequate income and quality of life for their providers. Federal policies have often upset this balance, leaving local rural populations with no nearby place at which to obtain care. Once local health care delivery systems are destroyed, few rural towns are able to redevelop their local access.

BACKGROUND

Rosenblatt and Moscovice[4] characterize the evolution of rural health into five periods:

- *The colonial period and advent of industrialization (1625–1850).* The agrarian era of the apprentice-trained country doctor gives way to increasing urbanization and formal urban-centered training.
- *Industrial growth and the pre-Flexner era (1850–1910).* Industrialization fuels greater urbanization, medicine becomes institutionalized in urban settings and begins to embrace the new science, and rural medicine wanes, although

rural populations remain generally healthier than their urban counterparts.

- *Flexner era to World War II (1910–1940)*. Dr. Abraham Flexner's report acts as a catalyst for transforming the medical training system into its present form, rural public health grows rapidly, and larger urban hospitals flourish, while over 700 rural hospitals close during the Depression and the shortage of health providers within rural areas grows acute.

- *From the Hill-Burton program to the War on Poverty (1940–1970)*. The Hospital Survey and Construction Act—Hill-Burton program—acts as a catalyst for rural hospital construction; physician specialization continues as the rural physician supply remains critically low; and, by the period's end, the federal government takes significant steps to insure and provide health care to the elderly and poor (e.g., Medicare, Medicaid, Community Health Clinics, and National Health Service Corps).

- *The technological era—the current rural health care crisis (1970 to the present)*. Great strides in and dependence on medical technology occur throughout the period and focus on large urban facilities; the federal government implements programs enacted at the end of the previous period and enacts new programs to improve rural health care; family medicine physician training spreads rapidly and is accompanied by an increased primary care emphasis on general internal medicine and pediatrics; and the general crisis in rural health facilities, technology, and personnel persists.

The decade of the 1970s can also be characterized as a decade in which emphasis was placed on access to health care for underserved rural and urban populations, especially the poor. Much of the decade's concern, federal programs, and research were devoted to access issues, with what is often considered limited success.

The era since 1982 can be characterized as the era of health care cost control. The 1980s and 1990s have seen the federal and state governments emphasize attempts to slow increases in the costs of health care, especially as regards governmental expenditures. These attempts have dramatically altered the health care delivery landscape. For instance, the implementation of the Prospective Payment System (PPS) to pay hospitals for inpatient Medicare services was a dramatic change in payment policy and was one of the principal causes behind the closing of 10 percent of the nation's rural hospitals. Further changes have involved the managed care revolution, which has greatly changed the way in which medicine is practiced. The spread of managed care to many rural areas has been slow.[5] However, it is clear that, while the ostensible impetus to managed care was to constrain health care expenditures, its implementation has been accompanied by reduced access and services in both rural and urban settings.

Most recently, the Balanced Budget Act of 1997 (BBA97) was enacted, with many provisions directed at controlling Medicare expenditures. The BBA97's Medicare provisions have far-reaching effects on rural health care. Most notably, they dramatically reduce Medicare payments for home health care services, nursing home care, and hospital outpatient services. These are the very services into which rural hospitals, which survived the reductions in inpatient reimbursement of the 1980s, diversified during the 1990s. If the BBA97's provisions go unchanged, many rural hospitals and providers will face fiscal catastrophe, and rural residents will face severe problems in obtaining access to medical care. The passage of the patchwork Balanced Budget Refinement Act of 1999 (BBRA99) does provide some minor relief for the rural health care delivery system from the detrimental provisions of the BBA97. However, for the most part, the BBRA99 only delays the full implementation of BBA97 provisions. The BBA97 is a classic example of a federal policy that is aimed primarily at solving urban health policy problems. Meanwhile, many of the rural issues of the previous periods persist (e.g., provider maldistribution and shortage; poor access to care for the medically indigent and racial/ethnic populations; and lack of equity).

EMERGENCE OF RURAL INTERESTS AT THE FEDERAL LEVEL

The concerns of the late 1960s and early 1970s about access to care led to the enactment and implementation of such federal programs as Medicare, Medicaid, Community Health Centers, the National Health Service Corps, and Area Health Education Center programs. These programs were indicative of a federal interest in providing fiscal support, training, and actual services to address the significant disparities in the nation's health care delivery system (Table 6-1). However, as the 1980s began, the problem of access to medical care in rural areas remained severe. The implementation in 1983 of the federal Medicare Prospective Payment System (PPS) and other federal cost-cutting policies acted as a catalyst for the organization of rural interests at the national level. The National Rural Health Care Association, American Rural Health Association, and American Small and Rural Hospital Association were formed during this period and then combined in 1987 to form the National Rural Health Association (NRHA). The NRHA has grown and has become an advocate at the federal level of rural health care interests. Although it remains a relatively small association by national standards, its activities include advocacy work with both houses of the Congress, the executive branch, the agencies of the Department of Health and Human Services (DHHS), the Health Care Financing Administration (HCFA), and the federal courts. The NRHA has also been supportive of rural health care research (e.g., it is a sponsor of the *Journal of Rural Health*). When the interests of their memberships have overlapped, the NRHA and other associations—such as the American Academy of Family Physicians (AAFP) and National Association of Community Health Centers (NACHC)—have collaborated in their congressional efforts.

During the rural health care crisis of the 1980s, the Senate Rural Health Caucus (1985) and the House Rural Health Care Coalition (1987) were formed to better address rural health care issues within the Congress. In 1987, the federal Office of Rural Health Policy (FORHP) was established within the Health Resources and Services Administration (HRSA). The FORHP has worked with other agencies of the DHHS, the secretary of HHS, and the Congress to provide them with a rural perspective on policy and program activities. In addition, the FORHP has administered federal programs, most recently the State Rural Hospital Flexibility Grant Program, which includes Critical Access Hospitals, and has promoted rural health care research and policy analysis. The first federally funded rural health research centers received grants from FORHP in 1988. FORHP has also helped to promote and establish state offices of rural health across the nation and has staffed the National Advisory Committee on Rural Health, which was established in 1990 to advise the secretary of HHS on rural policies.

In 1993, the Rural Policy Research Institute (RUPRI) was organized to provide timely expert advice to the Congress on the rural implications of legislative proposals and newly enacted laws. RUPRI's policy briefs and interaction with congressional players have influenced policy decisions. Likewise, in 1997 the Capital Area Rural Health Roundtable was developed. It provides information on contemporary rural health policy issues to congressional staff members and national associations with rural interests. Its principal vehicle is topically relevant policy seminars held on Capitol Hill. For another description of the federal rural health emergence and the related rural programs of the last few decades, see Samuels.[6]

The FORHP and other federal agencies such as the Department of Defense, Department of Education, and the National Library of Medicine have invested in research and demonstrations in telehealth during the last decade. The FORHP was critical in funding rural demonstrations and, along with the NRHA and others, in providing the information that led to the 1996 passage of the Universal Services Fund, which

Chapter 6   The Emergence of Federal Rural Health Policy in the United States

TABLE 6-1   SELECTED MAJOR MILESTONE EVENTS INFLUENCING RURAL HEALTH CARE—1946 TO 2000

1946	Hill-Burton Act facilitates the planning and building of rural hospitals.
1965	Medicare provides health insurance coverage for elderly.
	Medicaid provides health insurance coverage for indigent.
	Health Professions Educational Assistance Act provides for training and loan forgiveness for health professions in shortage areas.
1966	Comprehensive Health Planning Act establishes Community Health Centers and Migrant Health Centers.
1970	National Health Service Corps established.
1971	Comprehensive Health Manpower Training Act establishes Area Health Education Centers (AHECs).
1977	Rural Health Clinics (RHCs) Act authorizes RHCs.
1978	Organization of National Rural Primary Care Association (NRPCA), which later (1984) changes name to the National Rural Health Care Association (NRHCA).
1980	Funding of Community Health Care Center (CHC) program starts establishment of CHCs.
	American Rural Health Association (ARHA) is organized.
1983	Hospital Inpatient Prospective Payment System (PPS) Reimbursement is initiated.
1984	NRPCA and ARHA agree to jointly publish the *Journal of Rural Health.*
1985	U.S. Senate Rural Health Caucus is formed.
1986	American Small and Rural Hospital Association (ASRHA) merges with NRHCA.
1987	First research and policy agenda setting national conference held in San Diego.
	Establishment of the federal Office of Rural Health Policy (FORHP) of the Health Resources and Services Administration (HRSA).
	NRHA and National Association of Community Health Centers joint rural task force to coordinate mutual concerns is established.
	NRHCA and ARHA merge to form National Rural Health Association (NRHA).
1988	Rural health research centers are funded through FORHP.
1989	U.S. House Rural Health Care Coalition is formed.
1990	Federal funding for establishment of state offices of rural health.
	Release of Office of Technology Assessment (OTA) report entitled *Health Care in Rural America.*
1993	Rural Policy Research Institute (RUPRI) is started.
1996	Universal Services Fund establishment through the Telecommunications Competition and Deregulation Act of 1996.
1997	Balanced Budget Act of 1997 (BBA97).
	Capital Area Rural Health Roundtable started.
1998	Establishment of Office for the Advancement of Telehealth.
1999	Balanced Budget Refinement Act of 1999 (BBRA99).
2000	Second rural research agenda setting conference held.

SOURCE: Adapted from *National Rural Health Association Historical Highlights: 1978 to 1998,* July 14, 1998, provided by Ms. Donna M. Williams, Executive Vice President of the NRHA.

is intended to subsidize the telehealth phone line costs of remote rural health care providers. In 1998, the federal Office for the Advancement of Telehealth (OAT) was established within HRSA to take a lead position in telehealth development.

FEDERAL POLICYMAKING: MEDICARE EXAMPLE AND IMPEDIMENTS TO GOOD RURAL POLICY

It is beyond the scope of this chapter to describe in detail the process of legislation and how it specifically functions relative to rural issues. Redman[7] has called this the "legislative dance" and provides an excellent description. A good example of the process around the specific issue of the Community Health Center Program is available.[8] Samuels[6] provides policy development background on some rural programs not discussed in this chapter [e.g., Area Health Education Centers and Essential Access Community Hospital and Rural Primary Care Hospital (EACH/RPCH) programs]. However, the current process and the parameters that limit its sensitivity to the rural implications of legislation and regulation are well illustrated here by Medicare policy and regulation.

Development of Policy

We have chosen Medicare policymaking to illustrate federal health care policy development for two reasons. The first is that Medicare is the federal program with the greatest influence on health care, including rural health care. In rural hospitals, Medicare pays for the majority of inpatient days[9] and Medicare payments are 22 percent of total outpatient revenues.[10] Medicare's Graduate Medical Education policies have arguably been the major determining factor biasing the nation's physician workforce toward urban-based specialists and away from adequate supplies of primary care and rural-based physicians.

The second reason is that Medicare expenditures are a significant and growing percent of total federal expenditures. During much of the 1980s and 1990s, Medicare outlays were increasing much faster than the general inflation rate. The Medicare Trust Fund, despite increases in the payroll taxes which feed it, is forecast to be exhausted just about the time the baby-boom generation starts to swell the number of Medicare beneficiaries. In 1995, there were 38 million Medicare beneficiaries and $184 billion in Medicare expenditures, which were 2.5 percent of the gross domestic product (GDP) and 21 percent of Personal Health Care Expenditures (PHCE; 12.1 percent of GDP).[11]

The particular question addressed here is as follows: Why, in developing major Medicare cost-control measures, have federal policymakers used a "one size fits all" design that is a particularly bad fit for rural providers? Two major Medicare cost-control measures were enacted into law in recent years. The first was the inpatient Prospective Payment System (PPS—i.e., Diagnosis Related Groups, or DRGs) passed in 1983. The second, BBA97, legislated three additional prospective payment systems—for hospital outpatient, home health care, and skilled nursing facility services.

These national prospective payment systems can be extremely detrimental for rural providers unless adjustments are made. The majority of rural providers are low-volume providers. For example, in 1995, some 50 percent of rural hospitals had an average daily census of 15 or fewer patients.[12] Because low-volume providers have fewer cases across which to spread their fixed costs, their per-unit costs cannot be expected to be as low as those of the average-volume efficient provider, on which prospective payment systems are based. Also, small rural hospitals lack the number of units of care needed to be able to reliably average in high-cost cases and come out with an average cost per unit that is at or near the Medicare DRG payment amount. As DRGs are bundles of many services, there is considerable variability in costs across patients in a given DRG. Furthermore, because rural providers are often the only providers for Medicare beneficiaries within areas that are remote from care alternatives, discontinuing unprofitable but critical services is often contrary to their institutional missions, detrimental to beneficiary health status and quality of life, and costly to elderly ill beneficiaries in terms of travel time, cost, and comfort.

Federal Budget Politics

Federal expenditure levels are always too high in the eyes of many politicians. And from 1980 through 1998, there were large federal budget deficits—the result of record defense expenditures and large tax cuts. These deficits constrained domestic spending and were seen (especially by Republicans) as requiring cuts in domestic programs, including Medicare, in order to reduce the deficits. The 1983 and 1997 Medicare cost-control measures were enacted during periods of high Republican influence in the federal policy process. In 1983, a Republican, President Ronald Reagan, was in the White House, and the Republicans controlled the Senate. In 1997, Republicans were in control of both houses of Congress. However, it is important to note that there was continuing broad support in both parties for measures to control the steep rate of increase in Medicare expenditures.

THE PLAYERS

The major players in federal policy formation are the two houses of the Congress, the administration (the White House and the Cabinet departments), and the interest groups. Rural health policy scholars and analysts have a secondary though important role in policy formation.

THE CONGRESS

Congressional power over Medicare policies lies largely in the committees—the Senate Finance Committee and the House Ways and Means Committee and Commerce Committee. When there are major, pressing Medicare policy issues on the table, such as "saving the Medicare trust fund," rural health care is not a priority consideration in these committees. Another reason for rural health care's place on the Medicare back burner is the usual dominance of the committee and subcommittee chairs by members from urban states. In 1999, for example, the three chairs were from the urban states of Delaware, Florida, and California.

However, congressional members concerned about rural health care have joined together to exert their collective influence in the policymaking process. On the Senate side, the Senate Rural Health Caucus was formed in 1985, shortly after Medicare DRG payments began to impair rural hospitals. As most senators have substantial ru-

ral constituencies, a large majority of the senators are members of the Rural Health Caucus: 79 percent in 1999. Members of the House of Representatives with rural constituencies soon followed the Senate's lead and formed the House Rural Health Care Coalition. As fewer members represent rural districts, the House Coalition is proportionally smaller: its 134 members in 1999 represent 31 percent of the House. The two caucuses have often worked together, and have a record of success in correcting major Medicare policies *after their enactment into law* and in gaining passage of programs targeted specifically at rural people and rural providers. Their most notable success in recent years was the inclusion in the BBA97 of the Medicare Critical Access Hospital (CAH) reimbursement program. The CAH program allows the smallest of rural hospitals to be reimbursed on a cost basis if they meet program requirements.

THE ADMINISTRATION

During the last two decades of the twentieth century, there have been no outspoken advocates for rural health care in the White House or the highest levels of the Department of Health and Human Services (DHHS). The only unit of the executive branch charged with speaking out for rural health care is the federal Office of Rural Health Policy—a small office situated at the bottom of the bureaucratic structure, far removed from the secretary of the DHHS. This office has a staff of 10 professionals. The location of this office and the size of its staff tell the story of the priority given to rural health care matters within the DHHS.

INTEREST GROUPS

The interest groups most powerful in shaping Medicare policies are the national associations of insurance companies, pharmaceutical companies, health plans, hospitals, and physicians. Although the associations of hospitals and physicians have rural members, these associations seldom lobby for special provisions favoring rural interests because they must speak for all of their members. In the constrained budgeting process where there is a fixed pot of funds, a favor for one subgroup within an association has to come out of the funds for all the other members of the association. In the development of policies on purely rural health care matters, the principal organization representing rural health care interests to the Congress and the administration is the National Rural Health Association, a relatively small association with limited resources.

EXPERTS

Health policy researchers and analysts with expert knowledge of rural health care can have an important role behind the scenes in the development of policies. There are two important groups of rural health policy experts outside the federal government. Most prominent is the eight-member expert health panel of the Rural Policy Research Institute (RUPRI), composed almost entirely of university-based scholars from across the nation. The RUPRI panel members contribute their time to develop analyses of proposed and enacted national health policies from a rural perspective, apply recent rural research findings, and provide expert assistance to congressional members and staff in the development of legislative bills. The second group is composed of the rural health research centers. The five rural health research centers funded by the federal Office of Rural Health Policy, HRSA, target their research and analytic capabilities on understanding important national and regional issues in rural health care access and quality. Research findings are disseminated directly to the policymaking audience as soon as they are completed in short "briefs" and in longer working papers. And center staff are frequently called upon for expert assistance by congressional staff members, HCFA civil servants, and policymakers in their own states and regions. As a group, these rural health research centers now constitute a solid subdiscipline within the larger field of health services research. In addition, a handful of other rural researchers who are scattered across the nation and located mostly at universities also make a significant contribution to rural research and policy analysis. These researchers and those in the rural health research centers also produce research results that are relevant and influential in areas such as medical education, program evaluation, clinical care, and state policy issues.

Within the federal government, the single largest group of experts on rural health care policy is the professional staff of the federal Office of Rural Health Policy, in the HRSA of the Department of Health and Human Services. They are frequently called upon for expert assistance by the HCFA and congressional staff members.

The Process

When federal policymakers are developing major Medicare cost-cutting measures that will cause pain to most providers, they are often likely to employ strategies that minimize the opportunities of interest groups to shape the policies. A small group of congressional or administrative staff members may work in secret to develop the legislative proposal. For example, the first Medicare (inpatient) prospective payment system was developed very secretly by a small group of top civil servants working directly with the secretary of health and human services (Pat Taylor, unpublished research). Then, when the PPS reform package was sent to the Congress by the secretary of HHS, it was deliberately attached to a bill that was already moving rapidly toward enactment, another strategy to limit the access of interest groups into the policy development process.

The Content (One Size Does Not Fit All)

The two major Medicare PPS cost-control policies have been "one size fits all." The bill writers' intentions were to spread the impact across all providers as well as to simplify the work of administering these new policies. Also, federal policymakers have been slow to learn that Medicare PPS needs special rural adjusters in order not to fiscally damage rural providers. The decade following the implementation of inpatient PPS witnessed first their punishing impact on rural providers (hospital closures, negative operating margins) and then the passage of a series of adjustments to protect essential rural hospitals from PPS. But by 1997, as the BBA97 was being written, few of Washington's top health policy specialists, including HCFA bureaucrats, remembered the painful rural lesson of the 1980s: that the "one size fits all" inpatient PPS was inappropriate for low-volume rural providers. And the members of Congress and staff members of the key committees for Medicare were largely newcomers with no memory of the devastating impact that inpatient PPSs had on rural hospitals. The result was the legislation of three new Medicare PPSs without any special provisions for rural providers.

During late 1999, several rural "corrections" to the BBA97's three subacute care prospective payment provisions were being pushed for congressional passage by those who speak for rural health care—the two congressional rural health caucuses, the National Rural Health Association, the Office of Rural Health Policy, the Rural Health Policy Research Institute, and the Rural Health Research Centers—and, for the first time, the American Hospital Association (AHA). The AHA has joined in the battle because the damage projected for rural hospitals will be felt by other major groups of hospitals—e.g., teaching hospitals—except that it will be the worst for rural hospitals.[13] While rural advocates were not satisfied with the fruits of their labors, the passage of BBRA99 does provide minor relief to rural providers and delays parts of the implementation of BBA97.

Policy Implementation (Simpler Is Not Necessarily Better)

The Health Care Financing Administration (HCFA) is the agency of the DHHS responsible for carrying out the Medicare laws. The first step in policy implementation is development of the regulations—the detailed rules and procedures that translate a law into action. The sec-

ond step is the carrying out of the rules and procedures. Drafting of new Medicare regulations takes place behind closed doors. HCFA staff, including experts in Medicare, in regulation writing, and in legal matters, collaborate in the drafting. The regulation writing team pays close attention to the letter of the law as well as the congressional committee reports written as the bill moved through the Congress. These often spell out in detail the intent of the legislation's authors. By virtue of its authorizing legislation, the federal Office of Rural Health Policy has a seat on the Medicare regulation development teams working on rules that influence rural providers. As the FORHP seat is only one of many, FORHP influence in the rule making is limited to the ability of the FORHP staffer to persuade other members of the team to accept the rural-friendly positions being proposed. Involvement of interest groups is strictly controlled by HCFA staff; interest groups may be consulted only for expert information. HCFA staff have not historically understood the special issues of rural providers. However, there have been some recent initiatives by HCFA to train and sensitize its staff better along these lines (e.g., more contact between staff and rural health research center staffs).

When organizations and citizens are unhappy with various aspects of the Medicare program, they often unfairly blame the HCFA. If the complaints are about the substance of Medicare policies, the blame probably belongs to the Congress, to those who wrote the law. If the complaints are about the long time which HCFA takes to act, much of this blame also lies with the Congress and the White House for their serious underfunding of HCFA's staffing needs. This agency, which has the responsibility of managing the expenditure of more than $350 billion a year (1999), is critically and perennially short of the staff needed to handle these enormous responsibilities. Because of these staffing problems and the need to keep Medicare administrative overhead at a minimum, there is intense pressure to keep administrative policies as simple and universal as possible.

Results

Despite these efforts to keep regulations relatively simple and universal, later congressional and administrative adjustments to Medicare over the years have created a very complex reimbursement system. Many federal programs have been extremely detrimental to the rural health care system, as described above. The BBA97 has already caused substantial fiscal distress to rural hospital home health care and reduced the number and complexity of services to rural patients.[14] Unless major adjustments are made to BBA97's outpatient payment policies, many rural facilities that do not qualify as Critical Access Hospitals will certainly face a reduction in services and perhaps closure. However, the long-term effects of the described policy process permeate not only Medicare provider policies but those in other important areas relevant to rural health care delivery, such as the funding of graduate medical education.

ROLE OF RESEARCHERS

It became increasingly apparent in the early 1980s that the lack of relevant and objective rural health research at the federal level hampered those advocating federal policies. This made it difficult to argue for or against policies on the basis of objective and representative information. As a result, the advocacy process was often reduced to debates and arguments about quantified cost savings to the federal budget through program change versus anecdotal stories about the consequences of such actions.

Rural health care research had significantly lagged behind the rest of health services research, although researchers such as Roemer, Hassinger, Hein, and Sheps pioneered the way and inspired a second generation of rural researchers. These researchers and those of the late 1970s and first half of the 1980s—such as Cordes, Moscovice, Coward, Christianson, and Rosenblatt—provided the first documentation of the special rural circumstances of health care

delivery, access, and other problems. Much of this work is summarized in the rural health care text *Rural Health Care.*[4]

The year 1987 marked two significant milestones for rural health care research. The first was the inclusion in the congressional funding of HRSA's new federal Office of Rural Health Policy (FORHP) of funds for the establishment of rural health research centers. This program provides ongoing core funding for policy-relevant research. Research centers have competed for this funding over the last 12 years and the program continues into the twenty-first century. The various centers have copiously contributed to the policy-relevant research base used by policymakers, program administrators, and educators. As the critical mass of rural research has increased, many researchers and other federally funded centers have also contributed to this new age of rural research. For instance, the FORHP center funding, along with the critical rural health care problems, also helped spawn rural health research center programs funded by the Agency for Health Care Policy and Research (AHCPR), the National Institute on Aging (NIA), the National Institute for Mental Health (NIMH), and the National Institute of Occupational Safety and Health (NIOSH). The latter two center programs remain active. Across this entire period, foundations, most notably the Robert Wood Johnson and Kellogg Foundations, have funded rural health research and demonstration projects that have often made significant contributions to our understanding of rural health issues and that sometimes would not have been funded by federal funding agencies.

The second milestone was the 1987 Rural Health Services Research Agenda Conference, which took place in San Diego and was sponsored by the NRHA and the Foundation for Health Service Research and funded by the National Center for Health Services Research and Health Care Technology Assessment (NCHSR/ HCTA) and HCFA. This conference marks a date when rural health research came of age and reached the critical mass to become a more dynamic and contributing factor in rural health care federal policy formation, planning, debate, financing, and education. The conference policy agenda papers have been influential over the last decade.[15] A second national rural research agenda setting conference is scheduled for August 2000 to take stock of what had been learned and to help chart the research course into the first decade of the twenty-first century.

Three notable research/policy developments occurred during the 1990s. First, the Office of Technology Assessment published *Rural Health in America*. This encyclopedic volume has been a high-quality reference source for a decade. Second, in 1993, RUPRI began providing timely policy feedback to those interested in current congressional policies through quick qualitative interview methods and by applying the findings from the rural and other research literatures, including the most recent results. Last, in 1999, the five FORHP funded rural health research centers produced *Rural Health in the United States*.[1] This publication updates some *Rural Health in America* information by a decade and provides policy-relevant overviews of key aspects of rural health care, including such federal programs as Medicare and Medicaid.

As never before, current high-quality rural research and policy analysis covers a broad range of relevant topics. Studies of the influence of the BBA97 and BBRA99 are in progress. Research centers are involved in refining proposed federal adjustments to the Health Professional Shortage Area (HPSA) designation criteria. The results of an FORHP, Department of Agriculture, and research center collaborative project have created a new subcounty definition of rural (i.e., the Rural-Urban Commuting Areas, or RUCAs) for use in better targeting federal and state rural program funds.[17,18] Many other policy-relevant studies—in rural mental health, rural public health, women physician and physician assistant recruitment and retention within small rural towns, managed care in rural areas, and the like—are all in progress.

Although anyone involved in the legislative process, policy development, and regulation re-

alizes that much more is involved than just having relevant and objective research results, such results are important and can facilitate decisions that are less arbitrary and parochial. There is now a cadre of well-trained and active rural health researchers who focus on policy and other issues of rural health care. The challenge is to sustain this capability across time so that research and policy results can be available when critical needs arise.

ISSUES IN RURAL HEALTH CARE FOR THE FIRST DECADES OF THE TWENTY-FIRST CENTURY

It is not possible to predict all of the issues in rural health care policy that will be dealt with at the federal level during the first decades of the twenty-first century. However, most of the detailed federal policy questions posited by Patton[19] and by Hersh and Van Hook[20] are still relevant today and into the next decades, albeit there are twists on them and some new ones occasioned by such changes in the system as managed care and the BBA97. In the short term, there are critical questions surrounding the effects of the multifaceted BBA97 and BBRA99 in such areas as home health care and hospital outpatient service reimbursement, but it is important that issues related to access and quality also be addressed. While a long list of potential issues could be produced, we limit our focus to just five areas of policy that we believe will be especially important.

Workforce

One of the true constants during this century in the rural United States has been the shortage of appropriate health care providers in many rural areas. As illustrated in Chap. 3, the shortage and maldistribution of physicians remains dramatic, even after three decades of federal and state initiatives aimed at ameliorating this problem. Likewise, maldistribution and shortages of physician assistants, nurse practitioners, other nurses, dentists, and all other types of health workers are typical and recurrent. While federal programs have addressed these problems, they nonetheless remain. Some programs, such as the NHSC and the CHCs, have provided care in many rural areas where it would not otherwise have been available.

As illustrated in Chap. 3, there are many factors—such as the trends in urbanization, specialization, and managed care—that make it difficult to attract physicians to rural areas. Other trends, such as the increasing numbers and percentage of medical school graduates who are female, present new challenges. Graduating women physicians are significantly less likely to locate in rural locations than their male counterparts, and the smaller the rural town, the less likely women are to locate there.[21] This is also true for physician assistants.[22] An even more pressing problem relates to the BBA97. The reduction of graduate medical education (GME) funding and creation of a much less fiscally favorable rural health care delivery milieu is likely to cause some rural providers to leave rural practice and new graduates to avoid rural towns, especially those remote and smallest towns where they are most needed.

Many rural training programs have been successful at producing practicing rural providers.[23] At the same time, there are very real barriers to training rural physicians within rural places, such as federal GME financing policy and residency review committee (RRC) rules.[24] See Chaps. 22, 23, and 24 for detailed discussion of predoctoral, graduate, and continuing medical education related to rural practice.

There are many questions about health care providers and the rural health care delivery system that will need to be answered during the first decades of the twenty-first century.[25] For instance, will there be large losses of rural providers associated with the provisions of the BBA97 and will this adversely influence both provider scope of practice and quality of care? Will the burgeoning number of nurse practitioners translate into increased local access to generalist providers within rural areas?[26] Will

decreases in funding and the change in federal Medicare reimbursement adversely influence the amount and quality of training that takes place in rural locations? What role will the National Health Service Corps, J-1 visa waivers, and state loan repayment programs play in providing health care in rural shortage areas? How will the trend toward performance-based accreditation influence the quality of care and availability of rural providers?[27] Will better methods and data allow federal and state health provider training and placement programs to better target rural locations where there is need?

Hospitals

The early years of the 1990s saw a reversal of the widespread financial difficulties experienced by rural hospitals in the 1980s—difficulties rooted in changing technologies, outmigration of local residents to larger hospitals, and the Medicare inpatient PPS. External and internal factors contributed to this turnaround. Rural hospitals responded to their changed environment by expanding outpatient services, diversifying into new services, and increasing the efficiency of their inpatient services. In 1990 Congress acted to end the 25 percent differential in Medicare PPS payments to urban and rural hospitals, improving rural hospital Medicare payments approximately 40 percent on average.[9] Also, the 250-odd rural hospitals that closed between 1988 and 1997 likely included many of the weakest ones. By 1996, fewer than 1 percent of rural hospitals had losses greater than 10 percent of revenues during two consecutive years, compared to 4.6 percent in 1990, and net margins had more than doubled between 1987 and 1996—from 1.7 to 4.5 percent.[9]

However, rural hospitals have become increasingly reliant on Medicare and are now especially vulnerable to changes in Medicare payment systems. In 1996 Medicare was, on average, the payer for 60 percent of inpatient and swing bed days and 47 percent of total outpatient charges in rural hospitals.[9] In many states, such as Iowa, dependence on Medicare reimbursement is much higher. When Congress acted to control Medicare expenditures in the BBA97, tremors of fear reverberated through the rural hospital world. BBA97 aimed Medicare cost-reducing policies at the very sectors into which rural hospitals had diversified—outpatient services, skilled nursing care, and home health care.[28] New prospective payment systems were ordered for these three sectors of care. Seventy-two percent of rural hospitals will be affected by two of the new PPSs and 21 percent by all three.[9]

Many health policy analysts understand that prospective payment systems in their pure form are inappropriate for low-volume providers, since their small number of cases means that they are unable to average out high-cost cases and have relatively high fixed costs per patient service. However, BBA97 did not include any PPS protections for these low-volume, mostly rural facilities. Even with the enactment of BBRA99, the future of rural hospitals is uncertain as the twenty-first century begins. Their increased efficiency and diversification will not be enough to assure their future financial well-being. Rather, that will depend importantly on federal policy. To what extent will the federal government act to cushion low-volume rural hospitals and those hospitals essential for rural access from the unfair impact of the three new subacute care payment systems? How will rural hospitals evolve during the next 20 years and to what extent will rural residents be forced to travel long distances to receive their hospital-related services? And how will this influence their health? If rural hospitals close in many small towns, will their role as the centralizing base of the local delivery system be filled? And how will the absence of a hospital influence local economic development? How will Critical Access Hospitals influence the quality and long-term viability of care in small rural communities? These and a cornucopia of other questions hang in the balance as the twenty-first century begins. The answers are not clear, but it is certain that the answers will profoundly influence the

access to care, health status, quality of life, and economic well-being of rural populations.

Telehealth

Over the last decade, technology has developed rapidly to produce more economical and higher-quality telehealth technology (see Chaps. 15 and 16 for discussions of rural medical informatics and telehealth). With these developments, the federal government (through such sources as HRSA's Office of Rural Health Policy and the Department of Defense) has funded a large number of telehealth demonstration projects. In 1998, HRSA established the federal Office for the Advancement of Telehealth (OAT), which is currently funding over 40 telehealth demonstration projects. Although a few payers have started to reimburse providers for telehealth services, the norm continues to be that they, including the federal government, do not. Although it is certain that the technology is available to perform telehealth services and there are reasons to believe that care can be of good quality, there remain many uncertainties. For instance, there are significant problems related to interstate licensure, widespread insurance reimbursement, and standardization/quality criteria (e.g., how many pixels on an x-ray are enough for quality radiographic interpretation?). Questions about the quality of clinical care and how it differs across specific medical conditions and circumstances are just starting to be addressed. Ironically, for those places with the greatest relative need to overcome isolation (e.g., the smallest rural towns or where the providers are in short supply), the question is whether financing will be available for these low-volume telehealth users. Furthermore, in these circumstances, can telehealth become standard if it does not save the time of already overworked providers, regardless of whether it saves the patient time and resources or provides other improvements?

There are many other questions that will need to be answered during the next decade. While costs will continue to decrease for a relative unit of this technology, how far and fast will telehealth spread and how will this influence the rural health care system? How will clinical telehealth be combined with other services that use the technology—such as medical education and hospital and clinic administration? Some argue that these other uses should carry the cost load and that clinical uses can be thought of as an extra benefit. How successful will telehealth system designers be at integrating telehealth clinical care into the normal routine of rural providers and remote specialty physicians, and how readily will rural providers adapt to these new technologies?

It seems inevitable that there will be a dramatic diffusion of telehealth services across the rural and urban U.S. landscape, almost as a technological imperative. However, the question is in what form, doing what, and at what costs (both fiscal and in terms of personal care relationships and the like)? Will these technologies result in more or less rural providers? And what will be their net influence on the health and satisfaction of rural residents?

Safety Net

There are 10 million uninsured rural Americans[29] and there were easily that number of underinsured in 1999, with numbers still climbing. Will rural providers be able to meet the increasing need for free and low cost care? Can they meet the need now?

The multiplying millions of Americans without meaningful health insurance represent a national crisis, but a crisis with different dimensions in rural communities. The nation's large towns and cities have health care safety nets of publicly subsidized clinics and hospitals. These providers are badly overtaxed by the growing demand for their services; but should public policymakers choose to act, there is an obvious policy solution to the problems of urban safety net providers: increase their public subsidies.

Community and migrant health centers provide critical care for the rural indigent in many areas. These centers face severe fiscal challenges.

A new research agenda regarding them was recently outlined that focused on outcomes, managed care and finance, and service delivery issues and research.[30]

However, most small rural towns do not have any publicly subsidized clinics and hospitals. Here much of the safety net is an informal one—of private practitioners who give away care to the medically needy. Policymakers have yet to appreciate this rural difference, let alone formulate any policies to bolster this informal safety net. The question for rural communities is how long and how widely private practitioners will be willing and able to serve as the "safety net" when the demand keeps growing and reimbursement policies continue to tighten.

Almost nothing is known about the willingness and capacity of rural practitioners to provide care to the medically needy in rural communities. A first study of the informal rural safety net began in 1999, as a collaborative project of the federal Office of Rural Health Policy (FORHP) and four rural health research centers with FORHP funding. Preliminary findings are that there is a high percentage of medically needy—25 to 50 percent of working-age people and their families are without meaningful primary care insurance—and that most rural small town private practitioners, though not all, provide much of the care needed by this sizable population at low or no charge. Low-income minority populations in rural areas appear likely to encounter the greatest difficulty in obtaining care. What portion of the rural population will not have access to health care a decade from now and how will this influence their health and the very fiber of rural life?

Financing of Services

The mass closures of rural hospitals in the 1980s was followed by a relatively prosperous period during the 1990s for rural hospitals. BBA97 again threatens the remaining rural hospitals and many of their services, such as home health care and skilled nursing care. In addition, the move during the 1990s toward managed care is also having profound influences on rural health care providers, although rural managed care seems to have stalled and is even retreating from some rural areas.[5]

A sobering question to ask during these debates regarding rural health care reimbursement is whether there is much to be saved by programs that are miserly in their rural financing. Are there consequential HCFA dollars to be saved from rural providers? This is especially significant when one considers that the effects of such cuts in rural reimbursement often result in rural residents not obtaining care or being forced to obtain their care in distant, expensive, and intensive urban venues. Because of the great reliance of most rural providers on Medicare funds, decisions regarding Medicare reimbursement levels for rural providers are pivotal. Besides the obvious consequences of low payments already listed, low reimbursement will have negative long-term effects on the quality of the facilities within rural areas and subsequently on the availability of providers. The savings of federal cost-cutting programs must be weighed against the costs borne by local rural residents in terms of personal health status and other costs, such as those related to lengthy travel.

Few believe that the present reimbursement system is the definitive one or even a long-term one. There is a large array of proposed and possible reimbursement adjustments and alternative systems that are being proposed. The most important question facing Congress and rural residents is the extent to which federal and state policymakers will invest in the rural health care delivery system. Will the average elderly rural residents of a remote small town obtain nearly all of their medical care in a distant urban center in 2010, including primary care, or will they have local access to care? Irrespective of the perceptions of many policymakers, a recent state analysis shows that the rural elderly receive the vast majority of their care within rural areas.[31] Many other questions will be answered during the next decade. For example, will managed care dominate the rural health care deliv-

ery system? To what extent will the growing administrative overhead (e.g., paperwork related to quality assurance, fraud, and abuse monitoring) and reimbursement regulations make small rural practices (i.e., few providers or low volumes) economically impractical? See Chaps. 17, 18, and 19 for detailed discussions of managed care, the economics of rural practice, and practice management.

CLOSING COMMENTS

Federal health policy has a dramatic influence on local rural health care delivery. For structural reasons, congressional policies and regulatory rules are often detrimental to rural health care delivery systems. Over the last 20 years, there has been a significant emergence of a rural interest infrastructure that can act on the federal stage to exert influence for more effective and humane policies for small rural towns and their residents. Nevertheless, rural interests are not as effective as they could be. For instance, the great diversity of those with rural interests sometimes puts them on opposite sides of issues or in situations where they are required to compete for the same limited resources. Even in the best scenario, the structure of federal policymaking is such that there will probably always be the "insensitive rural policy followed by fixes" syndrome to legislation.

A true policy conundrum for federal congressional and regulatory leaders is to produce effective and efficient health care policies given the marked variation across the U.S. rural landscape and its inherent divergence from the majority urban milieu. However, a first step in the direction of developing such policy is to understand the fundamental differences and similarities between rural and urban health care delivery. The responsibility of rural providers, citizens, researchers, and policy analysts involved in rural health care is to assure that these federal policy leaders have the necessary information to understand rural health care delivery and the consequences of various policy initiatives. Lest it is overlooked, it is also critical that local rural residents and providers coordinate their community's available resources to provide as optimally cost-effective and high-quality care as they can manage.[32] The rest of this book is dedicated to this end.

REFERENCES

1. Ricketts TC III (ed): *Rural Health in the United States.* New York, Oxford University Press, 1999.
2. Ricketts TC III, Johnson-Webb KD, Randolph RK: Populations and places in rural America, in Ricketts TC III (ed): *Rural Health in the United States.* New York, Oxford University Press, 1999, pp 7–24.
3. Hassinger EW, Hobbs DJ: Rural society—the environment of rural health care, in Straub LA, Walser N (eds): *Rural Health Care: Innovation in a Changing Environment.* Westport, CT, Praeger, 1992, pp 178–190.
4. Rosenblatt RA, Moscovice IS: *Rural Health Care.* New York, Wiley, 1982.
5. Rural Policy Research Institute: *Implementation of the Provisions of the Balanced Budget Act of 1997: Critical Issues for Rural Health Care Delivery.* P99–5. Columbia, MO, University of Missouri, Rural Policy Research Institute, July 29, 1999.
6. Samuels ME: Policy initiatives and issues in rural health services development, in Beaulieu JE, Berry DE (eds): *Rural Health Services.* Ann Arbor, MI, AUPHA Press/Health Administration Press, 1994, pp 57–83.
7. Redman E: *The Dance of Legislation.* New York, Simon & Schuster, 1973.
8. Sardell A: *The U.S. Experiment in Social Medicine: The Community Health Center Program, 1965–1986.* Pittsburgh, PA, University of Pittsburgh Press, 1988.
9. Moscovice I: *Rural Hospitals: Accomplishments & Present Challenges.* Minneapolis, MN, University of Minnesota, Rural Health Research Center, 1999.
10. Mohr PW, Blanchfield BB, Cheng CM, et al: *The Financial Dependence of Rural Hospitals on Outpatient Revenue.* Bethesda, MD, Project HOPE Walsh Center for Rural Health Analysis, August 1998.
11. *Health Care Financing Review.* Medicare and Medicaid Statistical Supplement, 1997, tables 2 and 6.
12. Blanchfield BB, Franco SJ, Mohr PE: *Critical Access Hospitals: How Many Will Qualify?* Bethesda, MD, Project HOPE Walsh Center for Rural Health Analysis, November 1998.
13. Lewin Group: *The Balanced Budget Act and Hospitals: The Dollars and Cents of Medicare Payment Cuts.* Falls Church, VA, Lewin Group, May 10, 1999.
14. WWAMI Rural Health Research Center: *An Initial Report on the Impact of the Balanced Budget Act on Small Rural Hospitals.* Policy brief. Seattle, WA, WWAMI Rural Health Research Center, September 1999.
15. A rural health services research agenda. *Health Services Res* 23(6):special issue, 1989.
16. U.S. Congress, Office of Technology Assessment: *Health Care in Rural America.* OTA-H-434. Washington, DC, U.S. Government Printing Office, 1990.
17. Morrill R, Cromartie J, Hart G: Metropolitan, urban, and rural commuting areas: toward a better depiction of the U.S. settlement system. *Urban Geog* 20(8):727–748, 1999.
18. Hart G, Morrill R, Cromartie J: *A Health Care User Guide to Rural-Urban Commuting Areas: A New Tool for Targeting Rural Programs.* Working paper number 50. Seattle, WA, WWAMI Rural Health Research Center, May 2000.
19. Patton L: Setting the rural health services research agenda: the congressional perspective. *Health Services Res* 23(6):1003–1051, 1989.
20. Hersh AS, Van Hook RT: A research agenda for rural health services. *Health Services Res* 23(6): 1053–1064, 1989.
21. Doescher M, Ellsbury K, Hart LG: The distribution of rural female physicians in the United States. *J Rural Health.* In press.
22. Larson E, Hart LG, Goodwin MK, et al: Dimensions of retention: a national study of the locational histories of physician assistants. *J Rural Health.* In press.
23. Geyman JP, Hart LG, Norris TE, et al: Physician education and rural location: a review. *J Rural Health.* In press.
24. Saver B, Bowman R, Crittenden RA, et al: *Barriers to Residency Training of Physicians in Rural Areas.* Working paper number 46. Seattle, WA, WWAMI Rural Health Research Center, April 1998.
25. Council on Graduate Medical Education: Tenth Report: *Physician Distribution and Health Care Challenges in Rural and Inner-City Areas.* Washing-

ton, DC, U.S. Government Printing Office, February 1998.

26. Cooper RA, Laud P, Dietrich CL: Current and projected workforce of nonphysician clinicians. *JAMA* 280(9):788–794, 1998.

27. Moscovice I, Rosenblatt RA: *Quality of Care Challenges for Rural Health.* Minneapolis, MN, Rural Health Research Center, University of Minnesota, January 1999.

28. Rural Policy Research Institute: *Taking Medicare into the Twenty-first Century: Realities of a Post BBA World and Implications for Rural Health Care.* P99-2. Columbia, MO, University of Missouri, Rural Policy Research Institute, February 10, 1999.

29. Schur CL, Franco SJ: Access to health care, in Ricketts TC III (ed): *Rural Health in the United States.* New York: Oxford University Press, 1999, pp 25–37.

30. Mueller KJ, Curtin T, Hawkins D, et al: Building a research agenda: responding to the needs of community and migrant health centers. *J Rural Health* 14(4):289–294, 1998.

31. Hart LG, Rosenblatt RA, Lishner DM, et al: *Where Do the Rural Elderly Obtain Their Primary Care?* Seattle, WA, WWAMI Rural Health Research Center. In press working paper.

32. Amundson B: Myth and reality in the Rural Health Service crisis: facing up to community responsibilities. *J Rural Health* 9(3):176–187, 1993.

PART TWO

Special Clinical Problems and Approaches in Rural Health Care

R ural health care differs from other primary care in many ways. Perhaps the most important differences lie in the area of the actual provision of clinical care in rural settings. Among the distinctions that pervade all aspects of clinical care are the following:

- Distances and lack of population density
- Distance from (or complete absence of) medical and surgical specialists
- Paucity (and frequent "turnover") of well-trained ancillary medical personnel
- Scarcity of other types of health care providers (such as dentists, psychologists, physical therapists, etc.)
- A small primary care provider work force (often without the "depth" created by multiple providers who are not often on call)
- Lack of extensive laboratory, imaging, blood banking, and other similar resources
- Limited (or absent) hospital resources
- Limited (or absent) capacity for transportation of sick and injured patients
- A large presence of uninsured patients who cannot afford to travel to obtain care
- A practice that probably has a higher percentage of older and sicker patients than one might typically find in an urban or suburban primary care setting

These circumstances, both singly and in concert, create significant challenges for the provider of clinical care. Many of these hurdles can be overcome through innovation, anticipation, and adequate advance planning and preparation. The chapters in this section focus on areas in which the rural health care team is likely to encounter unique concerns, situations, and predicaments (often as a result of the factors noted above). Topics were chosen based either on the frequency or the severity of their occurrence. With this in mind, we highlight the rural clinical aspects of emergency care, obstetric care, perinatal care, surgery, home care, mental health care, and dental care. Although many additional topics could have been selected, the approaches applied to these common problematic areas illustrate methods that can be applied to a wide variety of clinical situations in rural settings.

Thomas E. Norris

CHAPTER 7

Emergency Care

HAROLD A. WILLIAMSON, JR.

Case 1: A Family Outing Gone Awry

A family of four return to their farm home after an evening of church services. The road home is familiar but narrow, poorly marked, not crowned, and without a shoulder or guard rails. An oncoming car, perhaps not able to see road markings in the rain, crosses the center line. The family's car swerves and rolls over several times down an embankment.

- Why are motor vehicular accidents more often fatal in rural areas?
- How much time will elapse before an emergency crew reaches the family?
- Should the most seriously injured be taken to the local hospital, 20 miles away, or to the designated trauma center, 60 miles away?

Case 2: An Earache

On a Thursday evening, after returning from work at a fast-food restaurant, a single mother is confronted by her 2-year-old daughter, who complains of an earache following a week of upper respiratory infection. The child is febrile and irritable but playful and eating well. Her mother decides to take her to the local emergency department.

- Is this an emergency?
- What is the relationship between primary care access and emergency department utilization?
- How will the emergency department services be paid for?

Case 3: A Man with Chest Pain

A 54-year-old hardware store manager develops crushing substernal chest pain while at work. He drives himself to the local emergency department. His doctor is seeing patients in her office 2 miles away. A nurse obtains an electrocardiogram, which shows ST-segment elevations in leads V_4 through V_6.

- How are current care standards for myocardial infarction implemented in rural emergency departments?
- Should this man be cared for in his community or transported to a tertiary care center?
- How will his community hospital's relationship with a distant tertiary care center affect his outcome?

*F*or many rural residents, emergency care is the raison d'être for rural hospitals and health systems. And why not? Emergency care is the high-profile function for rural health systems. Even though a population base of 10,000 may generate only one true emergency a day, the handling of these cases distinguishes the priorities, resources, and skills of one community from the next.

In the early peacetime history of North America, an emergency medical system was probably the doctor with the fastest horse. As we know them, emergency medical services

Part Two   Special Clinical Problems and Approaches in Rural Health Care

(EMS) evolved because of better roads and transportation as well as medical advances that made rapid access to care worthwhile. The growth of hospitals in the early twentieth century evolved from the needs created by advances in surgical and emergency care. Most of these hospitals were in cities and were founded to serve as the focal point of medical advances and nursing care.

Federal Hill-Burton legislation created a series of new rural hospitals, and their attached emergency medical systems, in the 1950s and 1960s. The coordination and capabilities of these rural hospitals were at best fragmented and uneven. The National Highway Safety Act of 1966 authorized the U.S. Department of Transportation (DOT) to set guidelines for EMS and support development of EMS systems. Perhaps most importantly, this act allowed DOT to establish the Emergency Medical Technician (EMT) as a new health professional.

The Emergency Medical Systems Act, 1983, aimed to improve poor rural emergency services. Many rural communities used these funds to train EMS prehospital providers and to improve transportation and communication systems. The hoped-for outcome of the EMS Act—to improve and standardize rural emergency care—was not realized by 1991, when the Act expired.

During the 1980s, state governments became responsible for oversight and development of EMSs. During the 1980s and 1990s, the development of rural EMSs centered around better and more efficient communication technologies, transportation in ground-based and air vehicles, improved training for EMTs, and standardization of care for life-threatening emergencies— especially trauma and cardiac emergencies. The overall trend of hospital system acquisition and consolidation has also affected rural emergency services by creating de facto clinical affiliations. Vertical integration of small rural systems with larger tertiary care centers has created both problems and opportunities for EMSs.

RURAL EMERGENCY MEDICAL SERVICES

The successful rural EMS system is integrated and seamless but has several distinct characteristics:

- Rapid and easy access for the public
- A central, coordinated communication system
- A trained response team, quickly dispatched to a site
- Rapid transportation appropriate to the emergency
- A well-trained and committed health personnel team
- A capable hospital and emergency department
- Efficient connections to higher levels of care

Urban emergency systems have evolved rapidly in the past 20 years. Rapid-response teams using a "scoop and run" method are linked to large emergency departments staffed by specialized physicians, nurses, and technicians. This system is, in turn, backed up by subspecialty physicians and care teams as well as hospital operating rooms and intensive care units. Translating this successful evolution into a rural EMS context has had benefit, although it is limited. Special circumstances in rural areas require special solutions:

1. Long rural distances translate into long transport time, the enemy of successful emergency care.
2. Financially marginal rural hospital systems must subsidize EMSs, which often do not pay for themselves.
3. Emergency medical personnel, from dispatchers to physicians, are in short supply, and emergency medical care is often a "second job."
4. Communication over long distances is often spotty, resulting in poor coordination and command functions.
5. The relatively small populations in rural areas make it unlikely that anyone in a rural

community has substantial experience with a specific life-threatening emergency.

The solutions to these rural challenges are varied, in both implementation and success. Systems that work in rural areas of the eastern United States are based on interhospital distances of 20 to 30 miles. In frontier areas of the intermountain West, such distances are commonly 60 to 100 miles. Tax structure, community tradition, and state laws each influence local solutions to the EMS puzzle. It is gratifying to see the individualized and successful adaptations that overcome these disadvantages.

THE RURAL EMS: PREHOSPITAL PHASE

Setting

Rural areas are characterized by long distances, isolation, geographic barriers (rivers and mountains), poor roads, and bad weather.

Communication and Control

A coordinated communication system, such as "911," facilitates rapid and coordinated response. Such systems are spreading across the rural United States but are not yet available in all rural areas. Radio "dead spots" still hamper effective communication even when there is an effective system in place. Continuing improvement in the communication technology in rural areas will diminish somewhat the effect of long distances and geographic isolation. Nonetheless, the rural EMS will still need to contend with much longer transport times than those of urban areas; the benefit of a coordinated 911 system in rural areas may not be incrementally as great as it is in urban areas.

Personnel

An effective rural EMS requires numerous personnel, ideally working in a coordinated, controlled, prearranged fashion.

Dispatchers are essential to receive news of an emergency, locate appropriate personnel, and pinpoint the geographic location of the emergency. Ambulance drivers need to be familiar with regional addresses and be capable of traversing local terrain. Dispatchers in rural systems are often filling similar roles for police and fire departments; ambulance drivers are often volunteers.

"First responders" in rural areas may be more important than in urban areas because of the dearth of qualified emergency medical personnel. These first responders may include trained or untrained citizens, police, or fire personnel.

EMTs represent the core of trained prehospital attendants in rural areas. Training requirements for these individuals vary from state to state and over time. Standardized curricula for training EMTs are now widely utilized. As a general rule, the standard prehospital personnel in rural areas are as outlined below.

EMERGENCY MEDICAL TECHNICIAN—BASIC (OR "AMBULANCE")
For short, this is EMT-B or EMT-A, requiring about 100 hours of training. Skills include basic victim assessment, managing an airway and delivering oxygen, basic cardiopulmonary resuscitation, control of bleeding, and extrication techniques. Some EMTs are trained to use defibrillators. These EMTs are the most common personnel in rural areas.

EMERGENCY MEDICAL TECHNICIAN—INTERMEDIATE
The EMT-I receives about 150 hours of additional training. His or her capabilities include those of the EMT-B plus initiating and continuing care under a physician's direction as well as inserting intravenous lines, administering some medications, and using pneumatic trousers.

EMERGENCY MEDICAL TECHNICIAN—PARAMEDIC
The EMT-P receives about 700 hours of training. In addition to having the skills listed above and

skills in advanced life support, the EMT-P functions under verbal or standing written orders. Such technicians are rare in rural communities.

Acquisition of EMT skills is difficult in many rural areas. The vast majority of rural EMTs are volunteers in situations where cost and distance to training are barriers to advanced certification. Turnover rates are very high. Nonetheless, these dedicated volunteers form the backbone of EMSs in the rural United States. Their success, against considerable odds, has been remarkable.

In most rural communities, local physicians supervise EMSs. These physicians may or may not have advanced training in emergency care and, like most emergency personnel in rural areas, are usually volunteers. Physicians may function "on line," meaning in direct radio contact with ambulances and ambulance crews. They may also function "off line," playing a role in assuring proper training and equipment, policies and procedures, and standing orders for prehospital transportation.

Transportation

The workhorse of the rural EMS is a life-support-level ambulance. The capabilities of these transportation units range from basic to advanced life support and to mobile intensive care units. In rural areas, a high proportion of transportation may be for nonemergent, facility-to-facility transportation. This is particularly true of the transportation of elderly patients from nursing home to hospital and back.

Urgent transportation from rural hospitals or emergency departments to tertiary care centers is often by helicopter. Usually, these runs are for trauma, cardiovascular emergencies, and perinatal complications. The effective range of helicopter transport from a tertiary care center is 150 to 200 miles. Most air transportation is from a rural hospital to a tertiary care center rather than from the scene to the tertiary care center. Fixed-wing vehicles are used in areas where greater distances require more rapid transportation. Most medical air transport systems are owned and/or operated by large medical centers.

TABLE 7-1   REASONS FOR RURAL AMBULANCE RUNS: THREE STUDIES[a]

	Georgia	South Carolina	Texas
Medical (noncardiac)	45%	30%	48%
Trauma/injury	33%	23%	38%
Cardiovascular	10%	10%	15%
Ob-gyn and neonatal	7%	2%	2%
Mental health	2%	3%	3%
Unclassified/other	4%	24%	20%

[a]More than one condition was present for some runs.

SOURCES: Data from *Special Report*[1] and Morrisey et al.,[2] with permission.

Scope of Prehospital Emergency Medical Services

A substantial portion of ambulance runs are for trauma/injuries and cardiovascular problems, but a wide variety of other health problems require a broad range of capabilities for the rural EMS (Table 7-1).[1,2] As an example, many rural EMTs will use a defibrillator only once every 2 or 3 years. An urban paramedic uses a defibrillator 8 to 10 times a year.

A different method of characterizing ambulance runs (in urban versus rural Nebraska) showed that 70 percent of rural ambulance calls involved the elderly and 36 percent were identified as "routine" (as opposed to emergent) transfers; both of these are roughly twice as frequent as in an urban comparison.[3]

RURAL EMERGENCY SERVICES: THE EMERGENCY DEPARTMENT

Facilities

Rural emergency departments vary from large, state-of-the-art facilities capable of handling 30,000 to 35,000 visits per year to small basic-care facilities with 4000 to 5000 visits that are staffed only intermittently. Most rural hospitals do not have the capability of caring for severe trauma, for high-technology cardiovascular services, or for burns and complex problems related to environmental exposures. Most rural hospitals do serve a triage function for these more complex medical problems.

The American College of Surgeons has recommended categorization of all hospitals based on their ability to respond to trauma. This movement has, in turn, created a more precise concept of "regionalization." Responsible EMSs have taken careful stock of their capabilities and resources and accordingly arranged for timely referrals to more comprehensive centers.

Personnel

The traditional staffing of the rural emergency department had been a rotating call system utilizing local physicians. Quality-of-care issues, regulations, and concerns about overburdening local physicians have precipitated a new system of salaried, visiting physician coverage, even in the smallest hospitals. During the 1980s and 1990s, rural emergency department coverage shifted from local physicians to visiting physicians, sometimes hired directly by the hospital and sometimes contracted from an emergency physician service. These changes have resulted in increased costs, which must be borne by the rural hospitals.

The vast majority of physicians who staff rural emergency departments are not trained in emergency medicine residencies. In fact, one-third are not board-certified at all.[4] Some have extensive training and/or experience, others do not. It is unclear whether the capabilities of the average rural emergency department have been improved or diminished by contracting for outside physician coverage.

The capabilities of the hosting rural hospital often dictate the capabilities of its emergency service. The presence of surgeons and anesthesiologists, for example, expands considerably the repertoire of small hospitals in dealing with moderate levels of trauma.

Who Uses the Rural Emergency Department and Why?

A study of 5722 patient visits to 17 rural Mississippi hospitals helps characterize the role and scope of these units.[5] The mean age was 36 years; 9 percent were less than 2 years old and 18 percent were over 60. Visits were most common on weekends and evenings but were distributed evenly across the four seasons. Of patients seen in rural emergency departments, less than 1 percent died, 14 percent were admitted to the hospital, 6 percent were referred to another medical center, and the remainder returned home. The elderly were more likely to be admitted to the hospital (34 percent). Diagnostic categories in rural hospitals were dominated by injuries (30 percent) but encompassed the breadth of medical practice.

TRAUMA IN RURAL AREAS

Trauma death rates are nearly twice as high in rural areas as in urban.[6] But even within rural areas, there is substantial geographic variation. Some of this variation is explained by lower socioeconomic status, differences in occupational and other environmental exposures, quality of roads, and access to EMS systems.

Some research has provided a look at the natural history of trauma in rural areas. Only about 10 percent of motor vehicle accidents investigated by police lead to an EMS dispatch.[7] Once activated, the average response time in rural areas (dispatch to scene time and dispatch to hospital time) is about twice as long in rural (17 versus 8 minutes) as in urban areas.[8] Only about 3 percent of rural trauma victims have severe multisystem injury [injury severity score (ISS) greater than 20], and another 14 percent experience severe trauma to a single body system (ISS 10 to 19).[9] Death from rural accidents may occur at the scene, en route, and in hospital. The death rate is much higher when the response time is 30 minutes or more.

Fortunately, severe trauma is not a commonly seen occurrence for a rural trauma team and a rural hospital emergency department. Unfortunately, this means that each individual on the EMS team may be exposed to severe trauma less than once a year; rural health care personnel are less experienced with life-threatening injuries than their urban counterparts.

Cales and Trunkey have described the trimodal distribution of trauma deaths.[10] About 50 percent of such deaths occur within seconds to minutes of the accident, 30 percent occur within the first 2 to 3 hours, and 20 percent occur after days to weeks of hospitalization, usually from secondary complications. The 30 percent that fall in the middle group are those most likely to benefit from acute medical interventions and are the target group for EMSs. This period, between 2 and 3 hours after the accident, has been called "the golden hour" of trauma care. The appropriate assessment, stabilization, and transport of patients within this hour are the keys to survival.

The role of the rural hospital in serious trauma is unresolved and controversial. The "scoop and run" procedure utilized in urban areas is designed to ensure that injured victims reach a definitive source of care as quickly as possible. The extension of this concept into rural areas suggests that small rural hospitals should be bypassed. On the other hand, scoop and run in a rural area may mean an hour or more of transport time from the scene to a trauma center. Proponents of expanded roles for rural hospitals suggest that ambulance runs from the scene to the rural hospital allow the stabilization and triage of patients, some of whom can then be evacuated by air to a definitive trauma care center. Evidence favoring each of these approaches has been presented, but none is yet definitive.[11,12]

A number of severity assessment scales have been developed for different trauma situations. Some relate to the overall trauma status of the patient (the ISS); others relate to changes in mental status suffered during an injury (the Glasgow Coma Scale). Still others are applied specifically to the prehospital phase of emergency care (the Prehospital Index). These scales have been developed primarily for research regarding the care of traumatized patients. The clinical use of these scores has been helpful to rural emergency personnel as they decide which intervention steps must take priority.

States have taken various routes to a more or less generally accepted trauma designation system. Originally, this system accounted for three potential levels of care:

Level 1 is reserved for tertiary care centers with frequent trauma experience and 24-hour availability of the most comprehensive services.

Level 2 centers require 24-hour availability of an advanced but intermediate level of care.

Level 3 centers have 24-hour availability of basic emergency services as defined by the American College of Surgeons and the American College of Emergency Physicians.

Originally, most rural hospitals were intended to be designated at level 3. However, many rural hospitals could not meet established guidelines for this level of readiness. In recognition that some smaller rural hospitals had been excluded—both in terms of designation and in terms of fitting into a system—some states have now designated level 4 and 5 trauma centers.

Evolving knowledge about trauma and its treatment raises serious questions for care given in rural areas. On the one hand, serious trauma is a relatively infrequent experience for the rural EMS. This forces consideration of the amount of precious resources expended on relatively rare events. On the other hand, timely assessment, stabilization, and transport lead to improved survival and decreased disability among rural accident victims. This combination of features suggests that rural emergency personnel must function under well-considered protocols and guidelines because their individual experience will only rarely be adequate to guide the evaluation and treatment of a trauma victim.

Courses such as the American College of Surgeons' course in advanced trauma life support are important. An open and well thought out relationship with a regional trauma center and a smoothly functioning prehospital EMS system will optimize results. Finally, research about the best way of dealing with rural trauma is sorely needed. Under what circumstances is a scoop and run protocol superior? What characteristics of rural counties, from roadways to EMS teams, can be changed to decrease crashes and improve survivability? What is the optimal training for rural prehospital and hospital-based emergency personnel?

CARDIAC EMERGENCIES

Cardiovascular disease is the leading cause of death in the United States. More importantly, advances in medical technology have allowed improvement in survival and quality of life when certain treatments for heart patients are delivered in a timely fashion. Ischemia and infarction can lead to fatal arrhythmias and shock. In survivors, the death of heart muscle leads to disability and a decreased life span.

Techniques to deal with life-threatening cardiac arrhythmias, especially ventricular fibrillation and tachycardia, can save lives. Unfortunately, survival rates well under 10 percent have been the norm, with even lower rates in less population-dense rural areas.[13] Recently, improvements in technology have made it possible for minimally trained individuals to deliver a defibrillation shock by using an automatic external defibrillator (AED). There is hope that with the increasing presence of these devices in emergency vehicles, airplanes, and other places, more effective resuscitation of individuals suffering ventricular fibrillation may be realized. In many areas, rural ambulance crews may use AEDs after certain levels of training. However, although an urban-based emergency medical technician might have occasion to use a defibrillator monthly, most rural EMTs will do so less than once a year.

Other technological developments in cardiovascular care capitalize on our ability to reverse cardiac ischemia before the heart muscle has been damaged. Two such methods currently exist on an emergency basis.

The development of powerful thrombolytics that dissolve the fibrin portion of clots in coronary arteries (and elsewhere) have led to their early use in myocardial infarction. These intravenous medications are reasonably safe and can be given by anyone able to establish an intravenous access. Ambiguities, cost, and misunderstanding have contributed to their limited use in rural emergency settings.

Cardiovascular specialists are able to restore adequate blood flow through a coronary artery in many individuals. Angioplasty and related procedures can be done only by highly trained individuals in centers where supportive services are available. These procedures have the added advantage of defining precisely the nature of the coronary artery disease before treatment.

Both of these techniques have supporting research and proponents. Both need to be delivered within a few hours of the onset of myocardial ischemia in order to achieve reversibility. Most rural centers defer to the closest cardiac referral center in deciding which of these two technologies to use. Unfortunately, ambiguous communications have often led to the underutilization of these procedures. For small rural hospitals, keeping a stock of the expensive thrombolytic drugs may be difficult, particularly when regional cardiologists prefer that patients be sent elsewhere for angioplasty. However, in many circumstances, the rapid delivery of a clot-dissolving drug is preferable to prolonged transport times and the possibility of performing an angioplasty too late.

It behooves rural systems and their cardiovascular consultants to develop clear protocols and lines of communication and authority. Often patients may suffer unnecessary loss of cardiac muscle because of unclear treatment protocols. When rural systems elect to use thrombolytics, local expertise must be ensured.

PEDIATRIC EMERGENCY CARE

Nearly one-third of visits to rural emergency departments involve children and adolescents, who also constitute about 10 percent of patients receiving prehospital EMS care. Agriculture is generally considered the most dangerous occupation in North America, and children make up a relatively large share of the agriculture work force. Motor vehicle accidents and injuries due to farm machinery remain important causes of fatal and disabling injuries among rural children and adolescents.

The usual difficulties of rural communication, access, and transportation are compounded by the relative infrequency with which EMS prehospital personnel and hospital-based caregivers encounter pediatric emergencies. Trauma rates are higher for rural than for urban children, and survival after cardiac arrest in rural areas is about 15 percent. Within rural settings, the availability of a county hospital with 24-hour emergency services and the presence of advanced life support prehospital care is associated with a lower death rate. Children living in poorer counties are at higher risk for traumatic death.[14] One rural education intervention project demonstrated improved knowledge and confidence of emergency care personnel in the management of acutely ill and injured children.[15]

FINANCING AND GOVERNANCE OF RURAL EMERGENCY MEDICAL SYSTEMS

In urban areas, emergency medical systems (EMS) are usually encompassed within one hospital system. Public access—via 911 and public dispatchers—quickly shunts calls to integrated, fully competent emergency and trauma systems.

In contrast, the ownership and control of the rural EMS is often fragmented, making it look and behave more like a hybrid of private industry and public utility. Public access and commu-

nication systems are usually sponsored by the municipality or county in rural areas; ambulance systems may be county-owned, town-owned, hospital-owned, or a combination. Medical direction of the EMS is usually provided by a volunteer physician who is often in private practice. The hospital, whose governance may be separate from that of the county, controls the emergency department and the services provided by the hospital, which usually owns and controls the transport system. The systems that operate tertiary care backup are controlled from distant cities. It is therefore no mystery that the rural EMS is often disjointed. In the best systems, well-intentioned public and private enterprise work closely together with a focus on providing the best care. In the worst systems, inadequate resources are protected in a colloquial, uncoordinated fashion.

The financing of the rural EMS is particularly problematic. From a financial standpoint, the rural EMS operates as a collection of unrelated elements rather than as a system. The tax base of urban and suburban areas is usually better able to support the infrastructure essential for a high-quality EMS. There is large variability in the resources available to rural systems, but many of the poorest rural counties lack capital to support the emergency infrastructure.

The cost of operating an ambulance service is about 25 percent of the total system cost. Personnel costs represent the remainder. The rural EMS, with low utilization and an unfavorable payer mix, has relatively high fixed costs for its infrastructure. The ability of a system to recoup expenses is largely a function of billing practices and payer mix, the latter of which is beyond the control of most rural governance systems.

The staffing and maintenance of a 24-hour EMS vehicle is estimated to cost a quarter of a million dollars a year. Only a few percent of the runs of such a vehicle will be truly emergencies and another 15 percent can be considered urgent; only one medical emergency per day will be generated per 10,000 population. Because the fixed costs of the EMS are so high and rural utilization is low, the rural EMS often operates at a very low level of efficiency and is very expensive on a per capita basis.

From the hospital's standpoint, these difficulties are often compounded by reliance on the emergency department for routine primary care. Insufficient primary care capacity in rural counties means that many visits better suited to a physician's office will be cared for in the emergency department.

FUTURE TRENDS

The future of the rural EMS will largely be a function of our ability to merge medical and surgical advances with distance and time. Rapid advances in trauma care, life support, and cardiac interventions will continue over the next decades. Bringing rural patients in contact with these new developments will require either faster transport of rural patients to urban areas or systems that allow technology and service to be brought to the rural patient. In turn, bringing the patient and the technology together will require better systems of financing and governance, possibly accelerated by the rapid consolidations and "vertical integration" of the late twentieth and early twenty-first centuries.

REFERENCES

1. *Special Report: Rural Emergency Medical Services.* Congress of the United States, Office of Technology Assessment, Congressional Board of the 101st Congress. Washington, DC, US Government Printing Office, November 1989, pp 18–19.
2. Morrisey MA, Ohsfeldt RL, Johnson V, et al: Rural emergency medical services: patients, destinations, times, and services. *J Rural Health* 11(4): 286–294, 1995.
3. Stripe SC, Susman J: A rural-urban comparison of prehospital emergency medical services in Nebraska. *J Am Board Fam Pract* 4(5):313–318, 1991.
4. McGirr J, Williams JM, Prescott JE: Physicians in rural West Virginia emergency department: residency training and board certification status. *Acad Emerg Med* 5(4):333–336, 1998.
5. Bross MH, Wiygul FM, Rushing SK: The role of the rural hospital emergency department. *Family Med* 23(5):351–353, 1991.
6. Baker SP, Whitfield RA, O'Neill B: Geographic variations in mortality from motor vehicle crashes. *N Engl J Med* 316:1384, 1987.
7. Grossman DC, Hart LG, Rivara FP, et al: From roadside to bedside: the regionalization of trauma care in a remote rural county. *J Trauma* 38(1):14–21, 1995.
8. Grossman DC, Kim A, Macdonald SC, et al: Urban-rural differences in prehospital care of major trauma. *J Trauma* 42(4):723–729, 1997.
9. Smith N: The incidence of severe trauma in small rural hospitals. *J Fam Pract* 25(6):595–600, 1987.
10. Cales RH, Trunkey DD: Preventable trauma deaths: a review of trauma care systems development. *JAMA* 254:1059–1063, 1985.
11. Veenema KR, Rodewald LE: Stabilization of multiple-trauma patients at level III emergency departments before transfer to a level I regional trauma center. *Ann Emerg Med* 25:175, 1995.
12. Young JS, Bassam D, Cephas GA, et al: Interhospital versus direct scene transfer of major trauma patients in a rural trauma system. *Am Surg* 64:88, 1998.
13. Stapczynski JS, Svenson JE, Stone CK: Population density, automated external defibrillator use, and survival in rural cardiac arrest. *Acad Emerg Med* 4(6):552–558, 1997.
14. Svenson JE, Spurlock C, Nypaver M: Factors associated with the higher traumatic death rate among rural children. *Ann Emerg Med* 27(5):625–632, 1996.
15. Smith GA, Thompson JD, Shields BJ, et al: Evaluation of a model for improving emergency medical and trauma services for children in rural areas. *Ann Emerg Med* 29(4):504–510, 1997.

CHAPTER 8

Obstetric Care

David A. Acosta

K.H. is a 17-year-old young woman, gravida 2, para 0 (1 prior termination of pregnancy) with an intrauterine pregnancy at 32 weeks gestation by the best estimate of her last menstrual period. She has had no prenatal care because of lack of transportation and the fact that she has to travel 90 minutes from home to any doctor's office or hospital; she has no medical insurance. She arrives at your rural emergency department complaining of lower abdominal pain that is cramping in nature and seems to "come and go." This all started 2 hours earlier, when she awoke from her sleep in a pool of water. The pain has now increased in intensity and she is scared. Her past medical history is significant for the following: she smokes a half pack of cigarettes per day and has smoked for the last 5 years; she is single and the father of the baby is no longer involved since she found out that he was using intravenous drugs; she occasionally smokes marijuana; and she thinks she has been told in the past that she has herpes. She is placed on the fetal heart monitor (FHM) and is having regular contractions every 2 to 3 minutes. The fetal heart rate is 170 beats per minute and there is poor beat-to-beat variability. The FHM is starting to show late decelerations with each contraction. The patient's cervical exam reveals that she is 3 cm dilated, the fetus is in the vertex position at −2 station, and her membranes are definitely ruptured. An active herpetic-like lesion is seen on the right labium. You decide that the patient needs a stat cesarean section. Unfortunately, you are informed that there is another case in the operating room, which will not be available for another 30 minutes. The nearest regional perinatal center is 1 hour away by ground ambulance and 45 minutes away by helicopter.

There are many issues facing the primary care provider who practices obstetrics in a rural setting. They are varied and diverse and are political, economic, social, and ethical, as well as clinical in nature. The provider who is aware of these issues and who has developed the skills to resolve them will be successful. Chapters 8 and 9 draw from the literature and from the author's personal experience in rural practice. This chapter defines these issues, their prevalence, their impact on patient care and the provider, and strategies that have been used successfully by others in grappling with these common issues.

DEMOGRAPHICS OF RURAL PREGNANT WOMEN

Over 3.8 million infants were born in the United States in 1996, and 20 percent of those represented births to rural mothers. Overall, a larger proportion of rural mothers were teenagers or in their twenties in comparison to urban mothers, where the majority were in their thirties. When stratified by race, over 25 percent of all rural black infants were born to teenagers, in comparison to 15 percent of all rural white infants.[1]

Since 1980, the percentage of births to teenage girls below age 15 has remained constant in both rural and urban areas. The percentage of births to older teens decreased in both rural and urban areas from 1980 to 1988 and then increased slightly in 1990; it has since remained stable. Since 1980, an increase in births has consistently been seen in those above age 30 for both rural and urban areas.[1] The rural provider should be well versed in the unique obstetric conditions that each of these "younger" and "older" maternal age groups present. For the adolescent pregnancy, preeclampsia, preterm labor, substance abuse, noncompliance with prenatal care, poor nutrition, poor or excessive weight gain, low birth weight, and social dysfunction are all prevalent conditions. The conditions that are more commonly seen among older mothers include preeclampsia, low birth weight, congenital anomalies, Down's syndrome, and spontaneous abortion.

Maternal mortality is greater among rural than among urban women, but mortality rates for both have declined over time. In 1980, 334 U.S. women died from conditions related to complications of pregnancy and childbirth. In that year, maternal mortality rates were 23 percent higher in rural than in urban areas (10.2 versus 8.2 maternal deaths per 100,000 live births). By 1986, the total annual number of U.S. maternal deaths had declined to 272. In 1986, maternal mortality rates were still slightly higher in rural than in urban areas, but the highest rates were seen in the most densely populated urban areas. In metropolitan areas, the death rate (per 100,000) was 4.51, as compared with 7.40 in nonmetropolitan areas.[2]

Rural women are more likely than urban or suburban women to have had three or more children. They are less likely to be nulliparous.[2]

For rural women, rates of early initiation of prenatal care are lower than the rate for suburban women but higher than the rate for urban women. Following the same pattern, more rural than suburban women had delayed initiation of prenatal care ($\geq$5 months), while urban mothers had the highest proportion of late initiation of prenatal care.[1] Studies have shown that there are several reasons why rural women delay the initiation of prenatal care, including transportation difficulties, greater distance to travel to obtain prenatal care, shortage of providers who offer obstetric care, and lack of medical insurance.[2]

Insurance status among women in their childbearing years differs substantially between rural, urban, and suburban populations. Rural women are less likely than either urban or suburban women to be covered by health insurance provided by their employers. Rural married women are more likely than their urban or suburban counterparts to purchase their own insurance or be enrolled in Medicaid. Rural unmarried women are less likely than urban women but more likely than suburban women to be enrolled in Medicaid. More unmarried rural women than unmarried urban or suburban women are covered under a parent's health insurance policy.[1]

Similar patterns are seen with payment sources for women's most recent labor and delivery charges. Only a small proportion of rural women had full insurance coverage for obstetric care. Rural women are slightly more likely than either urban or suburban women to pay out of pocket (in part or in whole) for costs associated with labor and delivery. Rural women were less likely than urban women but more likely than suburban women to have labor and delivery charges covered under Medicaid.[1]

OBSTETRIC PROVIDERS

Less than 11 percent of the nation's physicians practice in rural areas. A majority of those physicians (54 percent) are in primary care specialties—family practice, general practice, pediatrics, general internal medicine, and obstetrics/gynecology (Fig. 8-1). According to the Council on Graduate Medical Education (COGME, 1994), family physicians were three times as likely as general internists and five times as

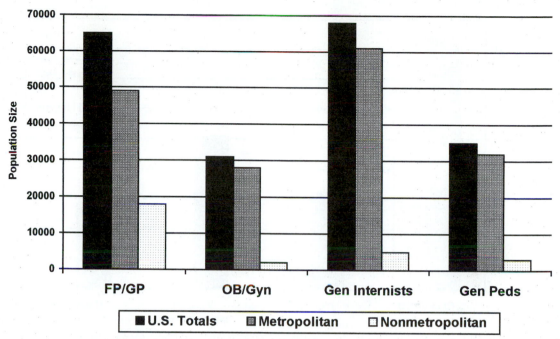

FIGURE 8-1 Location of primary care physicians in the United States by population, 1989. (Modified from Federal Office of Rural Health Policy: Facts about Rural Physicians. Health Resources and Services Administration. *Washington, DC, US Department of Health and Human Services, September 1997.)*

likely as general pediatricians to practice in rural areas.[3]

There is a continuing crisis in the United States regarding the provision of obstetric care in rural areas. The majority of maternal services in rural communities are provided by family physicians. There has, however, been a dramatic decline in the number of family physicians practicing obstetrics over the past 15 years.[4] In 1994, only 35.2 percent of family physicians were practicing obstetrics. More rural family physicians were practicing obstetrics than their urban counterparts (42 versus 22.3 percent, respectively). In addition, more rural family physicians were performing routine obstetric deliveries, doing high-risk and complicated deliveries (e.g., vacuum-assisted and low-outlet forceps deliveries), and performing cesarean sections than their urban counterparts (Fig. 8-2). In the United States, 25 percent of rural family physi-

cians include complicated deliveries in their obstetric practice, as compared with 9.3 percent of urban family physicians. High-risk obstetrics is practiced by 16 percent of rural family physicians versus 5.5 percent of urban family physicians. Cesarean sections are performed by 14.4 percent of rural family physicians as compared with 2 percent of urban family physicians.[5]

The level of obstetric care provided by rural family physicians varies according to the geographic location of the physician's practice (Fig. 8-3). Rural communities located in the East North Central, West North Central, Mountain, and Pacific regions have the most family physicians performing routine deliveries. By comparison, those rural communities located in the Middle Atlantic, South Atlantic, and East South Central regions have the least number.

In the United States, 50.8 percent of all practicing family physicians are located in metro-

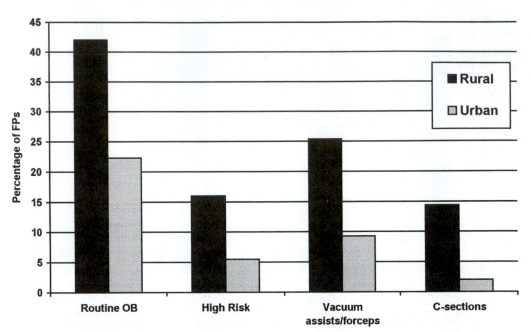

FIGURE 8-2 *Types of patient care in hospital practices of family physicians by census division and practice location, May 1994. (Data from American Academy of Family Physicians:* Facts about Family Practice 1995. *Kansas City, MO, AAFP, 1995, with permission.)*

politan areas and 23.5 percent are located in nonmetropolitan areas.[5] In contrast to family physicians, 90.4 percent of all obstetricians practicing in the United States are located in metropolitan areas and only 9.6 percent are located in nonmetropolitan areas.[3] Urban areas attract far more obstetricians. Differences in physician income, reimbursement differential for services rendered, available technology, hospital facilities, available call coverage, the number of "like" colleagues practicing in the same community, and the volume of patients have all been cited as reasons for this disparity.[6] In the United States there are only approximately 8.3 practicing obstetricians per 100,000 population in rural settings. As Fig. 8-4 shows, the number of obstetricians substantially decreases as the population base decreases.[7]

Conditions found in rural practice have contributed to the decline of rural obstetrical providers: the lack of coverage for time off, limited consultation opportunities, and difficulties with referrals to larger hospitals.[2] Nationally, the decision to limit or discontinue obstetric care appears to be associated with increasing physician age, solo practice, time concerns, and liability concerns.[8] The high cost of premiums for medical malpractice insurance coverage and fear of lawsuits have been cited as major factors contributing to the decline.[2] Malpractice concerns are greater in states with high malpractice insurance premiums and for physicians performing small numbers of deliveries.[9] The majority of those family physicians who discontinued obstetrics were in group practices, HMOs, or similar settings and were more likely to practice in larger communities (population >50,000).[10]

Characteristics of rural family physicians who continue to deliver maternity care have been identified. Family physicians who work in group practices and in physician-owned practices provide more obstetric care. Family physicians who are located in less populated counties, with fewer practicing obstetricians and other family physicians who are doing obstetrics, are more likely to provide maternity services. Family physicians who were more recently trained and who were fulfilling service obligations were also characteristic of those family physicians continuing obstetric practice.[11] In California, more than 70 percent of family physicians continuing to offer obstetrics do so largely because of personal satisfaction. More than 30 percent felt it was a responsibility to their community, while 25 percent felt obstetrics was a practice enhancer. Twenty-five percent of family physicians felt it was integral to their specialty.[10]

Obstetricians who migrated out of a rural community had their own unique features. Those who left were more likely to be between

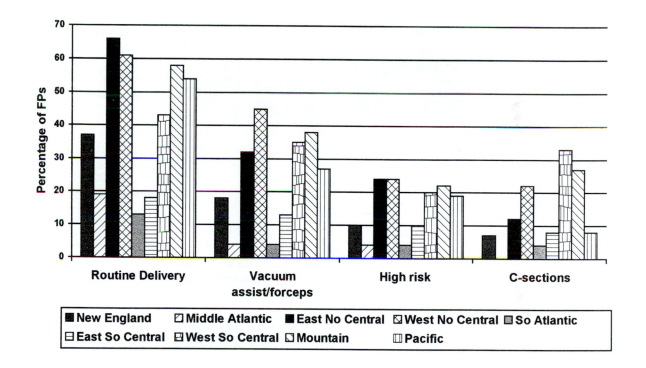

Regions:
New England: *Connecticut, Maine, Massachusetts, New Hampshire, Rhode Island, Vermont*
Middle Atlantic: *New Jersey, New York, Pennsylvania*
East North Central: *Illinois, Indiana, Michigan, Ohio, Wisconsin*
West North Central: *Iowa, Kansas, Minnesota, Missouri, Nebraska, North Dakota, South Dakota*
South Atlantic: *Delaware, District of Columbia, Florida, Georgia, Maryland, North Carolina,
    South Carolina, Virginia, West Virginia*
East South Central: *Alabama, Kentucky, Mississippi, Tennessee*
West South Central: *Arkansas, Louisiana, Oklahoma, Texas*
Mountain: *Arizona, Colorado, Idaho, Montana, Nevada, New Mexico, New Mexico, Utah, Wyoming*
Pacific: *Alaska, California, Hawaii, Oregon, Washington*

FIGURE 8-3 *Level of obstetric practice of rural family physicians by census division and practice location, May 1994. (Data from American Academy of Family Physicians:* Facts about Family Practice 1995. *Kansas City, MO, AAFP, 1995, with permission.)*

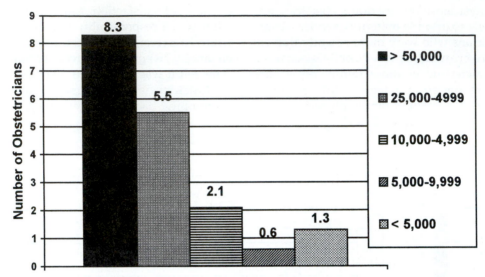

FIGURE 8-4 Number of obstetricians per 100,000 population by county size, 1988. (Data from Federal Office of Rural Health Policy: Rural Health Professions Facts. *Washington, DC, Health Resources and Services Administration, US Department of Health and Human Services, 1988.)*

the ages of 31 and 40 years. Rural areas with larger populations (and therefore larger volumes of patients) were more likely to attract and retain obstetricians.[6] In part, this may reflect the perception that an adequate practice volume is necessary to maintain skills. The American College of Obstetrics and Gynecology (ACOG) has recommended that its members should perform 160 deliveries per year in order to maintain their skills. Counties that had more community resources available (programs that support obstetric access) were also more likely to attract more obstetricians.[6] Areas that were able to increase their reimbursement for services and those that offered financial incentives were more likely to attract and retain obstetricians.[12]

It has been recognized that family physicians and obstetricians do differ in their approaches to maternity care. Family physicians offer a more family-centered approach to obstetrics (emphasizing continuous emotional support from family, friends, and staff for the patient), while obstetricians follow a more traditional medical approach.[13] Family physician behaviors

during labor and delivery are also affected by the environment in which they practice. These influences are dependent on the involvement of an obstetrician in the care of a pregnant patient, the facility (tertiary care), and the technology available.[14] The quality of maternity care in terms of obstetric outcome provided by family physicians in rural areas has been shown to be no different from that provided by obstetricians.[15,16] Smaller rural hospitals in Washington State have been demonstrated to have lower cesarean section rates, fewer instrumented deliveries, lower use of epidurals, and lower rates of induction while providing comparable outcomes.[13,16,17]

RURAL-URBAN DIFFERENCES IN MATERNITY CARE

There are many published studies examining rural and urban differences in the delivery of perinatal care. These differences cover a wide range of topics, including access to maternity care, the provision of obstetric services by rural hospitals, regionalization and outreach services, neonatal outcomes, economy and insurance coverage, financial reimbursement for services, nursing support, and the utilization of mid-level practitioners.

Access to Maternity Care

Access to maternity care for women is a problem that still plagues rural America. It has been well documented that pregnant women residing in rural areas do not have the same access to prenatal care as is available to most urban women. Several studies have tried to explain this disparity: absolute shortages of obstetric providers available in their communities; shortages of obstetric providers who will accept Medicaid or agree to see the uninsured; a lack of insurance coverage and an inability to pay for maternity services; a decline in the number of hospitals equipped and staffed to provide delivery services; geographic isolation from services; poor access to regional perinatal systems; and great distances to travel for obstetric services, usually out of the patient's area of residence.[2] Access to care is especially problematic for the poor, the uninsured, publicly insured low-income women, and teenage mothers.

What this means for the rural provider is that he or she must be prepared for the associated risks, complications, and increased maternal and neonatal morbidity/mortality that result from this lack of accessibility of services. Available evidence suggests that fetal, infant, and maternal mortality are somewhat higher and that late prenatal care is more of a problem in rural than in urban areas.[2] Declining access to maternity care in rural areas of Florida adversely affected the state's ability to reduce its infant mortality.[18] Maternity patients who must travel from rural areas to regionalized perinatal centers for prenatal care and delivery have more complicated deliveries, higher rates of prematurity, and higher costs of neonatal care.[19] Decreased access to maternity care in rural areas of Indiana resulted in an increase in infant mortality.[20] Rural pregnant women in Missouri who presented late for prenatal care were twice as likely to have had a low-birth-weight infant in the year after their local rural hospital closed.[21] Clearly, the rural provider must be prepared to deal with high-risk pregnancies that include maternal problems such as preterm labor, preterm rupture of membranes, and intrauterine growth retardation.

Several studies have confirmed that easy access to prenatal and perinatal care improves birth outcomes and justifies community efforts to assure service availability.[19] Many innovative programs have been developed to improve access to maternal care for rural women. Hueston describes the development of a hospital-sponsored maternity clinic to primarily extend obstetric care to the indigent women of eastern Kentucky, utilizing family physicians as the primary obstetric providers, with surgical and consultative backup provided by staff obstetricians.[22] Another strategy to improve access has been the increasing use of certified nurse midwives (CNMs), whose effectiveness has been demonstrated among special population groups. Bahry and colleagues reported on a university-based program (graduate nurse-midwifery education) that utilized a multidisciplinary health care team (comprising a physician, nurse-midwife, health educator, social worker, nutritionist, pediatric nurse practitioner, and patient case manager) in a decentralized service model (community health clinic) with central referral and management of high-risk problems at the university medical center.[23] Baldwin and associates described Washington State's implementation of a comprehensive Medicaid expansion program that included the expansion of eligibility from 90 to 185 percent of the federal poverty level; provision of maternity support services including nursing, psychosocial, nutritional, and case management services to all high-risk women; and increased reimbursement to providers for obstetric services.[24] The Colorado State Department of Health subsidized perinatal programs comprising contracted private physicians, social workers from local hospitals, and the county's health department, who provided risk assessment and prenatal classes by the public health nurses.[25]

THE PROVISION OF LABOR AND DELIVERY SERVICES IN RURAL HOSPITALS

The problem of access to maternity care for rural women has been compounded by the geographical scarcity of labor and delivery services in rural hospitals. Rural hospitals continue to face the threat of closing or the elimination of delivery services. Many reasons have been cited for the discontinuation of obstetric services in rural hospitals: decline in obstetric providers; increasing malpractice insurance costs; inadequate Medicaid reimbursement for services; capital expenses required to staff and equip obstetric units with state-of-the-art technology; competition with larger urban hospitals providing more specialization on perinatal care; and outmigration of rural women to urban facilities.[26–30] In addition, small rural hospitals located in communities with low socioeconomic status may have neither sufficient local revenues nor resources to pay for such services, nor the ability to garner outside support using outreach services. Isolated rural areas often lack the necessary resources or volume to support specialists such as surgeons.[31] In contrast to their urban counterparts, rural hospitals have fewer admissions, lower average daily census/occupancy rates, shorter lengths of stay, higher proportions of uncompensated care patients, and higher expenses than patient revenues.[2,31,32]

There are significant differences between counties and hospitals that do and do not offer obstetric services in rural areas. Almost 65 percent of rural hospitals in southern counties of the United States did not offer obstetric services. One in six rural hospitals in the West did not provide obstetric services, and 1 in 15 rural hospitals in the Northeast did not offer them. Overall, counties without hospital maternity services are smaller in both population and land area, have lower socioeconomic status, and have fewer health care resources.[27] In contrast, urban hospitals are located in more affluent counties.[17] Second, small rural hospitals were less likely to offer maternity services if they were located in counties with high unemployment rates. Third, the higher the percentage of the county's population that was white, the higher the probability that its hospital offered obstetric care. Last, hospital ownership had a strong impact on whether maternity services were provided. Government-owned hospitals were more likely to provide maternity services (55 percent) than not-for-profit and for-profit hospitals (38 and 7 percent, respectively).[27]

There are other obstetrically related differences between rural and urban hospitals. In contrast to urban hospitals, rural hospitals that offer obstetric services rely predominately on family physicians to provide maternity care.[17,26,29] In Washington State, even the small urban hospitals (defined as those with <500 deliveries per year) have more obstetricians and pediatricians on their staffs than they do family physicians. By contrast, even the largest rural hospitals (those with >500 deliveries per year) are predominantly staffed by family physicians.[17]

Outmigration of rural residents to urban areas for medical care, a well-known phenomenon to rural providers, is especially notable among pregnant women who are delivering their babies in more distant urban hospitals. Rural women utilizing local hospital services tend to be to be less affluent, less likely to have private insurance, but more apt to have identified a local personal provider.[31] The reasons cited for outmigration among rural women are multiple. Sometimes outmigration of pregnant women occurs because a community hospital has stopped offering delivery services, while other reports cite a decline in the number of physicians available to deliver babies. Other women have chosen to obtain maternity care in more distant hospitals because of the greater access to medical technologies and to gain access to family-centered birthing rooms.[2] Small rural hospitals tend to offer up to 30 percent fewer services than their urban counterparts.[31] In Washington State, most of the prenatal technological capabilities were available in more than 90 percent of all the hospitals in the state, no matter how small the hospital was or how few deliveries the hospital performed.[17] Additional reasons cited included referrals made to distant hospitals, perceptions that needed services were unavailable locally, and perceived deficiencies in local quality of care.[17] Nesbitt and associates reported that communities with a high outflow of women were smaller and closer to more sophisticated facilities and that they had fewer health care resources.[19]

REGIONALIZATION AND OUTREACH SERVICES

The majority of rural providers with small obstetric practices will not encounter complications. However, there will always be a number of presumed "low-risk" deliveries that have unanticipated complications. Overall, studies have reported that of all the 4 million U.S. women that give birth each year in both urban and rural areas, approximately 12 percent will have at least one major complication of pregnancy and 11 percent will have a major complication of labor; nearly 20 percent of the deliveries will occur by cesarean section; and about 4 to 6 percent of all the newborns will require intensive care.[2]

Rural hospitals that offer maternity services are much less likely than their urban counterparts to offer specialized services. Regional systems of perinatal care have been developed in some rural areas in order to assure access to specialized care when complications do arise in the rural hospital. High-risk patients can be selectively targeted and triaged utilizing outreach services that are set up within the rural community. These systems provide easier access for those rural women who require perinatal consultation and avoid the necessity of traveling great distances to obtain care. Most perinatal regional centers are located in metropolitan areas, and it is not unusual for these centers to be responsible for outreach systems in a number of the rural and urban counties that surround them.

NEONATAL OUTCOMES

The overall fetal (before birth) and neonatal (first 28 days of life) mortality has decreased steadily since 1980 for both rural and urban populations (Table 8-1). These decreases are thought to reflect better accessibility and quality of obstetric and neonatal care. Table 8-2 presents the fetal and neonatal mortality rates among urban and rural populations for the year 1992. Several things are important to note. Fetal deaths and neonatal mortality occurred at about the same rate for urban (6.1 and 4.3 percent, respectively) and rural whites (6.7 and 4.5 percent, respectively), but both fetal and neonatal mortality rates for blacks were higher than for whites for both urban (13.1 and 11.0 percent, respectively) and rural areas (14.1 and 10.0 percent, respectively).[1] However, the neonatal mortality rate for blacks was lower in rural than in urban areas.[2] For the black population, fetal death rates were significantly higher in rural areas, while neonatal mortality rates were higher in urban areas. For both the white and nonwhite populations, fetal death rates have remained higher in rural areas since 1980.[1]

TABLE 8-1 TRENDS IN FETAL AND NEONATAL MORTALITY RATES IN THE UNITED STATES, 1980 TO 1992

	1980	1992
Fetal death rate		
Metropolitan	9.0	7.3
Nonmetropolitan	9.9	7.6
Neonatal mortality rate		
Metropolitan	8.6	5.4
Nonmetropolitan	8.1	5.2

Source: Data from Clark et al.,[1] with permission.

TABLE 8-2   FETAL DEATHS AND NEONATAL MORTALITY
RATES IN THE UNITED STATES, 1992

	United States, Rate per 1000	Metropolitan, Rate per 1000	Nonmetropolitan, Rate per 1000
Fetal deaths			
Total	7.4	7.3	7.6
White	6.2	6.1	6.7
Nonwhite	11.6	11.4	12.4
Black	13.3	13.1	14.1
Neonatal mortality			
Total	5.4	5.4	5.2
White	4.3	4.3	4.5
Nonwhite	9.2	9.3	8.7
Black	10.8	11.0	10.0

SOURCE: Data from Clark et al.,[1] with permission.

ECONOMICS AND INSURANCE COVERAGE

Women of childbearing age (15 to 44 years) living in nonmetropolitan areas are more likely to be poor than their metropolitan counterparts.[26] In one significant way, access to maternity care in rural areas is not unlike that in urban areas—it is determined by the patient's income and insurance coverage.

Rural communities are disadvantaged in three ways with regard to insurance coverage: (1) rural residents have a greater likelihood of having no insurance coverage; (2) if insured, rural residents are more likely to have individual insurance coverage with high premiums (as opposed to employer-provided group coverage); and (3) those who have insurance coverage have policies that offer fewer covered services and generate more out-of-pocket costs (copayments and deductibles).[33]

Rural states traditionally have had the most restrictive Medicaid programs. Rural poor families frequently fail to qualify for Aid to Families with Dependent Children (AFDC) because of the program's exclusion of working two-parent families. Restrictive state Medicaid eligibility policies have resulted in many potentially eligible women remaining uncovered because their states have not exercised the option to cover them. In 1987, Medicaid reached only 25 percent of the rural poor. Rural states also have often failed to pursue additional Medicaid eligibility improvement options for pregnant women. In 1988, only 6 of the 15 most rural states had adopted the Medicaid option to extend eligibility to all pregnant women with family incomes below 185 percent of the federal poverty level. Many states require that Medicaid applications be filed in person and that face-to-face interviews occur. Often rural states have failed to take advantage of the program's design option, known as outstationing, that eases access to benefits. Outstationing is a relatively common practice at large urban hospitals, but it is a rarity in rural states. Because of the long distances involved and the lack of transportation, many rural women who are actually eligible for benefits are frequently not enrolled.[26]

Rural families typically have lower incomes than urban families[33] and are less able to afford private insurance coverage. However, rural residents were only slightly less likely to be insured than urban residents in 1989.[34] Rural farm families who buy medical insurance have less coverage than urban families, and a higher proportion of their income is required to pay for insurance premiums.[35] Those who are not self-employed are more likely than their urban counterparts to work in small firms. Smaller firms are less likely to offer health insurance benefits than larger firms, and rural residents are therefore less likely to obtain insurance from an employer. Among those who purchased insurance through an employer, rural residents had fewer covered benefits than urban residents. A greater proportion of rural residents bought their own private individual (nongroup) policies in spite of their low incomes. As a result, they were more likely to be underinsured.[33,34]

REIMBURSEMENT FOR SERVICES AND MALPRACTICE INSURANCE

The low reimbursement rates paid by many public and private insurers for maternity care and the high volume of uncompensated care may make obstetric practice unaffordable for the rural provider. A number of Medicaid expansion programs are starting to reverse that trend. Family physicians provide the majority of maternity care for women who are uninsured or on Medicaid in rural areas.[2]

Unfortunately, the cost of malpractice premiums paid by the rural provider still poses a problem. Family physicians delivering obstetric services often pay malpractice premiums that are two to three times higher than those of their urban counterparts who do not practice obstetrics. There is a huge variance in the cost of malpractice premiums by region in the United States. In some states, insurers are beginning to adjust premium rates for the number of deliveries performed by the physician. Where such adjustments are not made, malpractice continues to be a greater burden not only for some family physicians but also for certified nurse midwives (CNMs) because these providers generally have fewer obstetric patients over whom to spread the cost. In addition, physicians who provide backup for CNMs often have to pay additional malpractice premiums.[2]

NURSING SUPPORT

Providers who are new to the rural hospital milieu will encounter several surprises that they would not have anticipated. Rural America is also suffering from a shortage of nursing personnel, both registered nurses (RNs) and licensed practical nurses (LPNs). Recruitment and retention issues also plague this group of health professionals, much as they do physicians and midlevel providers. Hospital demands for nurses have increased faster than the supply. Factors shaping the increased demand include changes in the way medicine is practiced, increases in level of patient acuity, increased levels of nursing education, and increases in the financial pressures under which hospitals operate.[36] Coward and associates reported on the characteristics of nurses working in rural hospitals in comparison with those of nurses working in medium-sized and larger hospitals. These include: It was found that the former were older, reported lower annual personal incomes, were more likely to be LPNs, were least likely to be single, and had lived in their communities much longer.[37]

Rural providers must adapt to working with the level of nurses present in most rural hospitals. Because of the shortage of RNs in rural areas, it is not unusual to have a model in which one RN acts as supervisor for one or two LPNs, who provide most of the nursing care in the acute hospital setting. It is also not unusual to have two or three nurses aides also working as part of the team. The majority of these nurses will have a medical-surgical background and may lack any further obstetric or neonatal training than what they had during nursing school. In metropolitan hospitals, where most providers have received their medical school and residency training, physicians are accustomed to having a nursing staff that is specialized. For example, in the urban hospital it is not unusual to have a nurse solely trained for the intensive care unit (ICU), the emergency room (ER), or labor and delivery (L&D). Most nurses do not "cross the line"—e.g., an ER nurse never covers for an L&D nurse, and so on. In rural hospitals, it is the norm for the nurses to cover throughout the whole hospital at any given moment. For example, it is not unusual for the RN covering the medical-surgical floors to cover the ER or to provide nursing care for the labor rooms.

What does this mean for the rural provider? Physicians and midlevel providers must take on the role of educating the hospital staff in areas where additional training is needed. This could include fetal heart monitoring and strip interpretation, troubleshooting problems with the pressure monitor when a uterine pressure monitor is in place, tocolysis, administration of magnesium sulfate, amnioinfusions, and obstetric triage. It may also mean that the physician may have to monitor oxytocin infusion drips personally during inductions or augmentation.

Physicians play an instrumental role in developing policy and procedural protocols for the nurses in rural settings to follow. Implementation of these protocols via nursing in-service training is critical to their success. The rural provider should also support the existing nursing staff by finding ways to reinforce their job satisfaction. Care must be taken not to allow the provider's frustrations to disaffect the nursing staff. This may include encouraging the hospital administration to offer competitive compensation and benefits packages in order to recruit and retain quality nurses.

On a positive note, job satisfaction is a pivotal element in nurse retention. Nurses in small rural hospitals (up to 49 beds) reported the highest mean job satisfaction scores. In addition, nurses in rural hospitals reported the most positive attitudes about their professional status, the tasks that they were required to do, the organizational policies in their work settings, and their autonomy. However, these same nurses reported the most negative attitudes about their pay scales.[37]

Even with the best of efforts, the rural provider must be aware that good-quality nurses may be recruited by larger hospitals or practices, or they will decide to advance their skill levels and return to training.

ROLE OF MIDLEVEL PRACTITIONERS

Access to adequate prenatal and obstetric care has become difficult for rural residents, partly because rural providers and hospitals are decreasing their scope of services. Although many providers in the past cited malpractice and liability issues as the major reason for abandoning obstetric practice,[38–40] other factors have begun to surface that also contribute to this trend. Such factors include the large indigent population of women in rural areas, concerns about the adequacy of training in obstetrics, and lifestyle issues. The introduction of physician assistants (PAs), nurse practitioners (NPs), and certified nurse midwives (CNMs) has been described as a vital and unique solution to the problem of providing adequate access to quality health care in rural America.

Nonphysician providers are more likely to be employed in rural and medically underserved areas. Shi and associates reported that the majority of nonphysician providers are employed by community health centers throughout the United States. Among the 243 rural community health centers surveyed, 77 percent currently employ nonphysician providers. Most of these rural centers are located in the South and the Midwest regions of the United States.[42] Previous studies have confirmed the efficacy of these nonphysician providers. PAs and NPs often give care equivalent to that provided by physicians,[2] including low-risk prenatal care. CNMs are considered to be effective in providing access to prenatal care and delivery service in rural and poor communities[41] and manage low-risk pregnancies as well and as safely as physicians.[2] Although nonphysician providers may be only part of the solution to poor access to maternity care in rural areas, they do have recognized limitations. This cooperative, two-tiered system of care strategy and others are further discussed below.

The role of NPs, PAs, and CNMs in rural care is crucial and appropriate to the needs of rural communities. However, there are disturbing trends that may make these professionals more likely to prefer practice outside of the small rural communities where they are needed the most. The distribution of these practitioners has begun to resemble that of physicians and other clinicians, with heavy concentrations in urban areas and a growing shortage in rural and underserved areas. Market forces, rather than the health care needs of America's small and rural communities, have driven the distribution of these providers. The attraction of specialization that has occurred among physicians is repeating itself in these professionals. In addition, the demand for generalists is equally strong in urban and suburban areas (e.g., HMO practices, private practices).[41] A 1988 survey by the American Academy of Nurse Practitioners reported that nurse practitioners practicing in small communities were more commonly family nurse practitioners (FNPs) than other specialized nurse practitioners, with 33.8 percent of FNPs located in small communities (20.5 percent in communities with 1000 to 50,000 people).[2] The number of PAs in primary care practice has declined substantially, from 74 percent in 1978 to 65 percent in 1986. It appears that PAs often have a tendency to practice in specialty areas or with specialists performing specialized tasks. In 1985, the American Academy of Physician Assistants indicated that 30 percent of all PAs were practicing in rural areas or small towns with a population below 25,000. Conflicting evidence has been reported by the Institute of Medicine regarding the tendency for CNMs to practice more in urban areas than in rural areas.[43]

Because of the decreasing trend of family physicians practicing obstetrics and because of a lack of obstetricians choosing to locate to rural areas, new and innovative approaches are needed to provide personnel for the delivery of prenatal and obstetric care in the rural environs. A cooperative venture with midlevel practitioners could help fill some of this void and also help the family physician avoid the abandonment of obstetrics in his or her practice. Some of the strategies cited above have already met with success.[22,23]

The role of the NPs and PAs has been expanded to include performance of obstetric triage during the usual office hours. This task can be performed both at the hospital and at the office with the physician available for consultation if needed. The physician is therefore available to continue to see his or her patients in the office. NPs and PAs have also been granted privileges at hospitals to provide shared call coverage with the family physician. They participate by taking "first call" and triaging all obstetric patients. In addition, this model has the NP/PA participating in the provision of continuity of care with the physician in the office. Either prenatal visits can be alternated with the patient's physician throughout the pregnancy or the patient can be scheduled with the physician at specific times during pregnancy that are deemed as critical (i.e., at 26 weeks, 34 weeks, and all visits after 37 weeks). NPs have been noted to have received better training in communication, interviewing, and counseling skills than some physicians.[42] These are skills that are particularly important during the prenatal period. With this expertise, NPs can often function as prenatal educators for rural practices. However, this model has some limitations: dilution of continuity of care, the necessity for the development of protocols of obstetric care that NPs and PAs must adhere to, the additional requirement placed upon the physician supervisor to ensure that these protocols are followed, regular chart review, and the inability of the NP or PA to provide delivery service.

CNMs can lessen the burden for the busy rural physician who is providing obstetric care. This offers a unique advantage for the family physician over having just NPs and PAs, since the CNM can actually decrease the number of deliveries for which the physician has primary responsibility. Most successful models describe the CNMs as providing care for all low-risk pregnancies, including prenatal care, delivery, and postnatal care. The rural physician would be responsible for providing backup and accepting the responsibility for the high-risk pregnancies that do not require transfer. The family physician would be available to perform instrumented deliveries and/or cesarean sections if these were within his or her scope of practice. Hueston describes a three-tier model that was successful for his practice in rural northeastern Kentucky.[44] This successful model describes the CNMs and the family physicians providing care together for all low-risk pregnancies and referring all high-risk pregnancies and surgical backup to the specialists. One of the key factors in the success of this model was frequent meetings with obstetric consultants to discuss all high-risk patients and develop a care plan.

Another option for incorporating the use of midlevel practitioners into a rural obstetric practice is to create outreach prenatal clinics in outlying areas. NPs and PAs can provide continuity and prenatal care for the designated rural population and then transfer their patients at 36 weeks to the care of the CNM or physician (depending on risk factors) for care until delivery. The obvious advantage of NPs and PAs over CNMs is their ability to provide newborn care and well-baby visits for the same population.

Although the use of midlevel practitioners was intended to increase access to primary care services for rural residents, this function has been limited by legal and reimbursement issues. Legal constraints include the placement of restrictions on their services by various state professional practice acts, including supervision requirements, prescription authority, hospital privileging, etc. The rural provider must be cognizant of his or her state's rules and regulations regarding the supervision required for a midlevel provider. State requirements differ and the supervising physician must be aware of them. This information can be obtained from the state's government. Some states require written documentation of the type of medical conditions for which the midlevel provider is authorized to provide care. Some regulations require a specific percentage of the medical charts to be reviewed using quality improvement criteria. Others require that the supervising physician cosign all progress notes written by the midlevel practitioner within a designated time period. Finally, the supervising physician must identify what services performed by the NP or PA are reimbursable by third-party payers, including Medicare and Medicaid. This varies between insurance plans and regions.

EDUCATION AND TRAINING FOR RURAL OBSTETRICS

The Family Medicine Residency Review Committee (RRC) requires that family practice residency programs offer a minimum of 2 months of obstetric training over 3 years. However, the actual amount of obstetric training offered varies considerably from program to program across the nation. Residency programs providing more months of obstetric training tend to place more of their graduates in rural areas, especially those programs offering more than 4 months of obstetrics.[45] The level of training provided also varies considerably from program to program. Some programs offer training only in low-risk obstetrics while others offer training in high-risk and operative obstetrics. Programs that have a rural mission offer more training in obstetrics than those that do not[45] and are more likely to train their residents in operative obstetrics. Some residents from these programs are graduating with the skill level and competency to obtain privileges in performing cesarean sections.

Neither the RRC nor the American Board of Family Practice has delineated an absolute number of deliveries that residents should have performed in their training. Hospital obstetric privileges are generally granted to physicians who have performed at least 50 to 100 deliveries. However, this is also variable and is dependent on the region of the country where a physician decides to practice. It has been recommended that residents who are interested in including obstetrics in their rural practice should receive training in all of the obstetric skills shown in Table 8-3.[46]

Most rural family physicians practicing obstetrics felt they were adequately prepared to provide normal prenatal care, management of preeclampsia, and newborn resuscitation. However, 40 percent felt that better training in the management of multiple gestation and gestational diabetes would have been helpful during their residency.[47]

Many family physicians report that they feel comfortable performing cesarean sections. In Washington State, 59 percent of rural family physicians reported that they performed cesarean sections. Most (66 percent) learned how to perform cesarean sections during residency training. Most felt either very comfortable (59 percent) or extremely comfortable (35 percent) in performing the surgery, and reported that they performed on the average over 30 cesarean sections during residency training.[48] Another study of family physicians who perform cesarean sections found that the average number of cesarean sections completed in training was 46, with a range of about 25 to 100. The number of

cesarean sections performed per year among this group ranged from 5 to 22.[49] There is no recommendation from the AAFP regarding the number of cesarean sections that a resident in training or a family physician should perform in order to achieve competency. There have been no recommendations concerning volume of surgeries, scope of training, and experience that family physicians should acquire to competently perform cesarean sections.

Fellowship programs in obstetrics and rural family medicine are recent innovations providing family physicians with an opportunity to both enhance their obstetric skills and develop new technical skills. Presently there are 42 obstetric fellowship programs for family physicians and 16 rural family medicine fellowship programs in the United States. Each program has unique features, but most provide postresidency training in high-risk and operative obstetrics. The 5-year experience of one program has shown that all of its fellowship graduates have been able to obtain obstetric privileges and 75 percent of them have been granted cesarean section privileges.[50]

Residents, rural family physicians, and CNMs can also hone their skills through continuing medical education, including an annual perinatal course that is sponsored by the American Association of Family Physicians (AAFP). Advanced Life Support for Obstetrics (ALSO) was developed to enhance and sharpen the emergency obstetric skills of family physicians, including the management of shoulder dystocia, malpresentation, uterine bleeding, fetal distress, the interpretation of fetal heart monitor strips, use of vacuum extractors and outlet forceps, and so on. Information about the ALSO course can be found on the *AAFP Home Page* on the Internet at http://www.aafp.org.

TABLE 8-3   RECOMMENDATIONS FOR THE PREPARATION OF RESIDENTS IN TRAINING INTERESTED IN OBSTETRICS

Routine prenatal, intrapartum, and postpartum care
Early recognition of complications of pregnancy and labor
Procedures:
 OB ultrasound
 Outlet forceps
 Vacuum extraction
 Cesarean section
 Dilatation and curettage
 Postpartum tubal ligation
 Colposcopy
Management of dystocia
Management of breech presentations
Management of uterine bleeding

Source: Data from American Academy of Family Physicians,[46] with permission.

INFORMATIONAL RESOURCES ON MATERNITY CARE

There are several resources of obstetric information that may interest the reader. A number of

TABLE 8-4   INTERNET RESOURCES FOR MATERNITY CARE FOR THE RURAL PROVIDER

Internet Web Site	URL Address
Cochrane Library Database	http://www.updateusa.com/clib/CLIBNET
OBGYN.Net	http://www.obgyn.net
Journal of Reproductive Medicine	http://www.jreprodmed.com
American Journal of Obstetrics and Gynecology	http://www1.mosby.com/Mosby/Periodicals/Medical/AJOG
Web Path	http://www-medlib.med.utah.edu/WebPath
Medical Matrix	http://www.medmatrix.org
University of Iowa FP Handbook	http://indy.radiology.uiowa.edu/Providers/ClinRef/FPHandbook
Obstetric Ultrasound—A Comprehensive Guide	http://home.hkstar.com/~joewoo/joewoo

interesting and helpful Internet web sites have been developed to function as information resources for the busy rural provider who practices obstetrics (Table 8-4). The *Cochrane Library Database* is an updated obstetric resource providing evidence-based data on pertinent obstetric clinical topics. *OBGYN.Net* is an obstetric network that offers comprehensive reviews on clinical topics, editorial reviews of recently published articles, links to MEDLINE, and a large image library that houses some incredible graphics (most notable are the obstetric ultrasound scans and pathology photos). *Web Path* is sponsored by the University of Utah and has an excellent library of obstetric pathology photos. *Medical Matrix* and its obstetrics section provide a number of useful links to obstetric web sites on the Internet. The *University of Iowa FP Handbook* provides a comprehensive table of contents with complementary text on useful clinical obstetric topics.

Many journals are now online, and some provide their tables of contents and abstracts while others provide full text articles. Some of the journals online charge a user's fee, charge per journal article, or require that the user become a subscriber to the site.

For the rural provider who would like to enhance his or her obstetric ultrasound skills, a good resource is *Obstetrical Ultrasound,* created by Mark Deutchman, M.D., a hands-on interactive CD-ROM program that takes the user step by step through the principles and technique of obstetric ultrasound. One should also review *Obstetric Ultrasound—A Comprehensive Guide* on the Internet. This is an award-winning web site with both ultrasound images and links to informational resources.

CONCLUSION

All rural providers of obstetric care will encounter a number of challenges that impact the way they provide maternity care in the rural setting. It is important that the rural provider be aware of these issues in order to develop the necessary strategies to tackle them successfully.

A larger proportion of rural mothers are adolescents or in their twenties. Maternal morbidity among rural women is greater than it is for urban women. Poor access to maternity care plagues rural America because of transportation difficulties, greater distances needed to travel to obtain prenatal care, shortage of obstetric care providers, and lack of adequate medical insurance coverage.

Rural areas continue to face a shortage of obstetric care providers. Family physicians are most likely to be the providers of obstetric care in rural areas, but their numbers are in decline. The level of obstetric care (routine delivery, instrument-assisted delivery, high-risk obstetric care, C-section capability) that family physicians and other midlevel practitioners can provide differs from that offered by obstetricians because of past training, liability concerns, and hospital privileging.

Rural hospitals continue to face the threat of closure or the elimination of obstetric services. The decline in obstetric care providers, increasing liability costs, inadequate reimbursement for services, capital expenses for staff and specialized equipment, and outmigration of rural women to urban facilities have all contributed to this problem.

Strategies have been developed to handle patient volume, to improve better access to maternity care, and to improve perinatal morbidity/mortality, including the utilization of midlevel practitioners (nurse practitioners, physician assistants, and certified nurse midwives) to share prenatal care for low-risk pregnancies, the development of outreach maternity services, and the establishment of linkages with both local obstetricians and regional perinatal centers.

Overall, there is an ongoing need for more providers of maternity care in rural areas. Thus, it is important to encourage rural providers to include obstetrics in their practices. Providers who want to practice obstetrics in rural areas should be aware of the training opportunities available to them and the specific training they should acquire. In addition, there are many resources of obstetric information available on the Internet to help rural providers maintain their medical knowledge base and update themselves on the rapid changes in obstetric care.

REFERENCES

1. Clark SJ, Randolph RK, Savitz LA, et al: *A Quantitative Profile of Rural Maternal and Child Health.* Working paper no. 60. Chapel Hill, NC, North Carolina Rural Health Research Program. Cecil G Sheps Center for Health Services Research, 1997, pp 1–23.

2. Office of Technology Assessment: *Health Care in Rural America.* (OTA-H-434). Washington, DC, US Government Printing Office, 1990.

3. Federal Office of Rural Health Policy: *Facts about Rural Physicians.* Health Resources and Services Administration. Washington, DC, US Department of Health and Human Services, September 1997.

4. Caudle MR, Clapp M, Stockton D, et al: Advanced obstetrical training for family physicians: the future hope for rural obstetrical care. *J Fam Pract* 41(2):123–125, 1995.

5. American Academy of Family Physicians: *Facts about Family Practice 1995.* Kansas City, MO, AAFP, 1995.

6. Ricketts TC, Tropman SE, Slifkin RT, et al: Migration of obstetricians-gynecologists into and out of rural areas, 1985 to 1990. *Med Care* 34(5):428–438, 1996.

7. Federal Office of Rural Health Policy: *Rural Health Professions Facts.* Washington, DC, Health Resources and Services Administration, US Department of Health and Human Services, 1988.

8. Rosenblatt RA, Weitkamp G, Lloyd M, et al: Why do physicians stop practicing obstetrics? The impact of malpractice claims. *Obstet Gynecol* 76:245–250, 1990.

9. Institute of Medicine: *Medical Professional Liability and the Delivery of Obstetrical Care.* Washington, DC, National Academy of Sciences, 1989.

10. Nesbitt TS, Kahn NB, Tanji JL, et al: Factors influencing family physicians to continue providing obstetric care. *West J Med* 157:44–47, 1992.

11. Pathman D, Tropman S: Obstetrical practice among new rural family physicians. *J Fam Pract* 40:457–464, 1995.

12. Baldwin LM, Hart GL, Rosenblatt RA: Differences in the obstetric practices of obstetricians and family physicians in Washington State. *J Fam Pract* 32(3):295–299, 1991.

13. Hueston WJ: Specialty differences in primary cesarean section rates in a rural hospital. *Fam Pract Res J* 12(3):245–253, 1992.

14. Carroll JC, Reid AJ, Ruderman J, et al: The influence of the high-risk care environment on the practice of low-risk obstetrics. *Fam Med* 23:184–188, 1991.

15. Larson EH, Hart LG, Rosenblatt RA: Rural residence and poor birth outcome in Washington State. *J Rural Health* 8(3):162–170, 1992.

16. Hart LG, Dobie SA, Baldwin LM, et al: Rural and urban differences in physician resource use for low-risk obstetrics. *Health Services Res* 31(4):429–452, 1996.

17. Rosenblatt RA, Saunders GR, Tressler CJ, et al:

The diffusion of obstetric technology into rural U.S. hospitals. *Int J Technol Assess Health Care* 10(3):479–489, 1994.

18. Larimore WL, Davis A: Relation of infant mortality to the availability of maternity care in rural Florida. *J Am Board Fam Pract* 8(5):392–399, 1995.

19. Nesbitt TS, Connell FA, Hart LG, et al: Access to obstetrical care in rural areas: effect on birth outcomes. *Am J Public Health* 80:814–818, 1990.

20. Allen DI, Kamradt JM: Relationship of infant mortality to the availability of obstetrical care in Indiana. *J Fam Pract* 33:609–613, 1991.

21. Taylor J, Zweig S, Williamson H, et al: Loss of a rural hospital obstetric unit: a case study. *J Rural Health* 5(4):343–352, 1989.

22. Hueston WJ: Impact of a family physician-staffed maternity center on obstetric services in a rural region. *J Fam Pract* 32(1):76–80, 1990.

23. Bahry VJ, Fullerton JT, Lops VR: Provision of comprehensive perinatal services through rural outreach: a model program. *J Rural Health* 5(4):387–396, 1989.

24. Baldwin LM, Greer T, Hart LG, et al: The effect of a comprehensive Medicaid expansion on physicians' obstetric practices in Washington State. *J Am Board Fam Pract* 9(6):418–421, 1996.

25. Main DS, Tressler CJ, Calonge N, et al: A subsidized perinatal care program in a rural Colorado county. *J Rural Health* 5(4):397–411, 1989.

26. Hughes D, Rosenbaum S: An overview of maternal and infant health services in rural America. *J Rural Health* 5(4):299–319, 1989.

27. Lambrew JM, Ricketts TC: Patterns of obstetrical care in single-hospital, rural counties. *Med Care* 31:822–833, 1993.

28. Lawhorne L, Zweig S: Closure of rural hospital obstetric units in Missouri. *J Rural Health* 5(4):336–342, 1989.

29. Lawhorne L, Zweig S, Tinker H: Children and pregnant women. *J Rural Health* 6(4):365–377, 1990.

30. Hart LG, Pirani MJ, Rosenblatt RA: Causes and consequences of rural small hospital closures from the perspectives of mayors. *J Rural Health* 7(3):222–245, 1991.

31. Lishner DM, Amundson BA, Hart LG: The WAMI rural hospital project: Part 2. Changes in the availability and utilization of health services. *J Rural Health* 7(5):492–510, 1991.

32. Hicks LL: Availability and accessibility of rural health care. *J Rural Health* 6(4):484–505, 1990.

33. Hartley D, Quam L, Lurie N: Urban and rural differences in health insurance and access to care. *J Rural Health* 10(2):98–108, 1994.

34. Frenzen PD: Health insurance coverage in U.S. urban and rural areas. *J Rural Health* 9(3):204–214, 1993.

35. Krawlewski JE, Liu Y, Shapiro J: A descriptive analysis of health insurance coverage among farm families in Minnesota. *J Rural Health* 8(3):178–184, 1992.

36. Szigeti E, Laxdeal S, Eberhard BJ: Barriers to the retention of registered and licensed practical nurses in small rural hospitals. *J Rural Health* 7(3):266–277, 1991.

37. Coward RT, Horne C, Duncan RP, et al: Job satisfaction among hospital nurses: facility size and location comparisons. *J Rural Health* 8(4):255–267, 1992.

38. Nesbitt TS, Scherger JE, Tanji JL: The impact of obstetrical liability on access to perinatal care in the rural United States. *J Rural Health* 5(4):321–335, 1989.

39. Gordon RJ, McMullen G, Weiss BD, et al: The effect of malpractice liability on the delivery of rural obstetrical care. *J Rural Health* 3(1):7–13, 1987.

40. Chappell JL, Cianciolo MS, Harris DL, et al: A survey of obstetric malpractice in western frontier areas. *Fam Med* 22:226–227, 1990.

41. Institute of Medicine: *Preventing Low Birth Weight: Summary.* Washington, DC: National Academy Press, 1985.

42. Shi L, Samuels ME, Konrad TR, et al: The determinants of utilization of nonphysician providers in rural community and migrant health centers. *J Rural Health* 9(1):27–39, 1993.

43. Ricketts TC: Education of physician assistants, nurse midwives, and nurse practitioners for rural practice. *J Rural Health* 6(4):537–543, 1990.

44. Hueston WJ, Murry M: A three-tier model for the delivery of rural obstetrical care using a nurse midwife and family physician copractice. *J Rural Health* 8(4):283–290, 1992.

45. Bowman RC, Penrod JD: Family practice residency programs and the graduation of rural family physicians. *Fam Med* 30(4):288–292, 1998.

46. American Academy of Family Physicians: *Special Considerations in the Preparation of Family Practice*

Residents Interested in Rural Practice. Reprint no. 289-A. Kansas City, MO, AAFP, 1997.

47. Norris TE, Coombs JB, Carline J: An educational needs assessment of rural family physicians. *J Am Board Fam Pract* 9:86–93, 1996.

48. Norris TE, Reese JW, Pirani MJ, et al: Are rural family physicians comfortable performing cesarean sections? *J Fam Pract* 43:455–460, 1996.

49. Deutchman ME, Connor PD, Gobbo R, et al: Outcomes of cesarean sections performed by family physicians and of the training they received: a 15-year retrospective study. *J Am Board Fam Pract* 8:81–90, 1995.

50. Norris TE, Acosta DA: A fellowship in rural family medicine: program development and outcomes. *Fam Med* 29(6):414–420, 1997.

CHAPTER 9

Special Medical Problems in Perinatal Care

DAVID A. ACOSTA

R ural providers who practice obstetrics find themselves confronted with medical situations different from those of their urban colleagues. Many of these issues affect patient care, especially when the hospital facility and/or the providers cannot supply the appropriate care for the needs of their obstetric patients. This may necessitate the stabilization of the pregnant woman and subsequent transport to another facility for care. This chapter focuses on the accessibility of cesarean section, what anesthesia support is available in rural communities, and how these factors affect the obstetric provider's treatment strategies. In addition, rural providers are faced with the care of women who may pose sensitive issues calling for treatment strategies that will protect confidentiality, such as elective and therapeutic abortions, the care of HIV-infected women, and substance abuse. Finally, this chapter discusses several approaches to the care of the obstetric patient at risk for delivering a low-birth-weight infant or an infant requiring neonatal resuscitation.

CESAREAN-SECTION ACCESS

J.T., 28 years old (gravida 2, para 1), has been in active labor for 12 hours and had been progressing normally for the first 10 of these. She is now having contractions every 2 to 3 minutes and her cervical exam reveals that she is still dilated to 8 cm, 100 percent effaced, vertex position, 0 station. Her exam has not changed for 2 hours. A few minutes ago, the fetal heart monitor showed two consecutive late decelerations and a decrease in the baseline fetal heart rate (FHR), from 135 to 90 beats per minute, with a slow return to baseline and poor beat-to-beat variability. Now the FHR is showing a decrease in beat-to-beat variability between contractions. There is also meconium staining. The mother is placed in the Trendelenburg position and oxygen is given at 6 L/min by nonrebreather mask. A fetal scalp electrode is placed and confirms the late decelerations. Fetal scalp stimulation reveals good reactivity. The rural physician feels that a cesarean section may be indicated if the decelerations do not improve. However, the nursing staff informs him that there is a surgical trauma case in the operating room at this time and it will be another 30 minutes before the room will be available.

In the United States, the general expectation is that all hospitals providing obstetric services should be capable of performing cesarean section services and be able to provide these within a reasonable time (traditionally 30 minutes). A number of unpredictable complications requiring emergency interventions may develop despite risk assessment, and these may challenge the rural hospital. The small hospital that cannot provide this level of service is highly unlikely to be able to provide perinatal care.[1]

The major limiting factor in providing cesarean section services for the rural hospital is often the physician. The rural providers most likely to provide cesarean section services are obstetricians, general surgeons, or family physicians who have received specialized training in operative obstetrics during their residency. In Washington State, the responsibility of performing cesarean sections fell to family physicians in 94 percent of the rural hospitals without obstetricians on their medical staff. By contrast, in those rural hospitals with obstetricians, only about one-half of the family physicians practiced obstetrics and fewer than one-half of those performed cesarean sections. The smaller the hospital, the more likely that family physicians performed cesarean sections.[2]

In 1994, the American Academy of Family Physicians (AAFP) reported that only 14.4 percent of rural family physicians were performing cesarean sections. This varies between regions in the United States. The largest number of rural family physicians performing cesarean sections are located in the West North Central, East North Central, and Mountain regions.[3] Elsewhere, rural physicians practicing obstetrics must rely on other providers to perform cesarean sections as needed. As discussed in Chap. 8, only 9.6 percent of obstetricians practice in rural areas. The proportion of obstetricians available to perform cesarean sections is directly related to the number of hospital beds and delivery volume. Family physicians who practice in smaller hospitals are not likely to have obstetricians available. The local general surgeon is the provider most likely to perform cesarean sections in rural areas in the absence of obstetricians or family physicians who perform cesarean sections. Although the general surgeons have the technical skill to perform cesarean sections, they are not routinely trained to do so and frequently prefer not to because of scope of practice and liability concerns.[1] The general surgeon also has not been trained to assess when a patient needs a cesarean section. The major emphasis of decision making is therefore placed upon the rural family physician, even if he or she does not personally perform cesarean sections. Typically the rural family physician will serve as the first assistant at surgery and will provide the majority of postoperative care for the patient when the cesarean section is done by a general surgeon (who is covering more than the one local hospital).

The decision-making process on when to do a cesarean section varies significantly between the rural and urban setting. Factors such as staff availability, anesthesia availability, local specialty expertise, and availability of equipment may necessitate more conservative decision making with an earlier choice of operative delivery. For example, one might decide to operate earlier because the only nurse anesthetist available has another case pending at another remote hospital. Surgery might be delayed because the nurse anesthetist who is on call is covering another operation (at another remote hospital). One might decide to operate sooner if there is a significant chance that the surgical suite may be occupied by an impending emergency. The availability of surgical nursing personnel may alter surgery plans. In general, most small rural hospitals operate only one surgical suite at one time, and there is usually only one on-call team. The availability of the local general surgeon may also dictate whether one operates earlier or delays the case.

Because most small rural facilities lack personnel with neonatal expertise and/or lack a neonatal intensive care unit (NICU), the appearance of early signs of fetal distress may dictate earlier operation in order to avoid a poor neonatal outcome or a situation requiring much neonatal stabilization. The lack of other equipment utilized to assess fetal distress (e.g., scalp pH analysis) might push the provider to operate sooner when faced with a few late decelerations. All of these factors may play a role and legitimately affect how the rural provider practices obstetrics.

MATERNAL STABILIZATION AND TRANSPORT

C.G., 16 years old (gravida 1, para 0) has an intrauterine pregnancy at 28 weeks gestation. She presents to the emergency department complaining of abdominal pain, which has been intermittent for the preceding 4 hours. She denies any vaginal bleeding or rupture of membranes. The nurse informs the physician that C.G. is having regular contractions (as indicated by the external monitor every 2 to 3 minutes) lasting 60 to 90 seconds, and that the fetal heartbeat is 140 per minute with good beat-to-beat variability. No decelerations are noted. On exam, the patient's cervix is 80 percent effaced, anterior, 2 to 3 cm dilated, and her bag of waters is intact. Her vital signs are normal. You make the diagnosis of preterm labor. Appropriate laboratory studies are ordered, including cervical and urine cultures and toxicology screen. One liter of intravenous normal saline is started and she is given terbutaline 5 mg subcutaneously. The regional perinatal center is called, the case is discussed with the perinatologist on call, and transport is arranged. It is 85 miles to the nearest referral center, and December snow flurries are in the air. There is one mountain pass with a 5500-foot elevation to cross. Because of the terrain and the weather conditions, the preferred mode of transportation at this time is by ground ambulance.

There is no longer any question about the benefits of maternal transport over neonatal transport if maternal transport is available and appropriate for the mother's condition. Maternal transport has improved neonatal morbidity and mortality with regard to the delivery and survival of infants of very low birth weight (defined as less than 1500 g) and premature neonates.[4-7] This fact is largely due to (1) an increase in the delivery of low-birth-weight (LBW) and very-low-birth-weight (VLBW) neonates in tertiary referral centers, (2) an increase in the delivery of neonates with birth weights above 2500 g in tertiary referral centers, and (3) a 91 percent survival rate of these neonates if born at the tertiary care center versus a 67 percent survival rate if they were born at a less specialized facility, stabilized, and then transported to a tertiary care center.[6]

Reasons for Maternal Transport from Rural Areas

The medical reasons for maternal transport[8] from rural communities do not differ signifi-

TABLE 9-1   MEDICAL REASONS FOR MATERNAL TRANSPORT

Preterm labor	Fetal distress
PROM	Multiple gestation
Premature PROM	IUGR
Preeclampsia	VBAC
Third-trimester bleeding	Prematurity

Key: PROM, premature rupture of membranes; IUGR, intrauterine growth retardation; VBAC, vaginal birth after cesarean section.

SOURCES: Data from Low et al.[8] and Ackmann et al.,[9] with permission.

cantly from those found in the urban setting (Table 9-1). Prematurity and premature rupture of membranes head the list as the most frequently cited reasons for transport.[9] Sometimes, transfers may not be due solely to medical reasons. Most rural-urban differences in morbidity and mortality are due to rural facility limitations (Table 9-2). These factors must be appreciated by the receiving consultants. In the rural setting, these conditions can occur unexpectedly, necessitating the transfer of the patient to the nearest facility with the capabilities to care for the patient. Nursing shortages refer not only to the absolute number of nursing staff available but also to the availability of nurses who have had training in maternity or neonatal care.

Typical rural hospitals have only one or two surgical suites. In addition to room limitations,

TABLE 9-2   OTHER REASONS THAT MAY REQUIRE MATERNAL TRANSPORT

Lack of available surgical personnel
Lack of available anesthesia personnel
Lack of available surgical suite
Lack of physician(s) with NICU[a] or neonatal expertise
Lack of NICU or intermediate care nursery equipment
Lack of nursing staff trained in obstetrics or NICU
Lack of available blood products

[a]Neonatal intensive care unit.

many rural hospitals have only one surgical team. In this situation, surgical triage policies are appropriate to ensure that emergent conditions are prioritized. Cephalopelvic disproportion without fetal distress may not be deemed an emergency in these settings, in spite of the fact that the mother has been pushing for 3 hours. A patient in labor who refuses a vaginal birth after cesarean section (VBAC) and is requesting a repeat cesarean section would not be considered an emergent case. A patient who has just spontaneously ruptured her membranes and has an active herpetic lesion would not take precedence over an acute abdomen.

Arranging the Transport/Transfer

There are several important factors that will confront the rural provider considering maternal transport: the proper mode of transport and its availability, availability of appropriate equipment, availability of trained personnel to accompany the patient, the composition of the transport team, the referral center that will be accepting the patient, their willingness to accept the patient, and legal constraints.

The mode of transportation used is determined by multiple factors, any of which can create limitations: the distance to be traveled, the number of available transporting units, weather conditions, terrain, the type of medical insurance coverage the patient has, and whether that insurance will adequately reimburse the responsible transportation service.

It is important for the rural provider to understand the advantages and disadvantages of different modes of transportation (Table 9-3).[10] The rural provider must weigh the advantages and

TABLE 9-3   *ADVANTAGES AND DISADVANTAGES OF DIFFERENT MODES OF TRANSPORTATION FOR MATERNAL TRANSPORT*

Ground Ambulance	Helicopter	Fixed-Wing Plane
Advantages	*Advantages*	*Advantages*
Universally available	Rapid transport times	Rapid transport time over
Lots of room	Ability to reach inaccessible areas	long distances
Ability to divert transport		Ability to fly above inclement weather
		Cabin pressure
		Adequate cabin size
		High speed available
Disadvantages	*Disadvantages*	*Disadvantages*
Increased transit time when distances are long	Adequate unobstructed landing site is required	Need airport with adequate runway length
Mobility is limited by roads and weather conditions	Multiple transfers if landing site not near hospital	Multiple transfers if airport not near hospital
Not enough available units	Limited fuel capacity restricts range	High maintenance costs
	More prone to weather restrictions	
	Cabin space is limited	
	Noise and vibration interfere with monitoring	
	No cabin pressurization	
	High maintenance costs	
	Safety may be an issue	
	Relatively low speed	

SOURCE: Data from Academy of Pediatrics Committee on Hospital Care,[10] with permission.

disadvantages of transporting the patient by ground ambulance, fixed-wing aircraft, or helicopter. In some cases, the choice will be obvious, while in others it will be more difficult. The best choice will depend on the patient's condition, the expertise of the transport team, the availability of the services needed, and the receiving consultant's preferences.

The availability of proper equipment during transport is also key. The physician must understand that all needed equipment will not be consistently available. This situation requires some sensitivity and judgment on the part of the provider. For example, equipment limitations may include intravenous pumps for administering tocolytic agents and magnesium sulfate infusions or fetal heart monitors. In addition, telecommunications with the ambulance personnel may be limited due to radio frequency "dead spots," presenting difficulties for both the referring provider and the receiving hospital (particularly if there are significant changes in the patient's condition during transport).

Transports may also be limited by the availability of trained personnel. Many ambulance services in rural areas are staffed with "pre–hospital care providers" who are volunteers from the local communities who may or may not have any medical background. These volunteers usually have only basic levels of training and may often rely on a philosophy of "scoop and run." They are not necessarily trained in handling obstetric emergencies. The most common human resources include emergency medical technicians (EMT I or IIs) or paramedics. EMTs usually have basic life support (BLS) training and cannot insert intravenous lines or administer intravenous medications. They can administer oxygen, but they usually have no training in obstetric emergencies. Some rural hospitals may have paramedics on their local transport teams. Paramedics are usually BLS- and advanced cardiac life support (ACLS)-certified and have some training in obstetric emergencies. They can initiate and maintain intravenous infusions and administer some intravenous medications. Unfortunately, there is a profound shortage of paramedics in rural areas, due to

low salary, poor reimbursement for their services, and inadequate patient volume to maintain their skills. Rural emergency providers also have difficulty maintaining specialized skills to manage obstetric emergencies because of low volume. Thus, the rural provider must maintain contact with the transport personnel while en route or consider accompanying the transport team.

The two most common models of maternal transport are one-way and two-way transport systems (Fig. 9-1). In one-way transports, staff from the referring rural hospital accompany the patient during transport to the regional center. During two-way transports, the regional center staff travel to the referring rural hospital, where they assume responsibility for the patient and provide care during the transport back to their regional center. Since one-way transports decrease overall transport time to the regional center,[8] rural hospitals are more likely to utilize one-way transports. For the transport system to succeed, both parties (the consultant at the referral center and the referring rural provider) must understand that the rural transport team (one-way transport system) may not have expertise comparable to the referral center's transport team (two-way transport system) in maternal transport. The expectations of each party, especially of the consultant at the referral center, must be adjusted to the model used. With this understanding in place, appropriate communication with the rural transport team may be optimized. The rural provider must inform the receiving consultant of the limitations of the transport team at the time of the initial discussion. At this point the consultant may opt to send the regional center's transport team if it is the most appropriate.

It is critical for rural providers to establish a working relationship with a perinatal referral center. Sometimes reluctance to accept the rural patients may be encountered based on lack of insurance coverage or liability. The majority of pregnant women are uninsured or are covered by Medicaid, causing some reluctance among some consultants and referral centers to accept these patients. It has been reported that obstetri-

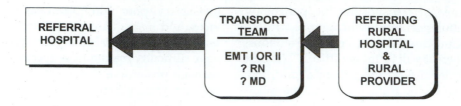

The Rural Model – One-way Transport System

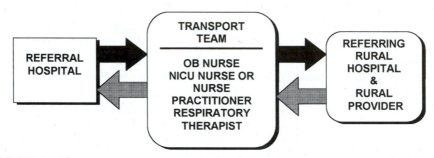

FIGURE 9-1 *The one-way transport system, in which the transport team comes from the referring rural hospital, is the model most likely to be utilized by the small rural hospital (rural model). In the two-way transport system, the transport team comes from the regional perinatal center (referral hospital), picks the patient up at the referring rural hospital, and then transports the patient back to the regional center once the patient is stabilized. The regional center's transport team provides ongoing care en route back to the referral center. Regionalized perinatal services are most likely to utilize the two-way transport system. (Data from Ackmann C, Russano G, Hobart J: Ten years of maternal-fetal transport.* Crit Care Clin *8(3):565–581, 1992, with permission.)*

cians in both urban and rural areas were far less likely than rural family physicians to accept Medicaid patients.[11,12] Some consultants and hospitals may also be reluctant to accept high-risk patients. Thus, the rural provider may be faced with sending patients to a referral center outside of the region and not meeting the patients' preference. The rural provider must also understand the legal constraints on the transfer of care.

Federal Laws Regulating the Transferring of Patients

The Consolidated Omnibus Budget Reconciliation Act (COBRA) was enacted in 1986. The in-

tent of COBRA was to prevent hospitals from "dumping" patients who were unable to pay for their care. It imposes regulations on all hospitals in the United States that receive Medicare funding (98 percent of hospitals in the United States). The Health Care Financing Administration (HCFA) is the agency charged with enforcing this law. COBRA has undergone two revisions (1989 and 1990) and the Emergency Medical Treatment and Labor Act (EMTALA) has been developed. EMTALA imposes two sets of duties: (1) it requires that all hospitals with an emergency department must provide an appropriate screening examination to any patient requesting treatment (the purpose is to determine whether an emergency medical condition exists), and (2) if an emergency medical condition is diagnosed, either the hospital must provide treatment sufficient to stabilize the patient or it must transfer the patient to another facility in an acceptable fashion. Once the patient's emergent medical condition is stable, the hospital has met its obligation under EMTALA. Specific provisions under EMTALA are included in Table 9-4. A critical component of EMTALA is that any evaluation received by a patient must be equal to that received by any patient presenting to the same facility regardless of gender, age, race, insurance coverage, or financial status.[13]

In essence, the transferring rural provider and hospital must ensure that the patient's transfer is medically appropriate, that the expected benefits of treatment at the other hospital outweigh the risk of transporting the patient, and that the receiving hospital can care for the patient adequately. If the one-way transport system is utilized, the sending physician and hospital are responsible until the patient arrives at the receiving hospital. In this situation, the rural provider must avoid patient abandonment. The concept of abandonment is defined as "the unilateral termination of a physician-patient relationship by the physician, without the patient's consent and without giving the patient sufficient opportunity to secure the services of another competent physician."[14] If the two-way transport system is utilized, the perinatal and/or neonatal transport team and the consulting perinatologist and/or neonatologist assume the responsibility once they have stabilized the patient and begin transport back to the receiving hospital.

Failure to comply with COBRA or EMTALA can result in (1) a fine, (2) suspension from providing services under Medicare, (3) a lawsuit by the patient for any injury suffered by a violation of COBRA, or (4) a lawsuit for the damages by the receiving hospital for patient dumping. For physicians, there is a $25,000 fine for each violation and prohibition from providing Medicare services. For hospitals, there is a $50,000 fine for each violation and possible suspension or termination from participation in the Medicare program for any violation.[15]

In HCFA region IX (Washington, Alaska, Idaho, Oregon), there were 43 investigations of possible COBRA/EMTALA violations during the period between 1986 and 1992. Of the confirmed violations, 67 percent occurred in rural hospitals while the rest occurred in urban facilities. The majority of the investigations (76 percent) were for failure to provide an appropriate screening evaluation. Only 5 percent of the investigations involved patients without medical coverage and only 5 percent involved patients on Medicaid. In all of the violations, patients felt that they had been treated with rudeness and lack of concern by the staff. Nursing personnel were involved in 77 percent of the confirmed violations and were chiefly responsible in 44 percent of the cases.[16]

The most common deficiency cited by HCFA is the lack of adequate documentation. Specific deficiencies mentioned include the inadequate

TABLE 9-4   PROVISIONS OF THE EMERGENCY MEDICAL TREATMENT AND LABOR ACT

1. The facility must be a participant in the Medicare program.
2. The individual patient involved must request to be evaluated.
3. The facility cannot delay evaluation and treatment to inquire about the patient's financial status.
4. The patient must receive an evaluation that is:
   Appropriate to the nature of the presenting complaint.
   Sufficient to determine the presence or absence of an emergency.
5. If an emergency is determined to exist, the patient must be treated and stabilized within the capability and capacity of the facility.
6. If the facility cannot provide stabilizing treatment, the patient must be transferred, accompanied by the appropriate personnel and equipment, to an accepting facility.
7. The risk and benefits of transfer must be explained and documented along with the patient's written consent for transfer.

SOURCE: Data from Diekema,[13] with permission.

documentation of incoming and discharge vital signs, pertinent physical findings, changes in the patient's status, and lack of physician countersignatures. Utilization of a standardized transfer form including the following information is recommended: reasons for transfer, signed request for transfer, description of the risks and benefits, countersignature by the consulting physician (within 24 hours), and the time and content of the contact with on-call physicians (see Fig. 9-2 for an example of such a form). Additionally, if the patient refuses treatment or transfer, the provider should document not only the refusal but also the patient's rationale and the recommendations of the provider.

Other Transport Issues for the Rural Provider

There are several other transport issues that the rural provider may encounter. For example, providers who have recently completed training or who have limited experience in rural areas may experience problems with the decision on appropriate timing for transfer. Inappropriate transfers may affect one's self-esteem and respect and decrease trust from the consultants. There may be fear of transporting patients too early ("overcalling a case") or not transporting soon enough ("undercalling a case"). The situation is further complicated by the fact that many obstetricians and perinatologists do not have a good grasp of the capabilities of rural family physicians.

Another common situation occurs when the rural provider feels "out of the loop" after the transfer. The consultant's approach to the patient's care may differ significantly from that of the rural provider because of different philosophies of training. The treatment plan may undergo a significant revision over that originally discussed with the consultant and the patient. This may affect the trust between the rural provider and the consultant and may also affect the patient-physician relationship for the rural provider.

A third problem area arises when communication between the rural provider and the consultant becomes problematic. The rural provider may not receive updates from the consultant on the patient's condition or outcome. Written correspondence may not be received in a timely manner. It is not uncommon for rural providers to see the patient back for follow-up before receiving copies of the consultant's discharge summary or discharge medication list. Failure to arrange follow-up appointments with the primary care provider is yet another problem that the rural provider may experience. Either the consultant does not refer the patient back to the primary care provider or the patient prefers to follow up with the consultant instead. Rural providers have at times felt that there was no encouragement from the consultant for the patient to follow up with the primary care physician.

To avoid these pitfalls, it is imperative that the rural provider develop a meaningful relationship with the consultant(s) at the referral center and establish functional communication linkages. It is critical for the rural provider to establish clear understandings with the consultant regarding continued involvement, patient follow-up, and what written documentation will be provided. It is also important for the rural provider to improve the consultant's awareness of the rural physician's training and skills. Similarly, the rural provider must be sensitive to the expectations and needs of the consultant. Collaboration can improve the quality of care delivered to the patient. Other strategies include inviting the consultant and the transport team to provide training for the rural hospital staff on the preparation of patients for maternal transport. The rural provider and the rural hospital administrator might also visit the regional perinatal center and arrange for the purchase or the loan of any necessary equipment that either the hospital or the EMS may need to assist in the stabilization and transport of perinatal patients. The rural provider can play a large role in encouraging the development of collaborative efforts between the rural hospital and the regional perinatal center that are required to

PHYSICIAN'S CERTIFICATE OF TRANSFER

I hereby certify that, based on the information available to me at the time of the transfer, the medical benefits reasonably expected from the provision of appropriate medical care at another medical facility outweigh the increased risk to the individual, and in the case of labor to the unborn child, from effecting the transfer.

This certification is based on the following:
Benefits: _____
_____
_____

Risks: _____
_____
_____

All transfers have the inherent risks of traffic delays, accidents during transport, inclement weather, rough terrain or turbulence, and the limitations of equipment and personnel present in the vehicle.

Physician's name: _____ Date: _____ Time: _____
Physician's signature: _____

IF NO PHYSICIAN IS PRESENT:
Nurse's name: _____ Date: _____ Time: _____
Nurse's signature: _____
On verbal orders of Dr. _____ received on (date) _____ Time: _____
PHYSICIAN MUST COUNTERSIGN WITHIN 24 HOURS
*   *   *

CONSENT TO TRANSFER

I hereby consent to transfer to another facility. I understand that it is the opinion of the physician responsible for my care that the benefits of transfer outweigh the risks of transfer. I have been informed of the risks and benefits upon which this transfer is being made. I have considered these risks and benefits and consent to transfer.

Signature of patient or responsible party: _____
Date: _____   Time: _____

Witness: _____   IMPRINT OF PATIENT
Witness's signature: _____   INFORMATION
Date: _____   Time: _____

Modified from reference 15.

FIGURE 9-2 Standardized transfer form. (Modified from Frew SA, Roush WR, LaGreca K:
COBRA: implications for emergency medicine. Ann Emerg Med 17(8):835–837, 1988,
with permission.)

establish a proper maternal transport system that will meet the needs of both parties and will be cost-effective.

Other Transport Issues for the Rural Patient

Rural patients may be reluctant to be transferred to a regional perinatal center. There may be a number of reasons for this reluctance. First, rumors from other rural residents regarding their past experiences of poor birth outcomes at the referral center may abound in the rural community. Second, the patient's reluctance may stem from a lack of a clear understanding on the need for transfer. Third, the patient may have an unexpressed need to stay close to family and children because of inadequate respite care. Fourth, there may be no means of transportation for other family members to visit if the patient were to be hospitalized. The rural provider may have to sift through these myths and concerns to answer the patient's questions, doubts, or fears. Support given in this manner enhances the patient's quality of care and may also create an opportunity to inform the patient of what to expect with regard to further diagnostic testing and treatment. The rural provider must be sensitive to all of these reasons and must be prepared to develop strategies to manage them.

ABORTIONS

K.L., 19 years old (gravida 2, para 0, abortus 1), has noticed that she is 3 weeks late for her menses. She is sexually active and has been using the withdrawal method of contraception. She had a positive home pregnancy test last night that her boyfriend does not know about yet. Her parents are also unaware of her pregnancy. You have been providing care for K.L. and her family for the past 5 years and you had prescribed birth control pills to K.L. about a year ago (and assumed that she was still using them). She often forgets to take them. She wants to have an elective abortion, and she wants you to perform the surgery as soon as

possible. She does not want her parents to know about this situation.

Abortions are virtually unavailable to rural women in the United States.[17] Ninety-four percent of nonmetropolitan counties in the United States have no legal provider willing to provide abortion services. In general, rural women wanting this service must travel significant distances. Rosenblatt and colleagues[18] reported that only 3.6 percent of rural providers (including family physicians, obstetricians, and general surgeons) in Idaho perform abortions. Only 4 of 44 rural communities had local abortion services for women. Providers' reasons for not performing abortions are presented in Fig. 9-3.

Physicians reported that they do not provide abortions because of their own moral objections to the procedure and because of local community opposition. However, 65 percent of these physicians referred their patients requesting abortions to another provider outside of their area despite their personal objections to abortions. Medical malpractice concerns and lack of training were not significant factors in preventing physicians from performing abortions. The "morning-after pill" was prescribed by 46 percent of family physicians and 89 percent of obstetricians. Interestingly, 26 percent of providers morally opposed to abortions indicated interest in using RU-486 when it became available (25 percent family physicians, 33 percent obstetricians).[18]

Findings in this study of rural Idaho physicians are likely representative of other rural areas of the United States. Abortions present an ethical dilemma for all rural providers, and the decision on how to approach this service must be carefully balanced with personal values and beliefs, the standard of care in the community, the treatment options available to the patient, and the associated benefits, risks, and potential outcome of each option. The rural provider must be aware of and sensitive to the traditional beliefs and values of the community. Decisions that rural providers make will certainly affect

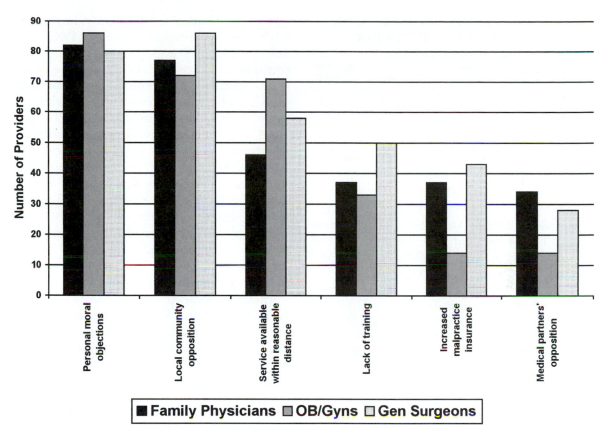

FIGURE 9-3 Reasons why physicians did not perform abortions, 1994. (Modified from Rosenblatt RA, Mattis R, Hart LG: Access to Legal Abortions in Rural America: A Study of Rural Physicians in Idaho. *Working paper no. 30. Seattle, WA, WAMI Rural Health Research Center, 1994, with permission.)*

their future practice and may reflect on their staffs, many of whom live in the local community.

HIV AND PREGNANCY

Since you are covering "no-doc" (patients without a local physician) admissions to the hospital, the nursing staff calls you to attend an imminent delivery. The patient, 28 years old (gravida 5, para 3), was just passing through town. At 38 weeks gestation, she has arrived at the hospital in active labor having had spontaneous rupture of membranes an hour earlier. She is having contractions every 2 minutes, and is 6 to 7 cm dilated, 90 percent effaced, vertex presentation. She has had late prenatal care but informs you that she knows that she recently tested positive for HIV. She denies any history of intravenous drug use but admits that her boyfriend uses intravenous drugs. She denies any history of opportunistic diseases, and does not know whether she has ever had her CD4 count checked. She is on no medications.

Between 1990 and 1995, the overall incidence of AIDS increased in the United States, but rates were lower in rural than in urban areas. However, the gap between urban and rural narrowed substantially over the period studied. The same

TABLE 9-5   TRENDS IN AIDS CASES, 1990 VERSUS 1995 (RATES PER 100,000 POPULATION)

AIDS Cases	1990	1995
Metropolitan	21.91	27.25
Females ages 13–34 years	7.80	13.81
Nonmetropolitan	4.65	7.29
Females ages 13–34 years	1.65	4.52

SOURCE: Data from Clark et al.,[19] with permission.

pattern is evident for AIDS cases among women aged 13 to 34 years. In 1993, the prevalence of HIV infection in women giving birth in the United States was 1.6 per 1000.[20]

The rising incidence of AIDS among women of childbearing age is an area of great concern. Since 1990, over 90 percent of new cases of pediatric AIDS in the United States were caused by transmission from mother to infant (Table 9-5).[19] The probability of transmission from an untreated mother to fetus or infant is about 25 percent. Perinatal transmission of HIV can occur during pregnancy (as early as 8 weeks gestation) or through breast-feeding. The majority of transmissions ($\geq$50 percent) occur during labor and delivery.[20]

Although HIV is still considered by some rural providers as a rare occurrence in the rural population, provider awareness of maternal HIV status is critical for those providing maternity and neonatal care. According to 1995 data,[19] utilization of HIV testing differs among rural and urban women in their childbearing years (Table 9-6). Overall, considerably fewer rural women had ever been tested for HIV. More urban women had been tested for HIV in the previous 12 months than rural women. Additionally, rural women were less likely to seek HIV testing to find out whether they were infected. In comparison to urban women, rural women were more likely to be tested by their providers for HIV during their prenatal care or hospitalization. Rural providers should counsel their patients and recommend testing for all women who are pregnant or who are seeking pre-pregnancy counseling.

Factors associated with an increased risk of perinatal transmission for mothers who are HIV-positive include low CD4 counts ($<$200/ mm^3), high viral loads, events that increase exposure of the fetus to maternal blood (amniocentesis, fetomaternal hemorrhage, placental abruption, use of fetal scalp electrode, instrumented deliveries, episiotomy), prolonged rupture of membranes (ROM) (recent data show an increased risk of infection with ROM greater than 4 hours), and premature delivery.[20]

A large multicenter trial[21] demonstrated that zidovudine (ZDV) can significantly reduce the perinatal transmission in pregnant women with

TABLE 9-6   HIV TESTING AMONG WOMEN AGE 22–44 YEARS, 1995

	Metropolitan	Nonmetropolitan
Total population	18,550	12,347
History of HIV testing (%)		
Never tested	48.7	56.8
Tested in the previous 12 months	21.3	14.6
Reason for testing (%)		
Hospitalization	6.0	7.9
Prenatal care lab (routine)	22.2	25.5
Finding out if infected	44.6	36.5

SOURCE: Data from Clark et al.,[19] with permission.

CD4 counts above 200/mm³. The transmission rate was 8.3 percent among 180 children whose mothers began taking ZDV between 14 and 34 weeks gestation compared to 25.5 percent among 183 children whose mothers took placebo.

Management Strategies for the Pregnant Patient Testing Positive for HIV

ANTEPARTUM

1. Obtain CBC, CD4 count, quantitative HIV-1 RNA (viral load), SGPT, and creatinine initially. Follow CD4 count and viral load every trimester. If not done as part of their routine prenatal care, then obtain toxoplasmosis IgG, cytomegalovirus (CMV) antibody screen, hepatitis BsAg, hepatitis C antibody, herpes simplex virus Western blot (HSV antibodies). Screen for tuberculosis with a PPD test.
2. Obtain infectious disease and perinatology consultations.
3. Begin ZDV 100 mg five times daily (initiate after 14 weeks gestation) and continue throughout the pregnancy. Alternative dosing regimens include ZDV 200 mg tid or 300 mg bid, which may improve compliance.
4. If the CD4 count is below 200/mm³, begin trimethoprim-sulfamethoxazole double strength (DS) one tablet daily for *Pneumocystis carinii* prophylaxis. If the CD4 count is <100/mm³, refer to ophthalmologist for a baseline funduscopic exam to rule out CMV retinitis.

LABOR AND DELIVERY

1. Avoid artificial rupture of membranes (AROM), fetal scalp electrode placement, intrauterine pressure catheter (IUPC) placement, fetal scalp sampling, forceps and vacuum extractor, or cutting an episiotomy if possible.
2. Administer loading dose of ZDV 2 mg/kg IV and run in over 1 hour, followed by a continuous infusion of ZDV 1 mg/kg/h until delivery.

POSTPARTUM

1. Avoid breast-feeding. This has been associated with an increased rate of transmission by 10 to 20 percent.
2. Consult infectious disease specialist regarding triple drug therapy for the mother.[20]

Guidelines for perinatal care and HIV patients are rapidly evolving. There are a number of excellent resources that the rural provider can utilize for updated recommendations. The CDC HIV/AIDS Hotline can provide information on any HIV issues 24 hours a day, as well as patient education materials. It can be reached at 1-800-662-4357 or at http://www.cdc.gov/epo/mmwr. The AIDS Clinical Trial Information Services is a national information hotline and can be reached at 1-800-874-2572 or at http://www.actis.org.

NEONATAL RESUSCITATION

You are called in "stat" by your partner to evaluate and help resuscitate an infant born to a 22-year-old woman (gravida 2, para 1) at 41 weeks gestation who just delivered vaginally after an extended pitocin induction for prolonged rupture of membranes. Membranes have been ruptured for 18 hours and the amniotic fluid is without meconium. The patient is negative for group B strep (GBS). She had an antenatal temperature of 100.5°F about 2 hours prior to delivery. Intravenous ampicillin and gentamicin were started. The infant was noted to be "floppy" upon delivery, without any respiratory efforts. The mother had not received any narcotics or sedatives during labor. When you arrive, two nurses are resuscitating the infant on the infant warmer. One nurse is performing positive-pressure ventilation with 100% inspired oxygen by a bag-mask device with a nonrebreather. The infant appears mottled, pale, and hypotonic; he is making no respiratory effort on his own. You also notice that the chest is not rising with each breath. The heart rate is 80 beats per minute. You begin to operate the bag-mask device, get an adequate seal around the nose and mouth, and see that you have a good chest rise with each breath. The infant's color turns pink within minutes, the heart rate rises to 120 beats per minute, and you pause in your bagging efforts to see whether the infant will breathe on its own. There is no cry and no respiratory effort despite added tactile stimulation. You begin bagging the infant again and prepare for intubation. Meanwhile, you have one of the nurses call the neonatal intensive care unit (NICU) response team from your perinatal regional center and arrange for transfer.

Rural physicians who provide obstetric care should possess the skills needed for neonatal resuscitation. Courses such as the Neonatal Resuscitation Program* (formerly known as Neonatal Advanced Life Support, or NALS course) can help the provider attain and maintain that skill. Most rural hospitals do not have pediatricians or neonatologists on staff to aid in newborn resuscitation. Thus, rural hospitals depend on their nursing staff to have some training and skill, in addition to the providers. The rural provider should be well versed in stabilizing the infant in these critical cases until the neonatal transport team arrives. Needed skills may include the utilization of bag-mask devices, performing endotracheal intubations, as well as undertaking umbilical artery catheterization should this be necessary to administer fluids for an infant in shock.

Certain conditions will cause the rural provider who is doing the delivery to call for backup. Fetal and maternal conditions that warrant two providers are listed in Table 9-7. One provider should attend to the newborn, who may require intensive and extended care. The other provider should attend to the mother who just delivered. In some circumstances, one provider cannot provide adequate care for two sick patients simultaneously.

Again, it is critical to develop a working relationship with a regional neonatal center. Most centers have a NICU resuscitation team that will

TABLE 9-7 CONDITIONS THAT MAY WARRANT ADDITIONAL PROVIDER BACKUP FOR NEONATAL RESUSCITATION

Fetal Conditions	Maternal Conditions
Meconium staining of amniotic fluid	Postpartum hemorrhage
Prematurity	Large, bleeding laceration
Fetal distress	Cervical tears
Anticipated shoulder dystocias	Retained placenta
Instrumented deliveries	Instrumented deliveries
Apgar score below 7	Hypotension
Floppy infants	Inverted uterus
Twin gestation	

come to your hospital. It is important to anticipate problems early, before allowing them to progress. Transferring the fetus in utero has improved morbidity and mortality outcome, especially with LBW and VLBW infants born to rural mothers.[6]

SUBSTANCE ABUSE

I.M., 32 years old (gravida 3, para 2) presents with an intrauterine pregnancy of 36 weeks gestation at the rural emergency department. She has abdominal pain and has had bright red vaginal bleeding for 30 minutes. Her prenatal course was uncomplicated. She had no history of prior placental abruption, hypertension, preeclampsia, or drug abuse. On the fetal heart monitor, uterine irritability is noted; the fetal heart rate is 150 beats per minute with good beat-to-beat variability. On exam, she is writhing in pain and has a very tense uterus that is exquisitely tender on palpation, with obvious bright red blood per vagina. Her vital signs are blood pressure, 120/75; pulse, 90; temperature, 98.5°F; respiratory rate, 22. She does not have orthostatic hypotension. You diagnose a placental abruption. The surgical team has been called, and you order a stat CBC, and type and cross-match for two units of blood. Her hematocrit is 32, and, to your surprise, her preliminary drug screen is positive for cocaine.

* The Neonatal Resuscitation Program is cosponsored by the American Academy of Pediatrics and the American Heart Association. For further information on the course, call AAP Life Support Program at 1-800-433-9016 or email at lifesupport@aap.org.

Studies done in the United States have demonstrated that substance abuse during pregnancy is prevalent and continues to be a problem for both urban and rural areas. The National Pregnancy and Health Survey (NPHS),[22] conducted by the National Institute on Drug Abuse (NIDA) in 1992, estimated that 221,000 women who gave birth in 1992 used illicit drugs while they were pregnant. Marijuana and cocaine were the most frequently used illicit drugs. The survey also found a high incidence of cigarette and alcohol use among pregnant women. At some point in their pregnancy, 20.4 percent smoked cigarettes and 18.8 percent drank alcohol. The survey demonstrated a strong link between cigarette smoking, alcohol use, and the use of illicit drugs. Among those women who used both cigarettes and alcohol, 20.4 percent also used marijuana and 9.5 percent used cocaine.

Obstetric providers often screen only those patients who demonstrate high-risk behavior. Thus, they may actually miss a larger proportion of pregnant women who have used drugs during pregnancy. Studies have demonstrated that drug and substance abuse are present in every socioeconomic, ethnic, and racial group. All pregnant women in Pinellas County, Florida, who presented to prenatal care to a public or private sector health provider had urine samples screened for evidence of recent alcohol or drugs regardless of background, ethnicity, or financial coverage. Approximately 15 percent had positive toxicologic drug screens. There was no difference in the prevalence of recent substance abuse between those with private insurance and those who were medically indigent.[23]

Studies have documented the many adverse effects of cigarettes, alcohol, and illicit drugs. Cocaine use and cigarette smoking are associated with similar high rates of potential complications for the fetus and newborn. These include spontaneous abortion, preterm labor, intrauterine growth retardation, placental abruption, and intrauterine fetal death.[24]

Since 1990, there have only been two published studies in the literature regarding substance abuse in rural pregnant women. Yawn and associates[24] reported that substance abuse among rural women was uncommon in comparison with that found among urban women. They tested all pregnant women who were admitted to four rural Minnesota hospitals in preterm or term labor. Urine samples from the mothers and meconium samples from the newborns were collected irrespective of their demographics. A total of 956 paired samples were tested for the presence of cocaine, amphetamines, opiates, and marijuana. Overall, 3.2 percent of all urine screens were positive, predominantly for marijuana. Meconium samples were positive in 1.8 percent, predominantly for marijuana. By history, 24.5 percent of the women admitted to smoking during pregnancy. O'Connor et al.[25] found similar results in a rural population from central Missouri: 2.4 percent of meconium samples tested positive for illicit drug use (predominantly marijuana) during pregnancy. This is similar to reports from the 1995 National Household Survey on Drug Abuse (NHSDA) conducted by the Substance Abuse and Mental Health Services Administration (agency of the U.S. Department of Health and Human Services) and NPHS (Table 9-8). The NHSDA also revealed that rates of substance abuse were higher among women ages 15 to 24 than among those 26 to 44, higher among unmarried women, and highest among women in the first trimester of pregnancy.

Rural providers should routinely ask women about their use of cigarettes, alcohol, and illicit drugs during their prenatal checkups. Patients need to be educated about the health risks of these substances and their effects on the fetus. Universal screening and random urine screening should be considered a routine part of the prenatal risk assessment. The approach to the patient who has a positive screen should be one that is supportive and not punitive. The role of the provider is to quickly access appropriate medical intervention for their patients and get them into a drug treatment program if available. Unfortunately, substance abuse treatment programs are not as readily available in rural areas as they are in urban areas. There are several

TABLE 9-8   SUBSTANCE ABUSE AMONG PREGNANT WOMEN
AND REPORTED USE

Substance	Percentage of Urban Pregnant Patients Reporting Use in the Past Month, Ages 15–44	Percentage of Rural Pregnant Patients Reporting Use in the Past Month, Ages 15–44
Any illicit drug	3.2	3.7
Alcohol		
Any alcohol use	16.1	15.3
"Binge" alcohol		
use	1.6	2.0
Cigarettes	20.3	28.3

SOURCE: Data from National Institute on Drug Abuse,[22] with permission.

resources that the rural provider can explore to locate the nearest treatment program in his or her community: the National Directory of Drug Abuse and Alcoholism Treatment and Prevention Programs (a service of the Substance Abuse and Mental Health Services Administration) is a large database that the provider can search online through the Internet (http://www.health.org/treatmnt/index.html) and access listings of all federal, state, local, and private providers of alcoholism and drug abuse treatment and prevention programs in the United States; the Center for Substance Abuse Treatment National Drug and Alcohol Treatment Referral Service (1-800-662-HELP) can link the caller to a variety of hotlines that provide treatment referrals 24 hours; and the Alcohol Treatment Referral Hotline (1-800-ALCOHOL) provides 24-hour help and referrals for people with concerns about alcohol or drug use.

LOW-BIRTH-WEIGHT INFANTS

The poorest of obstetric outcomes in rural areas are the result of the birth of LBW infants. These infants are at the greatest risk for morbidity and mortality, and the majority of neonatal deaths occur in them. It is therefore imperative that the rural provider of obstetric care have a high index of suspicion and screen for any maternal risk factors associated with LBW. The provider should ensure that a woman with an anticipated LBW fetus is transferred and delivered in a technologically sophisticated facility and not treated in a small rural hospital.

An LBW infant is one weighing less than 2500 g; a VLBW infant is one weighing less than 1500 g regardless of gestational age. The overall incidence of LBW infants is similar between urban and rural areas (6.89 versus 6.49 percent, respectively) for all races. Of note, the incidence of LBW for black infants is more than twice that for white infants in both rural and urban areas (12.6 percent for urban black infants versus 5.6 percent for urban white infants; 11.7 percent for rural black infants versus 5.7 percent for white rural infants). Interestingly, the incidence of LBW for black infants is lower in rural areas than it is in urban.[17]

LBW in infants may result from several causes, including prematurity from preterm labor, premature rupture of membranes (PROM), intrauterine growth retardation (IUGR), or twin gestation. Preterm labor, PROM, and IUGR are discussed in further detail below. Practical management strategies for each of these entities in rural settings are also discussed; these may serve as an aid for the rural provider who will be providing care for these patients.

PRETERM LABOR

T.P., 20 years old (gravida 3, para 2), has an intrauterine pregnancy at 32 weeks gestation based on a 12-week ultrasound. She presents to the labor and delivery suite complaining of regular contractions that have continued for 3 hours. She denies any spontaneous rupture of membranes (SROM). She has a history of one preterm labor with her first pregnancy and delivered at 34 weeks. Her prenatal course has been relatively uneventful with the exception of one episode of bacterial vaginosis that was treated at 26 weeks and a urinary tract infection that was treated at 29 weeks. On the fetal heart monitor she is found to be having regular contractions every 4 to 5 minutes, lasting 60 seconds each, and the fetal heart rate is 135 beats per minute with good beat-to-beat variability. On exam, she has no evidence of SROM, and there is no vaginal discharge. Her cervix is 70 to 80 percent effaced, 2 cm dilated; there is a vertex presentation, which is ballotable. You admit the patient to the hospital, place her at strict bed rest, order the appropriate laboratory work, start an intravenous line with 1 L of normal saline, and administer fluids over the next hour. In 1 hour, her contractions have increased and are now occurring every 2 to 3 minutes, each lasting for 60 seconds. You give her terbutaline 5 mg subcutaneously.

Preterm labor (PTL) has been defined by the American College of Obstetrics and Gynecology as labor that has spontaneously begun prior to term gestation (<37 weeks). Preterm births occur at similar rates for both rural and urban women. Overall, the rate of PTL is 6.33 percent in urban and 6.21 percent in rural areas. However, the rate of PTL appears to be significantly different among black women. For whites, the rate of preterm births is 5.08 percent in urban and 5.20 percent in rural areas, but for blacks, preterm births occur at a rate of 11.88 percent in urban and 12.79 percent in rural areas.[17]

The key to the management of preterm labor in a rural setting is twofold: (1) stopping the labor completely at the local rural hospital or (2) stopping labor temporarily until a transfer to the nearest facility that has a perinatal center and NICU can be arranged for the patient.

In most cases of PTL, the cause is unknown. Demographic risk factors have included low socioeconomic status, nonwhite race, and maternal age below 18 years or above 40 years.[26] Some of the known predisposing factors of PTL are listed in Table 9-9 (the prevalence for some risk factors is listed where it has been reported). It is imperative that the rural physician discover any possible treatable causes. Risk scoring systems for PTL have not proven to be sensitive or predictive.[26] Management must be based on the most likely cause, realizing that the majority of the time the definitive cause will not be identified.

Treatment has not changed much in the past 10 years. Tocolysis with beta-adrenergic receptor agonists is the first tier of treatment. Two

TABLE 9-9   PREDISPOSING FACTORS OF PRETERM LABOR (PTL) (RISK OF PRETERM BIRTH IN PERCENT IF KNOWN)

History of 1 previous PTL (17–37%)	Premature rupture of membranes
History of ≥2 previous PTL (32–70%)	Multiple gestation (10%)
Spontaneous second-trimester abortions (≥1)	Polyhydramnios
	Placental abruption
No prenatal care	Cervical incompetence (15–28%)
Smoking	
Drug use (23%)	Abdominal trauma
Cocaine	
Methamphetamines	Bacterial vaginosis
	Gardnerella
	Trichomonas
Uterine anomalies	Cervicitis
Bicornuate uterus	*Chlamydia*
Uterine myomata	Gonorrhea
Submucosal	Colonization with group B strep (12.8%)
Subplacental	Urinary tract infection

SOURCE: Data from American College of Obstetricians and Gynecologists, Committee on Educational Bulletins,[26] with permission.

comprehensive reviews have been published[27,28] on the efficacy and safety of tocolytic agents that are currently used to treat PTL. Beta-adrenergic receptor agonists (terbutaline, ritodrine) have been found to stop premature labor effectively only for 24 to 48 hours (usually enough time to administer corticosteroids if indicated). Contraindications to the use of beta mimetics include maternal cardiac rhythm disturbances or cardiac disease, poorly controlled diabetes, thyrotoxicosis, or hypertension. The efficacy of magnesium sulfate as a tocolytic agent is controversial. Some studies have shown that magnesium sulfate is no better than placebo.[27,28] Calcium channel blockers (e.g., nifedipine) inhibit uterine contractions, but their role in stopping labor has not been defined. However, prostaglandin inhibitors (e.g., indomethacin) appear to be very effective in treating premature labor and seem to have relatively few adverse effects on the mother. In contrast, there is potential for some worrisome fetal and neonatal complications. The use of indomethacin has been associated with constriction of the ductus arteriosus, oligohydramnios, and neonatal pulmonary hypertension. Prior to 32 weeks gestation, the incidence of ductal constriction has been reported to be 5 to 10 percent. After 32 weeks gestation, the incidence increases to 50 percent after prolonged use of indomethacin for more than 48 hours. Fortunately, ductal constriction is usually transient and responds to discontinuation of the drug. Oligohydramnios can be common with the use of indomethacin, is dose-related, and is reversible. Additionally, in preterm infants below 30 weeks gestation, indomethacin has been associated with patent ductus arteriosus, intraventricular hemorrhage, and necrotizing enterocolitis.[26–28] Oxytocin antagonists (e.g., atosiban) are presently being studied, and early results appear promising. Small clinical trials have reported greater specificity for these agents and improved efficacy; larger clinical trials are under way. The current recommendation for when to use tocolysis is between 24 and 34 weeks gestation. Tocolytic treatment often gives the rural provider the time needed to stabilize the mother, administer corticosteroids (if indicated), and transport the mother to a suitable tertiary care center.

Two new tests may help the rural provider predict which patients will go on to deliver prematurely and which ones need to be transferred to a regional facility. Fetal fibronectin and salivary estriol levels are two of the latest tests that may make a difference in the management of PTL. These are discussed in more detail below.

The most common treatable causes of PTL that the rural physician will face are usually secondary to bacterial vaginosis (common causative agents being _Trichomonas_ and _Gardnerella_) and urinary tract infections (UTI). Metronidazole 500 mg bid for 7 days is used to treat most bacterial vaginosis. Metronidazole has not been found to be teratogenic in the second and third trimesters; the evidence regarding its safety in the first trimester is controversial. Side effects that patients should be aware of include abdominal pain, nausea, and GI upset. For those with recurrent vaginosis, a single 2-g dose of metronidazole for both patient and partner may be curative. Should this fail and the patient continue to have symptoms of bacterial vaginosis, a trial of clindamycin 600 mg tid may be in order. Routine screening for the existence of bacterial vaginosis at the initial prenatal visit has been recommended.[28] This is performed by obtaining a random swab of the vagina and sending it to the laboratory for Gram stain, seeking increased WBCs, the presence of clue cells, and bacteria. If these are found, treating the presymptomatic patient with the appropriate antibiotics has been recommended.

The most common causative agent for UTI in pregnancy has been _Escherichia coli_. It is usually sensitive to ampicillin 500 mg qid, amoxicillin 500 mg tid, or cephalexin 500 mg qid. Macrodantin 100 mg bid and trimethoprim-sulfamethoxazole DS bid can be used, but they are contraindicated in the third trimester of pregnancy. Recurrences require monthly screening of urine specimens to rule out UTI. If the patient has had an episode of acute pyelonephritis during pregnancy or has had at least two documented UTIs, low-dose antibiotic suppression daily (usually at one-quarter to one-third of the usual dose) may be in order for the rest of the pregnancy to prevent further infections.

Strategies for the Patient Who Is in Preterm Labor

1. Rule out rupture of membranes with a sterile speculum exam, and assess cervical dilatation.
2. Obtain wet prep, cervical cultures for *Chlamydia,* gonorrhea, and group B strep.
3. Obtain a urine sample (either a clean-catch midstream sample or a catheter specimen) and send for culture if indicated on the microscopic exam or if positive for leukocyte esterase and nitrites on the urinalysis dipstick test.
4. Assess gestational age—is dating reliable?
5. External fetal monitors if >26 weeks gestation.
6. Start an intravenous and run in 1 L of normal saline over 1 hour, then reassess.
7. If the patient is still having contractions but they are infrequent (e.g., ≥10 minutes apart) and there is cervical change (e.g., cervix is ≤50 percent effaced and/or ≤3 cm dilated), admit the patient to the hospital for further observation and treatment if delivery is not imminent. Consider administering 5 mg of terbutaline subcutaneously if the contractions increase in frequency and/or intensity and there are no contraindications.
8. If the patient is having frequent contractions (e.g., ≤10 minutes apart) and the cervix is showing advanced changes (>50% effaced and >3 cm dilated), give 5 mg terbutaline subcutaneously stat, keep the IV fluids running at 150 mL/h, and contact the nearest perinatologist to discuss transport to the nearest regional center. Assess the level of care that the patient should have during the transport (EMT, paramedic, RN, or physician).
9. Terbutaline 2.5 to 5 mg may be repeated every 4 hours until the contractions have stopped. Contractions should be monitored closely; therefore the patient should remain continuously on the external fetal heart monitor. Common side effects of terbutaline include agitation, tremors, anxiety, tachycardia, restlessness, and insomnia.
10. Magnesium sulfate may be used in certain circumstances, although its efficacy as a tocolytic agent has been questioned.[27,28] Conditions that may suggest its use over beta agonists include preterm labor in the face of marginal or partial placental abruption, placenta previa, or a previous hypersensitivity reaction to terbutaline. Contraindications include hypocalcemia, myasthenia gravis, and renal failure. Dosing should be as follows: 4 g IM initially, followed with 1 to 4 g IV. Adjust the infusion rate depending on the progression of labor. Reflexes and respirations need to be monitored frequently to avoid magnesium toxicity [blunted to absent reflexes and hypoventilation (<8 respirations per minute) suggest toxicity]. Other side effects may include burning at the intravenous site, somnolence, and depression. The measurement of serum magnesium levels is no longer recommended routinely provided that the above parameters are carefully followed by the nursing staff.
11. An alternative to magnesium sulfate is indomethacin. A loading dose of 100 mg in suppository form is given rectally (for more rapid absorption), followed by 25 mg every 6 hours orally for 24 to 48 hours. Alternatively, an initial 50-mg dose orally followed by 25 mg every 6 hours is also acceptable. Contraindications include maternal asthma, peptic ulcer disease, coronary artery disease, preexisting oligohydramnios, and renal failure. Common maternal side effects include nausea and GI upset. The amniotic fluid volume should be measured by ultrasound prior to the initiation of indomethacin and at 48 hours thereafter. Fetal contraindications to the use of indo-

methacin include growth retardation, oligohydramnios, renal anomalies, chorioamnionitis, and duct-dependent cardiac defects.

12. Nifedipine can also be used as an alternative. The initial dose is 20 to 30 mg orally, then 10 to 20 mg every 6 hours. Contraindications include maternal liver disease and concurrent use with magnesium sulfate. Common maternal side effects include transient hypotension.

Sampling the cervicovaginal mucus for fetal fibronectin may change the way that PTL is managed by the rural physician. The test is most valid between 24 and 34 weeks gestation, with intact membranes (amniotic fluid creates false positives), cervical dilation <3 cm (probability is higher that PTL will ensue when cervical dilation is ≥3 cm), no blood present (creates false positives), and when no digital exams have been performed before obtaining the specimen (lubricants create false negatives). A specific collection kit is required to obtain the specimen per vagina. If fetal fibronectin is positive, the relative risk is 25.9 (95 percent confidence interval 7.8 to 86) of delivering within 7 days.[29] If fetal fibronectin is negative, the patient has less than a 0.3 percent chance of delivering within 7 days.[30] False positives occur in the presence of sperm or blood. False negatives will occur in the presence of soap and lubricants. This test may help the rural physician decide who needs to be transferred to a regional perinatal center. Unfortunately it is not yet readily available at all medical centers, and it may require sending the sample to a central laboratory for analysis. Turnaround time of at least 48 hours thus limits its clinical usefulness. While its value as a clinical tool remains to be proven, it is worthwhile to be aware of this technology.

Sampling the saliva for estriol is another new technology that may affect the care of PTL in our rural population. Salivary estriol increases 2 to 3 weeks before the spontaneous onset of labor and delivery. If salivary estriol is positive, the patient is seven times more likely to deliver

within 7 days. If it is negative, the patient is unlikely to deliver.[31] The process of collecting saliva, compared to that for fetal fibronectin, is easier and can be performed in the office setting as well. This test is not yet readily available but may become a very useful tool in the near future.

The role of home uterine activity monitoring (HUAM) in the prevention of premature birth is controversial. HUAM is a monitoring system that records uterine contractions with a tocodynamometer. These recordings are transmitted by telephone to the health care provider for immediate evaluation. Patient education and daily telephone calls or home visits to offer support and advice can also be part of the monitoring system. The premise of HUAM is that the onset of early uterine contractions will be identified sooner (especially in women who may not recognize contractions), thereby allowing intervention to occur before the patient develops unstoppable preterm labor. Neither ACOG nor the U.S. Preventive Services Task Force[32,33] recommend HUAM, as there is insufficient evidence of its clinical effectiveness to recommend for or against it as a screening test for preterm labor.

PREMATURE RUPTURE OF MEMBRANES AND PRETERM PREMATURE RUPTURE OF MEMBRANES

H.B., 24 years old (gravida 3, para 1, abortus 1), has an intrauterine pregnancy at 30 weeks gestation by well-established dates and a 15-week ultrasound. She presents to labor and delivery after waking up in a pool of clear fluid in bed about 2 hours earlier. She denies any contractions, dysuria, or vaginal bleeding. Her prenatal course has been uneventful except that she still smokes about 3 to 5 cigarettes a day despite having been urged to quit. She is negative for group B strep. On the fetal heart monitor, no uterine irritability or contractions are noted. The fetal heart rate is 140 beats per minute with good variability. On sterile speculum exam, she clearly has vaginal pooling, is Nitrazine*-positive, and has ferning. Her cervix appears to be long, thick, and closed. A sample of her cervicovaginal secretions is obtained and sent for fetal fibronectin. She is admitted for further care.

Premature rupture of membranes (PROM) can be defined as spontaneous rupture of the amniotic membrane (SROM) at ≥37 weeks gestation, and preterm premature rupture of membranes (PPROM) is defined as rupture of membranes at less than 37 weeks gestation. The key to the management of PROM and PPROM is rapid and accurate diagnosis. Several tools can help the rural provider arrive at the diagnosis and aid in the management. One of the most significant management changes over the recent years is the approach to the prevention of group B hemolytic strep (GBS) transmission. In 1996, the Centers for Disease Control and Prevention published a new set of recommendations for GBS prophylaxis,[34] urging obstetric providers to screen all pregnant women at 35 to 37 weeks gestation for anogenital GBS colonization and offering intrapartum chemoprophylaxis to all identified GBS carriers. In addition, the recommendations call for a chemoprophylaxis strategy based on the presence of intrapartum risk factors (e.g., gestation <37 weeks, duration of SROM ≥18 hours, or temperature ≥38°C). New on the horizon is the utilization of the Fetal Lung Maturity (FLM) index in ascertaining fetal lung maturation, as it may be more predictive than the lecithin/sphingomyelin (L/S) ratio and the measurement of phosphatidyl glycerol (PG). In addition, there are new cervical "ripeners" (prostaglandin E_2 gel and misoprostol) that may help make inductions more successful. Still con-

troversial is the use of corticosteroids and antibiotics in the setting of PPROM—that is, if and when one should administer these agents in a rural setting. Practical strategies for the rural provider are reviewed below.

The incidence of PROM and PPROM in rural settings is not known, but it is assumed that there probably are no significant rural-urban differences. The cause of PROM and PPROM is unknown; however, there are a number of known risk factors associated with PROM and PPROM (Table 9-10).

Prompt diagnosis of PROM or PPROM is a crucial step, since any delay may be catastrophic for both the mother and the infant. Prevention of chorioamnionitis—and subsequent risk of endomyometritis and sepsis—is the key for the mother. For the infant, complications such as prematurity, LBW, VLBW, sepsis, respiratory distress syndrome, and necrotizing enterocolitis are just a few of the causes of high infant morbidity and mortality found in this situation.

The natural history of PPROM and PROM reveals the following outcomes: if PPROM occurs before 26 weeks gestation, 30 to 40 percent of patients will gain an additional week before delivery, and 20 percent will gain over 4 weeks; if PPROM occurs between 28 and 34 weeks gestation, 70 to 80 percent will deliver within the first week after rupture of membranes and 50 percent of these will deliver within 4 days; if PROM occurs after 37 or more weeks gestation,

---

* Nitrazine is a litmus paper test that evaluates the pH of a substance. Amniotic fluid is alkaline. Nitrazine paper will turn blue in the presence of amniotic fluid. False-positive Nitrazine results occur in the presence of alkaline urine, blood, vaginal infections that raise the vaginal pH (*Trichomonas vaginalis*), or cervical mucus. *Ferning* is a term used to describe the pattern that amniotic fluid assumes when it is air-dried on a glass slide and viewed under a microscope under low power.

TABLE 9-10   RISK FACTORS ASSOCIATED WITH PROM AND PPROM

Prior history of PROM (21%)
  Smoking
  Genital tract infections
    Cervicitis
    Vaginosis
Intrauterine infection (average 28%)
  Placental abruption (5%)
  Incompetent cervix

Key: PROM, premature rupture of membranes; PPROM, preterm PROM.

SOURCE: Data from Graham,[35] with permission.

80 percent will develop labor within the first 24 hours after rupture of membranes.[35]

Even with a well-documented history, a sterile speculum exam is required in all patients to document whether the membranes are truly ruptured. This will be the deciding factor that guides which management protocol the rural provider must choose. Documentation of vaginal pooling, positive Nitrazine, and positive ferning together are still pathognomonic. If the history is convincing for rupture of membranes but the sterile speculum exam is negative or only partly positive, there are a number of other possible approaches to clarifying the diagnosis. Having the patient do a Valsalva maneuver or cough during the exam may reveal leakage of fluid. If no fluid is visualized, the patient may be asked to sit in a semiupright position for 1 hour and then rechecked. Another strategy is to obtain a bedside uterine ultrasound to check for a low amniotic fluid index (AFI), defined as equal to or less than 5.

Accurate assessment of gestational dating is critical. If the patient does not have good menstrual dating, an early ultrasound may be very helpful. Obstetric ultrasounds can be particularly helpful for dating, especially when they are obtained before 18 weeks gestation. If the ultrasound is obtained between 5 and 12 weeks gestation (crown–rump length), dating can be as accurate as ±3 days. Dating using biparietal diameter measurements between 12 and 20 weeks gestation can be reliable to ±8 days, and between 20 to 24 weeks gestation to about ±12 days.

Amniotic fluid examination can help assess fetal lung maturity. Measurement of phospholipids that make up pulmonary surfactant in the amniotic fluid allows prediction of the risk of development of respiratory distress syndrome (RDS) in the neonate. About 2 percent of infants with L/S ratios equal to or greater than 2.0 develop RDS, compared with 60 percent of infants with ratios below 2.0. The presence of blood or meconium in the amniotic fluid will affect the L/S ratio accuracy, leading to unreliable values. It has also been shown that a mature L/S ratio

(e.g., ≥2.0) in the diabetic patient may not be reliable. The fetal lung maturity index [measurements of the L/S ratio, phosphatidyl glycerol (PG), and phosphatidylinositol (PI) together] offers a more reliable predictor of pulmonary maturity, especially in infants of diabetic mothers. RDS is rare when the L/S ratio is below 2.0 and PG is present. When the L/S ratio is below 2.0 and no PG is present, over 90 percent of infants develop RDS. If the L/S ratio is immature but PG is present, less than 5 percent of infants will develop RDS. Another advantage of using PG is that it is reliably detected even with contamination with vaginal secretions or blood.[35]

An amniotic fluid sample can be obtained by amniocentesis or collection from vaginal pooling. Frequently it is not possible to obtain a "stat" fetal lung maturity index in the rural hospital laboratory, since many smaller facilities lack the required equipment. Infrequent requests do not justify the cost of the equipment. However, the rural provider may have some other alternatives (Table 9-11) when a complete fetal lung maturity profile is not available.[35–37]

Strategies for the Patient Who Presents with PROM

1. Determine gestational age as accurately as possible.
2. Document rupture of membranes (ROM) by performing a sterile speculum exam. Check for vaginal pooling, positive Nitrazine test, and ferning.
3. Swab for GBS, and obtain cultures for herpes, *Chlamydia,* and gonorrhea.
4. Check prenatal records for GBS status.
5. If ROM is confirmed and gestational age is ≥37 weeks: Are there signs of labor? If yes, admit the patient. Is she GBS positive? If yes, follow GBS protocol (Table 9-12).[34]
6. If there are no signs of labor, then:

   • Option 1: ambulate for 1 to 2 hours, then reevaluate for labor. If no labor, send home if patient is reliable for follow-up. Place at

TABLE 9-11   RAPID SCREENING TESTS FOR THE ASSESSMENT OF
FETAL LUNG MATURITY

Test	Principle	Mature Level	Advantages	Disadvantages
Amniostat-FLM	Immunologic test with agglutination in presence of PG	Test positive with PG $\geq 0.5\ \mu g/mL$	Rapid, few falsely mature tests; not affected by presence of blood / meconium	Many falsely immature results
Shake test	Generation of stable foam by pulmonary surfactant in the presence of ethanol	After shaking a 1:2 dilution, a complete ring of bubbles at meniscus appears in 15 minutes	Few falsely mature tests; fast, easily performed	Concentration of reagents is critical; many falsely immature results; affected by presence of blood or meconium
Lumadex-FSI	Modification of manual foam instability index; stable foam in presence of increasing concentration of ethanol	≥ 47	Few falsely mature tests; fast, easily performed	Concentration of reagents critical; some falsely immature results; affected by presence of blood or meconium
Tap test	Unstable foam in the presence of HCl acid and diethyl ether	1 mL AF is mixed with 1 drop 6N HCl acid and 1.5 mL diethyl ether in a test tube and tapped 3–4 times. Readings at 2, 5, and 10 minutes. Bubbles from mature AF break down (<5 remain).	PPV for mature tests = 95%; fast, easily performed. Not affected by presence of blood or meconium	Concentration of reagents critical; PPV for immature tests = 40–60%

Key: PG, phosphatidyl glycerol; AF, amniotic fluid; PPV, positive predictive value.
SOURCES: Data from Gabbe[36] and American College of Obstetrics and Gynecology, Committee on Educational Bulletins,[37] with permission.

pelvic rest. Return when labor begins or within 6 to 12 hours if no labor.
- Option 2: admit. If cervix is favorable (Bishop's score >6; see Table 9-13),[38] begin oxytocin induction[38] (see Table 9-14 for dosing recommendations). If cervix is unfavorable, consider the use of misoprostol or prosta-

glandin E_2 gel if there are no contraindications (see Table 9-14 for dosing recommendations).

7. If ROM is not confirmed (in the presence of a good history for PROM by the patient) and gestational age is ≥ 37 weeks:

TABLE 9-12   PROTOCOL FOR INTRAPARTUM GROUP B HEMOLYTIC STREPTOCOCCUS (GBS) PROPHYLAXIS

Risk Factor	Treatment
One or more of the following: Previous infant with invasive GBS disease GBS bacteriuria this pregnancy Delivery <37 weeks gestation PROM ≥ 18 hours Temperature ≥ 100.4°F (38°C)	Penicillin G 5 million units IV initially, then 2.5 million units IV every 4 hours until delivery[a]
Prenatal screen for GBS at 35–37 weeks positive	Penicillin G 5 million units IV initially, then 2.5 million units IV every 4 hours until delivery[a]

[a]Alternative is ampicillin 2 g IV initially, then 1 g every 4 hours. If patient is allergic to penicillin, clindamycin 900 mg IV every 8 hours or erythromycin 500 mg IV every 6 hours until delivery.

SOURCE: Data from Centers for Disease Control and Prevention.[34]

- Place the patient in a semiupright position for approximately 1 hour to encourage the pooling of secretions, then repeat the sterile speculum exam. Have the patient do the Valsalva maneuver or cough when reexamined and check for leakage of fluid.
- Obtain a beside ultrasound and check AFI. If low, this is probably most consistent with PROM and you should proceed as above. If normal, there may have been a "forebag" leak and membranes have "resealed," or there has been no PROM and other causes of leakage of fluid should be considered (e.g., urinary incontinence).
- Consider admitting the patient to the hospital if she is unreliable and observe (and document) for further leakage of fluid. Monitor temperatures. Limit vaginal exams to prevent chorioamnionitis. If no further leakage is found, this could be con-

TABLE 9-13   BISHOP'S PRELABOR SCORING SYSTEM

Factor	Score			
	0	1	2	3
Dilatation (cm)	Closed	1–2	3–4	5 or more
Effacement (%)	0–30	40–50	60–70	80 or more
Station	−3	−2	−1	+1/+2
Position of cervix	Posterior	Midposition	Anterior	

SOURCE: Modified from Gabbe,[36] with permission.

TABLE 9-14   RECOMMENDATIONS FOR CERVICAL RIPENING AND INDUCTION OF LABOR

Product	Initial Dose	Interval Dosing	Maximum Dose	Side Effects
Prostaglandin E2[a] gel				Hypertonus, fetal distress, fever, SOB, hypertension, chest pain[b]
Intracervical	0.5 mg in 3.5 mL gel	6 h	2 doses	
Intravaginal	5.0 mg in 10 mL gel	6 h	2 doses	
Misoprostol[c]				
Vaginal	25 µg	4–6 h		Hypertonus, fetal distress, fever, SOB, hypertension, chest pain
Oral	50 µg	4–6 h		
Oxytocin				
Mercer et al.[d 39]	0.5–1.0 mU/min	1–2 mU/min q 30–60 min	40 mU	Hypertonus, uterine rupture, fetal distress, hypotension, SIADH
Muller et al.[40]	1–2 mU/min	1–2 mU/min q 30 min	40 mU	

Key: SOB, shortness of breath; SIADH, syndrome of inappropriate antidiuretic hormone.

[a]Contraindicated in patients with a history of asthma. Obtain a baseline external fetal heart monitor strip for 20 to 30 minutes before insertion; then repeat for 1 hour after insertion for 4 hours if any regular uterine contractions persist. Maintain patient in a lateral recumbent position for 30 minutes after each dose, then reposition for comfort. A minimum safe time interval between PGE2 administration and oxytocin has not been established. Oxytocin induction or augmentation may be initiated 6 to 12 hours after last dose.

[b]Give terbutaline 0.25 mg SQ for hyperstimulation with hypertonus and/or fetal distress.

[c]Obtain a baseline external fetal heart monitor strip for 30 minutes before administration of medication; then repeat 60 minutes postinsertion for fetal response; then repeat for 15 minutes every hour. Maintain patient in a lateral recumbent position for 60 minutes, then reposition for comfort. Oxytocin induction/augmentation may be initiated 3 to 6 hours after last dose.

[d]Recommendations of the American College of Obstetricians and Gynecologists.

SOURCES: Data from Gabbe[36] and the American College of Obstetricians and Gynecologists.[37,38]

sistent with a "forebag" leak where membranes have "resealed," or there has been no PROM and other causes of leakage should be considered, as above.

- Consider obstetric consultation for diagnostic amniocentesis with injection of indigo-carmine dye into the amniotic fluid. Leakage of any blue-colored fluid from the vagina on reinspection is consistent with PROM.

Strategies for the Patient Who Presents with PPROM (<37 Weeks Gestation)

1. Determine gestational age as accurately as possible.
2. Determine rupture of membranes by performing a sterile speculum exam as above. If there is vaginal pooling, consider collecting specimen for L/S ratio and PG.
3. Swab for GBS and obtain cultures for herpes, *Chlamydia,* and gonorrhea.
4. Check prenatal records for GBS status. Follow GBS protocol (Table 9-12).
5. If ROM is confirmed and gestational age is below 37 weeks gestation, determine whether there are any signs of labor. If yes, consider tocolysis and corticosteroids if justified by gestational age (Table 9-15)[41] and cervical dilation.

- If cervix is ≤3 cm dilated, start intravenous fluids (1 L of normal saline administered over 1 hour). Apply continuous external

TABLE 9-15   DOSING OF CORTICOSTEROIDS FOR PREMATURITY

Gestational Age	Corticosteroids?	Dose
24–28 weeks	Yes (controversial—although antenatal corticosteroids do not clearly decrease the incidence of RDS in infants born at this gestational age, they reduce its severity; they clearly reduce mortality and the incidence of IVH in these infants)	Betamethasone 12 mg IM, 2 doses 24 hours apart, or dexamethasone 6 mg IM, 4 doses 12 hours apart[a]
29–32 weeks	Yes	Same as above
32–34 weeks	Yes (controversial—lack of convincing evidence whether antenatal corticosteroids clearly decrease the incidence of RDS)	Same as above
34–37 weeks	No	—

Key: RDS, respiratory distress syndrome; IVH, intraventricular hemorrhage.

[a]Optimal benefits begin 24 hours after initiation of therapy and last 7 days.

SOURCE: Data from American College of Obstetrics and Gynecology, Committee on Obstetric Practice,[41] with permission.

fetal monitors. Administer tocolysis per protocol above. Give antibiotics per GBS protocol. Call perinatal referral center and prepare for transport. Discuss with the consultant whether you should administer corticosteroids (see Table 9-15) to the mother before transfer. Limit vaginal exams.

- If cervix is more than 3 cm dilated, start intravenous fluids as above. Apply continuous external fetal monitors. Give antibiotics per GBS protocol. Consider maternal transport. Call perinatal referral center and discuss case immediately. Determine if there is enough time before imminent delivery to allow transfer. If insufficient time, call NICU referral center and request neonatal transport team ASAP. Anticipate delivery and call for some backup coverage for resuscitating infant.

- If there are no signs of labor, then:

  Start IV fluids of 1 L normal saline at 125 mL/h

  Apply continuous external monitors

  Give antibiotics per GBS protocol (Table 9-12)

  Limit vaginal exams

  Consider sending amniotic fluid from

vaginal pool specimen for stat L/S ratio and PG for fetal lung maturity

Call perinatal referral center and discuss transport

Discuss the administration of corticosteroids (see Table 9-15) to the mother with the consultant[41]

INTRAUTERINE GROWTH RETARDATION

J.L., 19 years old (gravida 2, para 0, abortus 1), has had regular obstetric care since 10 weeks gestation. Her prenatal course has been uneventful. At her 35-week visit, it was noticed that she has had poor weight gain since 32 weeks gestation. An obstetric ultrasound reveals a growth discrepancy of approximately 3 weeks, an estimated fetal weight (EFW) of 2120 g (which is at the fifth percentile for weight), and an amniotic fluid index (AFI) of 12.5 (normal range: 5.0 to 20.0). The umbilical Doppler* is normal, and the placenta is a grade

---

* Umbilical Doppler flow studies of the umbilical artery are used to measure the systolic to diastolic blood pressure (S/D) ratio. Normal S/D ratio is <2.5 after 26 weeks gestation and <3.0 after 30 weeks gestation. Abnormal S/D ratio > 3.0 has been associated with significant perinatal morbidity and mortality.

TABLE 9-16   NEONATAL COMPLICATIONS IN LOW-BIRTH-WEIGHT INFANTS

Intrapartum asphyxia	Meconium aspiration
Hypoglycemia	Hypocalcemia
Hypothermia	Polycythemia
Hyperbilirubinemia	Thrombocytopenia
Pulmonary hemorrhage	Intraventricular hemorrhage (mostly preemies)
Sepsis	Respiratory distress syndrome (mostly preemies)

SOURCES: Data from Vandenbosche and Kirchner[42] and Bernstein and Gabbe,[43] with permission.

II.* A diagnosis of intrauterine growth retardation (IUGR) is made. An obstetric consultation (at the nearest referral center) is obtained over the telephone to discuss further strategies. The consultant recommends biweekly nonstress tests (NSTs) and an AFI weekly to assess fetal viability, and allow progression of the pregnancy to 37 weeks gestation if possible. He also recommends a follow-up ultrasound in 2 weeks to assess interval growth. Biweekly NSTs and weekly AFIs reveal good fetal viability. At 37 weeks, a repeat ultrasound reveals only a 300-g weight gain, a growth discrepancy of approximately 5 weeks, an EFW of 2435 (e.g., LBW defined as <2500 g), and an AFI of 14.6; the umbilical Doppler is normal. The placenta is now a grade III with multiple microcalcifications. A biophysical profile† is normal, with a score of 8/8. Your consultant recommends that the patient be admitted for an elective induction for IUGR.

---

* Placental grading describes the maturation of the placenta based on placental morphology as examined by ultrasound. Correlation of placental morphology and fetal lung maturity has been demonstrated. With the progression from the least mature placenta (grade 0) to the most mature placenta (grade 3), one observes increasing deposition of calcium within the placental septa.

† Biophysical profile (BPP) is an antepartum assessment of the fetal condition using real-time ultrasonography that measures the following parameters: fetal breathing movements (at least 1 episode of >30 seconds duration in 30 minutes of observation); gross body movement (at least three discrete body/limb movements in 30 minutes); fetal tone [at least one episode of active extension with return to flexion of fetal limb(s) or trunk]; amniotic fluid volume (at least one pocket of amniotic fluid measuring 2 cm in two perpendicular planes). Two points are awarded for each normal finding and 0 for anything less. Normal BPP is 8/8, and chronic asphyxia is suspect with a score ≤6/8.

IUGR is the second leading contributor to the perinatal mortality rate. Several studies have shown an association between decreased perinatal service availability and the frequency of LBW and VLBW infants.[44–46] It is critical for the rural provider to identify and provide proper antenatal surveillance for these cases in order to decrease neonatal mortality. Table 9-16 shows the associated neonatal complications that can occur in LBW infants.[42,43]

IUGR is a diagnosis indicating that the fetal weight is below the 10th percentile for its gestational age. Symmetrical IUGR implies intrinsic factors as a cause. By definition, there is a normal ratio of head circumference/abdominal circumference (HC/AC) in these cases. Intrinsic factors causing symmetrical IUGR include genetic disease or fetal infection, often indicating a poor prognosis. Asymmetrical IUGR implies extrinsic factors as a cause. By definition, there is an increased HC/AC ratio. This type of IUGR is caused by placental insufficiency and yields a better prognosis with appropriate treatment.

Causes of IUGR usually fall into two categories: fetoplacental etiologies and maternal etiologies. Fetoplacental etiologies include chromosomal abnormalities, congenital malformations, and the genetic syndromes (<10 percent of cases); infectious diseases (<10 percent of cases); and placental abnormalities (Table 9-17).

The majority of IUGR cases are associated with maternal factors. Risk factors should be reviewed with the patient; they include a prior history of a LBW infant. Women whose first

TABLE 9-17   FETOPLACENTAL CAUSES OF IUGR

Chromosomal abnormalities	Infectious diseases
Trisomy 13	Herpes (HSV-1 or HSV-2)
Trisomy 18	Cytomegalovirus
Trisomy 21	Toxoplasmosis
	Rubella
	Syphilis
Genetic syndromes	Hepatitis B
Cretinism (hypothyroidism)	HIV
Congenital malformations	Placental pathology
	Previa
	Abruption
	Infarction
	Twins

Key: IUGR, intrauterine growth retardation; HSV, herpesvirus.

SOURCES: Data from Vandenbosche and Kirchner[42] and Bernstein and Gabbe,[43] with permission.

pregnancy resulted in an infant with IUGR have a 1 in 4 risk of delivering a second infant below the 10th percentile for weight. After two pregnancies complicated by IUGR, there is a fourfold increase in the risk of a subsequent infant with IUGR. Other risk factors are listed in Table 9-18.[42,43]

Maternal weight gain and/or fundal height measurements lack sensitivity for detecting IUGR. The presence of risk factors should therefore prompt ultrasound estimation of fetal size and growth. Nevertheless, a discrepancy in fundal height measurements may be the only clinical sign that first presents to the rural provider. In general, a discrepancy of more than 3 cm measured consecutively (preferably by the same provider) over a 2-week interval is grounds for obtaining an ultrasound to validate the diagnosis of IUGR. Ultrasound examinations should include determinations of biparietal diameter (BPD), head circumference/abdominal circumference (HC/AC), estimated fetal weight (EFW), and amniotic fluid volume (AFI). Guidelines for the use of ultrasound in the diagnosis and evaluation of IUGR are given in Table 9-19.[43]

Once the diagnosis of IUGR is made, antepartum fetal viability testing should be instituted. Biweekly NSTs with weekly AFIs is recommended. Repeat ultrasounds for fetal growth every 2 to 3 weeks are also recommended. As long as there is continued fetal head growth and testing remains reassuring, no other intervention is necessary.

TABLE 9-18   MATERNAL RISK FACTORS FOR IUGR

Preterm labor	Low maternal prepregnancy weight (<90% IBW)
Chronic hypertension	Poor maternal weight gain
Preeclampsia	Substance abuse (drugs, alcohol)
Diabetes mellitus	Smoking
Twin gestation	Maternal anemia (Hb <10)

Key: IUGR, intrauterine growth retardation; IBW, ideal body weight; Hb, hemoglobin.

SOURCES: Data from Vandenbosche and Kirchner[42] and Bernstein and Gabbe,[43] with permission.

TABLE 9-19   *UTILIZATION OF OBSTETRIC ULTRASOUND IN THE DIAGNOSIS AND EVALUATION OF IUGR*

Parameter	Results	Plan
No IUGR		
BPD	Appropriate for dates (within 2 weeks of dates)	Repeat only if indicated
EFW	>10th percentile	
HC/AC ratio	In normal range	
AFI	Normal	
Probable asymmetrical IUGR		
BPD	Appropriate for dates (within 2 weeks of dates)	Repeat US every 2–3 weeks if not delivered
EFW	<10th percentile	Start antepartum surveillance and continue until delivery
HC/AC ratio	>95th percentile	
AFI	Low	
Probable symmetrical IUGR		
BPD	2 weeks or more; smaller than expected for LMP	Repeat US every 2–3 weeks if not delivered
EFW	<10th percentile	Start antepartum surveillance and continue until delivery
HC/AC ratio	In normal range	If IUGR present before 20 weeks, scan for anomalies
AFI	Normal or low	

Key: IUGR, intrauterine growth retardation; BPD, biparietal diameter; EFW, estimated fetal weight; HC/AC, head circumference/abdominal circumference; AFI, amniotic fluid index; LMP, last menstrual period; US, ultrasound.
SOURCE: Modified from Bernstein and Gabbe,[43] with permission.

If the patient has a nonreassuring NST, further testing must be done. This includes either an immediate biophysical profile (BPP) or a contraction stress test (CST).* If the BPP score is ≤6 or the CST is positive (defined as late decelerations following 50 percent or more contractions), delivery should be considered. Management should be discussed with either the obstetrician or perinatologist at the nearest regional center. The presence of oligohydramnios (AFI <5) is associated with a higher perinatal mortality in IUGR and may require induction and preterm delivery. Where the patient should deliver will be dictated by the gestational age and the hospital's capacity to care for the antici-

pated sick newborn. As mentioned, this discussion should be undertaken with the consultant from the perinatal regional center. Most cases will require maternal transport to ensure the lowest perinatal mortality.

ANESTHESIA SUPPORT

Most rural hospitals in the United States do not have physician anesthesiologists on their medical staffs and therefore rely on certified registered nurse anesthetists (CRNAs) as the sole providers of anesthesia services. In 1982, some 34 percent of hospitals in the United States relied solely on CRNAs for the provision of anesthesia service, and 85 percent of these hospitals were located in rural areas. The highest concentration of CRNAs is found in the West North Central region (North Dakota, South Dakota, Minnesota), the Mid-Atlantic region (Pennsylvania,

* Contraction stress test is a test for uteroplacental dysfunction. A dilute infusion of oxytocin is given to establish at least three uterine contractions in 10 minutes. If late decelerations are observed with each contraction, the test is positive. If only one deceleration is observed, the test is suspicious.

West Virginia, Tennessee), the Southeast region (Alabama, South Carolina), and Kansas. There has been a 44 percent reduction in the number of graduates from nurse anesthetist programs from 1980 to 1988.[17]

As valuable as CRNAs are to rural hospitals and communities, the rural provider may find some unexpected limitations to the care that they can provide, sometimes requiring that other alternatives be considered. For example, not all CRNAs have been trained in epidural line placement. For those CRNAs who have this training, the low volume of epidurals seen in rural areas may be insufficient to maintain this skill. As a result, epidural anesthesia may not be available for labor, cesarean sections, or postoperative pain control. The rural provider may be limited to the use of spinal anesthesia and general anesthesia for cesarean sections, both of which carry a significantly higher rate of maternal and neonatal complications. However, Rosenblatt and associates,[47] in their survey of 34 rural hospitals in Washington State, reported surprisingly that epidural anesthesia was available in 91 percent. This service was dependent on the volume of annual deliveries performed in the rural hospital, being found in 71 percent of hospitals with ≤99 annual deliveries, 79 percent of hospitals with 100 to 499 annual deliveries, and 100 percent of hospitals with ≥500 annual deliveries.

Another limitation may be the availability of the CRNA. In isolated areas, a single CRNA may provide services in as many as four hospitals.[17] CRNAs who do possess the technical skill and competence to place epidurals may opt not to, as it requires that they be in house or within a certain range of the hospital should complications occur. This may not be practical when they are covering multiple hospitals. Because of poor reimbursement for their time, it may not be cost-effective for the CRNA to stay in house to supervise a continuous epidural infusion. Thus, the rural provider may need to utilize other methods for analgesia and anesthesia for laboring patients, such as narcotics and sedatives given parenterally or pudendal blocks.

The rural provider's decision-making process during the management of labor may also be affected by both the type and availability of anesthesia services. This limitation especially influences the timing of a cesarean section. Rural providers may have to perform a cesarean section sooner, in anticipation that the only CRNA may be called away for another case. Elective cases may be transferred to another facility offering anesthesia services that are not available locally. For example, the patient with a previous cesarean section and severe asthma who refuses a VBAC may have a better result undergoing her surgical procedure under epidural anesthesia rather than under general anesthesia.

CONCLUSION

Special concerns for the rural obstetric provider include the accessibility of cesarean sections, the availability of anesthesia support, maternal stabilization and transport issues (e.g., the type of transport system, mode of transportation, and EMTALA limitations), and the lack of abortion services. The limitations that these conditions impose on the rural provider and the problem-solving skills that he or she must possess make these situations somewhat unique and challenging. In addition, the rural obstetric provider must develop the skills that are necessary to care for some of the difficult obstetric problems encountered, including HIV-positive pregnant women, substance abuse, LBW infants, preterm labor, and premature rupture of membranes. Neonatal resuscitation skills will be a benefit for the rural provider to possess given the high rate of morbidity and mortality associated with these sick infants.

REFERENCES

1. Deutchman M: Who ever heard of family physicians performing cesarean sections? *J Fam Pract* 43(5):449–453, 1996.
2. Norris TE, Reese JW, Pirani MJ, et al: Are rural

family physicians comfortable performing cesarean sections? *J Fam Pract* 43:455–460, 1996.

3. American Academy of Family Physicians: *Facts about Family Practice 1995.* Kansas City, MO, AAFP, 1995.

4. Cowett RM, Coustan DR, Oh W: Effect of maternal transport on admission patterns at a tertiary care center. *Am J Obstet Gynecol* 154:1098–1100, 1986.

5. Kollee LA, Verloove-Vanhorick PP, Verwey RA, et al: Maternal and neonatal transport: results of a national collaborative survey of preterm and very low birth weight infants in the Netherlands. *Obstet Gynecol* 72(5):729–732, 1988.

6. Miller TC, Densberger M, Krogman J: Maternal transport and the perinatal denominator. *Am J Obstet Gynecol* 147(1):19–24, 1983.

7. Tomich PG, Anderson CL: Analysis of maternal transport service within a perinatal region. *Am J Perinatol* 7(1):13–17, 1990.

8. Low RB, Martin D, Brown C: Emergency air transport of pregnant patients: the national experience. *J Emerg Med* 6:41–48, 1988.

9. Ackmann C, Russano G, Hobart J: Ten years of maternal-fetal transport. *Crit Care Clin* 8(3):565–581, 1992.

10. Academy of Pediatrics Committee on Hospital Care: Guidelines for air and ground transportation of pediatric patients. *Pediatrics* 78:943, 1986.

11. Baldwin LM, Greer T, Hart LG, et al: The effect of a comprehensive Medicaid expansion on physicians' obstetric practices in Washington State. *J Am Board Fam Pract* 9(6):418–421, 1996.

12. Hughes D, Rosenbaum S: An overview of maternal and infant health services in rural America. *J Rural Health* 5(4):299–319, 1989.

13. Diekema DS: Unwinding the COBRA: new perspectives on EMTALA. *Pediatr Emerg Care* 11(4):243–248, 1995.

14. Pon S, Notterman DA: The organization of a pediatric critical care transport program. *Pediatr Clin North Am* 40(2):241–261, 1993.

15. Frew SA, Roush WR, LaGreca K: COBRA: implications for emergency medicine. *Ann Emerg Med* 17(8):835–837, 1988.

16. Baier FE: Implications of the consolidated Omnibus Budget Reconciliation "antidumping" legislation for emergency nurses. *J Emerg Nurs* 19(2):115–120, 1993.

17. Office of Technology Assessment: *Health Care in Rural America.* OTA-H-434. Washington, DC, US Government Printing Office, 1990.

18. Rosenblatt RA, Mattis R, Hart LG: *Access to Legal Abortions in Rural America: A Study of Rural Physicians in Idaho.* Working paper no. 30. Seattle, WA, WAMI Rural Health Research Center, 1994.

19. Clark SJ, Randolph RK, Savitz LA, et al: *A Quantitative Profile of Rural Maternal and Child Health.* Working paper no. 60. Chapel Hill, NC, North Carolina Rural Health Research Program, Cecil G Sheps Center for Health Services Research, 1997, pp 1–23.

20. American College of Obstetrics and Gynecology, Committee on Educational Bulletins: *Human Immunodeficiency Virus Infections in Pregnancy.* ACOG educational bulletin no. 232. Washington, DC, ACOG, January 1997.

21. Connor EM, Sperling RS, Gelber R, et al: Reduction of maternal-infant transmission of human immunodeficiency virus type 1 with zidovudine treatment. *N Engl J Med* 331:1173–1180, 1994.

22. National Institute on Drug Abuse. Women and Drug Abuse: NIDA's National Pregnancy and Health Survey. *NIDA Notes,* 10(1):1995, http://www.nida.nih.gov/NIDA_Notes/NNVol1ON1/NIDASurvey.html.

23. Chasnoff IJ, Landress HF, Barrett ME: The prevalence of illicit drug or alcohol use during pregnancy and discrepancies in mandatory reporting in Pinellas County, Florida. *N Engl J Med* 322:1202–1206, 1990.

24. Yawn BP, Yawn RA, Uden DL: Substance use in rural midwestern pregnant women. *Arch Fam Med* 1:83–88, 1992.

25. O'Connor TA, Bondurant HH, Siddiqui J: Targeted perinatal drug screening in a rural population. *J Maternal Fetal Med* 6(2):108–110, 1997.

26. American College of Obstetricians and Gynecologists, Committee on Educational Bulletins: *Preterm Labor.* ACOG technical bulletin no. 206. Washington, DC, ACOG, June 1995.

27. Higby K, Xenakis EMJ, Pauerstein CJ: Do tocolytic agents stop preterm labor? A critical and comprehensive review of efficacy and safety. *Am J Obstet Gynecol* 168:1247–1259, 1993.

28. Keirse MJNC: New perspectives for the effective treatment of preterm labor. *Am J Obstet Gynecol* 173:618–628, 1995.

29. Iams JD, Coultrip L, Eriksen N, et al: Fetal fibronectin as a predictor of preterm birth in patients

with symptoms: a multicenter trial. *Am J Obstet Gynecol* 177(1):13–18, 1997.

30. Goldenberg RL, Mercer BM, Iams JD, et al: The preterm prediction study: patterns of cervicovaginal fetal fibronectin as predictors of spontaneous preterm delivery. *Am J Obstet Gynecol* 177(1):8–12, 1997.

31. McGregor JA, Jackson GM, Lachelin GC, et al: Salivary estriol as risk assessment for preterm labor: a prospective trial. *Am J Obstet Gynecol* 173(4):1337–1342, 1995.

32. American College of Obstetrics and Gynecology, Committee on Obstetric Practice: *Home Uterine Activity Monitoring.* ACOG committee opinion no. 172. Washington, DC, ACOG, May 1996.

33. US Preventive Services Task Force: Home uterine activity monitoring for preterm labor. *JAMA* 270(3):369–376, 1993.

34. Centers for Disease Control and Prevention: Prevention of perinatal group B streptococcal disease: a public health perspective. *MMWR* 45(RR-7):1–24, 1996.

35. Graham ADM: Preterm labor and premature rupture of membranes, in Hacker NF, Moore GJ (eds): *Essentials of Obstetrics and Gynecology,* 2nd ed. Philadelphia, Saunders, 1992, p 276.

36. Gabbe SG: Antepartum fetal evaluation, in Gabbe SG, Niebyl JR, Simpson JL (eds): *Obstetrics: Normal and Problem Pregnancies,* 2nd ed. New York, Churchill Livingstone, 1991, pp 409–415.

37. American College of Obstetrics and Gynecology, Committee on Educational Bulletins: *Assessment of Fetal Lung Maturity.* ACOG educational bulletin no. 230. Washington, DC, ACOG, November 1996.

38. American College of Obstetrics and Gynecology, Committee on Technical Bulletins: *Induction of Labor.* ACOG technical bulletin no. 217. Washington, DC, ACOG, December 1995.

39. Mercer B, Pilgrim P, Sibai B: Labor induction with continuous low-dose oxytocin infusion: a randomized trial. *Obstet Gynecol* 77:659–663, 1991.

40. Muller PR, Stubbs TM, Laurent SL: A prospective randomized clinical trial comparing two oxytocin induction protocols. *Am J Obstet Gynecol* 167:373–381, 1992.

41. American College of Obstetrics and Gynecology, Committee on Obstetric Practice: *Antenatal Corticosteroid Therapy for Fetal Maturation.* ACOG committee opinion no. 147. Washington, DC, ACOG, December 1994.

42. Vandenbosche RC, Kirchner JT: Intrauterine growth retardation. *Am Fam Physician* 58(6):1384–1390, 1998.

43. Bernstein I, Gabbe SG: Intrauterine growth restriction, in Gabbe SG, Niebyl JR, Simpson JL (eds): *Obstetrics: Normal and Problem Pregnancies,* 3rd ed. New York: Churchill Livingstone, 1996, pp 863–886.

44. Larimore WL, Davis A: Relation of infant mortality to the availability of maternity care in rural Florida. *J Am Board Fam Pract* 8(5):392–399, 1995.

45. Nesbitt TS, Connell FA, Hart LG, et al: Access to obstetrical care in rural areas: effect on birth outcomes. *Am J Public Health* 80:814–818, 1990.

46. Taylor J, Zweig S, Williamson H, et al: Loss of a rural hospital obstetric unit: a case study. *J Rural Health* 5(4):343–352, 1989.

47. Rosenblatt RA, Saunders GR, Tressler CJ, et al: The diffusion of obstetric technology into rural U.S. hospitals. *Int J Technol Assess Health Care* 10(3):479–489, 1994.

CHAPTER 10

Surgery

DANA CHRISTIAN LYNGE

A 23-year-old man was driving alone and on an icy road in rural eastern Washington in midwinter late on a Friday evening. While crossing a patch of black ice, the back end of his truck skidded out. He lost control of the vehicle, which ran off the road, rolled, and came to rest in the ditch. The accident, which took place on the outskirts of the county seat (a town of approximately 3000 people), was witnessed by a passing motorist. This citizen called 911 and the information was passed on to the local volunteer emergency medical technicians. They found the driver unrestrained and smelling of alcohol in the cab of his overturned truck. He was initially unresponsive, but breathing regularly and with a palpable pulse. They extricated him from the truck—being as careful to protect his spinal column as circumstances allowed—and placed him on a backboard with a C-collar. His initial vital signs: pulse 120, blood pressure 110/60, respiratory rate 30. The patient was arousable (by painful stimuli) but confused. He was transported to the local emergency department (travel time 10 minutes), where he was seen and examined by the family physician on duty, who had been called in 30 minutes earlier to evaluate a child with fever and emesis.

The family physician found the patient with a clear airway, breathing spontaneously at 35 breaths per minute. The patient's pulse was now 140 and blood pressure 100/60. The patient responded incoherently to painful stimulus but was otherwise somnolent. The physician called for 100% oxygen by mask and the intubation kit as well as blood draws (complete blood count, standard blood biochemistries, liver function tests, type and cross, toxicology screen, blood gas), x-rays (cervical

spine, chest, pelvis), and two large-bore intravenous lines to be placed while she completed her secondary survey. Her findings were as follows: tenderness over the left frontoparietal area, but no step-off; no hemotympanum; no cerebrospinal fluid rhinorrhea; pupils equal and reactive to light; extraocular movements within normal limits; midface and dentition intact, no tenderness over the cervical spine; no tracheal deviation, decreased breath sounds on the left with tenderness on this aspect of the chest wall; abdomen slightly distended and diffusely tender; pelvis stable, limbs intact; no step-offs over thoracic and lumbar spine; rectal exam: guiac-negative, no high-riding prostate; no blood at the meatus; downward plantar reflexes bilaterally.

Initial test results came back as follows: cervical spine, no obvious abnormality on lateral; chest x-ray, small left pneumothorax; pelvis, intact; first hematocrit (drawn prior to administration of intravenous fluids), 30 percent; laboratory studies otherwise normal except for an alcohol blood level of 0.31 and moderate respiratory alkalosis. The family doctor asked for a second hematocrit to be drawn, the general surgeon to be called in to evaluate the patient, and the nurse anesthetist and OR team to be called in. She asked for a tube thoracostomy kit and placed a 32 French chest tube at the left fifth intercostal place at the anterior axillary line. There was a good rush of air on placement and good movement of the water column on the Pleurovac when the tube was hooked up. She then intubated the patient because of his fluctuating mental status and suspicion that he would have to go to the OR for an exploratory laparotomy. The second hematocrit came back 25 percent just as the general surgeon arrived. The surgeon and family physician performed diagnostic peritoneal lavage—which was grossly positive—and called for the OR team. The patient received 2 units of packed red blood cells (the patient was fortunate in that his blood type was O positive and two on-call donors with this blood type were available to come in and donate) and broad-spectrum antibiotics. At operation, the patient underwent splenectomy for a pulverized spleen. By the end of the case the patient had increasing oxygen requirements and an on-table x-ray showed opacity in both lung fields (left side greater than right). While the surgeon performed the operation, the family physician made arrangements for an Airlift Northwest helicopter with a flight nurse to pick up the patient immediately after surgery and take him to Harborview Medical Center for neurosurgical evaluation and treatment as well as probable prolonged intensive care for his pulmonary contusions.

The patient was stable during the 1-hour flight to Seattle, where he was seen and evaluated by the trauma team in the emergency department. At that time, the patient was intubated and sedated. Vital signs and hematocrit were stable, but the patient's Pao_2 was decreasing. Computed tomography of the head revealed diffuse cerebral edema but no obvious bleed. The patient was transferred to the surgical intensive care unit, where he underwent placement of an intracranial pressure monitor by the neurosurgical team and was placed on a ventilator with sufficient positive end-expiratory pressure to improve his oxygenation. His hospital course was complicated by nosocomial pneumonia, which responded to appropriate antibiotic treatment.

The patient's chest tube was removed on hospital day 3, with no residual pneumothorax. His intracranial pressure monitor was removed on hospital day 7, when his pressures returned to normal and the neurologic exam normalized. His pulmonary contusions resolved with supportive care. He was extubated on hospital day 8 and transferred to the ward on hospital day 9. He was discharged from Harborview on hospital day 11.

*T*his case illustrates four salient features of surgery in the rural setting today: (1) the importance of the primary care provider

in facilitating rural surgical care, (2) the importance of having a well-trained general surgeon available in rural areas (otherwise the patient might have exsanguinated prior to reaching the level 1 trauma center), (3) the impact of modern transport, and (4) the role of the tertiary urban referral center. Each of these issues, as well as related topics, is covered in this chapter.

SURGERY IN THE RURAL SETTING: AN OVERVIEW OF THE CURRENT SITUATION

Rural Patients, Urban Surgery

It is estimated that 25 percent of the population of the United States lives in rural areas (*rural* is defined as including all the counties not located within the Metropolitan Statistical Areas as defined by the Office of Management and Budget). A large proportion of these more than 55 million people are elderly. Yet this population is served by less than 15 percent of the nation's physicians in general and 10 percent of its general surgeons in particular.[1] Just how much surgery is actually performed in rural areas is not known because of the paucity of data collection in this area. However, one of the salient developments of the past decade has been for more and more rural folk to receive their surgical care in urban centers as opposed to their local hospitals. No discussion of rural surgery is complete without addressing this apparent threat to its very existence.

Just as many rural folk now drive 40 miles to the nearest Wal-Mart rather than patronize their local hardware store, they now are more likely than ever before to drive to an urban medical center for their surgery. As of 1993, approximately 60 percent of surgical charges billed on behalf of people from rural areas were collected by urban hospitals.[2] In some cases this was because specific surgical services (e.g., cardiac surgery) were not available at rural hospitals. However, the same study from 1993 found that almost one-third of patients undergoing cholecystectomy (a basic procedure in the repertoire of a general surgeon, rural or urban) had their surgery at an urban medical center, bypassing local hospitals and surgeons. Undoubtedly, a few of these were patients with extensive co-morbidities and were appropriately referred by their rural surgeons to an urban hospital (with intensive care units, house staff, medicine consultants, etc.). The majority of them, however, represent a trend that has its roots in several different causes, including modern transportation, aggressive marketing by urban medical centers/managed care monoliths, the shifting preferences of patients, changing referral patterns, the shortage of rural surgeons, and rural hospital shutdowns.

Patients who require emergent major surgery for such problems as neurosurgical trauma, major pelvic trauma, and rupturing abdominal aortic aneurysm can now be transported from the hinterlands to a tertiary medical center in a short span, undoubtedly saving lives but also transferring procedures and dollars from the rural to the urban setting. On a more basic level, people in the western states who would have been close to housebound during the winter in the horse-and-buggy era can now travel in heated all-wheel-drive vehicles several hundred miles over mountain passes to urban hospitals to have their gallbladders removed electively. With managed care have come aggressive marketing campaigns to attract insured patients from rural areas, who may choose to go to a major urban clinic with its complement of "specialists" and sophisticated technology. This problem is compounded by the increasing tendency of recently graduated rural family physicians to bypass the local general surgeon and refer cases to urban centers, under the impression that even routine surgeries can be done better in a tertiary setting.[3] These factors, as well as several others to be discussed further on, have contributed to the relatively recent phenomenon of massive rural hospital closures. Approximately 10 percent of rural hospitals closed between 1980 and 1989, and nearly one-third of rural hospitals were found to be in serious financial trouble during that decade.[4] Fewer hospitals in rural areas means less surgery in rural areas (however, the presence of freestanding ambulatory surgicenters in rural areas has not been documented to any extent). Fewer hospitals and less surgery means more difficulty recruiting surgeons to practice in a rural area. The net result of this is the shift of surgical cases, surgical expertise, and surgical dollars to urban centers.

The Rural General Surgeon: An Endangered Species

As the preceding paragraphs make abundantly clear, surgery in rural areas is a threatened endeavor. The vast majority of surgery performed in these areas is performed by general surgeons. The number of general surgeons in rural areas has been declining over the past two decades for a variety of reasons, examined later in this chapter. This decline is unlikely to alter given the numerous projections for a nationwide shortage of general surgeons in the new millennium. This present and projected problem is compounded by the fact that the older generation of general practitioners, who included some surgery (e.g., hernias, appendectomies, hemorrhoids, etc.) in their practices, has now largely retired. The new cohort of family physicians in the United States no longer receive enough surgical training as part of their residencies to allow them to perform the surgical procedures mentioned above. It is interesting to note that additional training programs in surgery for family physicians have been proposed in some of the western Canadian provinces.[5] There is also evidence that, in the isolated parts of that country, general practitioners continue to provide some surgical services.[6] Unfortunately, any incentive for family physicians in this country to acquire and practice additional surgical skills has been quelled by the current climate of malpractice litigation. In short, rural general practitioners who perform surgery are rapidly becoming extinct and rural general surgeons are endangered.[7]

Rural general surgeons are an endangered species, not only because of their decreasing numbers but also because the type of surgical training needed to prepare them for their practice is extremely difficult to obtain in this country at present. The training that general surgeons receive at urban, university-based medical residencies equips them well for the kind of practice—largely restricted to operations on the breast, abdomen, and alimentary tract—they will have in an urban center. By contrast, there is abundant evidence that 40 to 50 percent of most rural general surgeons' case loads include operations and/or procedures—orthopedic, gynecologic, obstetric, urologic, endoscopic, and other—outside the realm of what is currently defined as general surgery by university-based academic surgeons and for which they receive no significant training during their residencies. A review of the operative logs of the graduating chief residents in 1995 found that they performed an average of 8 obstetric and/or gynecologic (ob/gyn) procedures and 5.3 orthopedic procedures during their residencies. Over one-half of the 206 programs surveyed did not have an ob/gyn rotation.[1] The older generation of true rural "omnisurgeons" is not being replaced.[3]

Even within the realm of what is defined as general surgery by current academia and including operations for which general surgeons receive adequate exposure during the course of their residency, there is debate about which procedures general surgeons should be doing in the rural setting. Most of this debate centers around trying to determine the number of cases of a specific operation performed by a given surgeon at a given hospital per annum that are necessary to result in an acceptable outcome (e.g., low morbidity and mortality). There is not much dispute concerning the performance of such "low-complexity" procedures as herniorrhaphy, cholecystectomy, and appendectomy.[8] There are, however, conflicting opinions on whether surgery for colon and rectal cancer (procedures that are an integral part of the training of any general surgeon) should be performed by surgeons in hospitals that do not see a large number of these type of cases each year.[9]

There is a large body of literature on this volume–outcome issue for a variety of surgical procedures, most of it inconclusive. The salient point, though, is that the ability of rural general surgeons to perform even those procedures that are well within the purview of their specialty and training is being questioned. In short, contemporary general surgeons who go into rural practice are no longer being trained to do subspecialty procedures which formed the bulk of the practice of their predecessors, and they may soon come under pressure (in the form of either policy or litigation) to not perform some of the more complex procedures which they are trained to do.

The one undisputed role of the rural general surgeon is that of traumatologist. General surgeons are the principal providers of trauma care outside metropolitan areas. Their role includes (1) coordinating local trauma care and educational [advanced trauma life support (ATLS)] programs; (2) working with the primary care practitioner on duty to ensure that patients are adequately resuscitated and stabilized in the local emergency department; (3) performing surgery at the rural hospital, either as the definitive intervention or as a lifesaving temporizing measure prior to transfer; and (4) deciding on and coordinating the transfer of patients to a referral trauma center when indicated.[10] Traumatic injury in the rural setting has a much higher mortality rate than in urban areas. Regional trauma systems have been developed in an effort to combat this problem. A survey of a regional trauma system in Washington State from 1993 found that 90 percent of patients were able to be well cared for at local hospitals.[11] Other studies support the efficacy of starting rural level II and III trauma center programs (in which the staff general surgeon is the principal player) in decreasing preventable deaths. These systems appear to be a win-win situation, resulting in fewer inappropriate transfers and more surgery performed at a local level.[12] There is also good evidence in the literature that rural general surgeons—trained in the basics of hepatic, vascular, and neurosurgical procedures—working in consultation with the relevant urban subspecialist can save the lives of many patients who would otherwise expire in transit.[13,14] A surgeon whose practice and training is restricted to hernias, appendectomies, and cholecystectomies will not be able to provide that kind of surgical expertise.

The Rural Surgical Subspecialist

The paucity of data and published material on the subject of rural surgery is particularly severe in the area of surgical subspecialists. A paper from the WAMI Rural Health Research Center at the University of Washington noted that the more highly specialized the discipline, the less likely its practitioners were to be found in rural areas.[15] A closer look at the data in that paper (which assesses the number and percentage of physicians graduating from American medical schools, 1976 through 1985, who were practicing in rural counties in 1991) reveals some interesting findings. Although general surgery was listed as the most prevalent surgical specialty in rural counties (17.5 percent of graduates); orthopedics (12.8 percent), urology (12.3 percent), ob/gyn (12.2 percent), ophthalmology (12.1 percent), and otolaryngology (11.5 percent) were not that far behind. Still, it must be remembered that these specialists are serving almost 25 percent of the country's population. The same paper shows data suggesting that although the proportion of general surgeons practicing in rural areas is declining, that of surgical subspecialists is not. Indeed, there are some data to suggest recent growth in the number of subspecialty surgeons in rural areas. This phenomenon may reflect the current relative oversupply of some surgical subspecialties in urban areas. However, surgical subspecialists require a much larger catchment than general surgeons to support their practice and are therefore often in solo practice in rural areas. They also often require expensive technology for their procedures, which is beyond the budget of many small rural hospitals. For these reasons and many others, rural areas are likely to remain undersupplied with subspecialty surgeons. A recent survey of Washington State's 42 rural hospitals revealed that although 62 percent had at least one general surgeon on staff, only 21 percent had a surgical staff that included a general surgeon plus at least one anesthesiologist, gynecologist, orthopedist, and urologist.[2] In an era when fewer rural general surgeons have the training to do subspecialty procedures (e.g., fractures, hysterectomies, transurethral prostatectomies, etc.), patients will be forced to either travel to urban centers for their surgery or rely on the services of itinerant surgeons.

The Itinerant Surgeon

The phrase *itinerant surgeon* has always carried with it a pejorative connotation in the opinion of the urban, academic surgical elite of this country. Nevertheless, surgeons in rural areas have, of necessity, historically traveled to outlying communities to provide clinics and consultation. In the present-day United States, it is probably most common that patients deemed to be in need of surgery during these "circuit riding" clinic trips return to the surgeons' locale for their procedure. In certain areas of Australia and Africa, where it is impractical for patients to come to the surgeon's hospital for their procedures (owing to either the vastness of the territory, the lack of transportation infrastructure, or the relative poverty of the inhabitants), the surgeon goes to the patients' communities and performs the procedures there with the assistance of the local medical staff. In Australia, two different approaches have been tried. The Flying Surgeon Service of Queensland comprises a pilot, a surgeon, and an anesthesiologist who travel to isolated towns in this vast province and perform surgery—major and minor, emergent and elective—at the local hospital with the help of the resident physician. The more recently formed University Rural Surgical Services in western Australia provides specialist consultations and day surgery services to the inhabitants of the small towns in this huge region.[16] Both systems have shown benefits in terms of savings of patient transportation costs, increasing availability of surgical services to people in remote areas, educational benefits for the resident physicians, and helping to preserve the viability of the rural hospitals. A similar itinerant "flying surgeon" experience in Zimbabwe describes the benefits in a country where travel for local people is extremely limited and it is not feasible to have a resident surgeon in every district hospital.[17] A recent paper from South Africa describes a successful itinerant cardiovascular surgery program in two rural hospitals.[18] Whether such elaborate schemes will ever come into demand in this country (given our wealth and consequent access to transportation) or whether they are even feasible (given our legal system) is unknown. The one thing that is certain is that no itinerant surgeon can provide the immediate, invasive surgical service that a patient's life often depends on when he or she presents in extremis because of trauma or intraabdominal catastrophe. Only a resident rural general surgeon can do that.

SPECIAL PROBLEMS AND SOLUTIONS IN RURAL SURGERY

Recruitment

There is, in the literature, abundant testimony concerning the uniquely positive aspects of rural surgery. Its practitioners cite independence, absence of "turf battles," and close relationships with their patients and community as its principal benefits. Other positive aspects include the slower-paced rural lifestyle, absence of crime, and access to outdoor activities. Studies done to determine what sort of medical practitioner ends up in rural practice reveal a positive correlation with the following factors: origin in a rural area, having done a rural rotation in medical school or residency, and a love of outdoor activities and occupations as well as an aversion to

urban living. Despite all of the above, the proportion of general surgeons in rural areas continues to decline.

The reality of rural surgical practice is that many practitioners are in solo practice. Even in areas where there is more than one surgeon, rural practitioners are on call more frequently than their urban counterparts. In an era when choosing an area of endeavor with a "controllable lifestyle" is a priority with graduating medical students, the long hours and "perma-call" reality of rural surgical practice ensure recruitment difficulties. Even if the surgeon and his or her family adapt to this reality, problems with residing out in the country can arise when it comes time for children to be educated or if the spouse cannot find suitable employment or other activities. Studies have shown that female surgeons are even less likely than their male counterparts to choose a rural environment. This may have a significant impact on the rural surgical workforce in an era when women make up around one-half of all medical students. Lack of call coverage also ensures that it is difficult for rural surgeons to attend important continuing medical education activities such as conferences and technical workshops designed to keep them up to date on current surgical practices and to prevent professional isolation. There is also evidence that, given the long hours they put in, rural general surgeons are underpaid compared to their urban counterparts. The rural patient tends to be older, poorer, and less likely to have adequate insurance coverage. There are more Medicare and Medicaid patients in these areas, and both systems pay only a fraction of what an urban surgeon receives from a reputable insurance company.[4] To compound the problem, in some states, Medicare pays urban physicians 25 percent more than rural physicians for the same service. Other principal reasons why rural general surgeons consider relocation and that might dissuade recently graduated surgeons from choosing rural practice include (1) liability issues, (2) lack of adequate numbers of complex cases to maintain skills, (3) lack of ancillary and nonsurgical specialist staff to ensure optimal patient treatment, and (4) possible rural hospital closures. These last two reasons are especially significant and are discussed further on.

Crucial Colleagues and Technologies

General surgeons in urban tertiary care centers are able to perform complex procedures and to care for patients with significant physiologic impairment in large part because of the support of specialist colleagues and the availability of sophisticated diagnostic and therapeutic machinery (not to mention the availability of house staff in the case of teaching institutions).

Radiologists increase the diagnostic sophistication of the facility they are attached to [particularly with their ability to interpret scans obtained by computed tomography (CT) and magnetic resonance imaging (MRI), which surgeons do not necessarily learn how to read]. Those with invasive capabilities can provide additional therapeutic (e.g., percutaneous drainage of abscesses) and diagnostic (e.g., CT-guided biopsy of certain lesions) procedures. Their presence enables the surgeon to handle more complex cases. A study from rural Colorado revealed that only 40 percent of hospitals listed radiologists on staff. In other more rural states (i.e., Wyoming, Montana, the Dakotas, etc.) the percentage is probably less.

On-site pathologists provide services such as the frozen section (to identify tissue types and the presence or absence of malignancy), which can be crucial to intraoperative decision making. Not having a pathologist on site can restrict the kind of cases a surgeon can do at a given facility. The aforementioned Colorado study found that only 20 percent of hospitals in that state had attending pathologists.

A recent survey of 62 rural hospitals in Montana revealed that only 24 had attending anesthesiologists; the remainder were staffed by nurse anesthetists. The administrators of these hospitals did not feel that the lack of an anesthesiologist adversely affected the amount of surgery performed at their institution.[19] However, comments in the literature from practicing rural surgeons make clear that they are often hesitant to undertake certain major surgeries (e.g., repair of abdominal aortic aneurysm) unless an anesthesiologist is available.

Other medical specialties that provide important diagnostic and therapeutic aid to the general surgeon include gastroenterology, pulmonology, cardiology, and nephrology. There is abundant evidence in the literature testifying to the rarity of breast-conserving surgery for breast cancer in rural areas. This is most likely due to the absence of radiation oncologists in these areas.

Specific services lacking at rural hospitals that are cited as reasons for transfer of surgical patients (particularly trauma patients) to urban hospitals are blood banks and intensive care units. Finally, lack of modern technology (particularly diagnostic imaging devices) as used by the surgeon and specialist is often a factor in such transfers. The prohibitive cost of such technology is frequently a factor in rural hospital closures.

Rural Hospital Closures

As previously mentioned, at least 10 percent of rural hospitals closed between 1980 and 1989 and nearly one-third of rural hospitals were found to be in serious financial trouble during the same period. This trend has not abated. Rural hospitals differ from their urban counterparts in that they have fewer beds, lower occupation rates, shorter lengths of stay, more limited services, and a higher share of Medicare patients. As alluded to earlier in this chapter, aggressive marketing on the part of urban hospitals and the prohibitive cost of modern technology have played a part in this process. Other factors include relative economic decline in rural areas (especially those where the economy is based on extractive industries, such as logging and mining); population decline in rural areas; relative poverty of rural inhabitants and consequent limited tax-raising abilities of rural municipalities; and increased proportion of uninsured, Medicare, and Medicaid patients, resulting in low reimbursement rates. The major factors in hospital closures listed by rural mayors in a survey published in 1990 were government reimbursement policies (specifically the government's differential funding of urban and rural hospitals for Medicare patients), general financial problems, physician shortages, and poor management.[20] A survey of rural physicians from the same period listed government reimbursement policies, poor management, and general financial problems.[21] Studies examining the factors which distinguish rural hospitals that close found profit status and limited services to be highly correlated with closure. Closure of these hospitals only compounds the problem of rural economic decline, because they are often the largest employer in small communities and their presence and viability is a prerequisite to attract other industries. The closures also reduce the access to health care of rural inhabitants in that routine needs (e.g., vaccinations, prenatal visits, etc.) can no longer be taken care of locally and catastrophic services (e.g., trauma stabilization and emergency surgery) are no longer available. It is interesting to note that studies concerning surgery in rural areas show a high correlation between the provision of surgical services and improved hospital financial viability.[2] Unlike more routinely provided obstetric and emergency services, surgical services tend to pay for themselves and can support other less lucrative but vital hospital services. The final picture is one of a vicious cycle: fewer rural hospitals means fewer rural surgeons, fewer rural surgeons means fewer rural hospitals.

Telemedicine

One glimmer of hope for surgery in the hinterlands is telemedicine. This technology is now frequently used by the military and prison systems. It lends itself well to areas of medicine that rely on visual or electronic information (e.g., dermatology, cardiology, and pathology). It is now starting to be used in the arena of nongov-

ernmental medicine and some areas of surgery. A study of the use of telemedicine in orthopedic care from North Dakota revealed high satisfaction on the part of the rural physician and the orthopedic consultant and no adverse outcomes in 91 cases performed over a 2-year period.[22] Orthopedic cases made up 22 percent of teleconsultations over this time period for this network. Telemedicine consultations for surgical problems appear to have several benefits: avoiding costs and problems of transfer/transportation, increased continuity of care and continuing medical education by allowing management and follow-up of the problem with the local physician where possible, and keeping hospitalization revenues within the rural community. There are already projects under way in the telementoring of surgery performed at a remote site (i.e., the surgical consultant guiding and observing the procedure in real time via telemedicine technology and providing instant guidance to the on-site surgeon). However, there are still impediments to the widespread practice of telemedicine in the form of liability questions and remuneration disputes. Also, good studies must be done to assess the suitability of specific surgical disciplines to accurate diagnosis via telemedicine, ensure that patient outcomes are acceptable, and determine whether there are true cost savings. Finally, although telemedicine may be useful for a variety of surgical problems, no remote telesurgeon can provide the lifesaving capabilities of the on-site general surgeon.

EDUCATION AND TRAINING

The Flexner Report of 1910 had the effect of centralizing medical education (previously a sort of apprenticeship held in a variety of private hospitals) in urban, university-based medical schools. Residency training programs based at these centers have come to dominate their respective disciplines. This trend has undoubtedly raised the scientific standard of medical practice in the United States and made it an international leader in medical research and technology. However, the central task of rural surgeons is service rather than science, and their training requires more breadth than focused depth. As documented previously in this chapter, operations outside the realm of what is commonly thought of as general surgery (e.g., orthopedics, obstetrics-gynecology, etc.) constitute up to 50 percent of the case load of the rural general surgeon. Yet few modern general surgery residencies (which focus on GI, abdominal, and breast surgery) provide adequate training in these areas. A recent study from Canada showed that a full 57 percent of community general surgeons felt that their training had been inadequate preparation for their practice needs.[23] Only 7 percent of surgeons practicing in tertiary urban centers felt similarly. Recently, there has been much discussion of this problem in the surgical literature, and the consensus is that a "rural track" in general surgery training should be offered. The proposed curriculum of this track would include a true rotating internship followed by 3 years of general surgery core rotations and finishing with a final year that offers senior-level operative and management experience with basic orthopedic, ob/gyn, and urological problems (presumably this would be done by decreasing service time on such rotations as transplant and burn surgery). Proposals are afoot to implement such programs at the University of South Alabama and Oregon Health Sciences University. In Canada, the Royal College of Physicians and Surgeons of Canada has approved a core curriculum for "surgery in general" which includes a flexible year for those destined to practice rural surgery, so that they can obtain experience in other surgical disciplines. Queen's University in Ontario offers a community surgery postgraduate fellowship that tailors the community surgeon's extra training to his or her community's needs. Hopefully, this new awareness of the problem and the newly proposed programs will translate into surgeons who are more prepared for

rural practice and consequently more attracted to it.

CONCLUSIONS

Articles written by rural general surgeons testify to the unique satisfactions of their practice: using their full range of surgical skills, really getting to know their patients, playing a vital role in their communities, and having easy access to outdoor activities. Certainly their presence in rural areas provides better access to surgical and critical care for the inhabitants of these areas. Surgical services also appear to be vital to the economic viability of the rural hospital. Finally, a 1993 conference on rural health care sponsored by the University of South Alabama came to the conclusion that the presence of general surgery was a requirement for adequate health care in the rural setting. They emphasized the importance of the primary care and general surgery team concept. The presence of the general surgeon provides essential backup for rural family physicians.

However, in an era of a shortage of general surgeons nationwide, the percentage of rural general surgeons appears to be declining. Difficulty in obtaining suitable training, poor relative remuneration, long call hours, and professional isolation all contribute to recruitment difficulties. Policymakers are often urban academics and politicians (more likely to be doctors of jurisprudence than medicine by training) who have little grasp of the realities of rural medical practice. If they are serious about correcting the problem of medically underserved rural areas, they must offer general surgeons real incentives to practice in these areas. Such measures would include paying off educational debt, guaranteeing salaries, ensuring that the Medicare payment schedule does not punish rural surgeons, support for continuing medical education, locum tenens support, and shared practice arrangements. More well-designed studies are needed in the areas of incentives for rural surgeons, training for rural surgeons, and volume/outcomes–related research for surgeries performed in rural areas in order to inform the actions of both policymakers and rural surgeons.

Finally, one could posit that, given the current trends toward rural depopulation and economic centralization, the small-town rural surgeon is no longer necessary. Like the small-town independent hardware store, these surgeons may become a thing of the past and their clients may then have to travel to the nearest HMO satellite supermarket of medical care for their surgery—both elective and emergent. The difference here is that on-site rural surgeons are not just a convenience—they save lives. They are, to quote J. A. Spencer (a general surgeon practicing in Fort Francis, Ontario), "the real thing": "a real person who goes to work daily, and sometimes at night, not with the knowledge that you will be applying a well-known cure to a well-diagnosed ill, but with the knowledge that you will do your best, and your best will be infinitely better than nothing or a messy death during a transfer." In partnership with the rural family physician, the rural general surgeon forms the backbone of rural health care. If the rural populace is to have anything approaching the same standard of health care as urban residents, the training, incentives, and professional development of rural general surgeons must be carefully studied and made a priority by both the medical establishment and the government.

REFERENCES

1. Landercasper J, Bintz M, Cogbill T, et al: Spectrum of general surgery in rural America. *Arch Surg* 132:494, 1997.
2. Williamson H, Hart L, Pirani M, et al: Market shares for rural inpatient surgical services. *WWAMI Rural Health Working Paper Series.* Working paper no. 21. April 1993.
3. Wexler M: Presidential address, 1993: the general surgeon through the looking glass: bright reflections from a tarnished image. *Can J Surg* 37:4, 1994.
4. Sandrick J, Sabo R: Surgical practice in rural communities. *ACS Bull* 79:4, 1994.
5. Inglis F: Presidential address, 1994: the community general surgeon: a time for renaissance. *Can J Surg* 38:2, 1995.
6. Chiasson P, Roy P: The role of the general practitioner in the delivery of surgical and anesthesia services in rural western Canada. *Can Med Assoc J* 153:10, 1995.
7. Spencer JA: An endangered species: the community general surgeon. *Ann R Coll Phys Surg Can* 27:5, 1994.
8. Williamson H, Hart L, Pirani M, et al: Rural hospital inpatient surgical volume: cutting edge service or operating on the margin? *WWAMI Rural Health Working Paper Series.* Working paper no. 19. January 1993.
9. Callaghan J: Colorectal cancer in a small rural hospital. *Am J Surg* 159(3):277, 1990.
10. Bintz M: Rural trauma care: role of the general surgeon. *J Trauma* 41:3, 1996.
11. Grossman D, Rivara F, Rosenblatt R, et al: From roadside to bedside: the regionalization of motor vehicle trauma care in a remote rural county. *WWAMI Rural Health Working Paper Series.* Working paper no. 24. October 1993.
12. Richardson J, Cross T, Lee D, et al: Impact of level II verification on trauma admissions and transfer: comparisons of two rural hospitals. *J Trauma* 42:3, 1997.
13. Rinker C, McMurry F, Groeneweg V, et al: Emergency craniotomy in a rural level III trauma center. *J Trauma* 44:6, 1998.
14. Clark D, Cobean R, Radke F, et al: Management of major hepatic trauma involving interhospital transfer. *Am Surg* 60:11, 1994.
15. Rosenblatt R, Whitcomb M, Cullen T, et al: Which medical schools produce rural physicians? *JAMA* 268:12, 1992.
16. Kierath A, Hamdorf J, House A, et al: Developing visiting surgical services for rural and remote Australian communities. *Med J Aust* 168(9):454, 1998.
17. Cotton M: Five years as a flying surgeon in Zimbabwe. *World J Surg* 20:8, 1996.
18. Klein M, Ramoroko S, Jacobs A, et al: The cardiothoracic outreach program—a pilot project. *S Afr Med J* 86:12, 1996.
19. Dunbar P, Mayer J, Fordyce M, et al: Availability of anesthesia personnel in rural Washington and Montana. *Anesthesiology* 88:3, 1998.

20. Hart L, Pirani M, Rosenblatt R, et al: Causes and consequences of rural small hospital closures from the perspectives of mayors. *WWAMI Rural Health Working Paper Series*. Working paper no. 9. September 1990.

21. Pirani M, Hart L, Rosenblatt R, et al: Physician perspectives on the causes of rural hospital closure, 1980–1988. *J Am Board Fam Pract* 6:6, 1993.

22. Lambrecht C, Canham W, Gattey P, et al: Telemedicine and orthopaedic care: a review of 2 years of experience. *Clin Orthop* 348:228, 1998.

23. Chiasson P, Henshaw J, Roy P, et al: General surgical practice patterns in Nova Scotia: the role of the "generalist" general surgeon. *Can J Surg* 37:4, 1994.

CHAPTER 11

Home Care

Ian R. McWhinney

Eve Smith, 68 years old, is a retired factory worker who has never married. She has always lived in the house in which she was born, in an isolated section of the county. She has many friends in her neighborhood. Miss Smith's income is $478 per month. She is a diabetic and is knowledgeable about her diabetic regimen. Miss Smith has always taken pride in her independence and her ability to help her neighbors when they were in need of help. Recently she was hospitalized for complaints of constipation, with signs and symptoms of a bowel obstruction. Surgical intervention became necessary because of the extent of her obstruction. She was diagnosed with colon cancer, and a colostomy was performed. She was referred to home health services to educate her for colostomy care and evaluate her response to chemotherapy. A referral was made to the home health agency by the discharge planning department of the hospital and a nurse made a home visit the day after Miss Smith's discharge. On arrival, the nurse found her patient in a cluttered, dirty house, tearful, and verbalizing anger concerning her new colostomy.

The nurse made telephone contact with the physician and obtained an in-depth medical history, reporting her concerns about the patient's condition and behavior.

With the patient's input and acceptance, it was decided that physical therapy, medical social service, and a home health aide were needed to help Miss Smith. Interventions and goals for the plan of care were made by the nurse, physician, therapist, medical social worker, home health aide, and patient. The visiting nurse made the appropriate referrals and gave a report to each service. The physi-

cal therapist, medical social worker, and home health aide talked with the nurse on a weekly basis to evaluate Miss Smith's progress. The physician was given telephone and written reports on the patient's progress. Using the Family Caregiver Model, the nurse assessed the patient's readiness to learn her care; educated her in colostomy care; and mobilized resources such as Miss Smith's neighbors, the American Cancer Society, Meals on Wheels, and the Ostomy Organization. An evaluation phase was included at the end of 2, 4, and 9 weeks of service that included input from all the team members. Miss Smith was discharged from the Home Health Service Program independent in her care, receiving assistance and support from her friends and neighbors.[1]

Miss Smith is fairly typical of patients who receive home care in the rural areas of the United States. She is elderly and lives alone. She has strong roots in her community and a supportive network of friends and neighbors. The home assessment was done by a home health agency nurse, who developed a plan of care after telephone consultation with the patient's physician. As a rural patient, Miss Smith was fortunate to have the services of a physical therapist and medical social worker as well as those of a nurse and home health aide. The visiting nurse coordinated the patient's care and gave regular reports to the physician.

Home care is the fastest-growing sector of the American health care system. The increase is driven by several factors: demographic, economic, and technological. Elderly patients are by far the highest users of home care services, and the number and proportion of persons 65 years of age and older is increasing each year. As the "baby boomer" generation enters this age group, this increase will accelerate. The over-80 population is expected to double in the next 20 years and triple in the next 40 years, with the over 85-group growing faster than any other cohort. One out of every four Americans lives in a rural area, and elderly persons make up 15 percent of the population in small towns of 2500 to 10,000 residents, compared with 12 percent of the metropolitan population.[2] As Medicare beneficiaries, elderly patients are eligible for six types of home care services provided that they are homebound, under the care of a physician, or in need of skilled nursing or physical therapy on an intermittent basis. The six types of service are skilled nursing service; home health aide service; physical, occupational, and speech therapy; and medical social work. The requirement that the patient be homebound may cause difficulty in rural areas. A patient who cannot drive in an area with no public transport is essentially homebound, even though a neighbor drives her periodically to the hairdresser or other appointments.

The drive to reduce costs by decreasing hospital length of stay has increased the need for postdischarge home care. The closure of rural hospitals has added to the pressure on rural home care services. A total of 206 rural hospitals closed in the first 9 years of the 1980s, and the process is expected to continue.[3] This not only obliges patients and their families to travel long distances to urban hospitals but also increases the likelihood that discharge planners will have little knowledge or understanding of their home and community resources.

Recent advances in technology have favored the dispersal of health services. The information systems and medical technologies of the 1960s and 1970s favored concentration of patients in hospitals. Radiology, pathology, intravenous therapies, and monitoring techniques required cumbersome equipment. Information could not be rapidly transmitted over a distance. With paper as the medium, it made sense to concentrate a seriously ill patient's record in one place—the hospital. Surgical techniques required admission to hospital and long periods of postoperative care.

Now, point-of-care information systems can monitor patients in the home and transmit data to a distant nursing station. Nurses and physicians can enter and access data in an integrated patient record through a laptop or hand-held computer or through a computer in a patient's home. Interactive video enables patients, caregivers, physicians, and nurses to see and talk to each other across a distance. A demonstration project in rural Kansas[4] provides full interactive video and audio capacity between elderly patients in their homes and a telemedicine nurse. The system allows monitoring of blood pressure, medication, diabetic condition, diet, hygiene, and mental health status.

The following case history provides an example of the system's potential:

A 65-year-old woman with diabetes, high blood pressure, and manic-depressive disorder had been hospitalized multiple times for either hyper- or hypoglycemia. Psychiatric problems usually followed each of these episodes. The patient has been in the telemedicine program since June 1996. The telemedicine nurse has been monitoring the patient's insulin injections morning, noon, and night. At the start of the visits, the patient's blood sugar readings ranged from 100 to 500 mg/dL. In the second week of her care plan, the range was 100 to 375 mg/dL. She is now averaging 225 mg/dL. There have been no further hospitalizations.

The system attained a visual quality sufficient for the reading of syringes, glucometers, blood pressure meters, and medication labels. Adequate sound quality was very important and was eventually achieved with some difficulty. The role of the telemedicine nurse is a new one, and nurses have experienced a mismatch between the telemedicine situation and standard nursing procedures and protocols.[4]

The new communication technologies are in the process of development, and the next few years should see much progress in this field. New portable technologies include subcutaneous infusion pumps for insulin or opioids; intravenous pumps for antibiotics, chemotherapy, or parenteral nutrition; tools for the self-monitoring of blood glucose and blood pressure; bedside blood biochemistry; pulse oximetry; and respirometry and respiratory support. Intravenous therapy is the fastest-growing sector of home care.

Thanks to new monitoring and therapeutic technologies, patients at risk for such conditions as preterm labor can be managed at home in a collaboration between the home care team and the tertiary care specialist.[5] Early thrombolysis given to rural patients with myocardial infarction, before transfer to hospital, can reduce the risk of death.[6] Advances in pain management—with skilled use of drugs by oral, rectal, or transcutaneous routes or by subcutaneous infusion—allow patients with advanced cancer to remain at home.

ASSESSMENT OF PATIENTS IN THE HOME

It is difficult to express in words the difference between knowing patients by their visits to the office and knowing them as a visitor to their homes. The home is where a family's values are expressed. It is in the home that people can be themselves. The history of the family—its story, its joys and sorrows, its memories and aspirations—is there on the walls. What one can learn in the home is often of real practical value. For this reason assessment in the home is different from assessment in the office or the hospital. Instead of asking about activities of daily living, we see patients in their own bedrooms, bathrooms, and kitchens; climbing their own stairs; and so on. When we review the medications, we can assemble them all, including those from the bathroom cabinet, by the bedside or on the kitchen table. We can sense for ourselves either the peace or the tension in the home. We can meet with the family on their own ground, where they are most likely to express their feelings. In the home, the patient can be in control of his or her own care, and this can be a powerful influence on healing. The word *ecology* is derived from the Greek word *oikos*, meaning "home," so ecology is the study of living things in their environmental home. A physician or nurse who works in the home is a practicing ecologist.

For rural physicians covering a wide area and scattered population, visiting patients in their homes poses formidable problems. The rewards, however, are great, even for a single visit: the relationship with patient and family may be deepened and enhanced; there is often a deeper understanding of the patient's illness; and the ground is laid for more effective communication between doctor and nurse.

All home care referrals should begin with an assessment in the home. The home care agency may have a standard assessment protocol that can be followed by any health care professional. The development of a common assessment protocol can save multiple assessments by professionals from different disciplines. Each of the professionals can add items from his or her own perspective. Hospital discharge planning can often be more effective if an assessment of the home can be done before the patient is discharged.

The following account of home care assessment uses a patient with advanced cancer as an example. Given a continuing relationship, the assessment may be done cumulatively, not necessarily all at once. However, to form a plan of care, it is important to cover all the following aspects. Some will need to be repeated as the patient's condition or circumstances change.

1. *Clinical assessment.* This follows much the same process as a clinical assessment in the hospital or office except that in the home one is teaching the family caregivers how to make their own assessment. The symptom review and physical examination will pay special

attention to pain, bowel function, sleep pattern, and condition of mouth and skin. Since patients often do not identify their suffering as pain, one must look for physical evidence of pain: the furrowed brow, the awkward position, the groaning or grimacing on movement. These are especially important when clouding of consciousness impairs verbal expression.

2. *Functional assessment: mobility and activities of daily living.* This can go hand in hand with an assessment of the layout of the home: the bedroom, bathroom, stairs, and kitchen, identifying hazards that can be removed or avoided. The functional assessment may result in modifications to the home (e.g., a bath rail) or a recommendation for reassignment of space (e.g., move patient's room to the ground floor to avoid stairs).

3. *Assessment of the patient's state of mind: cognitive function, mood, and feelings.* The ability of the patient to cope with changes and crises will depend on his or her understanding of the illness, peace of mind, and confidence in the caregivers. Deficiencies in these areas can result in avoidable readmission to hospital.[7] It is important to address patients' hopes and fears. Kay Toombs,[8] writing of her own experience with advanced multiple sclerosis, notes that fears are nearly always specific (e.g., fear of dying in pain rather than fear of dying) and can often therefore be laid to rest.

4. *Assessment of caregiver's well-being.* Caring for a loved one at home can be exhausting, both physically and emotionally. Exhaustion of the caregiver is a common reason for the failure of home care. Home care services in rural areas are often tightly stretched in comparison with those in urban areas. Rural patients and their families are more likely to depend on support from informal networks of care. Caregivers often have difficulty in articulating their needs or feel that they should not draw attention to themselves. It is important to ask: "How are *you* doing?" "What

support do you have?" "How much sleep are you getting?" "Are you getting some relief?"

5. *Assessment of the family's needs.* Caring for a loved one with a serious illness or disability at home is an emotional experience for the family. Difficulties may arise with relationships even in the closest of families: For example, difficulties of dealing with the patient's anger, or resentments over perceptions that some family members are not "pulling their weight." Family members with unmet needs may be those who are most inarticulate, such as the siblings of a disabled child or schizophrenic adolescent, or school-aged children of a dying patient. It is common for family members to have major misconceptions about the patient's diagnosis, prognosis, or therapy. A family conference in the home can be a way of identifying some of these problems and beginning to address them. It may be difficult, in a rural area, to have all members of the home care team present, but time spent in achieving this can be rewarded by a better home environment.

6. *Review of medications.* The family caregivers and (if possible) the patient should understand the purpose of each medication, the reasons for the dosage schedule, and the difference between "as needed" and regular medication. Assessment in the home provides the opportunity to identify and explain each medication to the caregiver.

7. *Nutrition.* The advantage of home assessment is that a review of diet can include checking of food supplies and the preparation area, education of the patient, and identification of need for supplements or Meals on Wheels.

8. *Assessment of resources.* In rural areas, the informal community resources will often be especially important. A knowledge of community resources is important for home care professionals, including such items as night sitters for dying patients, respite care, day care, and services for the blind. The availability of equipment such as commodes, wheel-

chairs, and walking supports can be a problem in rural areas.

THE PLAN OF CARE

Ideally, this should be formulated by the nurse or case manager and the patient's physician, each contributing from his or her own knowledge of the patient, the family, the home, and the resources. In patients with unstable or progressive disease, it should include clear directions for the caregiver about how to respond to sudden changes and crises and how to reach a nurse or physician. In situations of high caregiver stress—such as terminal illness, Alzheimer's disease, and schizophrenia—there should be an assurance of a home visit in response to calls for help. In such stressful cases it is preferable for the physician to make regularly scheduled home visits rather than visits only on demand. Caregivers often find it difficult to articulate their needs and often do not call for help, even when in despair. Under current conditions of staff shortages and financial constraints, these standards may be difficult to achieve. In practice, the plan is more usually developed by the case manager nurse and approved by the physician, who has not done a home assessment.

CLINICAL DIAGNOSIS IN HOME HEALTH CARE PATIENTS

Information about diagnostic frequencies is available from Medicare billings and from the 1996 survey of home health (HH) agencies and hospices conducted by the National Center for Health Statistics. The three most frequent admission diagnoses in home health agency patients were heart disease, musculoskeletal disorders, and diabetes mellitus[9] (Table 11-1). These accounted for 25 percent of all first-listed diagnoses, and 72 percent of the patients were over 65 years of age. Among hospice patients, 77 percent were admitted with a diagnosis of cancer and 8 percent with heart disease, while 78 percent of hospice patients received care at home. Although 27 percent of Medicare enrollees live in rural (nonmetropolitan) areas,[10] fewer than 20 percent of patients being served at the time of the survey were enrolled with nonmetropolitan agencies. Table 11-2 shows the top 13 primary diagnostic categories for Medicare patients in urban and rural areas in 1987, ac-

TABLE 11-1   CHARACTERISTICS OF PATIENTS RECEIVING CARE FROM HOME HEALTH AGENCIES AND HOSPICES IN 1996

	Home Health[a] Patients		Hospice Patients	
Current Patients[b]	2,427,500		59,400	
Patients aged >64 (%)	72.2%		77.7%	
Most frequent first-listed admission diagnosis	Heart disease	10.8%	Cancer	58.3%
	Musculoskeletal disorders	8.7%	Heart disease	8.3%
	Diabetes mellitus	8.4%		
Location of agency				
Metropolitan	80.4%		81.1%	
Nonmetropolitan	19.6%		18.9%	

[a]A few agencies provide both home health and hospice care.

[b]Current patients are patients who were on the rolls of the agency as of midnight on the day before the survey.

SOURCE: From Haupt,[9] with permission.

TABLE 11-2   PERCENT DISTRIBUTION OF HOME HEALTH USERS, BY DIAGNOSIS AND RESIDENTIAL LOCATION: 1987

Diagnosis	Overall	Rural	Urban
		Percent	
Total	100.00	100.00	100.00
Malignant neoplasm	10.62	10.08	10.81
Cerebrovascular diseases	7.95	8.12	7.89
Diabetes mellitus	6.14	7.61	5.67
Bone and hip fractures	8.11	6.81	8.57
Digestive system diseases	5.52	5.08	5.61
Ischemic heart disease	5.36	4.83	5.55
Arthropathies	4.80	4.47	4.92
Heart disease	3.35	3.63	3.25
Hypertension	2.92	3.60	2.68
Chronic obstructive pulmonary disease	3.20	3.07	3.25
Chronic ulcers of skin	2.70	2.92	2.62
Incontinence	1.48	1.65	1.41
Urinary tract infections	1.25	1.51	1.16
Other	36.59	36.62	36.59

SOURCE: From Kenney,[10] with permission.

counting for 63 percent of all first listed diagnoses.[10] Since the Medicare data include both HH agencies and hospices, malignant neoplasm is the most frequent diagnosis in Medicare patients, but not in the HH agency data alone. If the categories "ischemic heart disease" and "heart disease" in Table 11-2 are combined, heart disease becomes the second most frequent diagnosis in Medicare patients. Cerebrovascular disease, diabetes mellitus, and arthropathies are high on both lists. Twenty-five percent of the HH agency patients were under the age of 65. Urban Medicare patients are 26 percent more likely to receive home care for bone and hip fractures, and rural patients are 35 percent more likely to have a diagnosis of diabetes mellitus or hypertension. Although technology transfer from hospital to home accounts for some of the increase in home care, it is clear from Tables 11-1 and 11-2 that a great majority of patients have common clinical problems requiring skilled nursing and conventional medical care

rather than complex specialized care. Among less frequent diagnostic categories are some that make heavy demands on family caregivers and home care services alike. Alzheimer's disease in older patients and schizophrenia in young adults are notable in this regard.[10]

Although the elderly are by far the greatest users of home care services, we must not lose sight of the fact that younger adults and children with chronic diseases and disabilities also have significant needs for home care, sometimes involving complex technologies. For some categories of home care services—intravenous therapy, for example—younger adults are the prime users. For example, in the Hospital in the Home Program in Hawkesbury, Ontario, based on a 110-bed community hospital, only 44 percent of patients were over age 65 in 1993 and 65 percent received intravenous therapy. A need for acute care was one of the criteria for admission to the program, and the average length of stay was 8 to 12 days.[11]

COMPLEX TECHNOLOGIES IN THE HOME

Table 11-3 lists some of the complex technologies now available in the home.[11] These are complex because they require multidisciplinary teams, education of patients and family caregivers, and well-organized support, with assurance of a rapid response to crisis. Shortages of specialized personnel, long distances, and thinly spread emergency services can make it difficult to provide these services in rural areas.

Intravenous Therapy

In the United States, infusion therapy is the fastest-growing sector of home care, with costs increasing from $1.5 billion in 1988 to $2.6 billion in 1990. Home intravenous antibiotic therapy is widely available in the United States, but lack of specialized personnel can create difficulties in rural areas. Programs typically involve a team that may include intravenous nurse specialists, clinical pharmacists, infectious disease specialists, and social workers. Patients are trained in aseptic technique and recognition of drug reactions. Twenty-four-hour emergency care is a requirement for this service. Home care is not always provided by these programs, in

TABLE 11-3   COMPLEX HOME CARE TECHNOLOGIES

Intravenous therapy
Blood transfusion
Drug delivery systems: pumps for administering drugs for diabetes mellitus, cancer therapy, or pain
Home parenteral nutrition
Home enteral nutrition by nasogastric tube
Respiratory therapy: oxygen concentrators and cylinders, mechanical ventilation, tracheostomy management
Renal and peritoneal dialysis

which case patients have to attend outpatient clinics.

Home Parenteral Nutrition

Home parenteral nutrition (HPN) has been made possible by developments such as the long-term indwelling Silastic catheter and has been shown to be cost-effective.[11] Patients usually infuse solutions during a 10- to 12-hour period at night. HPN is organized through hospitals and a home assessment is carried out to ensure that strict hygiene is observed. Training of patients in the technique takes place in the hospital. The main indications for HPN are as follows:

- Short bowel syndrome
- Nutrition combined with cancer chemotherapy
- Inflammatory bowel disease
- Chronic fistula of digestive tract
- Scleroderma of digestive tract

HPN may be a long- or short-term therapy. It has been growing rapidly in the United States, where companies marketing nutritional support products have become involved in assessing, educating, and treating patients and in monitoring the quality of care. Nutritional support teams are well established in the United States and typically consist of nurses, physicians, nutritionists, and pharmacists.

Home Enteral Nutrition

Home enteral nutrition (HEN) is also an increasingly common service in the United States. In 1987, almost 8000 people were receiving HEN, most of them over age 65. HEN can be applied to a wider range of patients than HPN; it is also easier to administer and less costly. Tubes can be changed by patients, caregivers, or nurses.

HEN has been estimated to be growing by 25 to 30 percent annually.[11]

Oxygen Therapy

Oxygen therapy is widely available at home, by either cylinder or oxygen concentrator, and is commonly prescribed for chronic obstructive pulmonary disease (COPD). Mechanical ventilation in the home is used for respiratory failure due to spinal cord injury or neuromuscular disease. It can be provided either through a tracheostomy, by external pressure to the chest wall, or by intermittent positive pressure through a nasal mask. France has a national home respiratory care program. There, 28 regional organizations serve over 50,000 people with respiratory problems, of whom, in 1986, some 1200 required prolonged ventilation assistance and 12,000 received respirator care for 12 to 24 hours a day. Ventilator-dependent patients and their families are vulnerable people and require well-organized support, with the assurance of a rapid response to crises. There is no margin for error either in the equipment or in the support system.[11]

Dialysis

Dialysis for end-stage renal disease (ESRD), either renal or peritoneal, can be carried out in the home. However, home renal dialysis is possible only for the limited number of patients with the necessary home environment and family support.

SERVICES IN THE HOME: RECENT TRENDS IN HOME VISITS BY NURSES, PHYSICIANS, AND OTHER HEALTH PROFESSIONALS

The increase in home care services began in the 1980s and has continued into the 1990s. Figure 11-1 shows the number of visits paid to the home by nurses, physicians, and all health care

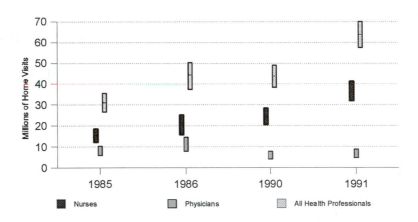

* From the National Health Interview Survey, National Center for Health Statistics, U.S. Department of Health and Human Services; 95% confidence interval ($p = 0.05$). Analysis of visits by nurses and physicians carried out in the Centre for Studies in Family Medicine, University of Western Ontario, on data supplied by the National Center for Health Statistics.

FIGURE 11-1 Home visits by health professionals, 1985–1991. (From McWhinney IR: Fourth Annual Nicholas J. Pisacano lecture: the doctor, the patient, and the home: returning to our roots. J Am Board Fam Pract 10(6):430–435, 1997, with permission.)

professionals in the years 1985, 1986, 1990, and 1991. The numbers are derived from the National Health Interview survey and includes all age groups. Visits by all health care professionals doubled from 31 million in 1985 to 63.6 million in 1991. Visits by nurses increased from 15.4 million to 36.5 million. Home visits by physicians were not significantly different at 8 million in 1985 and 6.7 million in 1991.[12]

The low numbers of home visits by physicians has been confirmed in studies using other sources of data. In a national questionnaire survey of physicians in 1991, family physicians reportedly made an average of only 21.2 home visits per year, and 35 percent did not make any. General internists made even fewer visits. Rural practitioners, however, made more home visits than urban practitioners and referred more patients to home health agencies.[13]

A study based on claims for home visits to Medicare patients not enrolled in HMOs showed that only 0.88 percent of Medicare patients received home visits in 1993.[14] Those in rural areas and in areas with a high ratio of physicians to population had an increased likelihood of receiving a home visit.[14] Billings to Medicare for physician home visits declined 31 percent from 1988 to 1993 and 12.3 percent between 1993 and 1996. The decreasing involvement of physicians in home care in the United States is in contrast to the situation in Europe, where general practitioners in most countries make several home visits a day. In England and Wales, 10 percent of general practitioner services are provided in the home.[15]

Although physicians in the United States make fewer home visits, they are still obliged to make referrals to home care agencies and expected to collaborate with case managers and home care nurses in formulating care plans for their patients. They are also responsible for prescribing and for making clinical judgments about patients. To perform these functions effectively, physicians should be skilled in assessing patients in the home and knowledgeable about their patients' home circumstances and community resources. In practice, home health agency personnel often develop the home care plan of treatment on their own because the physician is insufficiently familiar with the patient's home care needs or with home care regulations.[16]

Lack of physician involvement in home care has some potentially serious consequences. Without a medical assessment in the home, elderly patients may be transported long distances to emergency departments or admitted to hospital.[17] If patients cannot be moved, clinical decisions may be based on secondhand information, which may compromise the quality of care. The declining rate of home visits is probably attributable to two causes: inadequate training of physicians in the skills of home care and low rates of remuneration for home visits. Rural physicians, who often have to travel long distances to patients' homes, are especially vulnerable to economic factors.

SERVICES IN THE HOME: RURAL AND URBAN DIFFERENCES

Elderly patients in rural areas use home care less than their urban counterparts; but when they do, they have more visits than urban users. Rural patients receive more skilled nursing and home health aide visits and fewer visits by physio-, occupational, or speech therapists or by medical social workers (Table 11-4). The latter observation still holds true after controlling for primary diagnosis (Table 11-4). The range of services is more limited in rural areas, and within any one service, rural residents have fewer alternative forms from which to choose.[18] Rural residents place more reliance on informal helpers such as family, friends, and neighbors. Whether this is an advantage for rural patients or a response to deficiencies in formal services is difficult to say. Deficiencies in specialized home care services in rural areas have been found in specific conditions such as diabetes, suggesting that these deficiencies may have an effect on outcome.[19]

TABLE 11-4   MEAN NUMBER OF VISITS PROVIDED, BY RESIDENTIAL LOCATION: 1987

Type of Visit	Mean		Rural Mean Divided by Urban Mean
	Rural	Urban	
Total visits	25.8	22.6	1.14
Skilled nursing	13.39	11.49	1.17
Home health aide	9.83	7.12	1.38
Physical therapy	2.02	2.93	0.69
Occupational therapy	0.16	0.42	0.38
Speech therapy	0.26	0.32	0.81
Medical social services	0.13	0.28	0.46

SOURCE: From Kenney,[10] with permission.

PATIENTS WITH SPECIAL NEEDS

Children

There are an estimated 1 million children in the United States with chronic diseases such as cystic fibrosis, muscular dystrophy, and cerebral palsy. Some of these are medically fragile and dependent on technology, such as mechanical ventilation, dialysis, or total parenteral nutrition. Such children are now much more likely than before to be cared for at home. In rural areas, the highly specialized care needed by such children is often not available, either nursing or medical care. To fill the need, nurses and physicians responsible for the child's care can be offered in-service training before the child is discharged from hospital. Good discharge planning is crucial. If the distance is not too great, community nurses, the family physician, family caregivers, and special education teachers can attend the planning meetings. For remote rural areas, an instructional videotape or a two-way video conference can be arranged. The process should include anticipatory planning for the handling of acute episodes and crises and for liaison between the tertiary care center and the home care team. When a rural area has several medically fragile children, periodic visits by the specialist team can enhance communication and collaboration.[20]

Modern neonatal care has increased the survival rate of preterm infants, who may be discharged home with special care needs. Zelle[21] has described a partnership between a hospital and six California counties for the follow-up of at-risk infants in the home. Planning for discharge and follow-up begins when infants are admitted to the nursery. A hospital-based clinical nurse specialist (CNS) plays a key role in consulting with the community home nurse (CHN) before and after the discharge. The CHN continues to support the family and monitor the infant's progress after discharge, with the CNS providing consultation and support as needed. Parents who have developed skills in caring for their own babies may become resources for other parents in their community.

Clarke[22] has described the challenges of a family physician caring for a technology-dependent infant in rural Alberta. The infant, born with oculoauriculovertebral dysplasia, was transferred from a level III neonatal unit to the community hospital at 10 weeks with an oropharyngeal airway and gastrostomy. It was here that the parents learned to manage the airway and tube feeding. Before discharge, the home was equipped with oxygen, suction equipment, room intercoms, wall charts showing cardiopulmonary resuscitation techniques, and an intravenous pole stand. The infant remained under 24-hour observation at home until the age of 22 months, with shift nursing provided by the health unit. The family physician had a central role in coordinating care, supporting the parents during the physical and emotional stresses of this time, and ensuring that they were fully informed and understood the consequences of each management decision.

Patients with AIDS

In the West, patients with AIDS, and services for them, tend to be concentrated in urban areas. Patients in rural areas, and their caregivers, are often isolated from support groups. A rural physician may have had little experience with AIDS; infectious disease specialists and nurses are often few and far between. Lacking the range of services available in urban areas, patients and their caregivers rely very heavily on their family physicians for care and support.

Chial and Elliott[23] interviewed 15 family and volunteer caregivers of patients with HIV/AIDS in the Duluth area of Minnesota. The caregivers relied on family physicians for education about the disease and for knowledge of community resources, such as housing, extended care, and AIDS organizations. They wanted physicians and nurses to acknowledge them as members of the team. None of the interviewers had participated in a caregiver support group. One outcome of the study was the formation of a support group in Duluth.

Patients with Advanced Cancer

Cancer patients in rural areas have long distances to travel for treatment in urban oncology units. This can be avoided if oncology services are regionalized, with branch clinics in areas throughout the region. When rural patients with advanced cancer become housebound, they rely on their family physicians for their medical care. The transition from care by oncologist to care by the family physician requires good communication throughout all phases of treatment. Frequently, this is not the case. After the initial referral to oncology, the family physician may lose touch with the patient and have difficulty picking up the threads when the patient becomes terminally ill.[24] The follow-up of most cancer patients is well within the capacity of generalist physicians working in collaboration with oncologists.

The Rural Poor

Poverty in rural households can pose special difficulties for home care services. In some areas of extreme poverty, few households have indoor plumbing and telephones, and some may have no electricity. These deficiencies obviously place limitations on complex home care. Lack of transportation may prevent others from attending for prenatal care, or from bringing their children for immunization. Visits by public health nurses are especially important for these vulnerable families.

MANAGEMENT AND INTEGRATION

A number of management issues face home care services, both urban and rural. The team providing care for a patient in the home requires leadership and coordination, whether it is a two-person team of nurse and physician or a much more complex team providing complex technological care. The usual approach to this is the designation of a case manager, usually a nurse, for each patient. The case manager may be one of the care providers but more usually is responsible for the initial assessment of the patient, "brokering" of services, ongoing coordination of the services, and communication with other agencies and with informal caregivers.[1] At another level of the agency, a manager is responsible for taking referrals, determining eligibility, and assigning case managers to patients.

Since medical services are often provided differently from home care services, referring physicians are usually outside the home care agency even though they are members of the home care team. In patients with stable clinical conditions and infrequent needs for medical services, the separation of the physician from the agency may not cause difficulties. However, among the increasing number of home care patients who have acute illness and complex clinical problems, communication between physician and agency can be a serious problem. By appointing a medical director, an agency can enhance communication with attending physicians, but this does not necessarily integrate physicians' services with those of others.

One approach to the integration of services is the type of organization known as the hospital in the home (HITH). This brings together the home care services and attending physicians into one organization, just as a conventional hospital integrates physicians with other services. The HITH may be set up as a department of an acute care hospital or as a freestanding institution. The HITH model is probably more appropriate for urban than for rural areas. One exception, however, is the New Brunswick Extramural Hospital, which serves the mostly rural population of a Canadian province.[25]

In rural areas, merging primary care centers and home health services has the potential for increasing administrative efficiency.[26] Liaison with the regional hospital can enhance integration. The creation of a common computerized record system has the greatest potential for integrating services.

EDUCATION FOR HOME CARE

If health care professionals are to be adequately prepared for home care, the home must be part of the environment of learning in health sciences education. Nursing has a long and unbroken tradition of home care, and nursing education has continued to make the home a part of the learning environment. Not so with medicine. The modern medical curriculum has produced a generation of physicians overwhelmingly trained in the hospital environment. It is not surprising that home health agencies find many physicians to lack the knowledge and skills necessary for home care. As some acute and complex care is transferred from hospital to home, primary care physicians are likely to find themselves ill equipped to meet their patients' needs. Residency programs in primary care, especially family medicine, should now be making home care an integral part of their clinical experience. For residents to make occasional home visits will not be sufficient. The question for future physicians will not be: "Do you make house calls?" but "Can you be an effective member of the home care team, assuming leadership of the team when appropriate, based on your clinical skills, knowledge of the patient and family, and mastery of home care technologies?"

ACKNOWLEDGMENTS

Lynn Dunikowski and the staff of the College of Family Physicians of Canada Library provided bibliographic support. Linda Boyd prepared successive drafts of the manuscript.

REFERENCES

1. Esposito L: Home health case management: rural caregiving. *Home Healthcare Nurse* 12(3):38–43, 1994.
2. Magilvy JK, Congdon JG, Martinez R: Circles of care: home care and community support for rural older adults. *Adv Nurs Sci* 16(3):22–33, 1994.
3. Hart LG, Amundson BA, Roseblatt RA: Rural health policy: is there a role for the small rural hospital? *J Rural Health* 6(2):101–117, 1990.
4. Lindberg CCS. Implementation of in-home telemedicine in rural Kansas: answering an elderly patient's needs. *JAMA* 4(1):14–17, 1997.
5. Vrbicky K, Hill WC, Lambertz EL, Jurgensen WW Jr: Home uterine activity monitoring in a rural setting. *Obstet Gynecol* 76(1)(suppl):82S–84S, 1990.
6. Vale L, Silcock J, Rawles J: An economic evaluation of thrombolysis in a remote rural community. *BMJ* 314:570–572, 1997.
7. McWilliam CL: From hospital to home: elderly patients' discharge experiences. *Fam Med* 24(6): 457–468, 1992.
8. Toombs SK: *The Meaning of Illness: A Phenomenological Account of the Different Perspectives of Physician and Patient.* Dordrecht, The Netherlands, Kluwer, 1992.
9. Haupt BJ: An overview of home health and hospice care patients: 1996 home and hospice care survey. *Advance Data* 297:4–9, 1998.
10. Kenney GM: Rural and urban differentials in Medicare home health use. *Health Care Fin Rev* 14(4):39–57, 1993.
11. McWhinney IR: *Physician Services in the Home: Planning for the Integrated Home Care of Acute and Complex Illness.* Working paper series no. 95-1. London, Ontario, Canada, Centre for Studies in Family Medicine, March 1995, pp 1–23.
12. McWhinney IR: Fourth Annual Nicholas J. Pisacano lecture: the doctor, the patient, and the

home: returning to our roots. *J Am Board Fam Pract* 10(6):430–435, 1997.

13. Keenan JM, Boling PA, Schwartzberg JG, et al: A national survey of the home visiting practice and attitudes of family physicians and internists. *Arch Intern Med* 152:2025–2032, 1992.

14. Meyer GS, Gibbons RV: House calls to the elderly—a vanishing practice among physicians. *N Engl J Med* 337(25):1815–1820, 1997.

15. Aylin P, Majeed FA, Cook DG: Home visiting by general practitioners in England and Wales. *BMJ* 313:207–210, 1996.

16. Boling PA, Keenan JM, Schwartzberg J, et al: Reported home health agency referrals by internists and family physicians. *J Am Geriatr Soc* 40:1241–1249, 1992.

17. Philbrick JT, Connelly JE, Corbett EC Jr: Home visits in a rural office practice: clinical spectrum and effect on utilization of health care services. *J Gen Intern Med* 7:522–527, 1992.

18. Coward RT, Cutler SJ: Informal and formal health care systems for the rural elderly. *Health Services Res* 23(6):785–806, 1989.

19. Cheh V, Phillips B: Adequate access to posthospital home health services: differences between urban and rural areas. *J Rural Health* 9(4):262–269, 1993.

20. Wheeler TW, Lewis CC: Home care for medically fragile children: urban versus rural settings. *Issues Comp Pediatr Nurs* 16:13–30, 1993.

21. Zelle RS: Follow-up of at-risk infants in the home setting: consultation model. *J Obstet Gynecol Neonatal Nurs* 24(1):51–55, 1995.

22. Clarke JE: Rural home care of a technology-dependent infant. *Can Fam Physician* 41:1051–1056, 1995.

23. Chial H, Elliott BA: Caring for persons with AIDS in greater Minnesota. *Minn Med* 80:43–45, 1997.

24. McWhinney IR, Hoddinott SN, Bass MJ, et al: Role of the family physician in the care of cancer patients. *Can Fam Physician* 36:2183–2186, 1990.

25. Ferguson G: Designed to serve: the New Brunswick Extra-Mural Hospital. *J Ambul Care Manager* 16(3):40–50, 1993.

26. Zuckerman HS, Smith DG: The merger of rural primary care and home health services. *J Rural Health* 7(1):39–50, 1991.

CHAPTER 12

Rural Mental Health

L. Thomas Wolff   John Dewar   Fraser Tudiver

"I don't know what to do with this guy," says a rural family physician. "He's got traits of obsessive compulsive disorder and panic attacks, so I put him on Paxil and he got worse. He went to see a private psychologist, but he doesn't think it's helping. It's costing an arm and a leg, and the psychologist won't tell me anything because of his overblown ideas of confidentiality, even though the patient asked him to. So I talked to the psychiatrist who's the director of the county mental health clinic. He told me about a couple of therapists on their staff who he thought could help, but when I called to set up an appointment with one of them, the clinic staff said I couldn't pick and choose a particular therapist—my patient just had to take the next one in turn. Meanwhile the guy drives 30 miles out of his way just because he can't stand to drive anywhere if the trip doesn't start at his own home. He's a painting contractor who is self-employed and doesn't have any insurance, so he can't afford to be spending his time in counseling, and if I send him to someone else who doesn't help, I think he'll just bag counseling altogether."

*T*he challenges in the delivery of rural mental health care are complex and mirror those of rural health care delivery in general. These challenges are availability, accessibility, affordability, appropriateness, adequacy, and acceptability. They may be perceived as barriers or as facilitators, depending on whether one is a patient, a health care provider, a policymaker, or an insurer. Each challenge may be different not only in rural versus urban settings but also *among* rural settings, reflecting the variability as well as the unique character of each community.[1] The complexity of the issue is well documented by Blank and associates.[2] They point out that addressing financial constraints as the principal barrier to accessing mental health services for rural persons is short-sighted. The current system is distant, unfamiliar, and unacceptable to many rural patients. The use of facility-based concepts derived from urban hubs seems of limited value in rural settings. General lack of knowledge about mental illness—its causes, consequences, and treatments—often leads to stigmatization and intolerance.

Assumptions and Perceptions

Several assumptions about rural communities that have affected the development (or lack thereof) of mental health services are challenged. First, it is assumed that rural health communities are more closely knit, offering more support and assistance to one another than urban centers. In actuality, however, factors such as the outmigration of young people,[3] reduced social support for rural elderly from their families,[4] and urban workers living in rural communities dilute the sense of community in many rural environments. Second, it is assumed that rural people have substantial ties to larger population centers or regional hubs and will therefore use centralized mental health services. This is true of urban workers living in rural centers but not of indigenous rural people.[3] Finally, rural populations are believed to be at low risk as compared with urban populations for mental health problems. Actually, however, rural populations are at no lower risk than urbanites and are less likely to use facility-based services.[5]

De Facto System

Rural Montana is much different from rural New York, but family physicians in either place are faced with patients who are most likely to bring all their health problems to their doorstep. The ''de facto mental health service system''[6] in rural areas—which includes primary physicians, ministers, and counselors not trained in mental health as well as self-help groups, family, and friends—has often precluded the development and use of mental health services.[2] Since this system exists in rural areas, persons without a mental health provider often experience difficulty in accessing mental health care.[7,8] Limited accessibility often stems from problems in availability and acceptability of mental health care.[2,9] There are shortages of mental health workers, especially in psychiatry, in rural areas.[7] Because of the stigma that mental health may carry, rural people are often unwilling to seek mental health care, even from available providers. In small towns where people know whose vehicle is parked by the mental health center, the stigma may even be perceived as greater. Ironically, people with serious and persistent mental illness are often cared for by the strength of smaller communities—that is, the network of strong family and social relationships as well as religious conviction.[10] Distances, poor road conditions, and travel problems further hinder accessibility for people in rural areas from obtaining mental health services. Geriatric age groups are especially affected. They make up a higher percentage of rural than of urban populations[9] and face the limitations of inadequate Medicare payments for services, particularly to psychologists and social workers, who make up the largest component of available mental health workers in these areas. Thus affordability becomes an issue.

HISTORY, PHILOSOPHY, AND PERCEPTIONS

Historically, what has been available to help the primary practitioner serve these patients has changed significantly over the past 30 years. In the 1950s and 1960s, severely mentally ill patients were often institutionalized and medications to help control behavior were limited. Over the next three decades, several programs were initiated based mainly on urban models, with varying degrees of success.[2]

The biopsychosocial model of integrating physical health with the patient's state of mind and environment has been recognized for many years, but it has not been integrated into our systems of care. This is especially important, since the ''rural mind-set'' significantly affects the way in which these people perceive themselves, others, and their health.

Federal Programs/Economic Impacts

The Community Mental Health Centers Act of 1963 created a new mechanism for organizing the majority of rural mental health efforts. Over the next 20 years, through direct federal funding to local communities, rural community mental health centers were made available with a broad range of mental health services. The Omnibus Budget Reconciliation Act (OBRA) of 1981 changed this dramatically. Direct federal funding to the communities was shifted to large block grants to the states. At the same time, programs to deinstitutionalize patients were being promoted. This changed the programmatic focus of a wide variety of community mental health services through the Community Rural Mental Health Centers toward an emphasis on persons with serious mental illness—a much narrower scope.[11] It resulted in a 25 percent reduction in federal support for mental health services[12] and lack of professional and community capacity to cope with this increased number of patients.[13,14] It placed an increasing emphasis on fee-generating services, which further limited access by the rural poor. The OBRAs of 1987 and 1989, however, increased access to psychologists and clinical social workers by allowing reimbursement for their services under Medicare and Medicaid. However, the payment schedules were often inadequate.[5] Through all these changes, the available rural mental health services were still inadequate compared with those available to the larger urban centers.[5,15]

Mental versus Physical Health

Mental health and physical health have historically been considered separate entities even though the biopsychosocial model of health is now well recognized. The linking of primary care and rural psychiatry has been the goal of many policymakers for over 30 years.[16] It remains a difficult goal not only because of inadequate numbers of psychiatrists and mental health workers in rural areas but also because of the views mental health and primary care hold of each other.[7] From a mental health perspective, primary care providers often either fail to detect mental illness or do not adequately treat it.[17,18] The rural primary physicians feel they are able to detect mental disorders, but often they do not formally diagnose them for various reasons: to protect patient confidentiality, because there are too few specialists with whom to consult, or because they cannot receive adequate reimbursement for their time.[19,20] These perceptions from within the provider community compounded by the perceptions of patients in the rural areas regarding mental illness make access to adequate mental health care even more difficult.

Rural Mind-Set

"I'm just sitting home waiting to die," says the 85-year-old widow. "Ever since Bill died, I've been this way. I don't see anybody. I don't speak to my sisters any more—they as good as told me that I stole my mother's things, and I was the one who took care of her all those years." I can remind her all I want that the offense by her sisters was many years past, and that her depressed mood preceded her husband's death, to no avail. Meanwhile my prescription for sertraline is sitting unused on her countertop, according to the reports from her nephew, and any suggestion to seek mental health counseling meets with angry rejection. "I'm not one of those crazy people who goes to psychiatrists!"

Country people are different from city people. That is clear to anyone who has lived in both kinds of communities. Among the common rural problems is the stigma of seeking help for mental illness, especially among the generations that grew up before the 1960s. Younger rural residents tend to be less hesitant to accept mental health treatment, perhaps reflecting the reduced isolation of rural communities in recent decades or the improved access to care since the advent of community mental health centers.[9] The farm crisis that grew to public prominence in the mid-1980s initiated a wave of depression and suicidality among displaced farmers. This segment of the population proved to be unwilling to seek mental health treatment, with sometimes devastating consequences. Apparently, character traits that were common among the farmers—individualism, independence, distrust of outsiders—prevented an appropriate and timely call for help.[21]

Although professional confidentiality is just as important among rural practitioners as elsewhere, it is far more difficult in a rural practice to keep information confidential. Patients encounter acquaintances and relatives in the doctor's waiting room, in the parking lot, behind the receptionist's desk. For this reason, some patients do not want to be seen consulting mental health providers.

Physicians in rural communities encounter, among many rural residents, a pattern of fear and distaste for urban centers, particularly among families who have lived in the country for generations. Referrals to an urban center can be complicated by the patient's resistance to going to the city, especially for mental health issues. The primary physician is likely to have to work with the local system, even if more specialized care is advisable. The general public in most rural areas still believes it is protected from the ravages of the substance abuse epidemic, although marijuana and cocaine are now available in every small town in America. This denial is largely due to the absence of aggressive sales and the use of illegal drugs in public places, and the relative invisibility of the organized crime element of the distribution network. As in other communities, most of the crime and violence in rural America is due to alcohol and substance abuse, and at least half of the automotive deaths are related to intoxication.[22,23] Some but not all studies have found that rural residents are less likely than their urban counterparts to seek help for substance abuse.[9]

The rural mind-set is not necessarily destructive in regard to mental health. The fact that other people know your business in a small town keeps you from starving alone if you are too mentally ill to care for your basic needs. Because of rural extended families, there tend to be fewer truly isolated persons, and there is a resilient social support network. The relatively strong rural religious institutions provide a cadre of clergy and laypeople who take an interest in their neighbors' welfare. The fabled rural self-reliance can lead to an unwillingness to seek help, but it also correlates with a willingness to attempt to make do by helping other members of the community who are in need.[24]

DEMOGRAPHICS/SCOPE OF PROBLEM

Nearly one-third of our states have over 50 percent of their population living in rural (nonmetropolitan) areas.[25] Rural Americans make up 25 percent of the nation's population (U.S. Department of Commerce, 1990) but comprise a disproportionate share of the aged, chronically ill, migrants, poor, uninsured, native populations, and dependent persons. All these groups have a greater risk and incidence of mental health disorders than the general population.[5,10] They have more problems with geographic isolation, lack of transportation, increased stigmatization, and confidentiality.[26,27] Rural areas have higher rates of depression than urban areas, and this is intensified by the economic vulnerability of rural areas.[25] Approximately 10 percent of rural residents need psychiatric care, but only 2 to 5 percent are treated.[28] In at least one study, functional impairment in a rural population was explained more by psychological distress than by severity of medical illness.[29]

Another study compared two rural primary care groups, one with strong mental health links, the other with weak consultative linkages and less available mental health care. The site with the weaker mental health linkages used more mental health services by primary care providers, had more ambulatory care visits with mental health and primary providers, and had higher mental health hospitalization rates.[8] All these suggest a need for more mental health services and better systems of access.

SYSTEM ISSUES

The major system issues that make delivery of mental health services in rural settings so difficult are inadequate resources and lack of support. Rural primary care physicians have too little time and too few accessible supports to conduct much of the needed mental health care. Some solutions exist and others are suggested. In recent years more family physicians have been better trained to deal with mental health problems, and there have been many examples of an emphasis in rural training on this specialty.

Human Resources

Rural areas suffer from lack of medical resources in general, and this is true also of mental health services. Some 73 percent of all mental health manpower shortages are in rural areas.[30]

The providers of mental health in our rural communities make up a broad array of disciplines. Some 10 to 20 percent of the general population consult a primary care physician for a mental health problem annually, and primary physicians see the majority of patients seeking care for mental conditions.[31,32]

However, getting a good picture of manpower issues in mental health is difficult. The types of trained professionals who work in mental health include clinical social work, clinical psychology, education and counseling, "mid-level" providers like nurse practitioners, clinical nurse specialists and physician's assistants, and medicine (both psychiatrists and other physicians). In addition, paraprofessionals (associate degrees) and lay people without any formal training may substitute for or complement formally trained and licensed professionals.[32] These providers have a broad and variable array of skills and competence, making the assessment of available resources difficult.

There are estimated to be approximately 337,000 certified mental health care workers in the United States. This does not include physicians other than psychiatrists who may have had some formal training in mental health. As shown in Fig. 12-1, there are about twice as many Ph.D. psychologists (69,000) as psychiatrists (33,000), twice as many social workers (125,000) as psychologists, and about an equal number of certified workers (110,000) as social workers. This last group consists of marriage and family counselors (46,000), general counselors (53,000), and clinical nurse specialists (11,000). Any given rural community could have a varying complement of these mental health professionals, making services quite adequate in one community in one area of mental health but really lacking in another.[32]

If we look at the 15 states that have more than 50 percent of their population in rural areas and compare their resources in the three major mental health personnel areas (psychiatrists, Ph.D. psychologists, and social workers), we see considerable variation. One state, Idaho, has less than average numbers in all three types, while another, Vermont, has more than average.[32] However, studies have shown that the majority of mental health workers are concentrated in urban areas, even in states with significant rural populations.[5,33,34] The identified benchmark ranges for determining need are quite wide. For psychiatrists alone, the need varies from one psychiatrist for every 6500 people [Graduate Medical Education National Advisory Committee (GMENAC) 1996] to one for every 12,000 people (HMOs). The range for all other mental health workers is so wide as to be difficult to interpret. This makes the targeting of future needs difficult or impossible.[34] However, even with these wide ranges, shortages of mental health workers have been identified and are overwhelmingly rural.[30,33]

Reimbursement Problems

The physician reviewer from the patient's insurance plan was polite but immovable—he would not approve inpatient detoxification from heroin. I explained that the patient showed physical signs of opiate withdrawal. He lived more than 100 miles from our detox unit, and state law did not allow me to prescribe methadone for withdrawal to an outpatient, even if a responsible family member could supervise medication administration. "I know that in some parts of the country it's routine to treat people like this as inpatients, but CHAMPUS (Civilian Health and Medical Program of the Uniformed Services) is a nationwide program and their policies apply to the whole country. They've

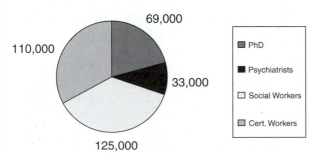

FIGURE 12-1 Comparison of numbers of mental health workers.

decided that those needing heroin detox can safely be treated as outpatients."

Reimbursement of physicians and other providers of rural mental health is a significant problem. Physicians are not generally reimbursed for mental health counseling services, so the only types of counseling that are practical in the physician's office are those that are brief enough to be provided free of charge. In a rural area, the time commitments for counseling sessions would generally be too great to allow a primary care physician to take time away from other commitments even if reimbursement were available. As the current shortage of rural primary care providers continues to improve, some rural physicians may have the time to engage in family therapy, marital counseling, and so on, but not if they cannot be paid.

The payment for mental health services in rural areas, although only part of a complex problem, is still a critical element in making services available and affordable. In a recent review,[35] the three most frequent payers noted by providers of mental health services in rural areas were Medicaid, private insurance, and self-pay sliding scale. Others included Medicare, self-pay full fee, workers' compensation, and federal, state, or local grants.

Medicaid appears to be the largest payer, and it has some problems. Medicaid does not pay enough for counseling to permit any private counselor to accept this form of insurance. When a primary physician needs to refer a Medicaid recipient for mental health counseling, the community mental health center is the only option. For the working poor and other uninsured patients, counseling is not affordable. Community mental health centers usually try to address this problem through the use of sliding fee scales. Since the Medicaid system operates on a "medical model" of specialized care, rural providers—facing chronic shortages of mental health professionals—experience great difficulty in meeting the standards of the Medicaid mental health clinic model. All care delivered must be ordered by a physician, and Medicaid

does not favor the use of midlevel mental health practitioners. Also, access to care in many rural areas has been enhanced or made possible by midlevel providers (e.g., nurse practitioners, physician's assistants, and nurse midwives). Medicaid does not reimburse master's level counselors or midlevel providers who often staff primary care and mental health services in rural areas. There are also cross-state variations that affect border communities (e.g., one state will reimburse only psychiatrists for patient assessments while the bordering state requires a psychologist to make such assessments).[35] Since Medicaid is a primary source of funding, these rules critically impede access for those people who often need care the most in rural areas.

The move to managed care by private insurers and the contracting to managed care of Medicaid have further compounded the problem. Most of these insurers have a "carve out" for mental health that further reinforces the "medical" model of separation of psychological and physical health. Not only are primary physicians not reimbursed for mental health diagnoses but access to mental health professions is often impeded or limited. Primary providers often "misdiagnose" major depression in order to bypass the reimbursement system or protect patient confidentiality.[19] Patients are often required to call a mental health access line where "anonymous" intake workers try to glean detailed mental health information by phone from the patient prior to authorizing or setting up service. The patient's reluctance to discuss these personal matters with someone on the phone who is not their health care or mental health care provider is understandable and sets up confidentiality issues. Additionally, the provider who would best deal with a particular patient's problems is often unavailable, either because he or she is outside the contractor's system or because "whoever is up next" gets the patient. Systems where these services are integrated and seamless have demonstrated overall improvement in patient outcomes and reduction in overall utilization of services as well as in costs.[8] However, the vast majority of reimbursement mechanisms have not adopted these principles.

SPECIAL POPULATIONS

A 44-year-old Native American man was referred to alcohol rehabilitation by a federal magistrate after he was arrested for smuggling illegal aliens across the Canadian border. Although he was a resident of a reservation that straddles the border between the United States and Ontario, he had little or no integration into native culture. His involvement with an extensive organized smuggling ring was his only close link to the native community. In an attempt to provide culturally sensitive treatment, his therapist encouraged him to become more involved with his own roots. Concepts included the "recovery medicine wheel"—a way of relating basic principles of alcohol recovery to native principles of unity with the natural world and personal balance. After discharge, he took a native name and began to learn his native language. He participated in a ritual known as the "sweat lodge" and gained a new understanding of the elders who were seeking to pass on tribal culture to members of his generation.

Rural areas often have a disproportionate share of people with special needs and problems. The vast majority of our native people and migrant workers live in rural areas. Additionally, groups often associated with inner cities—such as the poor, homeless, and uninsured—are also represented in significant numbers in rural areas. Moreover, the extreme lack of child and adolescent services provides unique challenges.

The mental health delivery system in rural America is distinct from its urban counterparts in several important ways. Delivery to special populations such as Native Americans requires unique knowledge and cultural sensitivities as well as special skills for managing problems such as substance abuse with little specialist support. In order to work effectively with other special rural populations—such as the rural poor, migrant workers, and adolescents— mental health care providers need an understanding of the rural mind-set, which includes the persisting stigma attached to mental illness, challenges related to maintaining confidentiality, and attitudes about treatment in urban settings.

Native Americans

Delivery of mental health care to certain populations in the rural United States requires knowledge that is not readily available to health care providers. For example, most providers have not worked with Native Americans. The nation's 557 Indian reservations are almost all located in rural areas. In their relative isolation, Native Americans tend to grow up considering the customs and mores of their people as the norm; they are sometimes as perplexed by the beliefs of the rest of the country as the majority is by Native American customs. The Indian Health Service furnishes most of the primary medical care on the reservations. Most of the physicians in these clinics are recent graduates fulfilling a service commitment early in their careers, although they are assisted by nurses and physician extenders who are often Native American and more experienced medically and culturally. Lack of sophistication and experience in Native American ways may therefore act as a barrier to the detection and treatment of mental disorders.

Substance abuse is a particular problem in reservation communities, although the scale of the problem varies from tribe to tribe and some Indian nations actually have less drug abuse than the general U.S. population. Where the drug problem is great, reservation society can resemble the worst areas of the inner city in the sense that drug sales are open and common, violent drug gangs intimidate the neighborhoods, and drug dealing dominates the economic activity. Studies of substance abuse treatment in Native American populations suggest that programs designed to be sensitive to Native American cultures are more likely to be successful than 12-step programs like Alcoholics Anonymous.[36] There are new programs adapted specifically to the traditions of an individual Indian nation, such as the "Red Road" programs for Lakotas. On some of the larger reservations, there are substance abuse programs developed by Native Americans themselves that use traditional tribal methods.[37] Prognosis is better for those Native Americans who are more integrated into both native and U.S. cultures, and worse for the "marginal men" who are alienated from both cultures.[38]

The Rural Poor

Poverty is common in rural America, with the associated problems of impaired access to care and increased mental health stressors, but rural poverty can differ from urban poverty in ways that are important for mental health care. The poor are less segregated from the rest of society in rural areas in the sense that there are few "exclusive communities" and no ghettoes outside of the metropolitan areas. The strong kinship network in rural communities includes many of the poor and binds together a large cross section of the population. The well off and the poor may live in closer proximity in rural areas, and this reduces the access problems for health care in general, which can be so difficult in cities.[39] A health care provider may be less inclined to turn away patients who are on public assistance when they are his or her neighbors or relatives.

Apart from the mental health care that can be provided in the primary care physician's office, the provider of last resort for the mentally ill rural poor is the community mental health center.[9] This usually takes the form of one or more county-run clinics that provide outpatient treatment, or a county may contract with a private corporation to provide these services. A psychiatrist director usually supervises a staff of counselors, social workers, and physician extenders. Budgets are determined by politically elected representatives through the county's department of social services or equivalent and supplemented by state and federal appropriations. Substance abuse treatment is usually provided in a separate office or location.

Community mental health centers have the advantages of governmental organizations: a stable work force that is provided with benefits, a mentality that is not driven by profit, and a publicly subsidized budget that prevents such centers from going out of business with economic downturns or changes in reimbursement. Disadvantages are many as well. Primary physicians are often frustrated by the lack of innovation in contrast to a private organization; by the lack of client focus at the organizational level, where the needs of the county legislature may dominate decision making; by difficulty finding providers after hours (except for crisis hotlines); and by long delays in getting new clients into the system. Community mental health centers produced a remarkable improvement in access to mental health care from the time they were first started as part of the Great Society programs of the 1960s; however, they may no longer be flexible or innovative enough for the 1990s and beyond.

Severe mental illness impoverishes its victims. The process of deinstitutionalization that has dominated mental health care in recent decades has emptied the state mental hospitals. Severely mentally ill patients have been moved into community settings. In the cities, this process has dramatically increased the numbers of the homeless mentally ill. In rural areas, this problem is not nearly as prominent. Patients who are not capable of basic self-care are housed adequately, in "family care" settings. These are private homes in which the household is paid by the state to care for one or more severely mentally ill individuals. Some daytime programming and transportation is provided to the patient, psychiatric medications are prescribed by the community mental health center staff, and primary medical care is reimbursed by Medicaid. The provision of primary medical care for these patients can be complex, but it does not approach the problems of caring for the street people of America's cities.

Migrant Farm Laborers

One segment of the rural poor that is particularly hard to serve is the migrant farm labor force that passes through rural communities following the harvests. The federal government maintains a network of clinics to serve migrants through the Migrant Health Branch, Division of Community and Migrant Health, of the Bureau of Primary Health Care. Little is known about the mental health problems of this population, but substance abuse seems to be a particular and increasing problem. It appears that there is a trend toward a higher proportion of unattached Hispanic males in this work force, and their lack of social and family support may predispose them to substance abuse.[40]

The primary physician assessing a migrant worker with mental illness is thus confronted with linguistic and cultural barriers, lack of continuity of care, devastating financial constraints, and the diagnostic problems of distinguishing mental illness, substance abuse, and the effects of neurotoxic agricultural chemicals.

Adolescent and Child Mental Health

A haphazard patchwork of providers—including primary care physicians, school psychologists, community mental health centers, and child protective caseworkers—makes up the rural network for the treatment of children and adolescents with mental health problems.[41] This system works fairly well for addressing routine problems like attention deficit disorder and various mild developmental problems. However, communication between providers and school districts remains the greatest problem, since there are usually no effective mechanisms in place to facilitate exchange of information.[41] Communications can be improved when a provider serves on a school district's special education committee, thus acting as a liaison between the school and providers.

Rural health care delivery systems rarely have the resources to care for children with major mental health problems. These cases require consultation with distant centers where child psychiatrists and other specialized experts are available. The same holds true for adolescents who require residential substance abuse treatment.

SPECIAL MENTAL HEALTH PROBLEMS

The management of special mental health problems in rural settings also calls for unique approaches. In rural areas, unlike the city, resources for treating alcohol and substance abuse problems or dual-diagnosis problems are few and far between. Expertise is often far away, rural physicians are left with challenges in communicating with urban-based specialists, and they are often left on their own.

Alcohol and Substance Abuse Issues

The infrastructure for substance abuse treatment is widely scattered or nonexistent in rural communities. Obviously, no rural area would have the population base to support the full range of services: crisis hotlines, school-based prevention programs, outpatient counseling, intensive outpatient rehabilitation, inpatient rehabilitation units, detoxification units, halfway houses, therapeutic communities, sobering-up facilities, and methadone maintenance programs. Occasionally, attempts to develop such facilities in a rural community can provoke political opposition.

Self-help groups like Alcoholics Anonymous (AA) and Al-anon are widely available throughout rural America, and primary physicians should be aware of contacts in these organizations. In some areas, AA is the only service for addictions, and groups tailored to the specific needs of women, gays, teens, professionals, and minorities are usually not available.

Methadone maintenance is one treatment modality that is completely unavailable in rural America. Historically, this was due to the onset of the opiate abuse epidemic in the inner city, but 30 years later, all methadone maintenance programs remain in urban areas. Rural opiate abusers are rarely enrolled in these programs, even though methadone maintenance has been shown to reduce the mortality rate by two-thirds. The main problem preventing more widespread use of this modality is excessive governmental regulation: the requirements for a program are so onerous that small rural hospitals or nonprofit corporations cannot hope to comply. A private physician is not permitted to manage methadone maintenance out of the office, even if it is coordinated with an outpatient substance abuse counseling program. As long as the current regulatory climate persists, rural opiate addicts will have no access to methadone maintenance in their hometowns.[42]

Treatment of substance abuse in the primary doctor's office can be crucial, but beyond the short-intervention technique adapted to primary care, the main caregiver for the substance abuser is the substance abuse counselor [the certified alcoholism counselor (CAC) in many states]. Relationships between counselors and physicians can be difficult in both rural and urban areas, but the primary physician in the country must learn to overcome difficulties while the city colleague may be able to avoid the issue by making a referral to a physician who has specialized in addiction medicine.

Dual Diagnosis

Patients with a "dual diagnosis"—that is, both mental illness and substance abuse—present special problems in both rural and urban areas. Typically both mental health and substance abuse counselors should be involved, and they may not communicate well or may not be located nearby. The primary care provider may be left as the only person who can understand all sides of a case and may not be adequately trained to handle these potentially difficult patients. Inpatient mental health care for these patients is not available in small communities and requires a distant referral.

Paradoxically, the rural setting can benefit dually diagnosed patients. The limited numbers of providers can be an advantage—continuity of care is more natural than in the multilayered specialty systems in larger communities. Communication among the doctors, counselors, social workers, and law enforcement personnel may be facilitated by the fact that they are often personally acquainted. In the words of one hospital social worker: "Our system isn't big enough for anyone to get lost!"

POTENTIAL SOLUTIONS

Many of the problems of getting mental health services to rural populations are centered around issues of manpower, models of practice that meet patient needs, adequate reimbursement for services provided, and the need to build supports and linkages to these rural practitioners, thus reducing their sense of isolation.

Various solutions are proposed for some of these system issues. More collaborative training programs, with a focus on developing effective networks between providers in different communities, are needed. Further, the enhancement of training of primary care physicians combined with the integration of primary care with mental health is suggested, with mental health workers providing basic care on site. Last, potential solutions for the reimbursement issues are presented. Barriers imposed by Medicare and managed care providers may be surmounted with improved access to mental health, with a seamless, integrated delivery system.

Human Resources

In assessing the manpower issue, one must consider training, recruitment, and retention. As noted earlier, a significant portion of rural people consult a primary physician for mental health care. Family physicians have integrated significant amounts of mental health care as a requirement of their residency training.[43] They also have a large portion of their graduates entering rural and small-town practice.[44] Mental health professions, especially psychiatry, have not had the same success in getting practitioners into the rural areas. One of the reasons for the success may be that many family physician training programs have emphasized rural care and promoted training of physicians in rural settings. Also, the federally sponsored Area Health Education Center (AHEC) program has supported interdisciplinary training in rural areas for over two decades and has had success in meeting rural health manpower needs. Often these programs are strongly linked to family medicine training programs.

Another key issue in the recruitment and retention problem is the sense of isolation and often lack of support available to the rural practitioner. This extends particularly to the boundary issues in relation to patients. Rural practitioners are more likely to care for their own family and close friends than their urban counterparts. They are often knowledgeable about more things than go on in the typical biomedical or mental health interview, which forces an integrative approach to medicine.[26] It also places them in often strained positions in both their personal and professional lives, with little or no linkage. Building bridges through collaborative training programs and setting up networks between providers in different communities can be helpful both in retention and in reducing this isolation; it can be a beginning to help solve these manpower problems.

MODELS OF PRACTICE

Living and working as a physician in a rural community produces a knowledge of complex psychosocial issues in individuals and families that is automatically incorporated into any care plan. The option of ignoring psychological issues, consciously or unconsciously, is not available.[26] This leads to a consideration of integrated models of primary care and mental health services. Efforts to foster such integration have been federal policy for over 30 years. As a result, many integration models have been developed that fall into one of four major categories. These are diversification, linkage, referral, and enhancement, which seem to exist mostly in some combination rather than as pure types.[35] The success or failure of these models often depends on available personnel, financing, and how well they meet community needs in availability and accessibility. *Diversification* involves the primary

care organization or practitioner directly hiring mental health personnel to provide mental health services at the primary care site. *Linkage* occurs when the primary care organization arranges to have an independent practitioner or an employee of another organization provide mental health services at the primary care site. *Referral* describes a variety of arrangements to assure that off-site mental health services are available to the patients of the primary provider. *Enhancement* is the expansion of training of primary providers to improve their ability to recognize, diagnose, and treat mental health problems independently. The dominant model appears to be a mental health worker placed at a primary care site to provide basic services as well as referral to off-site specialty care.[35]

The availability and integration of mental health services at the site of primary care has many advantages:

- It reinforces what is already known—the intuitive understanding that mental health and physical health are inseparable.[45]
- It enhances both the real and perceived level of confidentiality.[41]
- It leads to enhanced referrals and earlier identification of persons with mental health problems.[41]
- It provides for interaction between professionals, reducing the sense of professional isolation.[41]
- It can reduce operational cost because some overhead expenses can be shared.[41]

However, there are some cautions in establishing a truly collaborative practice.[26] Preparation of the community, office, and patients for such a close association is needed. The differences in the definition of confidentiality as well as methods of documentation for the physician and mental health worker must be addressed at the beginning. Finally, the issue of billing must be looked at carefully, since sustaining a therapist in this setting will probably not be budget-neutral.[26]

Overall, the benefits of integrated systems to

the community, its people, and its practitioners seem formidable.

Payment for Services

To improve the reimbursement system, several changes must be made. Primary physicians must be adequately paid for providing mental health services to their patients. They address the entire patient and do not separate the mind from the body, but the system pays adequately only for physical maladies. Changes in reimbursement codes need to be addressed to recognize this discrepancy. The payers must recognize the mental health worker's value. These workers must be adequately included in payment schemes so that they can bill appropriately for their services. In managed care systems, services need to be integrated and seamless and to eliminate "carve outs" that isolate both the patient and the payment. Integrated, seamless services have demonstrated overall improvement in patient outcomes, a reduction in the utilization of services, and reduced costs.[8]

SUMMARY

The provision of mental health services in rural areas is complex and challenging. An understanding of the issues, unique to rural lifestyle, involved in making service available, accessible, affordable, appropriate, adequate, and acceptable is critical. The potential solutions require a recognition of the fact that physical and psychological health are fully integrated, one affecting the other; to address the individual's needs adequately, the system of care must be integrated as well. Our training of health professionals must reinforce this model to develop linkages that support the providers already in place in rural settings and to make provision for the future. Payment mechanisms should support the primary providers of direct services as well as a variety of levels of other professionals to meet patients' needs. A well-financed, integrated system of care would go a long way toward solving the problems of meeting the mental health care needs of our rural people.

REFERENCES

1. National Consensus Panel: *Report on Community Based Health Care: Nursing Strategies. Rural America: Challenge and Opportunities.* Washington, DC, National Institute of Nursing Research, 1995, vol 7, chapter 2.
2. Blank MB, Fox JC, Hargrove DS, Turner JT: Critical issues in reforming rural mental health service delivery. *Community Ment Health J* 31(6):511–524, 1995.
3. Hill CE: *Community Health Systems in the Rural American South: Linking People and Policy.* Boulder, CO, Westview, 1998.
4. Kivett VR: The importance of emotional and social isolation to loneliness among very old rural adults. *Gerontologist* 34(3):340–346, 1994.
5. Human J, Wasam C: Rural mental health in America. *Am Psychol* 46(3):232–239, 1991.
6. Reiger DA, Goldberg ID, Taube CA: The defacto US mental health services system: a public health perspective. *Arch Gen Psychiatry,* 35:685–693, 1978.
7. Lambert D, Hartley D: Linking primary care and rural psychiatry: where have we been and where are we going? *Psychiatric Serv* 49(7):965–970, 1998.
8. Yuen EJ, Gerdes JL, Gonzales JJ: Pattern of rural mental health care—exploratory study. *Gen Hosp Psychiatry* 18:14–21, 1996.
9. Wagenfeld M, Murray J, Mohatt D, et al: *Mental Health and Rural America: 1980-1993.* Washington, DC and Rockville, MD, Health Resources and Services Administration, Office of Rural Health Programs and National Institutes of Mental Health, Office of Mental Health Research, 1994.
10. Kane CF, Ennis JM: Health care reform and rural mental health: severe mental illness. *Community Ment Health J* 32(5):445–462, 1996.
11. Hargrove DS, Melton GB: Block grants and rural mental health services. *J Rural Community Psychol* 8(1):4–11, 1987.
12. Andrulis DP, Mazade NA: American mental health policy: changing directions in the 1980's. *Hosp Community Psychiatry* 34:601–606, 1983.
13. Mechanie D: The challenge of chronic mental illness: a retrospective and prospective view. *Hosp Community Psychiatry* 37:891–896, 1986.

14. Ozarin LD: Community care. *Hosp Community Psychiatry* 37(2):184–185, 1986.

15. US Congress, Office of Technology Assessment: *Health Care in Rural America* (OTA-H-434). Washington, DC, US Government Printing Office, 1990.

16. Bird D, Lambert D, Hartley D, et al: Integrating primary care and mental health in rural America: a policy review. *Administr Policy Ment Health.* 25:287–306, 1998.

17. Rost K, Williams C, Wherry J, et al: The process and outcomes of care for major depression in rural family practice settings. *J Rural Health* 11:114–121, 1995.

18. Strum R, Wells KB: How can care for depression become more cost effective? *JAMA* 273:51–58, 1995.

19. Rost K, Smith GR, Matthews DB, Guise B: The deliberate misdiagnosis of major depression in primary care. *Arch Fam Med* 3:333–337, 1994.

20. Susman R, Crabtree BF, Essink G: Depression in rural family practice. *Arch Fam Med* 4:427–431, 1995.

21. Cecil H: Stress, country style—Illinois response to farm stress. *J Rural Community Psychol* 36(2): 51–60, 1988.

22. Kelleher K, Robbins J: *Social and Economic Consequences of Rural Alcohol Use.* Washington, DC, US Department of Health and Human Services, National Institutes of Health, National Institute of Drug Abuse, 1997.

23. Donnermeyer J: *The Economic and Social Costs of Drug Abuse among the Rural Population.* Washington, DC, US Department of Health and Human Services, National Institutes of Health, National Institute of Drug Abuse, 1997.

24. Fox J et al: Defacto mental health services in the rural South. *J Health Care Poor Underserved* 6(4): 434–468, 1995.

25. Sheldon DA, Frank R: Rural mental health coverage under health care reform. *Community Ment Health J* 31(6):539–552, 1995.

26. Farley T: Integrated primary care in rural areas, in Blount A (ed): *Integrated Primary Care.* Norton, 1998.

27. Hargrove DS, Fox JC, Blank MB, Eisenberg MM: Introduction to special issue: rural mental health theory and practice. *Community Ment Health J* 31(6):507–509, 1995.

28. Flax J, Wagenfeld M, Ives R, Weiss R: *Mental Health and Rural America: An Overview and Annotated Bibliography* (DHEW Pub. No. ADM 78-753).

Washington, DC: US Government Printing Office, 1979.

29. Thurston-Hicks A, Paine S, Hollufield M: Functional impairment associated with psychological distress and medical severity in rural primary care patients. *Psychiatric Services,* 9(7):951–955, 1998.

30. DeLeon P, Wakefeld M, Schultz A, et al: Rural America: unique opportunities for health care delivery and health services research. *Am Psychol* 44(10):1298–1306, 1989.

31. De Gruy F: Mental health care in the primary care setting, in McCubbins L, Figlay CR (eds): *Primary Care: America's Health in a New Era.* Washington, DC, National Academy, 1996, pp 285–311.

32. Ivey SL, Scheffler R, Zazzali JL: Supply dynamics of the mental health workforce: implications for health policy. *Milbank Q* 76(1):25–28, 1996.

33. Department of Health and Human Services, Health Resources and Services Administration: *List of Primary Medical Care, Mental Health & Dental Health Professional Shortage Areas.* Washington, DC, US Government Printing Office, 1997.

34. Eveland AP, Dever GE, Schafer E, et al: Analysis of health service areas: another piece of the psychiatric workforce puzzle. *Psychiatric Services* 49(7):956–960, 1998.

35. Bird DC, Lambert D, Hartley D, et al: Rural models for integrating primary care & mental health services. *Admin Policy Ment Health* 25(3):287–308, 1998.

36. Stubben J: Culturally competent substance abuse prevention research among rural American Indian communities. Washington, DC, US Department of Health and Human Services, National Institutes of Health, National Institute of Drug Abuse, 1997.

37. Marley A: *CSAP Resource Guide: American Indians and native Alaskans.* 498 Inventory #419. Bethesda, MD, National Clearinghouse for Alcohol and Drug Information, 1991.

38. Coggins K: *Alternative Pathways to Healing: The Recovery Medicine Wheel.* Health Communications, 1990.

39. Conger R: *The Special Nature of Rural America.* Washington, DC, US Department of Health and Human Services, National Institutes of Health, National Institute of Drug Abuse, 1997.

40. Watson J: *Alcohol and Drug Abuse by Migrant*

Farmworkers: Past Research and Future Priorities. Washington, DC, US Department of Health and Human Services, National Institutes of Health, National Institute of Drug Abuse, 1997.

41. Wagenfeld MO, et al: Mental Health Service Delivery in Rural Areas. Organizational and Clinical Issues. Rural Substance Abuse: State of Knowledge and Issues. Research Monograph No. 168. Washington, DC, US Department of Health and Human Services, National Institutes of Health, National Institute of Drug Abuse, 1997.

42. National Consensus Development Panel on Effective Medical Treatment of Opiate Addiction. *JAMA* 280(22):1936–1943, 1998.

43. American Academy of Family Physicians: *RAP Criteria for Excellence in a Family Practice Residency Program,* 4th ed. Family Practice Residency Program. Kansas City, MO, AAFP, 1998.

44. American Academy of Family Physicians: *Facts about Family Practice.* Kansas City, MO, AAFP, 1998.

45. Hill CE, Fraser GT: Local knowledge and rural mental health reform. *Community Ment Health J* 31(6):553–568, 1995.

CHAPTER 13

Dental Care

PETER M. MILGROM   DAVID TISHENDORF

H istorically, many rural areas of the United States have been inadequately served by dentists. This situation is not likely to change, primarily because the number of dentists being trained is decreasing and the options for newly graduated dentists are many. The large increases in the number of dental trainees during the 1970s and 1980s had little effect on the maldistribution of personnel.[1] State and federal efforts to place government-sponsored dental personnel in rural, underserved areas have not met with much success, and there is often resistance from dental associations. There is little documented effort by underserved communities themselves to recruit and keep dental personnel.

Nearly 1 in 4 persons in the United States lives in a nonmetropolitan county. In 1990, the Area Resource File defined 2249 counties in the United States as rural.[2] Based on the 1990 decennial census, these are counties with cities having fewer than 50,000 people or metropolitan areas with fewer than 100,000 people including urbanized areas having fewer than 50,000 people. These counties had an average population in 1990 of 21,900 and a range of 100 to 165,300 people. The counties averaged 1002 square miles, with a range of 48 to 17,182 square miles. Per capita annual income in rural counties averaged $14,438, versus $15,199 for the nation as a whole.

The primary goal of this chapter is to document the status of the rural work force in dentistry as well as to review the education and training of dental personnel for service in rural communities. The use of dental health services and the health status of rural communities are discussed. A second goal is to provide a guideline for medical personnel who may be called upon to provide dental emergency care in the absence of a dentist. The chapter concludes with a brief look at the future of dental care services in America's rural areas.

RURAL DENTAL WORK FORCE

Any evaluation of the rural work force should take into consideration the overall context of dental work force projections for the United States. The ratio of dentists to the population is expected to peak in 2000 and then drop sharply during the next decade. By 2010, the decrease is estimated to be the equivalent of the closing of more than 10 percent of all dental schools. There also remains considerable variation in the distribution of dentists across regions of the United States. Trends for dental hygienists are similar.

Within the overall dental trainee populations there have also been changes.[3] Consistent with the shifts to urban areas for the whole population, fewer applicants to dental schools come from farming or nonurban areas. Evidence suggests that there is a relationship between the size of the town where dental students were raised and their eventual choice of a practice location.[4] For the great majority of young dentists, this choice is made directly out of their initial professional training and is probably not affected greatly by the 1-year, general-practice residency programs that only one-third of dentists attend following dental school.[3]

At the same time the overall number of dentists is decreasing, the number of female trainees is increasing. Women represent more than a third of all current trainees.[3] It has been suggested that women dentists are more likely than men to select communities where salaried positions in multidentist practices are available. Whether women dentists are more likely to end up in urban settings or whether this is simply a stereotype is largely unknown.

Of much greater concern is the decreasing number of African-American trainees. The number of minority graduates of dental schools has increased during the past several decades,[3] but the number of African-American graduates dropped 20 percent, from about 213 in 1976 to 171 in 1993. At the same time, the proportion of African-American women graduating rose to more than 50 percent of all African-American graduates. In 1997 the enrollment of black and/or African-American students represented only 5.2 percent of all enrolled dental students. To the extent that historically African-American communities in the rural South have received their dental care from African-American dentists, there will be an increasing shortage in these areas as the number of dentists retiring or dying outstrips the number of new graduates. This problem may be further exacerbated if the female graduates follow a pattern of seeking urban rather than rural practice, as their majority colleagues do. Trainees from the Hispanic community represent 4.9 percent of all students, while Native Americans total less than 1 percent of enrolled trainees.[5] None of these groups is represented in schools of dentistry in proportion to their percentage of the U.S. population.

The proportion of dentist general practitioners is predicted to decrease as well.[6] The number of graduates enrolling in specialty training rose from about 1 in 5 in 1983 to 1 in 3 in 1993. Many rural communities cannot support specialist dentists. One encouraging note is that the number of pediatric dentists nationally has remained fairly stable.[7] However, 22 states had a decrease in the ratio of pediatric dentists to children during the past decade. Of particular concern are states with large numbers of agricultural workers.[8] Waldman has argued, however, that more dentists interested in children would locate and be successful in nonurban areas were it not for lack of accurate information on the opportunities available in these communities.[9]

The federal government defines shortage areas as those with 5000 or more persons per dentist. Typically, better-served areas have ratios of 3500 persons per dentist or better. More than 1000 areas of the United States have been designated shortage areas for dental health professionals, although relatively few dentists have actually been placed in them. Testimony before Congress regarding the fiscal year 1999 budget by the American Association of Dental Schools also indicated poor coordination between state and local officials and those responsible for designations at the federal level. A federal program that provides scholarships for dental training and offers loan forgiveness for those willing to practice in a designated shortage area does not appear to be living up to its full potential. Evaluation of the National Health Service Corps has found that this program has not had much impact on the maldistribution of primary care dental services.[6] In the federal appropriations for fiscal year 1998, Congress instructed the National Health Service Corps to increase dental participation, and participation is expected to increase slowly.

For rural counties, the number of dentists is directly related to the population of the county. In 1990, rural counties without a dentist averaged 11,459 people, versus 28,393 for counties with a dentist. Some 52 percent of the rural counties in the United States (1179 of 2249) had four or fewer dentists. In 1990, there were but 66 National Health Service Corps dentists assigned to these counties. Fewer are being assigned today, and 38 percent (856 of 2249) of the rural counties in the United States have no dentist. Similarly, counties without a dental hygienist averaged 14,227 persons, versus 34,607 persons for counties with a dental hygienist. In 62 percent (1397 of 2249) of counties, there was not a single dental hygienist. The average number of dentists per county was 8.5, with a range from 0 to 158 dentists. The average number of dental hygienists was 4 per county, with a range from 0 to 79. The ratio of dental hygienists to dentists was 0.5 in rural counties, slightly lower than the national mean of 0.58 in 1990.

Absolute levels of population, population change, population density, and levels of per capita income are all different for counties with no dentist. Table 13-1 displays these data.

As can be seen in Table 13-1, counties without dentists in 1990 had smaller populations and lower population density than counties with dentists. Also, counties without dentists, on average, declined in population during this decade, while those with dentists had small gains. This was true irrespective of the median age of the population. The proportion of blacks and Hispanics in the population also did not differ significantly between these counties. The average per capita income in 1990 for counties with dentists was slightly higher than income in counties without dentists ($14,557 versus $14,244). It appears that population size, growth, and density are better predictors of having a dentist than per capita income alone. Of course, dentists in urban centers in contiguous counties may serve residents of counties without dentists, although this increases the problems of transportation in areas where distances may be great and public transportation poor.

Regions of the United States varied in their dental manpower. Overall, the number of people per dentist in all rural counties was 3118. The population-to-dentist ratio ranged from 2409 for counties in the West to 3614 in the Northeast. The Midwest had a ratio of 3051, and the South had a ratio of 3382. The proportion of rural counties without a dentist also varied. The Northeast had 9.1 percent of counties without a dentist (8 of 88), while the South had 46.3 percent (465 of 1004) counties without a dentist. The Midwest had 31.3 percent (261 of 833), and the West had 37.7 percent (122 of 324) counties without a dentist.

Similar results are found for dental hygienists in rural counties. The Northeast had 13.6 dental hygienists per county, while the other regions had 3.5 to 3.8 dental hygienists per county.

Indian Health Service clinics have traditionally provided dental care in 430 primarily rural areas in the United States. In the period 1994–1997, however, significant downsizing occurred.[10] In the short run, this is exacerbated by the attempts of Native American tribes to take control of their own dental health services. Recruitment of adequately trained providers is a continuing and probably insoluble problem in an era of overall short supply.

According to the recent Office of Technology Assessment report, federal programs that might deal with rural dental services fall into four categories: programs that pay for direct services, block grants to states with resources that might fund and provide services, programs to aug-

TABLE 13-1   RURAL COUNTIES WITH AND WITHOUT DENTISTS

	Population, 1990	Population, 1980	Percent Change in Population Using 1980 as a Base	Population Density in 1990, Persons per Square Mile
Counties with at least one dentist (N = 1393)	28,393	27,593	1.6	44.6
Counties with no dentist	11,459	11,449	−1.9	21.4

ment health care resources, and health policy and research.[1]

Medicaid is the primary direct payer for many low-income rural people. Dental services for children are mandated under the Early, Periodic, Diagnosis, Screening and Treatment Program (EPDST), although states vary in the income eligibility criteria applied. The program requires states to recruit providers, locate and inform families about the availability of services, and assure that services are provided. Evidence suggests that only one in five eligible children receives screening services, and even fewer receive actual dental care.[11] The percentage of eligible children receiving services varies across states. These programs are underfunded and fail to reach most of the needy population. More affluent states also have adult dental programs under Medicaid. Many of these programs are underfunded, and access to dental care is poor. The proportion of adults served by these programs is likely to drop as eligibility is tightened under welfare reform. Medicare does not provide payments for dental services.

Maternal and child health block grants to the states as well as preventive health and health services block grants have been used to fund some dental services in rural and urban areas. These efforts have consisted primarily of periodic disease surveillance programs, water fluoridation, and fluoride rinse programs in elementary schools as well as pit and fissure sealant application programs, again associated with schools. However well meaning, these programs are small and underfunded. Little is known about their effectiveness.

The programs to augment rural health resources have also included dental care. The National Health Service Corps was discussed earlier in this chapter. Some populations—especially American Indians, Alaska Natives, and migrant workers—have poorer access to dental care than other groups, and it may be getting worse. According to Isman and Isman,[10] the proportion of Native Americans who had a single dental visit dropped 34 percent between 1994 and 1996, and less than 25 percent of the 1.4 million Native Americans living near or on

reservations received any dental care in 1996. Native Americans also have twice the rate of dental disease as the rest of the population.

The myriad other federal programs in the manpower area have also included dental components. These have included Area Health Education Centers (AHEC), Border Health Education Centers, and various special projects. AHEC funds have supported rotation of dental trainees to underserved areas in some states such as North Carolina. The focus has been broad, with little specific attention to rural populations. Little is known about the successes or failures of these dental programs.

Similarly, there is little evidence that programs designed to create federally qualified health centers and the rural health clinic programs have resulted in expanded access for rural underserved populations.[10] In 1988, there were 526 federally funded community health centers, of which 319 were in rural areas. There were also 118 migrant health centers,[1] many of which included dental care. By and large, these programs hire inexperienced recent dental school graduates who are ill equipped to provide the kinds of services required. Anecdotally, few of these programs attract pediatric specialists, even though their caseloads are full of children. Most important, these clinics are now competing for scarce Medicaid reimbursement dollars, and their built-in inefficiencies make them vulnerable to financial difficulties.

The research programs of the Agency for Health Care Policy and Research and the Office of Rural Health Policy have largely been nonstarters as far as rural dental care is concerned. Few research efforts have been supported, and it is very difficult to find any published data examining the special problems of dental care in nonurban areas of the United States.

EDUCATION AND TRAINING OF DENTAL PERSONNEL

There does not appear to be a concerted effort by colleges and schools of dentistry and dental hygiene to focus attention on the preparation of students for rural practice. Dental education is different from other aspects of health service in that dentists and dental hygienists in training are expected to provide actual services. Few rural areas have facilities available where trainees can work, and supervision of trainees by university staff is problematic. Increasingly, schools see their fixed-base clinics on the university campus as a major revenue source and are reluctant to assign their students to rotations that keep them out of the urban clinics and generate little or no income. This is particularly true for dental schools in private universities, but it is becoming equally true for publicly supported schools.

Some schools, such as the University of North Carolina School of Dentistry, have always rotated students for short-term clerkships that may include assignment to rural Appalachian clinics. The University of Colorado rotates its fourth-year students to clinical programs serving migrant worker populations. The University of Washington also rotates dental and dental hygiene students and pediatric dental residents to a farm workers' clinic system in the agricultural areas of Washington. Other schools appear to offer similar elective opportunities, some using mobile facilities. A small college dental hygiene training program in Ohio recently described its rotation of clinical students to programs in its rural communities.[12] These individuals were assigned to programs designed to reduce the incidence of early childhood caries.

There are general practice residency programs that include clinical assignments in underserved areas. Programs in New Jersey and Ohio include such rotations. These programs typically call for up to 2 years of additional general practice clinical training beyond the initial DDS degree. In testimony before the House Labor–Health and Human Services–Education Appropriations Subcommittee in January 1998, a dental school dean argued that 87 percent of general dentistry residents remain in primary care practice and that they treat 4 times the number of developmentally disabled, 6 times the number of medically compromised, and 26 times the number of HIV/AIDS patients as col-

leagues without this training (testimony of Russell J. Stratton given on the American Association of Dental Schools Web site, AADSOnline). The grants for these programs provide startup funds, but the programs are expected to be self-sustaining after 3 years. There is no accreditation requirement that these professional programs address the needs of rural America. Public health textbooks offer little to the prospective practitioner on the opportunities in these areas.

UTILIZATION OF DENTAL CARE

The proportion of persons with at least one dental visit in 1989 varied somewhat by place of residence.[13] About one-half (53.6 percent) of persons 2 years of age and older living in rural counties had at least one dental visit. This rate was similar to that for central city residents (54.9 percent) and less than that for metropolitan residents not living in the central cities (60.6 percent). Rural residents had the fewest number of average visits per person per year (1.7 visits). Both the proportion of persons having at least one visit and the number of visits varied by region of the country. The South had the lowest rates (52.2 percent having at least one visit, 1.8 visits per person). Rates were highest in the Midwest (61.5 percent, 2.1) and Northeast (60.7 percent, 2.2) and slightly lower in the West (57.8 percent, 2.4).

In general, most populations of low-income people in the United States follow the "role performance model of dental health." That is, an individual is considered healthy as long as he or she is able to work and carry out his or her role. Under these conditions, an individual is unlikely to seek preventive care. There are many studies documenting that such populations see no need for dental care even in the face of documented oral pathology.[14] In a study of low-income blacks in rural Georgia, only 38 percent of more than 700 persons surveyed had had a dental visit within the past year; 53 percent reported the primary reason for not seeking care was that it was not needed.[15]

HEALTH STATUS

Dental problems are epidemic in rural America. Young children suffer needless toothaches, lose time from school, and in the worst cases fail to thrive. Many rural workers lose time from work because of unnecessary dental problems. In Washington State, the dental health status of children is a function of family income and race. Children from low-income families and Hispanic children have dramatically poorer dental health. In a state like Washington, this translates into a rural health care problem because of the particular distribution of the Hispanic population in agricultural areas. This likely is true in other heavily agricultural states. Agricultural workers are unlikely to have dental insurance. In other areas, such as the Northeast, this problem may be concentrated in the inner city. Nationally, children from families in the lowest income groups and Mexican-American and African-American children have the poorest oral health of any group.[16] This same relationship to health status is true for other age groups as well.

DENTAL EMERGENCIES

Often the physician or physician surrogate in a rural area is called upon to manage dental emergencies. These emergencies are primarily a result of trauma or infection.[17] All of these situations require dentist follow-up.

Trauma

Younger children fracture or avulse teeth in falls. Older children are usually injured in sports. There will be bleeding if the gums are involved, and this area will need to be gently cleaned and debrided. Tetanus prophylaxis may be needed. Horizontal tooth fractures are most common and require no immediate treatment if the tooth is not sensitive. Sensitive teeth are typically managed by cleaning the area with water or saline and then placing a "bandage" over the fractured area. Glass ionomer cement is used. This type of cement can be obtained from the local dentist, and a kit consisting of the cement, a spatula, a plastic instrument, and a mixing slab can be kept in the office for such occasions. If the tooth is bleeding internally, the bleeding is stopped with local pressure and then glass ionomer is placed over the wound. Some dentists prefer the use of a premixed calcium hydroxide dressing, which is then covered with the glass ionomer cement. If the tooth is fractured vertically, it will have to be removed. The soft tissue should be debrided. Analgesics, such as children's acetaminophen, can be used to manage the emergent situation.

Primary incisors that are avulsed are not replanted. Permanent incisors in adults and children that are avulsed can be cleaned and replaced in the socket if this is done within 10 to 20 minutes of the accident. Such a tooth should be stored in milk packed in ice and then gently rinsed in milk or saline to remove debris before replanting. Replantation will be more successful in younger patients. There is no consensus on antibiotic coverage, but it may be advisable. If coverage is chosen, a broad-spectrum agent such as penicillin V (1 g initially followed by 250 to 500 mg q 6 h for 1 week) or doxycycline (100 mg initially followed by 50 mg q 12 h for 1 week) is appropriate. Tetanus prophylaxis is important. Most teeth that are replanted will become nonvital and will eventually require root canal therapy. If the tooth is merely displaced, it should be gently pushed back into its normal position and the patient instructed to maintain a soft diet until the dentist can splint the tooth temporarily. Often you will see a discolored incisor; this is caused by the internal bleeding that occurs when teeth are traumatized. Such teeth may eventually abscess and require root canal therapy.

Adults with tooth fractures and luxations from trauma, as from vehicular injury, can be treated much as children are. Replantation of avulsed teeth in adults can be attempted, but the success rate is likely to be low.

Infection

Tooth pain from inflammation of the tooth pulp tissue and abscess is common. Tooth wax can often be put in the damaged area to isolate it from mouth fluids and reduce the discomfort. Nonsteroidal anti-inflammatory analgesics and infiltration injections of long-acting local anesthetics are useful management tools. A rural physician might keep a dental aspirating syringe on hand as well as several cartridges of bupivacaine or etidocaine hydrochloride with epinephrine. A lesson on injection technique from the local dentist is required. Often, frequent intraoral rinses with warm water will encourage drainage and reduce the pain markedly. Placing packs on the outside of the face encourages drainage through the skin and is inadvisable.

Odontogenic infections can be severe and may require emergent care. Antibiotic coverage is needed where there is cellulitis, swelling, trismus, and fever. Rule out facial space infections that may compromise the airway. Most dental infections appear as gum boils in young children or more diffuse soft tissue swellings in older children and adults. A broad-spectrum antibiotic such as amoxicillin or penicillin V is appropriate when swelling is present, typically given as 1 g initially followed by 2 g per day for a week. The bacteria most commonly identified in dental infections are gram-positive cocci, such as alpha-hemolytic streptococcus, as well as anaerobic streptococcus species and gram-negative bacilli. In the case of marked swelling, incision and drainage may be required. With pain in the lower jaw and difficulty swallowing, a compromised airway should be suspected and the patient referred immediately. Consultation with the local dentist about his or her management preferences is recommended.

THE FUTURE

The demands on a dentist in a rural area are large. Many work long days. Dentists seeking to take holidays are rarely replaced; the concept of *locum tenens* is not well developed in dentistry. As dental care is primarily an out-of-pocket expense, many of these clinicians are at the mercy of dwindling rural economies. Those practices that see a heavily Medicaid population worry about the continued viability of these programs. Many dentists in smaller communities are worried, as are many of their urban and suburban colleagues, that they may never be able to sell their practices as the number of newly trained dentists continues to decrease.

Dentists, as a group, have done exceedingly well in the past decade. Incomes have never been higher, and the trend toward a smaller work force will accelerate incomes further. Predictions that universal fluoridation of water and toothpaste would erode incomes by reducing levels of disease or that auxiliary personnel would reduce the need for dentists have proved largely untrue. Similarly, dentists have largely escaped the trends toward managed health care. Most continue to derive their income primarily from direct payments.

Groups studying the future of the dental profession from the perspective of national health care needs have recommended a greater integration of dentistry with medicine. The prospect of doing this in rural communities seems good. Tying preventive dental care to prenatal care and well-child visits and immunizations after a child is born is an idea worth trying.[18] Outreach efforts will be needed.[19] Rural clinics and hospitals can and should include dental care. Few do so now. Although children's care is the most obvious example, the concept is valid throughout the age spectrum. This kind of integration of the health providers is also likely to create a better environment for attracting and maintaining dentists and for reducing the transportation and other logistical problems that can plague rural residents in seeking dental care. Head Start and school-based programs for older children also can be successful in reducing the burden of dental disease in rural communities if the programs are intensive and well managed. Such programs can use locally trained paraprofessionals.

Few rural communities have made broad-based efforts to attract dentists. One pediatric dental specialist strategically recruited to a rural center can provide care for several thousand children. Levels of community awareness about oral health problems need to be raised, and the business community as a whole needs to embrace making better oral dental health an important goal.

REFERENCES

1. Office of Technology Assessment: Health Care in Rural America. OTA-H-434. Washington, DC, U.S. Government Printing Office, 1990, pp 268–272.
2. Revised statistical definitions of metropolitan areas (MAs) and guidance on uses of MA definitions. *OMB Bulletin*, 96-08. Washington, DC, Office of Management and Budget, June 28, 1996.
3. Waldman HB: Rural and urban distribution of dentists, or is there still gold in them thar hills? *Illinois Dent J* 64(3):121–125, 1995.
4. More DM: The dental student. *J Am Coll Dent* 28:79–83, 1961.
5. Losing ground: underrepresented minority dental student enrollment shifts. *Bull Dent Ed* 31:2, 1998.
6. Field MJ (ed): *Dental Education at the Crossroads: Challenges and Change.* Washington, DC, Institute of Medicine, National Academy Press, 1995, pp 255–261.
7. Waldman HB: Are we maintaining the ratio of private practicing pediatric dentists to the number of children? *J Dent Child* 65:264–267, 1998.
8. Waldman HB: Invisible children: the children of migrant farm workers. *J Dent Child* 61:218–221, 1994.
9. Waldman HB: Children in rural areas: extending the horizons of pediatric dental practice. *J Dent Child* 61:289–292, 1994.
10. Isman R, Isman B: *Oral Health America White Paper: Access to Oral Health Services in the United States 1997 and Beyond.* Chicago, Oral Health America, December 1997, pp 15–16.
11. Brown JG, Inspector General, Department of Health and Human Services, Office of the Inspector General: *Children's Dental Services under Medicaid: Access and Utilization.* OEI-09-93-00240. San Francisco, Regional Office, April 1996.
12. Burger AD, Boehm JM, Sellaro CL: Dental disease preventive programs in a rural Appalachian population. *J Dent Hygiene,* 71:117–122, 1997.
13. Bloom B, Gift HC, Jack SS: Dental services and oral health: United States, 1989. National Center for Health Statistics. *Vital Health Stat* 10:183, 1992.
14. Gift HC: Utilization of professional dental services, in Cohen LK, Bryant PS (eds): *Social Sciences and Dentistry: A Critical Biography.* Vol II. London, Federation Dentaire Internationale, 1984, pp 238–239.
15. Strickland J, Strickland DL: Barriers to preventive health services for minority households in the rural south. *J Rural Health* 12:206–217, 1996.
16. Vargas CM, Crall JJ, Schneider DA: Sociodemographic distribution of pediatric dental caries: NHANES III, 1988–1994. *J Am Dent Assoc* 129:1229–1238, 1998.
17. Montgomery MT, Redding SW (eds): *Oral-Facial Emergencies. Diagnosis and Management.* Portland, OR, JBK Publishing, 1994.
18. Milgrom P, Weinstein P: *Early Childhood Caries: A Team Approach to Prevention and Treatment.* Seattle, University of Washington Dental Continuing Education, 1999.
19. Clarridge BR, Larson BJ, Newman KM: Reaching children of the uninsured and underinsured in two rural Wisconsin counties: findings from a pilot project. *J Rural Health* 9:40–49, 1993.

PART THREE

Organization and Management of Rural Health Care

T he differences between rural health care and that found in urban and suburban areas are not limited to the clinical aspects of the care itself. One also finds major differences in the organization and management of the entities providing care. An understanding of these facets of the rural health firmament is absolutely essential to building an optimal health care system. The purpose of this section is to help the reader understand the infrastructure of our system of rural care and to offer a few glimpses of what our future may hold. Foundational understanding will be aided by consideration of rural health care facilities and underpinnings as well as the micro- and macroeconomics that determine the course of these enterprises. Increased cognizance of current medical management practices will be found in the study of rural managed care, networks, quality management, clinical guidelines, and health services development. Foresight into likely future components of rural health care will be gained through consideration of telehealth services and informatics.

In sum, attention to these topics will help the reader to comprehend *why* rural health care is the way it is, *what* some of its current nonclinical characteristics are, and *how* it might change in the future. Too often we find ourselves so overwhelmed by the constant demands and complexities of "now" that we are unable to consider these questions thoughtfully. The authors of the chapters in this section have addressed these provocative subjects in ways that we hope will provide useful insights.

Thomas E. Norris

CHAPTER 14

Rural Hospitals, Consultation, and Referral Networks in Rural Practice

THOMAS S. NESBITT   CHRISTINA A. KUENNETH

Colusa Community Hospital is located in the rural town of Colusa, California—a community of 5000 and home to the only hospital in the county. Colusa County is mainly agricultural and has a population of approximately 15,000. The nearest metropolitan area is Sacramento, which is 75 miles away. The hospital has 38 acute care beds but currently averages a daily census of 12 patients, a significant improvement from several years ago. With the advent of the prospective payment system under Medicare in the 1980s, the hospital's revenue began to decline dramatically. In 1992, Colusa's hospital was within a year of closing because of operating deficits. At that time the medical staff consisted of three general practitioners, one surgeon, a radiologist, and a visiting pathologist. The hospital discontinued obstetrics in 1987 after local physicians decided they could not afford the malpractice insurance for that service. Members of the community viewed the hospital as "dying" and began seeking care outside of the community. As revenue continued to decrease, services and staff were cut. This is the classic "death spiral" that many rural hospitals face.

After hiring a new administrator, the hospital was able to make a dramatic turnaround while maintaining its independence. The size of the medical staff doubled as new physicians with specific skills needed in the community were recruited by using a combination of incentives, such as loan repayment. Some of the hospital's beds were converted to swing beds, creating a more consistent revenue stream. Services that had previously been discontinued, including obstetrics, were restarted, and the quality of care improved, using telemedicine, visiting specialists, reorganization of services, and the establishment of relationships with larger urban health systems and medical groups. Quality assurance and physician proctoring activities included support from a university health system. All of this was made visible to the community through various marketing campaigns, which subsequently helped reestablish local confidence in the care provided by the hospital.

Many of these organizational changes are relevant to rural hospitals across the United States. These issues and many others are discussed in this chapter.

RURAL HOSPITALS—INTRODUCTION AND OVERVIEW

During the past several decades, the community hospital has been a key component of rural health care. For many communities, rural hospitals represent a significant source of local employment. Although rural hospitals flourished through the 1970s, the 1980s introduced the era of Medicare reform and marked the advent of prospective payment. This change in health care financing disadvantaged rural hospitals for several reasons, including lower reimbursement, relatively high fixed costs, and fewer programs available to support early discharge. Problems related to inadequate numbers and diversity of medical staff and services, increased competition, aging facilities, and lack of access to state-of-the-art technologies also put many rural hospitals at risk. In fact, between 1980 and 1989, a total of 252 rural hospitals, or 10 percent, closed.[1]

Number of Rural Hospitals and Total Rural Hospital Beds

The American Hospital Association (AHA), in its 1996 annual survey, reported that there were 2514 nonmetropolitan short-term general and other special service hospitals in the United States (Table 14-1). A nonmetropolitan area, as defined by the AHA, is any area that does not match the definition of a standard metropolitan statistical area (SMSA). In its 1986 survey, the AHA reported 2638 nonmetropolitan hospitals. In contrast to the decrease in nonmetropolitan hospitals over the last decade, the total number of nonmetropolitan hospital beds, including swing and skilled nursing facility beds, has increased. In 1986, the AHA reported 223,422 nonmetropolitan hospital beds,[2] whereas in 1996, the AHA reported 226,688 hospital beds. Thus, the trend in rural health care appears to be toward reducing the total number of com-

munity hospitals while maintaining or even modestly growing the total number of available beds.

Average Number of Beds in Rural versus Urban Communities

In 1996, more than 70 percent of all nonmetropolitan hospitals had fewer than 100 beds (Table 14-1). Conversely, 68 percent of metropolitan hospitals had 100 or more beds. In contrast with nonmetropolitan areas, metropolitan areas were about 10 times more likely to have a hospital with 500 beds or more. Nonmetropolitan hospitals, on the other hand, were almost three times more likely to have between 6 and 24 beds when compared with metropolitan hospitals. In terms of the average number of hospital beds for all metropolitan and nonmetropolitan hospitals, metropolitan hospitals had more than twice the beds of nonmetropolitan hospitals: 219 versus 90. In 1986, the average number of beds was 248 and 85 for metropolitan and nonmetropolitan hospitals, respectively. Competition and consolidation in urban health care markets may ex-

TABLE 14-1   U.S. METROPOLITAN AND NONMETROPOLITAN HOSPITALS BY NUMBER OF BEDS, 1996

| Number of Beds | Metropolitan Hospitals | | | Nonmetropolitan Hospitals[a] | | |
	Number of Hospitals	Percent of All Urban Hospitals	Number of Beds	Number of Hospitals	Percent of All Rural Hospitals	Number of Beds
6–24	123	3.2	2,067	255	10.1	4,489
25–49	346	9.0	13,026	776	30.9	28,398
50–99	771	20.0	56,238	745	29.6	52,661
100–199	1,031	26.8	147,163	519	20.6	71,356
200–299	649	16.9	158,526	140	5.6	34,254
300–399	382	9.9	131,589	44	1.8	15,009
400–499	216	5.6	95,627	16	0.6	7,189
500+	331	8.6	238,424	19	0.8	13,332
Total	3,849		842,660	2,514		226,688
Average bed number			219			90

[a]Rural hospitals are those located outside a standard metropolitan statistical area (SMSA).

SOURCE: *Healthcare QuickDisk*. Chicago, Healthcare InfoSource, Inc., 1998.

plain some of the decline in the number of hospital beds in metropolitan areas.

HOSPITAL CAPABILITIES

Rural hospitals continue to face significant challenges that affect the future viability of rural health care delivery systems. To survive in the highly competitive, rapidly changing health care environment, rural hospitals must prepare strategies that integrate health service delivery systems across multiple levels of care. The continuum of services and programs ensures that rural hospitals are able to meet the range of health care needs presented by the communities they serve. By pursuing strategies that integrate care systems, community hospitals can better maintain their position as the focal point of the rural health care delivery system.

A number of clinical, operational, and structural strategies have been pursued by rural hospitals to sustain local service delivery in very competitive health care environments. These strategies include growing patient revenues by diversifying into ambulatory, nonacute, and primary care services; controlling operating expenses by consolidating resources; and achieving funded depreciation and cash reserve targets to access capital for equipment and facility upgrades.

For many hospitals, however, clinical and operational strategies may not be sufficient to sustain long-term competitiveness or meet capital requirements. As a result, rural hospitals may look to structural strategies, such as reduction in services, merger, affiliation, or alliance. Each of these strategies fundamentally changes the hospital's mission, level of autonomy, and role in the local health care delivery system. Structural strategies involve changes in ownership, control, and relationship to the communities served. Regardless of the strategic focus, the trend in rural hospital survival is toward maximizing existing resources and developing an integrated continuum of services and programs.

Programs and services that have supported these efforts are described below.

Scope of Care

The scope of hospital services is generally related to local demand, provider capabilities, access to technology, and the mission or market position of the hospital. Historically, rural hospitals have provided more long-term care to their patient populations to accommodate the higher proportion of elderly residents living in rural areas. Although many small rural hospitals with fewer than 50 beds may provide some emergency or obstetric care, many do not have the patient volume to support highly specialized services such as cardiac intensive care or complex surgical procedures. In 1996, the AHA reported that only 22 percent of nonmetropolitan hospitals with fewer than 25 beds had medical/surgical intensive care units (Table 14-2). Additionally, nonmetropolitan community hospitals with fewer than 300 beds were less likely than metropolitan hospitals of the same size to have specialized diagnostic technologies, such as computed tomography scanning (70 versus 81 percent), magnetic resonance imaging (MRI) (29 versus 48 percent), and cardiac catheterization (9 versus 39 percent).

MOST COMMON HOSPITAL SERVICES
As health care has become increasingly dependent on technology and financing has driven health services away from acute care, hospitals have universally come to rely on outpatient services. Rural hospitals have been adversely affected by this transition because the majority of their inpatient services, a crucial source of revenue, have shifted to outpatient settings. The technology issue, on the other hand, has driven the most acute rural patients out of their communities and into large urban centers for sophisticated diagnostic and therapeutic procedures. These two forces combined have caused inpatient volume in rural settings to drop precipitously.

TABLE 14-2   PERCENTAGE NONMETROPOLITAN COMMUNITY HOSPITALS WITH SELECTED INTENSIVE CARE AND DIAGNOSTIC/TREATMENT SERVICES, 1996

Service	Nonmetropolitan Hospitals						Metropolitan Hospitals
	6–24 Beds	25–49 Beds	50–99 Beds	100–199 Beds	200–299 Beds	All <300 Beds	All <300 Beds
Intensive care							
Medical/surgical ICU	22	39	59	74	86	53	75
Cardiac IC beds	14	18	24	34	48	25	37
Neonatal IC beds	1	1	2	7	15	3	16
Selected technologies							
Computed tomography scanner	34	63	73	86	95	70	81
Magnetic resonance imaging	6	16	30	47	66	29	48
Cardiac catheterization laboratory	1	1	5	22	50	9	39
Organ transplant	1	1	1	4	10	2	6
Open heart surgery	0	1	1	3	15	2	18
Extracorporeal shock-wave lithotripter	0	2	4	14	27	7	12

SOURCE: _Healthcare QuickDisk._ Chicago, Healthcare InfoSource, Inc., 1998.

The Essential Access Community Hospital Program evolved as an alternative to the traditional hospital-based model of health service delivery by emphasizing limits on health service delivery based on available resources and community need. Research has indicated that obstetric and newborn cases, although among the most common type of diagnosis-related group (DRG) treated in small rural hospitals, may not be appropriate for the abilities of most rural primary care hospitals (RPCHs).[3] Further studies are needed to know under what conditions obstetrics and surgery involving general anesthesia can be safely performed in the smallest rural hospitals.

Table 14-3 includes a list of common services available in community hospitals with fewer than 300 beds. These data show that most community hospitals, regardless of size, have an emergency department and outpatient surgery. It is interesting to note that roughly 50 percent of hospitals with fewer than 50 beds have a birth room or labor and delivery service, hospital-based outpatient care, home health services, and skilled nursing or long-term care. Ultrasound is available in only 49 percent of hospitals with 6 to 24 beds, but that proportion increases to 72 percent among hospitals with 25 to 49 beds. When all nonmetropolitan hospitals with fewer than 300 beds are compared with all metropolitan hospitals of the same size, there appears to be a slightly higher proportion of home health services and skilled nursing being provided in rural communities. This may be due to the fact that many rural communities have a disproportionate share of elderly as compared with urban areas.

EMERGENCY CARE

The availability of local emergency services is often listed as a top priority of rural hospitals and an important indicator of how local health care is viewed in a rural community. Certainly, the problems with providing 24-hour emergency service are well documented: inadequate physician pay, poor distribution of physicians, and too few to share on-call duty.[4] Others relate to how a specific hospital fits within a regional system and how to develop standards or guidelines for providing emergency services.

"Basic" emergency services are typically defined as triage, care for cardiac emergencies, resuscitation, stabilization, referral, and transfer as appropriate. Physician coverage may be available 24 hours a day but not necessarily on site. One study suggests that up to seven physicians are needed to provide a reliable on-call schedule, but for most community hospitals, it is up to the board to establish policy for emergency coverage.[5] For hospitals with 10,000 or fewer unscheduled emergency department visits, about 30 a day, "basic" emergency services are probably sufficient for the community.

When a community loses the emergency department of its local hospital, residents may experience new barriers to accessing essential services. If the next closest emergency department is 30 miles away, patients with emergent conditions, such as myocardial infarction, can die or experience a worse prognosis by traveling to a distant hospital than if services had been available locally.[6] For this reason, some health care policymakers are attempting to reopen hospitals as critical access facilities. Others, where closure is imminent, are examining ways of improving access to emergency services through the use of ambulances and emergency medical technicians so that patients may be attended by health providers while traveling to the nearest hospital.

SURGICAL SERVICES

Surgical services are regarded as an important element of local health care because they enhance patient convenience, provide needed health care revenue, and save the lives of trauma victims and those experiencing surgical emergencies. Nonetheless, local surgery is one of the areas where rural hospitals commonly reduce services. This is because any hospital that provides surgery has to maintain licensure standards in staffing, equipment, and facility safety. Hospitals with fewer than 100 beds generally perform only surgical procedures with low risk.

The appropriateness of providing surgical services in a rural community may depend on

TABLE 14-3   *PERCENTAGE OF COMMON SELECTED SERVICES AVAILABLE IN NONMETROPOLITAN COMMUNITY HOSPITALS WITH FEWER THAN 300 BEDS, 1996*

| Service | Nonmetropolitan Hospitals | | | | | | Metropolitan Hospitals |
	6–24 Beds	25–49 Beds	50–99 Beds	100–199 Beds	200–299 Beds	All <300 Beds	All <300 Beds
Emergency department	81	83	86	90	95	86	82
Outpatient surgery	71	81	87	91	95	85	85
Ultrasound	49	72	77	86	94	76	82
Physical rehabilitation outpatient services	45	56	67	74	85	64	71
Birthing room/labor and delivery room	36	48	63	79	86	60	59
Hospital-based outpatient care	51	53	57	69	76	59	66
Home health services	55	55	55	63	63	57	45
Skilled nursing or other long-term care	25	25	44	58	68	40	36
Patient education	23	28	39	55	68	39	51

SOURCE: *Healthcare QuickDisk*. Chicago, Healthcare InfoSource, Inc., 1998.

four factors: (1) disease incidence in a specific patient population; (2) willingness of physicians to operate; (3) proclivity of patients and physicians to bypass local care because of poor hospital or surgeon reputation; and (4) the "closeness" of a rural facility to a large urban referral center. A Washington State study of rural surgical services concluded that hospitals with low catchment populations, no local anesthesia services, and difficulty attracting or retaining competent surgeons may be better served by restricting surgery to the least complicated care and participating in a regional surgical referral program.[7]

OBSTETRICS

Local access to obstetric services in rural areas has been shown to have a positive impact on neonatal outcomes. However, like rural surgical services, maternity care is a medical specialty that has become highly regionalized, meaning that only the most sophisticated tertiary hospitals have the combination of specialists and technology to adequately treat high-risk women. One study showed that 5 of 11 urban hospitals with fewer than 500 deliveries annually provided 24 hours of care to newborns who weighed less than 2000 g; this figure compares to 2 of 27 rural facilities.[8] This suggests that rural hospitals prefer to refer high-risk women and babies to urban hospitals owing to the lack of specialists in their own facilities. Because of manpower and technology constraints, many rural hospitals are unable to provide accepted standards of care, such as epidural anesthesia, and must use general surgeons or other non-obstetric providers to perform cesarean sections. In cases such as these, community satisfaction with obstetric care may plummet.

The 1990 Office of Technology Assessment report *Rural Health Care in America* noted that more than half a million rural residents live in counties without a physician trained in obstetrics.[2] Indeed, obstetricians are choosing not to practice in rural areas for a variety of reasons, including the high cost of premiums for medical malpractice coverage, lack of coverage for time off, limited consultation, and difficulty making referrals to larger hospitals. Family physicians represent two-thirds of obstetric providers in rural areas. In fact, some estimates suggest that family physicians in rural locations are more than twice as likely to perform obstetrics than family physicians in urban areas.[2]

SKILLED NURSING FACILITIES AND SWING BEDS

Rural hospitals have pursued several clinical strategies to address patient care and revenue objectives, and one of the most frequently implemented of these is the conversion of acute care beds to swing beds or distinct-part skilled nursing services. Swing beds provide rural hospitals with the flexibility to designate a portion of their acute care beds for non–acute care patients. As a result, hospitals can expand the care continuum without costly changes in licensing status, facility modifications, or staffing requirements. This program has been particularly important in the management of Medicare patients. Hospitals with swing-bed programs are enabled to continue to manage the postacute phase of the patient's recovery outside of the financial constraints imposed by Medicare's prospective payment system (PPS).

Many rural hospitals have moved beyond swing beds and permanently converted acute care beds to accommodate distinct-part (i.e., hospital-based) skilled nursing services. As is the case with swing beds, skilled nursing allows the rural hospital to meet the care needs of patients from the acute through the subacute phase of recovery. Both swing-bed and skilled nursing are reimbursed based on the cost of services. However, skilled nursing services are unique in that they require licensure based on the availability of physical, occupational, and speech therapy services. Furthermore, modification of the hospital facility to accommodate separate dining and activity areas and the administrative support of a licensed long-term-care administrator are necessary.

The skilled nursing and swing-bed programs have proved to be effective clinical strategies for rural hospitals. However, the future of these programs is jeopardized by a proposed shift in Medicare reimbursement from the cost-based model to a prospective DRG-type model. Additionally, the reimbursement differential enjoyed by distinct-part skilled nursing services will be eliminated to create parity with freestanding long-term-care facilities. Rural hospitals are much more likely to support a separate long-term-care unit if they are relatively large in size. Indeed, the smallest nonmetropolitan community hospitals appear to have a higher proportion of skilled nursing facilities (SNFs) than long-term-care facilities: 28 percent of nonmetropolitan community hospitals with fewer than 24 beds had SNFs, whereas only 8.2 percent of these hospitals had long-term-care facilities (Table 14-4).

HOME HEALTH SERVICES

Home health has been a component of many hospital designations and has been included among the services that must be available or accessible to primary care hospitals for patients who are discharged to their homes. However, with pressure from the Health Care Financing Administration (HCFA) to increase requirements for staffing while reducing reimbursement for Medicare and Medicaid patients, rural hospitals are finding themselves in a difficult struggle between a decreasing supply of qualified home health professionals and an increasing demand for services. For instance, many hospitals lack both a full-time registered nurse (RN) director and appropriate instructors to conduct the classroom teaching mandated for all home health aides. At the same time, these hospitals are experiencing increasing pressure to refer their elderly, chronically ill patients to home health as quickly as possible following an acute episode of care.

RURAL HEALTH CLINICS

Hospital-based ambulatory care has been particularly attractive to rural areas owing to its need for limited capital, convenience for physicians, and ability to provide a source of surgical emergency care. Changes in patient volume and reimbursement, however, can make ambulatory care unprofitable. Another option for diversifying into primary care is to create hospital-based primary care clinics, which can serve the important function of providing backup assistance for physicians and removing administrative responsibilities from them. However, in other cases, rural physicians have seen these clinics as competitors, resulting in strained hospital-physician relationships in some communities.

TABLE 14-4   LONG-TERM CARE SERVICES PROVIDED IN NONMETROPOLITAN COMMUNITY HOSPITALS, 1996

Bed Size	Total Facilities	Total Separate LTC Unit	LTC, Percentage of Total	Total with SNF Unit[a]	SNF, Percentage of Total
6–24	207	17	8.2	59	28.5
25–49	718	91	12.7	178	24.8
50–99	688	320	46.5	300	43.6
100–199	494	272	55.1	271	54.9
200–299	115	91	79.1	92	80.0
300+	41	19	46.3	19	46.3
Total	2,263	810	35.8	919	40.6

[a]The number of hospitals with skilled nursing facility units is probably included in the number of hospitals with separate long-term-care units.

Key: LTC, long-term care; SNF, skilled nursing facility.

SOURCE: *Healthcare QuickDisk.* Chicago, Healthcare InfoSource, Inc., 1998.

Rural health clinics are discussed in greater detail in Chap. 19.

ALTERNATIVE MODELS

When a hospital cannot introduce all of these clinical strategies owing to lack of physician support, the competitiveness of the local market, or poor financial performance, several alternative models exist that allow the rural hospital to continue to provide a more limited scope of service to the community. Proposed alternative models of care must take into consideration seven components of health service delivery: (1) licensure and certification regulations, (2) reimbursement mechanisms, (3) staffing requirements, (4) staff training and scope of practice, (5) service requirements and configuration, (6) technical needs, and (7) relationships among rural hospitals. Failure to address fully any one of these areas may severely limit the degree to which the model is locally accepted and adopted within a rural community.

THE ESSENTIAL ACCESS COMMUNITY HOSPITAL/ PRIMARY CARE HOSPITAL. The Essential Access Community Hospital/Primary Care Hospital (EACH/PCH) model was developed in 1989 as an alternative health service delivery model. The original EACH legislation was part of the Omnibus Budget Reconciliation Act of 1989 (Public Law 101-239), with technical amendments enacted in 1990 (Public Law 101-508) and 1994 (Public Law 103-432). As of 1990, seven states had received grant awards from the HCFA for designating EACH/PCH facilities; these included California, Colorado, Kansas, New York, North Carolina, South Dakota, and West Virginia. Since May 1997, a total of 40 rural PCHs have been developed in six of the seven eligible states.[9]

The EACH/PCH model is based on two different types of complementary health care facilities. The PCH, which must affiliate itself with an EACH, is a hospital without critical care capabilities. It is equipped and staffed to meet the acute medical needs of patients who require a basic level of monitoring and support but

whose lives are not threatened. This means that PCHs must provide 24-hour emergency care but have no more than 6 inpatient beds—up to 12 if a participant in Medicare's swing-bed program—with a policy to keep patients for no longer than 72 hours. All PCHs have five essential components: (1) hospital-based primary care practice; (2) observation beds; (3) hospital-based ambulance service; (4) modern diagnostic services, which may not be in the hospital but must be locally accessible; and (5) formal clinical affiliations with secondary and tertiary providers. In addition, other essential services must be available to patients, including home health care, durable medical equipment, long-term care, pharmaceutical services, and outpatient surgery, which is optional based on community preferences for maintaining local surgery.

Hospitals eligible to convert to a PCH must have the following: an average daily census of 20 patients, a private-pay population of 10 or fewer patients, a primary service area of fewer than 10,000 patients, and a full-time resident staff of fewer than five competent physicians. It is interesting to note that distance to the nearest secondary care facility is not a factor, due to enhancements in transportation and telecommunications.

The PCH has not been widely accepted because traditional providers find it threatening. Reimbursement has been a problem because the conditions of being a PCH do not qualify it for receiving Medicare/Medicaid reimbursement. Additionally, private insurance companies have not taken a lead in developing systems for reimbursement. Licensure standards add another constraint, as existing rules and regulations for secondary care facilities do not fit the PCH model. Although the PCH can enhance the scope of practice and professional responsibility of midlevel providers, this cannot be accomplished in states that restrict the professional roles of nurse practitioners (NPs) and physician assistants (PAs).

The other half of the EACH/PCH program is the EACH. When a patient located in a PCH requires support or monitoring for more than

72 hours, he or she is transferred to an EACH. EACHs are larger than PCHs and must have at least 75 beds while being located more than 35 miles from any other hospital. EACHs are paid by Medicare as sole community hospitals (SCHs)—a designation used for hospitals that serve as the only local provider for some months out of the year based on weather and topography conditions. SCHs also include hospitals that serve at least 75 percent of all local residents and Medicare beneficiaries; hospitals that were designated SCH by Medicare before the implementation of PPS have kept their status as such.

CRITICAL ACCESS HOSPITALS AND MEDICAL ASSISTANCE FACILITIES.   Another type of model has been developed that has been the first alternative model to seek and receive funding from the HCFA under the Medicare Rural Hospital Flexibility Program. This program promotes a critical access model based on the combined experiences of the rural PCHs and the medical assistance facilities (MAFs) that have been piloted in Montana since 1987. MAFs are defined as health care institutions that offer inpatient care to ill or injured persons for no more than 96 hours by providing a combination of emergency and short-term acute care. MAFs can be staffed by midlevel practitioners, with physicians available within 20 minutes. A physician, however, must visit the facility at least once every 30 days. As of May 1997, 12 MAFs have been developed in Montana, generally though conversion of existing rural hospitals.[9]

Because of the success of the MAF pilot project in Montana, the federal Balanced Budget Act of 1997 authorized the development of Medicare-eligible MAF-like facilities, termed critical access hospitals (CAHs), in rural communities nationwide. The characteristics of the MAF model that have been retained by CAHs include distance of more than 35 miles from the nearest hospital; emergency department and inpatient services provided by physicians, PAs, and NPs; 15 or fewer inpatient beds; inpatient stay of 96 hours or less; and cost-based reimbursement.[10]

To support the feasibility analyses and assessments of the CAH model, the Rural Hospital Flexibility Program will offer support for local citizens, employers, and heath care providers to conduct community development activities. These may include but are not limited to planning community health assessments and designing systems of care to address local needs. For hospitals, this funding will provide technical assistance to (1) develop integrated networks of care, (2) examine the conversion to CAHs, (3) develop information systems and telehealth activities, (4) improve quality assurance activities, (5) conduct financial feasibility analyses, and (6) improve rural emergency medical systems.[11]

Hospital Organization and Administration

MEDICAL STAFF

The maldistribution of medical providers in rural versus urban areas has been a dynamic of the U.S. health care culture since the late 1960s, and it continues to challenge issues of access and quality. Rural hospitals have fewer than half the medical staff of urban hospitals with comparable numbers of beds, and those with fewer than 50 beds have roughly one-third of the medical staff of their urban counterparts. In 1990, the Office of Technology Assessment reported that more than 80 percent of nonmetropolitan hospitals with fewer than 50 beds were lacking at least one of the following medical specialties: pediatrics; obstetrics and gynecology; ophthalmology; anesthesiology; dermatology; emergency medicine; nuclear medicine; psychiatry; and orthopedic, plastic, or thoracic surgery.[2] The shortage of medical specialists in rural communities is discussed in greater detail under "Common Problems," below.

Midlevel providers have been used to allay some of the stress placed on rural health care. However, successful employment of NPs and PAs on a medical staff is contingent on the organization of medical services in the community and local acceptance of midlevel providers. Where small physician groups exist, NPs and

PAs are more likely to be employed; solo practitioners, however, may view midlevel providers as competing against them for rural patients. Midlevel providers are not widely employed on the staffs of rural hospitals, although both NPs and PAs are more likely to have hospital privileges than midlevel providers practicing in urban locations.

Certified nurse midwives (CNMs) and certified registered nurse anesthetists (CRNAs) are two other types of midlevel provider that are commonly used as physician substitutes in rural hospitals lacking obstetricians and anesthesiologists. In addition to providing gynecologic services, family planning, and prenatal care, CNMs can deliver babies, comanage high-risk pregnancies with physicians, and care for mothers and infants after pregnancy. CNMs can practice independently of physicians but only as providers who conduct consultations, provide collaborative management, and coordinate referrals. CRNAs, on the other hand, are baccalaureate-prepared RNs who have completed 24 to 36 months of additional training in anesthesiology and passed a national certification examination. Licensure and certification regulations require that CRNAs work under the supervision of a physician, but supervision by an anesthesiologist is not often necessary.

The supply of RNs working in rural areas has decreased since the 1980s; whether this trend is a function of supply or demand is still not certain. The RNs who are practicing in rural areas are selecting the most populated counties in which to work. According to 1990 data, only 8.7 percent of all RNs employed in nursing were located in counties of fewer than 50,000 residents.[2]

OWNERSHIP STRUCTURES

In 1996, nearly half (49 percent) of all rural community hospitals were owned by nonprofit organizations and church-operated groups; state and local government owned another 42 percent, and for-profit investors owned the remaining 9 percent (Fig. 14-1). State and local governments have traditionally owned hospitals of fewer than 50 beds; conversely, hospitals with 100 beds or more have been predominantly private nonprofit facilities. These trends hold for hospitals participating in both multihospital systems (Table 14-5) and alliances (Table 14-6).

Hospital districts have been important in parts of the United States where access to health care is limited and health service delivery unprofitable.[12] In 1987, a total of 31 states reported health and hospital expenditures by special districts.[13] Unlike for-profit hospitals or nonprofit

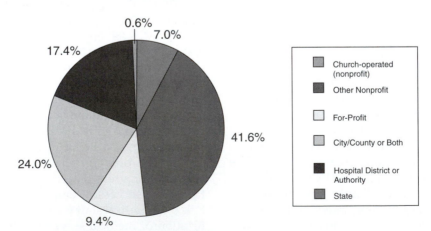

FIGURE 14-1 *Ownership of nonmetropolitan community hospitals, 1996. (From* Healthcare QuickDisk. *Chicago, Healthcare InfoSource, Inc., 1998, with permission.)*

TABLE 14-5   NUMBER AND PERCENT OF NONMETROPOLITAN COMMUNITY HOSPITALS WITH FEWER THAN 300 BEDS IN MULTIHOSPITAL SYSTEMS BY OWNERSHIP AND BED SIZE, 1996

| Ownership | Hospital Bed Size | | | | |
	6–24 Beds	25–49 Beds	50–99 Beds	100–199 Beds	200–299 Beds
Government	9 (25.0%)	43 (30.5%)	22 (11.0%)	8 (5.4%)	6 (15.4%)
Nonprofit	22 (68.8%)	84 (59.6%)	135 (67.5%)	93 (63.3%)	27 (69.2%)
For profit	2 (6.3%)	14 (9.9%)	43 (21.5%)	46 (31.3%)	6 (15.4%)
Total	32	141	200	147	39

SOURCE: *Healthcare QuickDisk*. Chicago, Healthcare InfoSource, Inc., 1998.

facilities, district hospitals are supported by local tax revenues and governed by a publicly elected board, thereby constituting a form of local government. Another source of publicly funded health care is the county hospital, which still exists in some rural areas. Here, the county board of supervisors has ultimate control over the facility, including the authority to hire and fire the administrator. Other government-owned hospital models include Indian Health Service hospitals, military hospitals, and city hospitals.

GOVERNANCE AND ADMINISTRATION
The majority of rural hospitals are governed by boards made up of local residents who are either elected, appointed by an elected body, or selected through a recruitment and nomination process. The governing board is responsible for a variety of tasks, including establishing and evaluating the hospital's mission; creating policies; appointing, supporting, and evaluating the chief executive officer (CEO); setting goals and objectives; assessing and improving the quality of care and service; strengthening financial viability; and complying with all legal and regulatory requirements.[14] The hospital administrator or CEO usually serves as an ex-officio member of the governing board.

One of the most important board responsibilities is the selection of the CEO. This can be a difficult task for rural hospital boards because of the competition from urban hospitals for talented managers. Rural hospital boards find it difficult to compete with the higher compensation packages larger urban hospitals can offer. As a result, some hospitals have turned to affiliation with a larger health system or contracted with a hospital management company for administrative services. CEO hiring decisions for

TABLE 14-6   NONMETROPOLITAN COMMUNITY HOSPITALS WITH FEWER THAN 300 BEDS IN ALLIANCES BY OWNERSHIP AND BED SIZE, 1996

| Ownership | Hospital Bed Size | | | | |
	6–24 Beds	25–49 Beds	50–99 Beds	100–199 Beds	200–299 Beds
Government	18 (54.5%)	88 (56.4%)	54 (36.5%)	43 (30.0%)	20 (35.7%)
Nonprofit	15 (45.5%)	64 (41.0%)	89 (60.1%)	98 (68.1%)	35 (62.5%)
For profit	0	4 (2.6%)	5 (3.4%)	3 (2.1%)	1 (1.8%)
Total	33	156	148	144	56

SOURCE: *Healthcare QuickDisk*. Chicago, Healthcare InfoSource, Inc., 1998.

rural hospitals that are owned by or affiliated with larger systems are usually made by the corporate board with the concurrence of the local board.

COMMON PROBLEMS

Physician Recruitment and Retention

A number of factors can weigh into a physician's decision to work in a rural community, including the experience of having grown up in a rural location, desire to live at a more relaxed pace, better air quality, and closer proximity to outdoor recreation. However, in addition to these lifestyle preferences, there may be concerns about geographic and professional isolation, spouse employment, quality of education for children, and proximity of cultural resources that may make the decision to live and work in a rural community more difficult.

Indeed, lifestyle issues are only half of the picture. Among professional concerns are working longer hours, practicing outside of a group-practice environment, seeing more patients each week than providers in urban communities do, and struggling to meet the demands and expectations of the community. Lack of access to the technology that allows providers to use the full scope of their medical training is a professional concern for many rural doctors, as is lack of professional backup for personal illness or vacation. One study showed that lack of planned time off adversely affected willingness to stay of 63 percent of rural physicians.[15]

Improving the professional lifestyle of rural physicians often depends on borrowing or using clinical and professional resources commonly housed in large urban hospitals. Some solutions have evolved for relieving professional stress and thereby increasing provider retention, including:

1. *Locum tenens.* These programs use temporary traveling physicians to staff emergency departments and to provide clinical coverage on weekends. This type of program is expensive, and many rural hospitals contract with locums companies to provide coverage.
2. *CME.* Traditionally, CME has been extended to rural areas by sending specialists and other health care providers into rural hospitals to provide educational programming on site. More recently, however, CME has been provided over videoconference to allow multiple rural sites to connect at one time to a large tertiary medical center for a CME program.
3. *Technical support.* Some tertiary care medical centers may take on consultative roles with community physicians in terms of reading fetal monitoring strips and interpreting x-rays.

Maintaining Scope of Services

Physicians have traditionally located their practices in areas where local health services already exist. Given this condition of rural practice for many physicians, the closure of small rural hospitals has had an even more devastating impact on physician supply. In order to maintain a simple menu of medical services, rural hospitals will frequently contract with large urban facilities for medical services provided by a visiting consultant. One study of rural and urban hospitals located in Missouri demonstrated that hospitals using hospital-based consulting were able to increase clinical hours in medical subspecialties by 61.8 hours or 1.24 FTE.[16] Cardiology, pathology, and oncology were the medical specialty areas provided to the largest number of hospitals.

Continuous Quality Improvement Issues, Credentialing, and Proctoring

Recruiting qualified physicians is often very difficult for rural hospitals, as noted above. Applicants for positions in rural communities may also have had difficulty in previous positions, leading them to seek more remote medical practices. Confirming qualifications and previous medical-legal or licensure problems takes hospital staff time and expertise, which is often unavailable in rural hospitals.

Also, with medical staffs that contain only one or two physicians in some specialties, it can be difficult to provide unbiased continuous quality improvement (CQI) activities and sometimes impossible to proctor physicians for procedures. In some cases when standards of care are not practiced due to lack of peer review, iatrogenic adverse outcomes may occur repeatedly. These are more visible in rural communities, damaging what is sometimes an already marginal community image of the local health care system.

Nursing and Midlevel Provider Recruitment and Retention

Recruitment and retention of nursing and midlevel providers involves many of the same lifestyle and professional issues that are related to physician retention. Midlevel providers have been the target for specific recruiting strategies as a means of alleviating provider shortages in rural areas. Indeed, research suggests that physician assistants can provide between 60 and 90 percent of the care that a family physician delivers.[17]

The types of services provided by NPs and PAs and how practices are structured are very important to job satisfaction and subsequent retention. Compared to NPs, PAs are more likely to provide services in emergency departments, to assist with surgery, to make nursing home visits, and to do inpatient rounds. Furthermore, PAs can take call for physicians. Nonetheless, great variation exists in the scope of practice for midlevel providers. In one study, fewer than 50 percent of hospitals said that their NPs and PAs had admitting and discharge privileges, although more than 80 percent said that their midlevel providers could prescribe medication.[18]

Practice autonomy plays a significant role in midlevel provider satisfaction. It has been noted that the PAs who practice in primary care settings with smaller numbers of physicians on staff are among the most satisfied, which sug-

gests that the PAs in small group practices enjoy a wider range of patient care responsibilities. It is important to note, however, that state law determines the scope of practice for PAs and NPs. In 1994, the Joint Commission on the Accreditation of Healthcare Organizations revised its policies relating to the organization of hospital medical staff, including whether clinical privileges could be made available to PAs or NPs.

Ancillary Staff

Ancillary staff—including radiology technicians, respiratory therapists, pharmacists, and physical therapists, among others—are also difficult to recruit to rural hospitals. Issues similar to those described for physicians and nurses also exist for these professionals; indeed, issues of overwork, lack of support, and limited opportunities for growth prevail. Working in a hospital where the scope of service is limited and advanced technology absent may also produce professional dissatisfaction. Last, financial constraints and patient volume may dictate lower salaries and the need to cover multiple areas. For instance, it is not uncommon for x-ray technicians to perform electrocardiograms (ECGs) and transport patients to and from the emergency department. This may become a vicious cycle as qualified physicians become dissatisfied with the quality of ancillary care that exists in the hospital. Ancillary staff issues can cause some rural hospitals to refer certain patients out of the community or in some cases can be cited as the principal reason for discontinuing practice in the community.

Facilities

The Hill-Burton program was enacted by Congress in 1946 as part of the Hospital Survey and Construction Act. This program provided federal matching funds to survey state needs, develop statewide plans for building nonprofit nongovernment hospitals, and building facilities. However, it was not until 1965 that the act was amended to address the modernization and replacement of facilities; standards for structure, design, and safety; and the provision of free care to the medically indigent.

It is important to note that about 30 percent of all hospitals built between 1949 and 1962 were created with Hill-Burton monies.[2] However, because the program was disbanded in 1974, many aging rural facilities have not had the financial support to make improvements in physical plant. This means that many rural hospitals have not been retrofitted to adapt to infrastructure needs to support emerging technology. For this reason alone, many rural hospitals have made the decision to convert to long-term or skilled nursing care, as this type of service delivery does not involve the technology burden of providing more advanced health services, such as emergency and intensive care or telemedicine, which may enhance ambulatory services.

Although many hospitals would like to update their facilities and many community residents would have a better opinion of local health care if the facilities appeared more modern and sophisticated, this is often very difficult for a hospital to do alone. Bond measures to finance improvements or build new facilities may be proposed and voted on by the community. However, in the absence of publicly proposed and funded renovation strategies, hospitals must generate the operating revenue and reserves to cover the capital costs of modernizing their physical plants. For many rural hospitals, this is virtually impossible to do without a business partnership.

Administration

The recruitment and selection of a qualified hospital CEO is a significant challenge for rural hospitals because of competition from urban hospitals for talented managers. Rural hospital boards find it difficult to compete with the higher compensation packages offered by larger urban hospitals. In addition to income disparity, rural CEOs face professional isolation and lack of specialized expertise. They have fewer sup-

port staff and a broader span of responsibilities and are more subject to board, medical staff, and community politics. As a result, administrative turnover is usually higher in rural hospitals than in their urban counterparts. To attract the most qualified candidates, some boards have turned to affiliation with a larger health system or contracted with a hospital management company for administrative services.

Governance

Members of hospital governing boards face numerous pressures in carrying out their strategic, policy, and fiduciary responsibilities. Competition, organizational realignment, declining reimbursement, managed care, access to qualified staff, and compliance with federal and state laws are just a few of the issues boards must confront. To govern effectively requires that board members share a clearly articulated vision and mission for the hospital; a thorough understanding of key strategic, operational, and financial issues; and a strong commitment to service to the community. Board deliberations and decision making should be based on clearly defined strategies and a thorough examination of alternative courses of action. Board decisions should be timely and provide clear direction to management.

A well-functioning board is critical to the success of the hospital. Factors that undermine governing board effectiveness include high turnover of board members; politically based decision making; and the absence of clearly defined roles, a mission, and an effective nominating and selection process. For public hospitals, governing boards must carry out their responsibilities in public forums because of open-meeting laws. This legal requirement puts public hospitals at a disadvantage to private, nonprofit, and for-profit competitors, who are able to gain access to the public hospitals' strategic and policymaking processes.

Although these factors can be found throughout the hospital industry, certain ownership and governing structures are more susceptible to them. Many rural hospitals are publicly owned either by the county or through legislatively approved hospital districts. In both cases, board members are either elected or appointed by an elected body. Publicly selected board members face conflicting demands from political groups, interest groups, and their constituents.

To survive the transformation of the health care industry brought on by changes in reimbursement, care delivery systems, managed care, and organizational restructuring, hospitals that previously were governed by counties or districts have decided to serve their communities by becoming part of larger hospital systems. In California, 13 of 74 hospital districts have consolidated their hospitals with other hospitals and health systems.[12] These affiliations bring about significant changes in hospital governance. In many cases, hospital boards are better able to carry out their duties because they have better access to information systems, health care industry resources, and hospital-specific trends while being less vulnerable to the influence of political and community-based factions.

Economics

Reimbursement Issues

In 1990, it was reported that approximately 44 percent of state spending for rural health care was funded by federal sources, primarily Medicare. On average, rural hospitals relied on Medicare for almost 41 percent of patient revenues, and Medicare accounted for at least half of revenues in 30 percent of rural hospitals.[19] Despite the significant role that Medicare plays in financing rural health services, many rural hospitals are faced with rates of reimbursement that do not cover the full cost of care.

As mentioned earlier, hospitals are reimbursed by Medicare through PPS. Under this system, the hospital is paid a set amount for treating each patient based on the primary diagnosis of the patient and the DRG to which the patient has been assigned. For efficiency's sake, costs are based on averages, and if a hospital is able to keep its costs lower than the average

DRG payment, it is allowed to keep the difference. However, because of declining patient volume, many rural hospitals are unable to meet their fixed costs. In the first 3 years of Medicare's PPS, 83 percent of hospitals with negative hospital margins were located in rural areas. In 1988, a total of 38 percent of all rural hospitals had negative total operating margins.[20]

The alternative hospital models, including the EACH/PCH and the SCH, have been established so that specific hospitals can qualify for special reimbursement. SCHs, which may be the only source of care in geographically remote areas, can receive PPS payments that are the highest of either the full federal PPS rate or 100 percent of a target amount based on the hospital's costs. Rural PCHs providing emergency and limited inpatient care receive cost-based reimbursement, and EACHs qualify for the SCH payment rules.

Medicaid reimbursement is also based on a prospectively set rate that is established either by selective contracting, hospital-specific negotiated rates, DRG-based methods, or past hospital costs. One difficulty with Medicaid reimbursement is that many rural residents do not qualify for assistance because they are self-employed or part of a two-parent family. In fact, it has been estimated that up to 30 percent of rural inhabitants have no health insurance.[20]

Economies of Scale

PPS has made survival difficult for many rural hospitals. This is because many rural hospitals receive a rate of reimbursement for services based on a system of cost averaging applied to urban hospitals, where system efficiencies and economies of scale allow fixed costs to be spread over a larger patient population. Rural hospitals do not have this advantage due to limitations in staffing, inefficiencies in aging physical plants due to the Hill-Burton program, and the smaller patient population they serve. Research suggests that hospitals reach their own least-cost output at 80 percent of capacity; small hospitals, however, operated at about 40 percent through the 1980s.[21] In the 1996 AHA survey, nonmetro-

TABLE 14-7   *SUMMARY OF COMMUNITY HOSPITAL SIZE AND UTILIZATION BY METROPOLITAN/NONMETROPOLITAN STATUS, 1996*

Characteristic	Metropolitan Hospitals	Nonmetropolitan Hospitals
Number of hospitals	2,649	2,263
Average number of beds	245	84
Occupancy rate (%)[a]	63	56
Average length of stay[a]	5.9 days	7.3 days

[a]Based on 2210 metropolitan hospitals and 1966 nonmetropolitan hospitals.

SOURCE: *Healthcare QuickDisk.* Chicago, Healthcare InfoSource, Inc., 1998.

politan hospitals averaged an occupancy rate of 56 percent (Table 14-7). Nonetheless, occupancy rates among hospitals with fewer than 50 beds remained under 40 percent (Table 14-8). Underutilization makes hospital closure a serious issue for many rural communities, especially when privately insured patients travel to urban locations for services, thereby leaving the local health care system to serve a largely publicly funded, medically indigent population.

MANAGED CARE

Managed care is primarily an urban phenomenon that is not easily transferable to rural communities owing to the absence of a coordinated medical system that includes a large panel of qualified specialists, computer technology, information systems, clinical protocols, and well-defined policies and procedures pertaining to administration and operations processes. Because of the absence of a clear health care "system" in rural areas, physicians commonly find themselves referring patients out of the community to urban medical centers that have developed this range of complex organizational features.

Nonetheless, rural hospitals are realizing that they must maintain a mix of primary care physicians and specialists in order to provide the level of service integration that is attractive to managed care. In fact, a survey of hospital CEOs indicated that managed care was the primary reason for developing affiliations with other hospitals and health systems.[22] Because rural markets do not have the population base to support a wide range of specialists, many are

TABLE 14-8   *UTILIZATION OF NONMETROPOLITAN COMMUNITY HOSPITALS BY HOSPITAL TYPE AND NUMBER OF BEDS, 1996*

Number of Beds	Number of Hospitals	Admissions per Hospital	Inpatient Days per Hospital	Occupancy Rate,[a] Percent	Total Admissions	Total Inpatient Days	Total Beds
6–24	178	434	2,163	33	77,274	384,995	3,213
25–49	611	974	5,292	39	595,241	3,233,587	22,451
50–99	596	1,881	14,275	55	1,120,824	8,508,099	42,401
100–199	436	3,864	30,475	60	1,684,725	13,287,062	60,105
200–299	108	7,647	56,494	64	825,878	6,101,377	26,233
300+	37	12,287	89,476	64	454,627	3,310,595	14,151
Total	1,966	27,087	198,175	56	4,758,569	34,825,715	168,554

[a]Occupancy rate = (total inpatient days/366)/total beds. (366 was used to reflect the 1996 leap year.)

SOURCE: *Healthcare QuickDisk.* Chicago, Healthcare InfoSource, Inc., 1998.

linking with large health systems. Additionally, because such a large proportion of the rural patient population is publicly insured through Medicare or Medicaid, hospital executives are recognizing the importance of keeping private paying patients in the local delivery system by using managed care. One hurdle is the small numbers of employees of rural businesses, which may not provide health benefits. Furthermore, larger local employers may hesitate to contract with a hospital for managed care if there is the perception that a small local facility lacks the information and financial systems necessary for producing sound pricing of medical services.

CONSULTATION AND REFERRAL STRATEGIES

Ownership of Hospitals by Larger Health Systems

The literature suggests that a number of rural hospitals have chosen to become part of multi-hospital or integrated health systems. The strategic advantage to affiliating this way is that a rural hospital can gain access to additional insured patients. This is especially beneficial if better reimbursement from payers can be secured by a hospital system than by individual rural hospitals. The disadvantage of an affiliation involving hospital ownership is that the hospital loses authority as a decision maker and must rely on the larger health system to provide the health services that meet local needs.

The ownership of a rural hospital by a larger health system constitutes a type of contractual arrangement. The distinction between purchasing and other types of contractual arrangements is the locus of ownership. The purchase of a rural hospital by a larger health system involves the loss of individual legal identity. This is in contrast with a lease or contract management arrangement, where the local rural facility maintains facility ownership and physical assets.[23]

There has been little evidence to suggest that joining a multihospital system preserves the viability of small rural hospitals. One study actually showed that investor-owned systems actually increased the probability of closure, while affiliation with a not-for-profit system or contract management had no effect.[24]

Affiliations with Larger Health Systems

Changes in the delivery and organization of health care services brought on by declining reimbursement, expanding technology, managed care, competition for physicians and hospital staff, and regionalization of services and providers have had a profound impact on rural hospitals. To survive, rural hospitals that had been independent county-, district-, or community-based providers are pursuing affiliations with larger private and public systems. These affiliations may take several forms.

1. *Acquisition,* where the rural hospital is purchased by another hospital or system and all assets are merged into the parent organization.
2. *Merger* of two or more hospitals to create a new system, where the rural hospital takes on a new identity, assets are joined, and governance is shared by the hospital partners.
3. *Alliance* with a health system to gain access to specialty programs and services. (In this mode, the rural hospital remains autonomous from the health system. The rural hospital may contract with the system for selected services.)
4. *Network participation* in joint purchasing, shared services, physician recruiting, or contracting.

The form of the affiliation and the selection of a partner or partners are based on the strategic, financial, and clinical needs of the rural hospital. Although the decision to affiliate may be made for many different reasons, the most common of these are to strengthen a primary care physician base; expand specialized clinical services and improve local access to specialists; secure capital and financial support for capital projects; gain access to managed care contracts; access management expertise, technologies, and information systems; and improve the local image of the hospital.

Regionalization of Specialty Services

Regionalization of health care is an attempt to increase the efficient use of intensive care services within a geographically defined population. Because only certain units are licensed to provide very expensive services, such as neonatal intensive care, duplication of services is reduced because only the sickest people enter the system through appropriate medical screening. In a regionalized health system, for example, family physicians and other providers of prenatal care screen pregnancies for medical and behavioral risk factors and refer the highest-risk pregnancies to the appropriate tertiary care center for labor and delivery. Family physicians and rural pediatricians may also screen high-risk babies in their practices and refer their patients for advanced care in tertiary care facilities when the needs of the patient cannot be met by the local hospital.

Trauma care is another area of health service delivery that has been regionalized. Like the regionalization of perinatal care, effective trauma regionalization is based on stabilization, appropriate referral, and transfer to a level 1 trauma center. Furthermore, although most community hospitals are designated level 3 trauma centers, some states have developed level 4 and level 5 centers for smaller hospitals based on a facility's ability to participate in staff training, develop quality assurance procedures, and implement guidelines for transfer.[25]

Any system of regionalized care demands ongoing support for clinical and educational linkages. This may take place through continuing medical education (CME) provided to nurses and physicians, the development of clinical protocols, and quality assurance activities that allow community hospitals the opportunity to have their performance in the regional system measured and evaluated.

Transfer Agreements

Transfer agreements essentially outline the responsibilities of the referring and receiving hospitals involved in transporting a patient who is unable to receive risk-appropriate care within his or her community. Transfer agreements often exist for trauma care and serve as a framework for assigning responsibilities related to providing medical records and documentation; securing consent from both the patient and participating physicians; arranging transportation; resolving disputes; and developing systems for providing outreach education, liaison selection, and continuous quality improvement activities.

Ownership of Medical Groups in Rural Communities

Hospitals are increasingly engaging physician groups in joint ventures to strengthen their referral base for inpatient services and outpatient specialty care. This strategy has been used by hospitals that compete against their staff physicians who have private practices in the community. Joint ventures may take the form of diagnostic imaging centers, laboratories, ambulatory surgery centers, and space leasing.

Physicians can gain significantly from these relationships through the centralization of accredited CME, communications with administration, and the availability of medical offices and staff support. Other incentives to joining a group include (1) subsidized malpractice insurance, (2) patient referrals from hospital satellite centers or through managed care contracts, (3) management services (i.e., billing, marketing), and (4) guaranteed income or incentive compensation.[2]

Visiting Specialists

The concept of the visiting consultant clinic represents the advent of private or market-driven "regionalization" in the health care delivery system. In the area of visiting consultant clinics, the most common medical and surgical specialties establishing outreach activities include cardiology, orthopedics, oncology, otolaryngology, and urology. Visiting specialists are particularly useful in providing nonemergency care for patients with chronic illness or complex conditions requiring in-depth specialty diagnostic expertise.

The oversupply of specialists in many urban and suburban areas has created incentives for specialists to establish community outreach as a component of their practices. This is compounded in areas with high penetration of managed care, which often limits urban and suburban patients' access to some specialists—a situation less common for rural patients. For rural providers, the principal disadvantage to referring patients to urban or suburban specialists for advanced surgical procedures—which may stimulate outmigration in other areas—is losing control of the patient's care once a specialist has taken the case out of the community. Local physician acceptance is therefore a key ingredient to ensuring the success of visiting specialist clinics.

Seven criteria should be considered before a visiting consultation clinic is established: (1) ensuring regular and dependable service; (2) selecting the physicians staffing the clinic; (3) establishing patient referral protocols; (4) defining specialists' responsibilities to local physicians and hospital staff; (5) managing competition among specialists; (6) specifying costs borne by the hospital versus visiting specialists; and (7) determining clinic marketing and scheduling.[26] The fulfillment of these criteria puts a large burden on the small staffs of many rural hospitals.

To relieve administrative strain, the urban providers and their associated hospitals must be cooperative about supplying necessary administrative paperwork and proactive at all levels of communication regarding the course of a rural patient's care. Because interfacility communication of this nature has not been formalized by many hospitals, it is important for both the rural and urban hospitals to consider developing communications systems between physicians and staff at both facilities to be certain that records and x-ray results are available to rural providers. This is especially important when patients self-refer or have more than one source of specialist care. Finally, regardless of whether the patient is cared for in the urban or rural setting by the specialist, it is critical that the responsibility for care of the patient be clearly defined after hours as well as at other times when the specialist is not available in the rural community. Clearly, issues can arise if the rural providers are not able to attend to the patient's needs due to lack of communication with the specialist about the condition, its treatment, and possible side effects.

University Health System Affiliations

Most academic medical centers have joint missions of patient care, education, research, and community outreach. These missions may be more compatible with the rural hospital and more conducive to its survival compared to relationships with health systems more focused on a financial "bottom line." The development of affiliations between academic centers and community hospitals is one way of solidifying a teaching hospital's commitment to outreach while at the same time supporting research, patient care, and education both on and away from the medical center campus.

University health system affiliations may begin with CME programs or medical student and resident training. From these activities may grow a variety of other joint ventures, including purchasing and contracting, strategic planning, telemedicine, library information systems, and medical informatics. By offering rural hospitals assistance with these activities, the university health system is able to strengthen the quality of care that is provided within its region while developing opportunities for medical student and resident training and research partnerships. The rural community hospital, on the other hand, gains needed expertise in a number of areas without losing its independence.

FUTURE TRENDS

Telemedicine

Telemedicine is strategically important for many rural hospitals and their urban partners as a referral linkage. Using any variety of tele-communications modalities, including remote interactive videoconferencing and still-image store-and-forward, telemedicine allows for the electronic importation of a full range of medical services to patients in their own communities, thereby preventing the erosion of the local health system's patient base. For participating susbspecialists, using telecommunications to deliver patient care reduces the opportunity costs of having to leave an urban medical center to attend clinic in a remote area.

Training Physicians for Rural Communities

Practice in a rural community is clearly different in many significant ways from practice in an urban or suburban community. These differences relate not only to the scope of practice (more often including obstetrics, surgical procedures, and orthopedics) but also to the practice environment, hospital medical staff organization, lifestyle, and other areas.

Preparing residents for all of these aspects of rural practice has been a priority for many family practice programs. This issue has been addressed using several methodologies. Some programs have purposely emphasized areas of training such as maternity care, orthopedics, and surgical assisting. In addition, programs have included both mandatory and elective rural practice rotations to expose residents to other aspects of rural practice. More recently, an increasing number of programs have created *rural training tracks.* In these programs, residents spend the majority of their second and third years in a rural community practice as part of a separately accredited residency program.

Although many rural communities have a need for certain specialists, the population base often does not exist for specialists to have a full-time practice. These needs can be met by visiting specialists. However, a new model is emerging that involves combining training programs in primary care and other specialties. The best-known combined training program is internal medicine and pediatrics (MED/PEDS), although it has produced few rural physicians and experienced limited success.

The concept of creating a family physician with a specific area of medical expertise has a great deal of appeal in many rural areas. One popular way of gaining this expertise is through fellowship programs, such as those available in sports medicine and geriatrics, which may result in a certificate of added qualification. One fellowship program enables family physicians to obtain additional training in obstetrics—an important skill set for physicians in communities that have limited access to obstetricians.

Another newer method of training is through an integrated combined residency. Examples include family practice and psychiatry, where board certification can be obtained in both specialties.[27] There are also combined obstetrics and family practice residencies mainly designed to supplement the obstetric training of a family physician. Under this program, the physician would be boarded in family practice with a certificate indicating extended training in operative obstetrics.

Urban Market Expansion

As urban areas become saturated with managed care, some organizations may look to more rural areas to increase their patient base. Although there has been limited entree of managed care into rural communities (see Chap. 17), managed care is likely to expand much more quickly to rural areas that are in close proximity to urban areas highly penetrated by managed care. There are clearly natural advantages in terms of utilization to enrolling rural patients in managed care plans. However, the onus will be on managed care organizations to provide reasonable geographic access to specialists and technology in order to compete for covered lives. Depending on the state, managed care organizations may even be required to demonstrate access in order to receive a license to operate in certain rural counties.

CONCLUSION

Several major issues of importance have been addressed in this chapter. First, we discussed the value of developing market niches in specific areas of care that reflect the increasing emphasis in health care financing on ambulatory and long-term care. Next, the importance of training, recruiting, and retaining health care providers of all types was introduced. Third, the centrality of developing hospital networks and systems that hinge on health service integration was described. And finally, the emergence of telemedicine and other technologies to facilitate information sharing was evaluated. These four themes will play a key role in the future vision of rural hospitals.

Information technology in all likelihood will have the leading edge in changing the way rural hospitals manage and deliver care. Just as the improvement of transportation in the twentieth century increased access for rural residents, the telecommunications and information technology available may bring many of the advantages of urban health care to rural areas. For this to occur, however, providers, services, and technology must be integrated in a synergistic fashion.

Already, models of health service delivery have been proposed in which midlevel providers serve as physician surrogates over telemedicine to increase access to medical care without requiring the full-time presence of a physician in the rural community, thereby allowing nonphysician providers an increased range of clinical responsibility. A strategy such as this, combined with the programs and policies that have already been established to promote the training of more primary care physicians, may significantly improve issues of rural access to health care.

Regarding local improvements in health service delivery, telemedicine may act as the catalyst that stimulates the development and maintenance of triage in emergency care, fetal monitoring in low-risk obstetrics, and CME in common inpatient surgical procedures. When these enhancements to existing services are not enough, contracts with urban teaching hospitals can be used to provide or supplement physician supply in the community.

Service integration between rural and urban hospitals will also benefit from a variety of medical informatics technologies, including the use of the electronic medical record. The bidirectional sharing of patient information facilitated by such technology should solidify hospital affiliations and partnerships through coordinated and streamlined systems of care that can be operationalized in diagnostic and treatment algorithms and transfer and referral protocols. Such systems will help ensure that best practices are implemented throughout all rural hospitals and associated physician practices.

Rural health care of the future will have to operate as a system rather than as clusters of independent health service providers. Federal policy will dictate the development of some systems through health care financing, as demonstrated in the Medicare Rural Hospital Flexibility Program, but many will grow from the ingenuity and resourcefulness of the clinical relationships that are driven by need and sustained by cooperation. Technology, which has the advantage of accommodating a variety of levels of sophistication and need, will be the essential connection that links the providers, services, and decision-making tools necessary to coordinate and standardize care between rural and urban locations.

REFERENCES

1. Hart LG, Pirani MJ, Rosenblatt RA: Causes and consequences of rural small hospital closures from the perspectives of mayors. *J Rural Health* 7(3):222–245, 1991.

2. Office of Technology Assessment: *Health Care in Rural America.* OTA-H-434. Washington, DC: US Government Printing Office, 1990.

3. Wellever A, Moscovice I, Chen MM: *A DRG-Based Service Limitation System for Rural Primary Care Hospitals.* Working paper no. 4. Minneapolis, MN, University of Minnesota Rural Health Research Center, December 1993.

4. Croll K: Emergency room services in rural hospitals. *Leader Health Services* 5(6):14–18, 1996.

5. Scott GWS: *Report of the Fact Finder on the Issue of Small/Rural Hospital Emergency Department Physician Service.* Toronto, Ontario Ministry of Health, Ontario Hospital Association, and Ontario Medical Association, 1995.

6. Reif S, DesHarnais S, Bernard S: *Effects of Rural Hospital Closure on Access to Care.* Working paper no. 58. Chapel Hill, NC, Cecil G. Sheps Center for Health Services Research, University of North Carolina at Chapel Hill, 1998.

7. Williamson HA, Hart G, Pirani MJ, Rosenblatt RA: Rural hospital inpatient surgical volume: cutting-edge service or operating at the margin? *J Rural Health* 10(1):16–25, 1994.

8. Rosenblatt RA, Saunders GR, Tressler CJ, et al: The diffusion of obstetric technology into rural U.S. hospitals. *Int J Technol Assess Health Care* 10(3):479–489, 1994.

9. http://ahec.msu.montana.edu/cah/.

10. McNeely GH: Evaluating alternative rural hospital models: what are we learning, in Straub LA, Walzer N (eds): *Rural Health Care: Innovation in a Changing Environment.* Westport, CT, Praeger, 1992.

11. Senator Max Baucus (D-MT): *Medicare Rural Hospital Flexibility Program Fact Sheet,* April 1998.

12. Franklin A: Doing it all in the public eye: a comparative analysis of California district hospital affiliations. *J Health Care Finance* 24(2):48–55, 1998.

13. Straub LA, Walzer N: Financing the demand for health care, in Straub LA, Walzer N (eds): *Rural Health Care: Innovation in a Changing Environment.* Westport, CT, Praeger, 1992.

14. Bumdenstock RJ: *So You're on the Hospital Board,* 4th ed. Chicago, American Hospital Association, 1992.

15. Hospital Research and Educational Trust, Section

for Small or Rural Hospitals, American Hospital Association: *Increasing Rural Health Personnel: Community-Based Strategies for Recruitment and Retention.* Chicago, American Hospital Association, 1992.

16. Hicks LL, Hassinger E, Taparanskas W: Effects of second office and hospital consulting practices of physicians on rural communities. *J Rural Health* 13(3):179–189, 1997.

17. Muus KJ, Geller JM, Williams JD, et al: Job satisfaction among rural physician assistants. *J Rural Health* 14:100–108, 1998.

18. Krein SL: The employment and use of nurse practitioners and physician assistants by rural hospitals. *J Rural Health* 13(1):45–58, 1997.

19. Reczynski DF: *Environmental Assessment for Rural Hospitals, 1988.* Chicago, American Hospital Association, 1987.

20. Damasauskas R: The case for keeping the rural hospital, in Straub LA, Walzer N (eds): *Rural Health Care: Innovation in a Changing Environment.* Westport, CT, Praeger, 1992.

21. Bauer JC: The primary-care hospital: more and better health care without closure, in Straub LA, Walzer N (eds): *Rural Health Care: Innovation in a Changing Environment.* Westport, CT, Praeger, 1992.

22. Hudson T: Rural priorities: hospital links and managed care contracts top the list. *Hospital Health Netw* 69(4):40,42,44, 1995.

23. McKay NL: Rural hospitals: organizational alignments for managed care contracting. *J Health Care Mgt* 43(2):169–184, 1998.

24. Halpern MT, Alexander JA, Fennell ML: Multihospital system affiliation as a survival strategy for rural hospitals under the prospective payment system. *J Rural Health* 8(2):93–105, 1992.

25. Esposito TJ, Lazear SE, Maier RV: Trauma care systems development: evolution and trends, in Maul K et al. (eds): *Advances in Trauma and Critical Care.* St. Louis, Mosby, 1991.

26. Tracy R: Considerations in establishing visiting consultant clinics in rural hospital communities. *Hosp Health Services Admin* 41:255–265, 1996.

27. Chapman R, Nuovo J: Combined residency training in family practice and other specialties. *Fam Med* 29:715–718, 1997.

CHAPTER 15

Medical Informatics and Information Access

SHERRILYNNE S. FULLER   DAVID MASUDA   PAUL GORMAN
DONALD A. B. LINDBERG

Today we are witnessing the early, turbulent days of a revolution as significant as any other in human history. A new medium is emerging, one that may prove to surpass all previous revolutions—the printing press, the telephone, the television—in its impact on our social and economic life.

—Don Tapscott, 1995

I n his 1995 book *The Digital Economy*, Don Tapscott characterized the digital age as the "convergence of computing, communication and content"—the result of the simultaneous and rapid evolution of two technologies that exponentially increase the power and significance of information.[1] According to Tapscott, convergence will bring a fundamental change to our society and economy. In medicine, convergence has the potential to introduce synergistic beneficial effects to both physicians and patients as computers and telecommunications networks enable us to create, store, exchange, and share all types of medical data and information. This growing availability of and access to digital medical knowledge can improve health care decision making, prevent dangerous oversights, increase access to care, and reduce unnecessary costs.[2]

The potential for this technology is especially promising in rural medical practice. This is true because of several fundamental differences between rural and urban medicine. Rural providers have, of necessity, learned to deliver skillful care in the face of limited information resources: small and sometimes outdated medical libraries, few specialist colleagues within the local community, and constrained access to sophisticated diagnostic technologies. What rural providers lack in technological advantage is often made up in other ways: close and personal relationships with patients often lasting for life, the ability to initiate care across a broad range of medical conditions, and the skills to play many and varied roles as a care provider. Given these significant differences, improved access to the newer information technologies has the potential to enhance the unique value inherent in rural practice.

Academic medical centers, where most health professionals train, are information-rich environments with the latest in computer technology and teaching and learning tools. In such settings there is abundance: a diversity of specialist colleagues and unequaled breadth and depth of medical library resources. Hospital information systems provide access to computer-based patient records, including laboratory results, medication lists, transcriptions, and a wealth of other patient-specific information. Moreover, artificial intelligence designed into such systems provides real-time decision support, such as drug alerts, preventive care reminders, and diagnostic aids.

Upon completion of their training in these information-rich centers, physicians who go on to practice in rural settings often feel isolated, as the academic resources and educational opportunities are no longer locally available. The lack of point-of-care information can be particularly troublesome, as rural practitioners are increasingly required to command a broad knowledge base across a growing spectrum of clinical problems. These include not only the diagnosis and triage of rare injuries and illnesses but also relatively mundane but highly complex tasks such as keeping abreast of the most current indications, contraindications, and dosages of a large number of drugs.

Emerging computer and communications technologies will aid significantly in alleviating this sense of isolation as they provide access to knowledge resources for rural providers. The technology itself is not years away; a computer linked to the Internet is an information tool that is functional, affordable, and available now in even the most remote parts of the United States.

This chapter provides an overview of how electronic information resources can enhance rural medicine, concentrating less on technology and more on information. We begin with a discussion of "clinical information." What is it, what are the clinical information needs that providers in rural settings face, and what are the barriers (perceived and real) to resolving these information deficits? The chapter continues with a discussion of the principal electronic resources currently available for meeting these needs, and it concludes with a summary of promising medical informatics research and development technologies and trends.

DATA → INFORMATION → KNOWLEDGE → WISDOM

On first blush, one might think that the clinical information needs rural providers experience are simply "keeping up with the literature and the current standards of practice in my specialty." The empiric evidence suggests, however, that they are considerably more diverse. A brief case study, in the form of clinical questions that arise in everyday practice, is illustrative.

THE CASE OF JOE B.

Joe, 64 years old, has insulin-dependent diabetes of long standing and moderately severe hypertension. He lives alone and has always been a "difficult" patient, poorly compliant with diet and medications. He stubbornly resists any changes in his lifestyle, which includes flying his small private airplane. He does see several specialists (ophthalmology, nephrology, and vascular surgery) for complications of his advanced disease; he is also a "frequent flyer" in the urgent care clinic.

Question 1.   Joe sees each of his specialists and me, his primary care provider, regularly, and each keeps a separate medical record of his or her findings, tests, and treatments. Given this fragmented delivery system, coordinating Joe's care is difficult. "How can I keep track of what each consultant is doing for my patient?"

Question 2.   There are many journal articles I see each week that describe various trials of therapy for diabetes—it is so hard to keep current. "What is the most recent scientific evidence regarding optimal drug regimen for an elderly, hypertensive, diabetic patient?"

Question 3.   Joe came to the office yesterday with a low-grade fever, slightly productive cough, and chills—the fifth patient this week to present with such symptoms. "Is there a new strain of flu virus going around?"

Question 4.   Joe is insured by a National Committee for Quality Assurance (NCQA)-accredited HMO that requires patient data from my practice for Health and Employer Data and Information Set (HEDIS) reporting. "What percentage of all the diabetics in my practice have had a retinal exam within the last year?"

Question 5.   Joe's health plan also controls referrals such that only "in-network" specialists are covered. "Where do I find a current list of approved specialists and the proper referral forms, and for which referrals do I need prior authorization?"

Question 6.   The local endocrinologist has developed a clinical guideline for treating complicated diabetics admitted to the hospital; however, this guideline varies in certain ways from the one published by my specialty society. "What is the standard guideline or care path in my hospital for patients admitted with uncontrolled diabetes?"

Question 7.   I heard recently on the radio about a clinical trial that was testing the use of two-way pagers to remind patients to check their blood sugar and to take their medications. "Are there any new techniques for increasing treatment adherence in noncompliant older patients?"

Summary.   How do I best care for an elderly hypertensive diabetic who won't always comply with my recommendations, and who insists on living alone and continuing to fly his airplane?

"Keeping up with the literature" will at best provide answers for only a few of these questions. Finding timely and accurate answers to the other questions can be a daunting and frustrating task. However, to practice medicine effectively requires all of the answers to be available and synthesized. Fortunately, medical informatics is beginning to provide such solutions.

TYPES OF INFORMATION USED BY CLINICIANS

In developing technology tools to help fill in these information gaps, it is important to understand not just when and where information is missing but also the various *types* of information that are missing. Table 15-1 provides a useful classification that further clarifies the nature of the questions that arise in Joe's case.

Patient data and *medical knowledge* are the most familiar types of information. In one sense, the essential function in the practice of medicine is to synthesize patient-specific information with formalized medical knowledge, bringing to bear what the physician has learned through study and experience with the specific signs, symptoms, and test findings for each individual patient so that evidence-based, patient-specific clinical decisions can be made.[4]

However, the remaining three categories are equally important, as any active practitioner would attest. *Population data* can be of two types. The first is "informal epidemiology," a personal knowledge of recent illness patterns in a community. Unfortunately, population data (e.g., public health data) are often not available on a local scale or in a timely fashion. The second is a result of the "outcomes movement," which has grown in the last several years. As we begin to better understand how to measure the clinical effectiveness of our practices, the need arises to be able to gather physician-specific information across a population of patients. For example, HEDIS reporting requires clinicians to be able to collect and report the results of their care not only on individual patients but also across the entire patient population.

Logistic information may be one of the most vexing problems in day-to-day practice. With each patient, the clinician must know how to schedule, how to bill, and how to refer. For each patient these can be different, resulting in a complex and growing situation in every clinic setting. And, since each physician may practice in multiple hospitals and across a dozen or more health plans, having the ability to retrieve logistic information is crucial.

Finally, *social information* comes from myriad sources and can include political, legal, managerial, and ethical components, being local, regional, or national in scope. Social information clearly affects how medicine is practiced and

TABLE 15-1   CATEGORIES OF INFORMATION NEEDED BY CLINICIANS

Question	Type of Information	Description	Examples	Usual Sources
1	Patient data	Information about a single person	The history and physical exam The problem list Laboratory data	Patient and family Hospital medical records Clinic medical records
2	Medical knowledge	The diagnosis and treatment of injury and disease	Original research Textbook descriptions Experiential knowledge gained in residency and practice	Textbooks Journals Consultants, colleagues CME
3	Population data	Aggregate patient information across populations	Summary data of patient population in a practice Recent patterns of illness Public health data	Public health departments Practice information systems Medical records
4	Logistic information	How to get the job done	Referral request forms Preauthorization lists Preferred provider lists Hospital formularies	Office staff, hospital personnel Policy and procedure manuals Managed care organizations Insurers
5	Social influences	How others get the job done	Implicit local practice patterns and expectations Explicit care paths and guidelines	Patients, families Colleagues, consultants Professional organizations Government agencies Lay media

SOURCE: From Gorman PN: Information needs of physicians. *J Am Soc Info Sci.* Copyright 1995 by John Wiley & Sons, Inc. Reprinted by permission of John Wiley & Sons, Inc.

explains a significant component of the known variation in practice. For instance, in Joe's case, what is the aviation licensing law with regard to patients with uncontrolled diabetes? Do I as a practitioner have a responsibility to report Joe's noncompliance with therapy to a flight licensing authority?

INFORMATION NEEDS AND BARRIERS TO ACCESS

Clearly, clinical information is diverse in nature. But what is the evidence on how or even if clinicians resolve these needs? Gorman has sug-

gested one approach that is illustrative. He has characterized four types of physician information needs: unrecognized needs, recognized needs, pursued needs, and satisfied needs[4] (Fig. 15-1, Table 15-2).

It should not be assumed that each information deficit is recognized by the clinician; many simply cannot be. For example:

- Patients for whom one or more medications have been prescribed by other physicians
- A clinical alert issued overnight by the National Institutes of Health on a potential adverse drug reaction

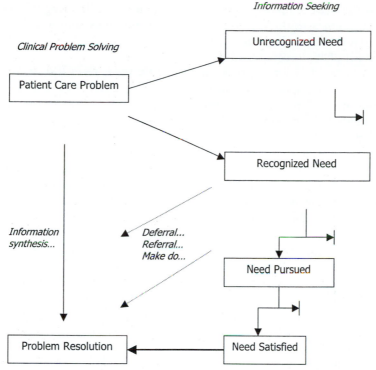

FIGURE 15-1 *States of information need. (From Wilson T (ed):* Proceedings of Second Information in Context Meeting. *Copyright 1998 by Taylor Graham Publishing, London, England. Reprinted by permission of Taylor Graham Publishing.)*

TABLE 15-2   STATES OF INFORMATION NEEDS

Type of Information Need	Description	Comment
Unrecognized needs	Clinician not aware of information need or knowledge deficit	Inferred from assessment of knowledge; external action required to correct (e.g., reminder systems, self-assessment programs)
Recognized needs	Aware that information is needed: may or may not be pursued	Articulated by clinician or inferred by observer
Pursued needs	Information seeking occurs: may or may not be successful	Observed or recalled information-seeking behavior
Satisfied needs	Information seeking succeeds	Recalled information-seeking successes

SOURCE: From Gorman PN: Information needs of physicians. *J Am Soc Info Sci.* Copyright 1995 by John Wiley & Sons, Inc. Reprinted by permission of John Wiley & Sons, Inc.

Obviously, if a clinician is unaware that an information deficit exists, a solution is unlikely without outside intervention. The most common informatics solution to unrecognized needs has been computer-based decision support. Active computerized decision support—including reminder systems, drug alerts, or self-assessment programs—have been shown to be very valuable in this setting.

Recognized needs are those known to the clinician.[5,6] When an information need is recognized, it may or may not generate a response by the clinician; the need may become a pursued need. Unfortunately, less than half of these needs are actively pursued. The busy clinician has alternatives. He may defer the search until some later date, he may refer the patient to a specialist (allowing the specialist to provide the answer), or he may simply "make do" and make the clinical decision in the face of missing information.

There is some evidence to suggest that clinicians do have a "triage" pattern. For example, one study suggests the three most common predictors of a need being pursued are whether the clinician believes an answer exists, whether an answer is urgently needed, and if the answer is specific to the care of the patient at hand.[4]

Finally, needs that are pursued may or may not be entirely satisfied. Studies indicate that, although clinicians pursue answers to only 30 to 40 percent of their questions, they succeed in finding answers to nearly 80 percent of those they pursue.

According to Gorman,[4] despite the variation in research methods of information needs analysis studies, two conclusions about clinician information needs can be made. First, questions about optimal patient care arise quite frequently, with many questions occurring each day for a typical physician. It is estimated that each patient encounter generates at least one question for which the clinician does not have an immediate answer. Second, many of the questions that do arise are never pursued; of those that are, some are never successfully answered. Arguably, this type of information

deficit is one that might be eminently amenable to informatics solutions.

CLINICAL INFORMATION NEEDS SUMMARY

In summary, what is known about clinician information needs? Smith offers a synopsis based on a review of 13 studies on the information needs of clinicians.[3] Although the evidence in this domain is limited, a number of constant findings emerge:

- Information needs arise very regularly in clinical settings. Each interaction between a patient and clinician is likely, on average, to generate at least one question and very probably more.
- Most commonly, the questions that arise are related to therapy, in particular drug therapy.
- While some questions are simple ("Does Norpace cause fatigue?"), many are often complex and multidimensional ("In an octogenarian with anemia, angina, and a history of transient ischemic attacks, with a normal creatinine, iron, and mean corpuscular volume, who refuses a bone marrow exam, what diagnostic and therapeutic options are there?")
- By far the most favored source of answers is dialogue with clinical colleagues. This suggests that for rural clinicians, information technology (e.g., electronic mail, televideo-consulting, and the telephone) that links them to colleagues in geographically distant settings may be a significant source of answers.
- Resolving these complex questions requires more than single source answers. It requires the synthesis of individual patient data and several diverse sets of medical knowledge in addition to social, logistic, and population information. Clinicians are not simply looking for medical knowledge, they are often looking for confirmation, guidance, explanation, commiseration, synthesis: in a word—judgment.
- Increasingly, physicians and health care providers are becoming overwhelmed with information resources that are, for the most part,

disorganized, noncontextual, and irrelevant in answering questions about the care of individual patients.

- From the perspective of medical informatics, perhaps the most important finding is that many of the questions generated by clinicians *can* be answered by the use of electronic resources. There are obstacles that persist: these tools are often time-consuming and relatively inefficient; using them requires information retrieval and management skills that many clinicians do not yet possess.

INFORMATICS SOLUTIONS TO RURAL INFORMATION NEEDS

Unfortunately, not all of the five types of information described by Gorman have equally compelling informatics solutions. Obtaining population data, logistic information, and social influence information by electronic means may remain problematic in rural locations for the foreseeable future.

There is, however, a rich and growing set of resources that can serve to satisfy needs for patient data and medical knowledge. In the next two sections, the major resources and developments with which rural clinicians should be familiar are described.

RESOURCES FOR MEDICAL KNOWLEDGE NEEDS

Mooer's law[11] states that an information retrieval system will tend *not* to be used whenever it is more painful and troublesome to retrieve the information than it is to act without it. In the past, medical libraries were the primary resource for information retrieval, yet they were often not equipped to provide rapid answers to clinical questions. Unless the clinician was fortunate enough to have access to a clinical librarian, locating particular articles often required a visit to the library and a search of *MEDLINE*. This search might mean paging through the print volumes of the *Index Medicus* or an online search of *MEDLINE* at a terminal in the library. Finally, the searcher would make a trip to the journal stacks to retrieve the articles. More often than not, the journal would not be in the local collection, so a phone call to a regional library would be necessary.

Fortunately, the advent of sophisticated information technology and databases that support instantaneous access to resources has resolved many of these difficulties. The medical library will remain the central resource for medical knowledge. Although it remains too expensive for most individual rural facilities to maintain a comprehensive print-based medical library, the arrival of the *digital electronic* medical library is a major advance. The digital electronic library—a computer linked to the World Wide Web—is an information tool that is now very affordable and available everywhere in the United States.

Many of the most important resources and databases have been developed by the National Library of Medicine of the National Institutes of Health (NIH).

The National Library of Medicine

The National Library of Medicine (NLM) in Bethesda, Maryland, is the world's largest medical library. It houses materials in all major areas of the health sciences. The collections consist of over 5 million items—books, journals, technical reports, manuscripts, microfilms, photographs, and images.

The NLM has an extensive and very powerful computer-based system for rapid access to this vast store of biomedical information. Today, via telecommunications networks, NLM search services are available everywhere in the world through a family of approximately 40 databases, of which *MEDLINE* (over 9 million references to articles published in 3900 biomedical journals since 1966) is the best known. In June 1997, NLM began offering free access to *MEDLINE* and several other NLM databases on the World Wide Web.

Training and Access—the National Network of Libraries of Medicine

The NLM is a resource for all U.S. health libraries through the National Network of Libraries of Medicine (NN/LM). This network consists of 4500 primary access libraries (mostly at hospitals), 140 resource libraries (at medical schools), and 8 regional libraries (covering all geographic regions of the United States). In addition to serving as a resource for libraries and librarians, the NN/LM serves all health professionals— clinicians, allied health professionals, researchers, administrators, students—who need access to biomedical information. The NN/LM reaches out to all health professionals, no matter where they are located, and provides options for their personal access to information.

Regional libraries can provide referrals to nearby librarians, who can assist in accessing information, getting answers to questions, and getting copies of articles and books. In addition, regional libraries offer classes and consultations on site, fact sheets, and other useful information resources.[12] Online information about the NN/LM can be found via the Internet at [http://www.nnlm.nlm.nih.gov/].

RETRIEVING REFERENCES TO THE LITERATURE

MEDLINE is by the far the most widely used database for medical information retrieval.[13]

The first Web-based search tool that NLM

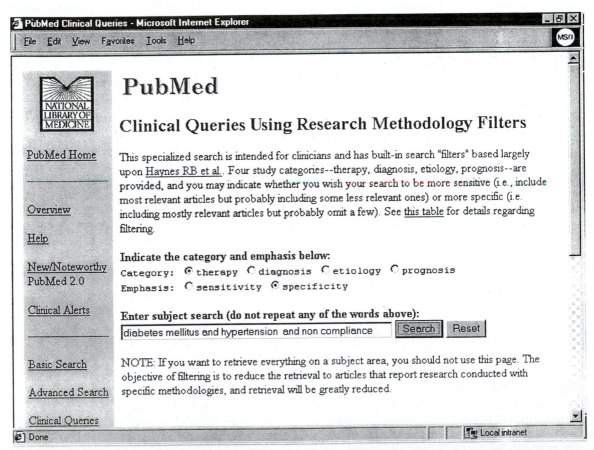

FIGURE 15-2 PubMed clinical query.

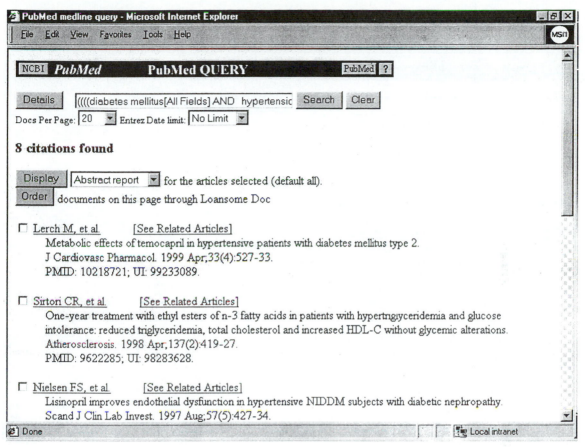

FIGURE 15-3 Clinical query result.

developed was Internet Grateful Med [http://igm.nlm.nih.gov/]. This tool was designed to make it easier for the clinician with little or no database-searching experience to search *MEDLINE* (and many other NLM citation databases) to retrieve pertinent citations.

PubMed [http://www.ncbi.nlm.nih.gov/PubMed/] (Figs. 15-2, 15-3, and 15-4) is the newest search technology now available from NLM. *PubMed* is an innovative web-based interface to *MEDLINE* that greatly reduces the complexity of searching by adding artificial intelligence pattern-recognition and matching capabilities. This technology allows a clinician to enter a search, review the list of retrieved citations, and indicate which articles are most relevant to the problem at hand. *PubMed* will then search the *MED-*

LINE database again, finding additional articles that are close topical matches to the initially selected articles. Another search aid built into *PubMed* is the "Clinical Queries" function. This feature allows the clinician to "filter" the search to retrieve citations limited to a specific *type* of article that answers a specific clinical question. The four available filters are diagnosis, etiology, therapy, and prognosis. Figure 15-2 shows a clinical query that will run a search for articles regarding diabetes, hypertension, and noncompliance and retrieve *only* the citations that cover the treatment (and not the diagnosis) of this condition. Figure 15-3 shows the retrieved citations that are the result of this search. Figure 15-4 shows the citations retrieved as a result of clicking on the "See Related Articles" button in

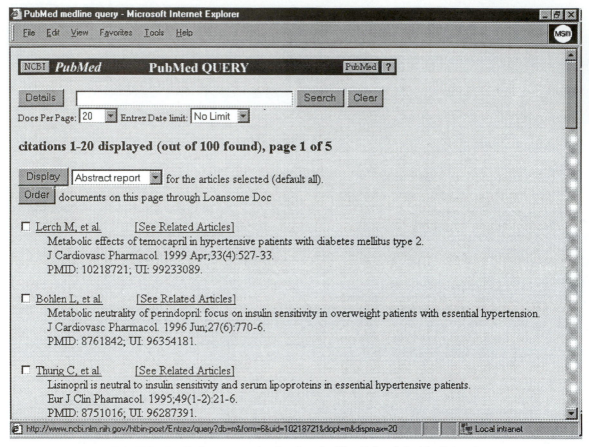

FIGURE 15-4 *References retrieved using the "See Related Articles" search.*

Fig. 15-2. This feature is a very useful one for refining a search once one finds the "perfect" article.

It is important to note that *MEDLINE* (and the other NLM bibliographic databases) contain information on article citations only. A *PubMed* search will retrieve the abstract of the article, not the full text for all articles. There are, however, several options to obtain the full text of an article. One of the most popular related features of *PubMed* is direct access to document delivery. This feature, named *LoansomeDoc,* enables a clinician to arrange with a medical library to have the full text of articles delivered to his or her doorstep. Once access arrangements with a chosen medical library have been made (including selection of payment options), a simple click on the order box will route the request from *MEDLINE* to the local library. This library will then obtain the article, using regional library assistance if it is not available locally. The retrieved article can then be mailed, faxed, or delivered electronically to the requesting clinician, often in 24 hours or less. In addition, *PubMed* is making arrangements with a number of medical journal publishers for direct access to their full-text electronic journals; if full text is available, a link to the full text will appear adjacent to the citation.

Increasingly, these full-text databases are becoming widely available. With this type of database, the entire article is available electronically—text, images, charts and graphs—and can be downloaded directly to the local computer. Some medical publications, such as the *British Journal of Medicine*, make full text available free of charge; others charge by the article or by annual subscription. There are also commercial ventures such as MDConsult that aggregate a number of online full-text journals and medical textbooks, allowing an individual physician to purchase access to a "virtual medical library." Clinicians affiliated with academic medical centers often have access to many full-text electronic journals through the academic health sciences library.

Other Online Databases

Although *MEDLINE* will likely fulfill the majority of clinical information needs relating to the published literature, it is by no means the only resource available to rural clinicians. In addition to the NLM databases discussed so far, there are numerous online databases of health sciences information that can provide rapid answers to health sciences questions. Many of them are accessible via the Internet. Table 15-3 provides a selected list of online databases useful in rural practice and their Web addresses. The "Type" column distinguishes between databases that

TABLE 15-3   SELECTED LIST OF ONLINE DATABASES USEFUL IN RURAL PRACTICE

Database	Type	Topic	Publisher	Web Address
AIDS drugs and AIDS trials	D	AIDS drug and clinical trials	NLM[a]	igm.nim.nih.gov/
BIOSIS	B	Biological research	BIOSIS	www.biosis.org
CancerLit	B	Cancer information	National Cancer Institute	cnetdb.nci.nih.gov
ChemId	D	Chemical dictionary file for over 339,000 compounds of biomedical and regulatory interest	NLM	igm.nim.nih.gov/
Current Contents	B	Health sciences—most recent clinical and research articles	Institute for Scientific Information	www.isinet.com
Genline	D	Peer-reviewed clinical genetics profiles	University of Washington	www.geneclinics.org/
HealthStar	B	Health services, technology, administration, and research	NLM	igm.nlm.nih.gov/
Helix: Genetic Testing Resource	D	Medical Genetics Laboratory directory and testing information	University of Washington	healthlinks.washington.edu/helix/
Online Mendelian Inheritance in Man	D	Catalog of human genes and genetic disorders	John Hopkins University and National Center for Biotechnology	www.ncbi.nlm.nih.gov/Omim/
Toxline	B	Toxicologic, pharmacologic, biochemical, and physiologic effects of drugs and other chemicals	NLM	igm.nlm.nih.gov/

[a]National Library of Medicine.
Key: B, bibliographic; D, data.

TABLE 15-4   *USEFUL WEB SITES BY TOPIC FOR RURAL PRACTITIONERS*

Topic	Organization/Service	Web Address
Rural health/rural issues		
	National Rural Health Association	www.nrharural.org/
	National Center for Farmworker Health	www.ncfh.org/
	National Drinking Water Clearinghouse	www.estd.wvu.edu/ndwc/
	National Rural Development Partnership	www.rurdev.usda.gov/nrdp/
Health meta-guides (provide broad access to health information)		
	Achoo-on-Line Healthcare Services	www.achoo.com/
	HealthSeek Health Information Resources	www.healthseek.com/
	HealthLinks—Connecting People with Knowledge	healthlinks.washington.edu
	Medical Matrix	www.medmatrix.org
	Doctors' Guide to the Internet	www.pslgroup.com/docguide.htm
	Virtual Hospital—University of Iowa	vh.radiology.uiowa.edu/
Continuing education		
	Continuing Nursing Education	www.springnet.com/ce/
	Continuing Medical Education	www.ama-assn.org/medsci/cme/cme.htm
	Continuing Dental Education	www.dental.washington.edu/conted/
	Doctors' Guide to Medical Conferences and Meetings	www.pslgroup.com/medconf.htm
Patient/consumer health information resources		
	The National Library of Medicine's consumer health site	www.nlm.nih.gov/medlineplus
	American Academy of Family Practice	www.aafp.org/family/patient/index.html
	Mayo Clinic Health	www.mayohealth.org/
	HealthFinder	www.healthfinder.gov/
Full-text books, journals		
	Harrison's Textbook of Medicine	www.harrisonsonline.com/ (subscription required)
	Journal of Family Practice	jfp.msu.edu/
	Evidence-Based Practice	jfp.msu.edu/ebp.htm
	AMA journals	www.ama-assn.org/
	British Medical Journal	www.bmj.com/
	Morbidity and Mortality Weekly Reports	www.cdc.gov/epo/mmwr/mmwr.html
	New England Journal of Medicine	www.nejm.org/content/index.asp

TABLE 15-4.   *Continued*

Topic	Organization/Service	Web Address
Reference/guidelines		
	Online Clinical Calculator	www.intmed.mcw.edu/clincalc.html
	Martindale's Virtual Reference Desk	www.virtualref.com/
	Primary Care Clinical Practice Guidelines	medicine.ucsf.edu/resources/guidelines
	National Guideline Clearinghouse (Agency for Healthcare Policy and Research)	www.guideline.gov/index.asp
Associations and societies	American Academy of Family Practice	www.aafp.org/
	American Academy of Pediatrics	www.aap.org/
	American Academy of Physician Assistants	www.aapa.org/
	American Association of Emergency Physicians	www.aep.org/
	American Association of Poison Control Centers	www.aapc.org/
	American College of Nurse Practitioners	www.nurse.org/acnp/
	American Medical Association	www.ama-assn.org
	American Public Health Association	www.apha.org/

provide citations, usually including abstracts, of the published literature and resources containing actual data—i.e., facts. Some are available at no charge; others require a subscription fee.

The Online World of Health Information—Medical Resources on the Web

The digital medical library as developed by the NLM has greatly increased the availability and accessibility of medical information in the form of the current medical journal literature and formal clinical databases. But another parallel development in informatics over the last 5 years has created an even larger universe of available medical information. This is, of course, the arrival of the Internet and the World Wide Web. Information regarding connecting to the Internet can be obtained from Internet Services Providers (ISPs). Two of the larger ISPs are American Online (AOL) and Microsoft Network

(MSN). Others can be located through your local telephone directory.

Accessing Health Sciences Web Resources—A Quality-Filtered List for Rural Practitioners

Many organizations and institutions are delivering valuable information on the World Wide Web. In fact, the very nature of the Web is such that literally anyone can become a "publisher of medical information." But what is gained in volume of information is offset by the fact that there is no central authority over its content and that the accuracy and reliability of the content is highly variable. Therefore reaching good, useful information is often like looking for a needle in a haystack.[14] Several efforts are under way to resolve this dilemma.

A number of organizations and institutions have developed *quality-filtered* links to useful sites for clinical practice information. Table 15-4 provides Web addresses of selected sites offering resources of particular value to rural practitioners.

Another option for assessing the accountability of health and medicine Web sites is embodied by the Health on the Web Foundation. This group, headquartered in Geneva, Switzerland, has developed a set of principles that can guide Web users to easily assess the medical responsibility of the owners of the site. In brief, the principles they espouse are that (1) medical advice will be given only by trained and qualified professionals, (2) the information is designed to support, not replace, the physician-patient relationship, (3) there is respect for confidentiality, (4) the information will be supported by clear references to source data, (5) any commercial support will be identified, and (6) the Web site will provide contact addresses for individuals seeking further information. Sites that adhere to these principles are given the right to display the Health on the Web Seal of Approval.

THE INTERSECTION BETWEEN MEDICAL KNOWLEDGE AND PATIENT-SPECIFIC DATA

Bringing Knowledge to the Point of Decision Making

Medical informatics can be defined as "the scientific field that deals with the storage, retrieval, and optimal use of biomedical information, data, and knowledge for problem solving and decision making."[15] The goal of medical informatics research and development is to coalesce data, information, knowledge, and tools necessary to apply those data and that knowledge in the decision-making process at the time and place that a decision needs to be made.

The various databases and Web resources described above are useful in retrieving "medical knowledge." Yet to optimize the actual delivery of care requires this medical knowledge to be combined with individual patient-specific information *at the point of care.* A number of critical medical informatics efforts have been undertaken in this area, including the computer-based medical record, clinical decision support, and clinical email.

Computer-Based Medical Record Systems

Computer-based medical record systems are beginning to be used widely in many distributed health care settings.[16-19] Such systems can provide distributed access to the complete patient record regardless of the location of the clinician or the patient. Moreover, they permit multiple providers to access the record simultaneously. Increasingly, these systems are providing linkages between detailed patient information and relevant knowledge resources in context. An example of such a system in current use throughout the University of Washington Medical Centers is shown in Fig. 15-5.[20] The problem list for the test patient is shown. Across the top are selectable "guidecards" to access the other components of the record. A click on the "I" icon in front of each problem links automatically to the National Library of Medicine's *PubMed* bibliographic retrieval system, as illustrated previously (Fig. 15-2). Note that an alert is shown at the top of the screen, indicating that the patient has reminders due. Figure 15-6 lists the reminders. Clinician reminder systems are increasingly being used to ensure timely testing and follow-up.[21]

The medications shown in Fig. 15-7 provide direct links to detailed drug information from the *U.S. Pharmacopoeia* (Fig. 15-8), including dosages, interactions, and adverse effects. All of these interactions with knowledge resources occur in the context of the computer-based medical record and provide knowledge resources at the point of decision making.

Clinical Decision Support Systems

Most of the information sources discussed in this chapter provide access to generalizable medical knowledge and require active pursuit of information by the clinician. Decision support

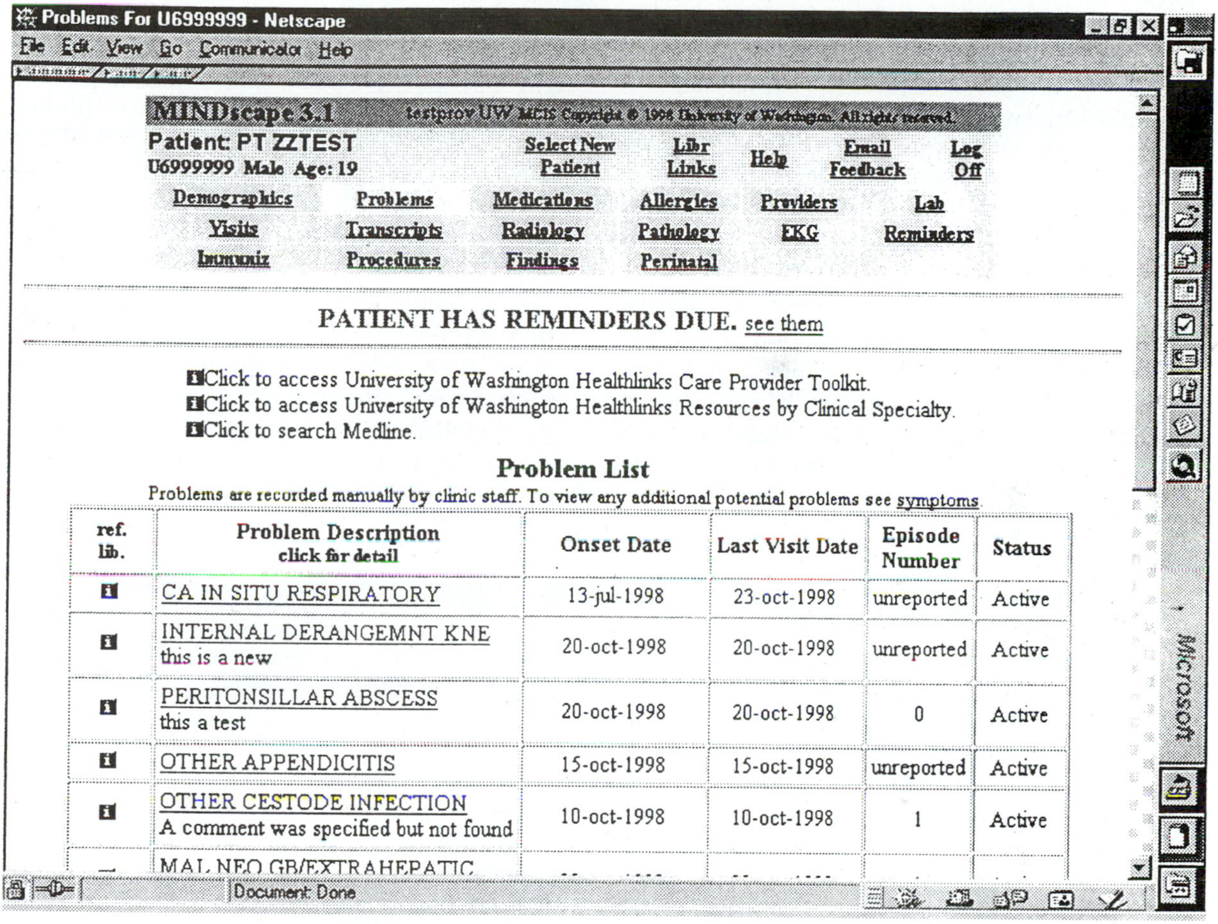

FIGURE 15-5 Mindscape—UW computer-based medical record.

systems go one step further, either by providing solutions that are specific to the context or case at hand, by actively offering information or assistance without requiring initiation by the system user, or both. Because so many of the questions that occur in primary care are about therapy, because drug prescribing errors are so common and important, and because some decision support systems have been shown to reduce errors and improve adherence to guidelines, these information systems have great potential to help clinicians improve their practices. A complete review of these systems is beyond the scope of this chapter, but we briefly describe four major categories of decision sup-

port that may benefit rural clinicians and their patients.

Diagnostic decision support software (DDSS) is available mainly as general-purpose, stand-alone systems, such as QMR[22] and DXplain.[23] Each of these systems contains a knowledge base consisting of four types of information: (1) diseases, drawn mainly from the domain of internal medicine; (2) findings associated with these diseases, such as patient history, physical examination, and laboratory information; (3) relationships between diseases and findings, with some measure of the strength of this relationship, such as the true-positive and false-positive rates; and (4) related information about complications and treatment. The information in these systems can generally be used in one of four modes: consultation, critique, simulation, and browsing. Consultation mode is used to solve a puzzling diagnostic dilemma. In this mode, the user enters information about a specific patient, adding history, physical, or laboratory data until the system is able to generate a differential diagnosis. Critique mode, which may be more efficient for the experienced clinician, allows one to begin with a working hypothesis about the diagnosis, obtaining suggestions about which other diagnoses to consider and what additional information might be useful. Simulation mode is meant to provide a learning experience, testing the user's diagnostic ability as he or she works through a case selected from the system's knowledge base. Finally, in browsing mode, the user can explore the knowledge base for information about a disease or finding. This is similar to using a textbook, but the DDSS gives the user more control over the information, harnessing the ability of the computer to rapidly navigate, sort, filter, or make calculations.

Therapeutic decision support systems range from simple prescription writing software running on hand-held or palm-top computers, to sophisticated pharmaceutical information services integrated into a hospital- or office-based electronic medical record. Excellent products exist that support each step in the therapeutic

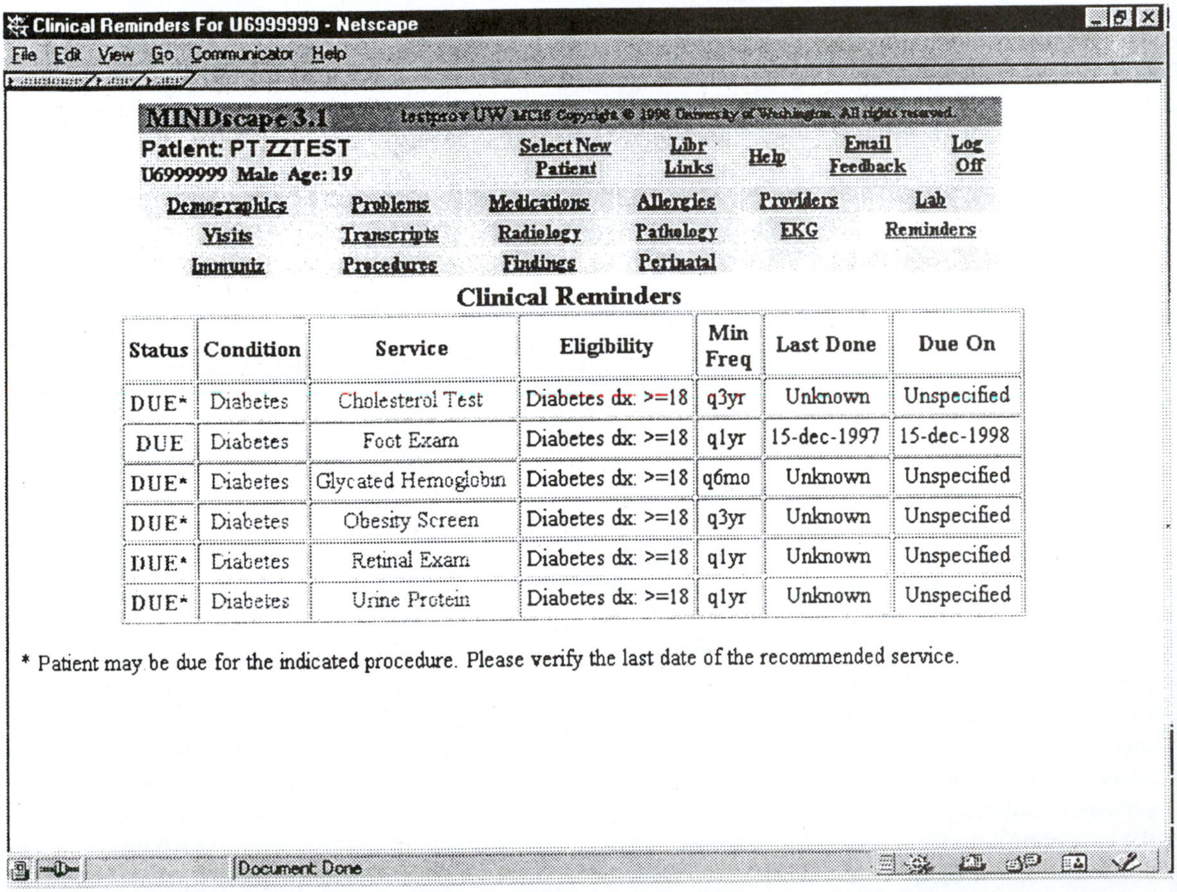

FIGURE 15-6 MINDscape reminders.

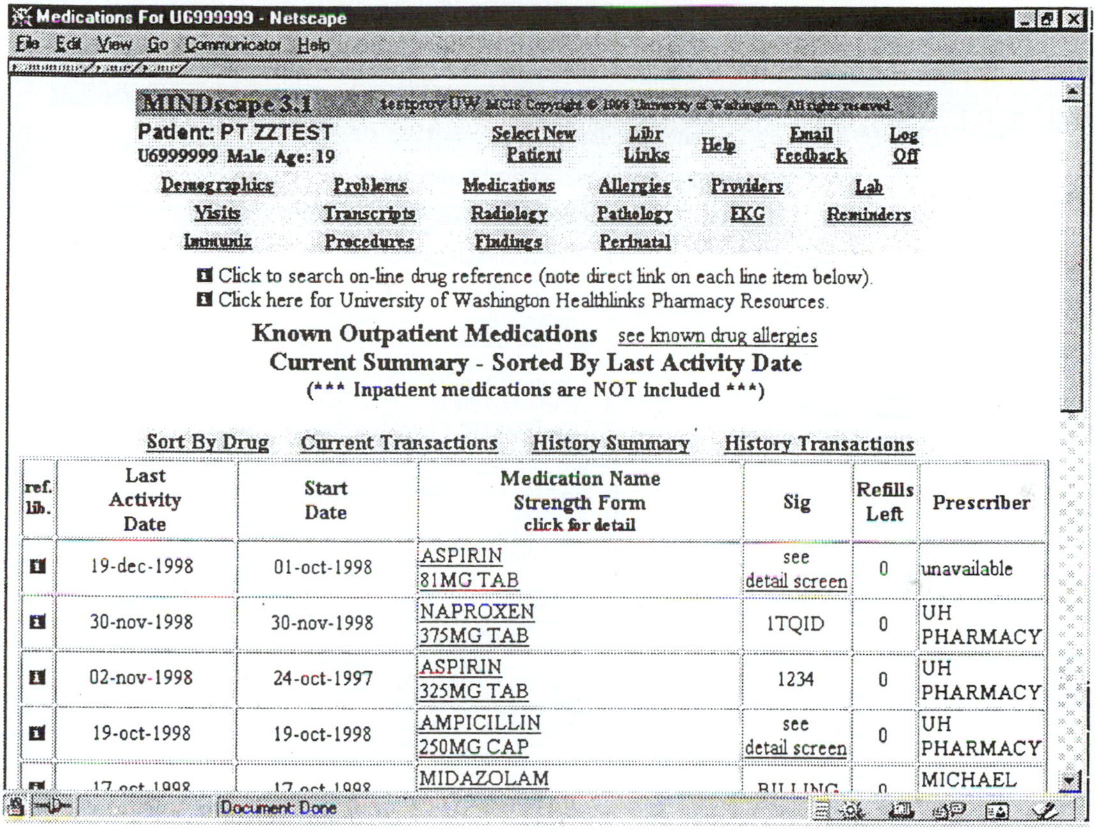

FIGURE 15-7 MINDscape medications list.

decision process: (1) choosing treatment, (2) obtaining basic drug information, (3) checking for drug interactions, (4) writing the prescription or order, (5) recording this information in the patient record, (6) providing patient education materials, (7) refilling prescriptions, and (8) reviewing prescribing practices for quality improvement. No single product is available that supports all of these tasks, and no single product will be helpful to all practices. Like individualizing the medication regimen for a patient with hypertension, choosing the right therapeutic decision support software involves tailoring the solution to individual circumstances and requires (1) having clearly defined, realistic objectives for the system; (2) recognizing which steps in the process are already well supported, such as Internet-based patient education materials or

a local pharmacist using drug interaction software; (3) identifying existing information systems in your setting with which the selected software must interact or be compatible; and (4) examining your practice style, interests, and tolerance for technology, so the new system can be adopted without causing major disruption. If you move from patient to patient without returning to your desk until the end of the day, a desktop computer–based product will be much less useful than something that fits in your coat pocket.

Do-it-yourself decision support refers to informal solutions developed to meet individual needs. Although fully developed commercial systems have the potential to provide great benefits, in many cases clinicians can meet their own unique needs with little effort, using relatively

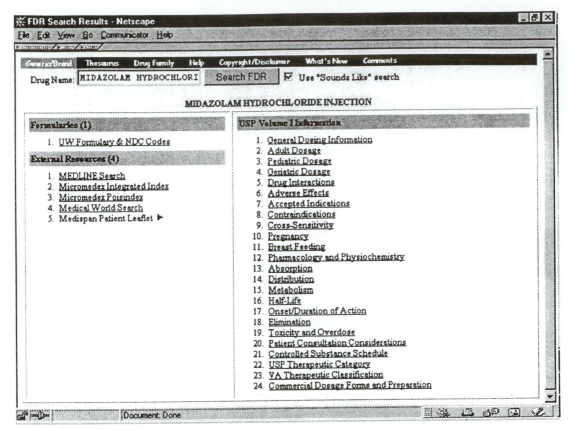

FIGURE 15-8 Drug Information Resource—U.S. Pharmacopoeia.

simple, widely available software. Examples abound. Using word processing software, many physicians have developed templates of their most common admission and discharge orders. They modify the orders as needed, print and sign them, and enter them in the hospital chart. Many physicians use simple spreadsheets found on virtually every desktop, laptop, or hand-held computer to perform useful but sometimes difficult-to-remember calculations. Everything from creatinine clearance or drug dose calculations to positive predictive values and the number needed to treat can be instantly computed in this way, promoting better clinical decision making with minimal time and effort.

Integrated decision support is the approach that informatics experts now believe will have the most impact on clinical practice. Most studies that have demonstrated benefits of decision support, such as reducing prescribing errors or increasing physician adherence to recommendations and guidelines, have involved the use of information systems that tightly integrate the decision support into the clinical process of care, in most cases providing not only needed information but also the means of enacting the recommended practice or procedure. Increasingly, this type of integrated decision support is being incorporated into commercial electronic medical record systems. However, whether one implements a full-featured commercial medical record system, chooses a stand-alone solution meant to address a specific need such as prescription writing or interaction checking, or develops individualized decision support for an individual practice, success depends largely on the extent to which the decision support is integrated into the process of care, providing the information needed to support improved clinical decisions and enabling these decisions to be enacted without excessively disrupting clinical workflow.[24]

A review of the effects of computer-based clinical decision support systems (CDSSs) on physician performance and patient outcomes reported that published studies of these systems are increasing rapidly and their quality is improving. The authors concluded that CDSSs can "enhance clinical performance for drug dosing, preventive care and other aspects of medical care but not convincingly for diagnosis."[25]

Clinical Email Communications: Clinician-Clinician and Clinician-Patient

As the research assessing clinician needs indicates, the first choice for an information source is another person. Use of electronic communications to contact other clinicians, patients, pharmacies, laboratories, and others is increasingly common. Robinson et al. examined the current status of interactive health communication (IHC) and proposed evidence-based approaches to improve the quality of such applications.[26] The conclusion is that such communications have great potential to improve health, but they may also cause harm. Robinson et al. believe that a rigorous evaluation of the safety, quality, and utility of these resources is vital. In particular, Spielberg points out that increased use of email by physicians and patients has the potential to reshape the current boundaries of relationships in medical practice, resulting in new expectations, practice standards, and potential liabilities.[27] Health professionals using email should recognize that email may be included in the patient's record and should discuss the ramifications of electronic communication with their patients. Spielberg believes that physicians should obtain documented informed consent before using email with their patients.

Special care must be taken to protect the patient's confidentiality and privacy. According to Spielberg, privacy measures for email use are fundamentally similar to those required in other situations where health information is communicated. However, according to Spielberg, the potential damage to the patient may be greater with email because of the potential widespread dissemination of written information gathered by unlawful email readers. Therefore the basic ethical duty is fundamentally the same regardless of the medium of communication. Spielberg concludes: "With sufficient precautions and vigilance, email can enhance patient dialogue and physician access without reducing the patient-physician relationship."[27]

The American Medical Informatics Association has published guidelines regarding patient-provider electronic mail.[28] The intent is to provide guidance concerning computer-based communications between clinicians and patients within a contractual relationship in which the health care provider has taken on an explicit measure of responsibility for the client's care. The guidelines address two interrelated aspects: effective interaction between the clinician and patient and observance of medicolegal prudence. Recommendations for site-specific policy formulation are included.

CONCLUSION AND DIRECTIONS FOR THE FUTURE

As medicine enters the twenty-first century, we can predict that the tools emerging from medical informatics will provide many of the answers to these problematic information needs. However, it is overly simplistic to argue that computers and the Web are easy or complete answers. As anyone who has used this technology in the last few years would attest, the current resources and tools, while promising, are still works in progress.

It is virtually impossible to look at any of today's media—paper or electronic, lay or professional—and not be inundated with predictions of how computers and communication will forever alter our world. In general these predictions are rosy. The touting of technology as a cure for all that ails us is a common phenomenon. We would suggest that a more balanced world view is in order, at least in the realm of rural medicine. It would be foolhardy to make grand predictions of just how medical informatics and rural medicine will coevolve over the next decade. This may be cooperative, but there will be unpleasant side effects. But with certainty, it will occur. Rural clinicians would be well advised to do some proactive planning. We would propose the following ideas for your consideration:

1. Unless you intend to retire from practice within the next 5 years, do not think that you can avoid or postpone becoming "wired."
2. Although there are many stories of grand failures in implementing information technology in medicine, there *are* clearly successful and valuable tools (email and *PubMed*) that are available today, easy to use, and very affordable. Make the commitment to learn to use them now.
3. Avoid adopting the perspective that informatics is a panacea—thinking that your practice must become completely computerized as a "paperless office." This is the "technology in search of a problem" dilemma. Begin to think strategically about what aspects of your practice might truly benefit from a judicious application of proven technology.
4. Think of computers in terms of what they do best (storing and retrieving volumes of facts) and not in terms of what they do poorly (synthesizing different and varied information to make a diagnosis).
5. Do not worry that you must become a computer expert. The tools that are of the greatest value are not difficult to learn, and help is available from your nearest medical librarian.
6. It is the nature of clinical information that the more widely shared it is, the more it is beneficial to everyone. Seek out the interested parties in your community—physicians, hospitals, payers, employers, and, of course, patients—and begin to consider how you can best develop and utilize information technology collaboratively.

REFERENCES

1. Tapscott D: *The Digital Economy: Promise and Peril in the Age of Networked Intelligence.* New York, McGraw-Hill, 1996.
2. Lindberg D, Humphreys BL: Computers in medicine. *JAMA* 273:1667–1668, 1995.
3. Smith R: What clinical information do doctors need? *BMJ* 313(7064):1062–1068, 1996.
4. Gorman PN, Helfand M: Information seeking in primary care: how physicians choose which clinical questions to pursue and which to leave unanswered. *Med Decision Making* 15:113–119, 1995.
5. Stross J, Harlan WR: The dissemination of new medical information. *JAMA* 241:2622–2624, 1979.
6. Williamson JW, German PS, Weiss R, et al: Health science information management and continuing education of physicians: a survey of U.S. primary care practitioners and their opinion leaders. *Ann Intern Med* 110:151–160, 1989.
7. Tang PC, Fafchamps D, Shortliffe EH: Traditional medical records as a source of clinical data in the outpatient setting. *Proceedings of the 18th Annual Symposium on Computer Applications in Medical Care,* American Medical Informatics Association, Philadelphia, PA, 1994.
8. Kassirer JP, Gorry GA: Clinical problem solving: a behavioral analysis. *Ann Intern Med* 89(89):245–255, 1978.
9. Osheroff JA, Forsythe DE, Buchanan BG, et al: Physicians' information needs: analysis of questions posed during clinical teaching. *Ann Intern Med* 114:576–581, 1991.
10. Gorman P, Yao P: Comparison of information needs of rural and nonrural clinicians. *American Medical Informatics Association Spring Meeting.* Philadelphia, PA, American Medical Informatics Association, 1998.
11. Lancaster FW: Effect of physical accessibility and ease of use, in *The Measurement and Evaluation of Library Services.* Washington, DC, Information Resources Press, 1977, pp 312–321.
12. Bunting A: The nation's health information net-

work: history of the Regional Medical Library Program, 1965–1985. *Bull Med Library Assoc* 75(3 suppl):1–62, 1987.

13. Lindberg DA, Siegel ER, Rapp BA, et al: Use of *MEDLINE* by physicians for clinical problem solving. *JAMA* 269(24):3124–3129, 1993.

14. Jadad AR, Gagliardi A: Rating health information on the Internet: navigating to knowledge or to Babel. *JAMA* 279(8):611–614, 1998.

15. Shortliffe EH, Perreault LE, Widerhold G, et al: *Computer Applications in Medical Care.* Reading, MA, Addison-Wesley, 1990.

16. McDonald C: The barriers to electronic medical record systems and how to overcome them. *J Am Med Inform Assoc* 4(3):213–221, 1997.

17. Sujansky W: The benefits and challenges of an electronic medical record: much more than a "word-processed" patient chart. *West J Med* 169(3):176–183, 1988.

18. Tarczy-Hornoch P, Kwan-Gett TS, Fouche L, et al: Meeting clinician information needs by integrating access to the medical record and knowledge resources via the Web: proceedings. *JAMIA* 4:809–813, 1997.

19. Goldberg H, Tarczy-Hornoch P, Stephens K, et al: Internet access to patients' records. *Lancet* 351(9118):1811, 1998.

20. Hagland M: Glimpses of a Web-enabled future. *Health Mgt Technol* 19(4):22–29, 1998.

21. Nilasena D, Lincoln MJ: A computer-generated reminder system improves physician compliance with diabetes preventive care guidelines. *Proc Annu Symp Comput Appl Med Care. JAMIA* Symposium Supplement:640–645, 1995.

22. Berner E, Jackson JR, Algina J: Relationships among performance scores of four diagnostic decision support systems. *JAMIA* 3:208–215, 1996.

23. Barnett G, Cimino JJ, Hupp JA, et al: DXplain: an evolving diagnostic decision-support system. *JAMA* 258(1):67–74, 1987.

24. Overhage J, Tierney WM, McDonald CJ: Computer reminders to implement preventive care guidelines for hospitalized patients. *Arch Intern Med* 156:1551–1556, 1996.

25. Hunt DL, Haynes B, Hanna SE, Smith K: Effects of computer-based clinical decision support systems on physician performance and patient outcomes: a systematic review. *JAMA* 280(15):1339–1346, 1998.

26. Robinson TM, Patrick K, Eng TR, et al: An evidence-based approach to interactive health communication: a challenge to medicine in the information age. *JAMA* 280(14):1264–1269, 1998.

27. Spielberg AR: On call and online: sociohistorical, legal and ethical implications of email for the patient-physician relationship. *JAMA* 280(15):1353–1359, 1998.

28. Kane B, Sands DZ: JAMIA Internet Working Group, Task Force on Guidelines for the Clinical Use of Electronic Mail with Patients. *JAMIA* 5(1):104–111, 1998.

CHAPTER 16

Telemedicine and Telehealth Service

THOMAS E. NORRIS

CASE 1

It was a cold Montana evening in February. There had been snow the night before, but the temperature during the daytime had risen to above freezing and melted much of the snow on the road. It was now well below freezing again. On a highway in northwest Montana at 11:00 p.m., a car crested a small hill and slammed on its brakes to avoid four mule deer standing in the middle of the roadway. The driver lost control and the car swerved into a snowbank at the side of the road, rolling twice before stopping in an inverted position. Another traveler found the driver, the sole occupant of the car, still belted into his seat but unconscious, about 10 minutes later. The local emergency medical team responded to the highway patrol's call and transported the driver, strapped to a spine board, to the nearby rural hospital. One of the three local family physicians was on call for the emergency department that evening and was called from home to see the patient, who was regaining consciousness. After a careful examination, the physician found the patient to be apparently uninjured with the exception of fairly severe neck pain and a severe headache associated with a scalp contusion. Before unstrapping the patient from the spine board, the physician obtained cervical spine films. The small hospital had no radiologist, and the family physician reading the films at 1:00 a.m. was uncertain whether a cervical fracture was present. In most circumstances, the physician would have been forced to combine clinical information with his interpretation of the C-spine films to determine how to manage the patient. Fortunately, this rural hospital was equipped with a telemedicine unit. Using a digitizer (an electronic device that digitizes radiographs—similar to a fax machine), the rural family physician was able to transmit the cervical spine radiographs to the trauma radiologist at the regional trauma center, over 500 miles distant. The trauma radiologist then looked at the digitized films and determined that several additional views were necessary. These views were obtained using telephoned instructions from the radiologist; they were then digitized and again transmitted to the trauma center. At this point the trauma radiologist was able to diagnose an unstable cervical fracture. The rural physician continued to keep the patient's cervical spine immobilized and transferred the patient to the care of a neurosurgeon in a larger Montana city 80 miles distant. There, the neurosurgeon was able to provide definitive care for the patient, and the patient recovered without residual neurologic deficit.

CASE 2

Most days the physician's assistant worked with a rural family physician in a small rural community in the northern Rocky Mountains. Several afternoons per week she traveled to an even smaller community, 30 miles distant, where the practice operated a "satellite clinic." The itinerant physician's assistant was the only health care provider for this tiny community. One of the patients, an elderly disabled miner, had seen the physician's assistant regularly for the past several months. The patient had a number of medical problems, but the one that had caused the repeated visits was a significant dermatologic eruption on his left hand. The physician's assistant had entertained several presumptive diagnoses and had discussed the case with her supervising physician. Several forms of therapy had been tried without success. The situation was exacerbated by the fact that the miner was uninsured and disabled. He refused to travel 75 miles to a larger community for a dermatologic consultation. He also refused to travel 30 miles to the practice's "base" site. He said to the physician's assistant, "I guess it's not gonna go away, and if it kills me, it kills me." The physician's assistant was quite concerned by this interchange, by the worsening condition, and by the lesion's failure to respond to therapy. She was worried that her experience with common dermatologic problems did not encompass the type of disease process that she was seeing on the patient's hand. She suggested to the patient that a biopsy be obtained, but he refused. Fortunately, the practice had recently begun participating in an experimental program with a regional medical school, using digital still photographs of dermatologic lesions to obtain consultations with academic dermatologists. At the next visit to the satellite clinic, the physician's assistant brought a small digital camera. The miner's lesions were photographed, and the photographic image was loaded into the computer at the practice site, attached to an email message containing details of the miner's history and physical examination as well as his past medical history and medications. This material was transmitted electronically to the telemedicine/telehealth service of the regional medical school. Later that day the dermatologist evaluated it, called the physician's assistant at the satellite clinic, and asked specific questions about the miner's exposure to heavy metals over the previous few years. Based on the miner's answers to the questions, coupled with the dermatologic photographs, the dermatologist was able to make a presumptive diagnosis of a lesion associated with a mining-related heavy metal exposure. A skin biopsy was obtained and appropriate treatment was then undertaken by the physician's assistant who had been providing the miner's care.

*T*he two cases above illustrate useful applications of electronic telehealth services for rural practices. This chapter is de-

voted to an exploration of telemedicine and telehealth; it includes a discussion of the possible applications of these new technologies to rural practice.

DEFINITION OF TELEMEDICINE

The Institute of Medicine defines telemedicine as "the use of electronic information and communications technologies to provide and support health care, when distance separates the participants."[1] This umbrella definition covers a number of derivative terms that can also apply to specific aspects of telemedicine, such as *teleconferencing*, *teleconsultation*, *telementoring*, *telepresence*, *telehealth*, and *telemonitoring*. Additionally, terms related to specific clinical fields—such as *teleradiology*, *teledermatology*, and *telepsychiatry*—are also included in this definition.

Although many health care professionals consider only interactive real-time video teleconferencing when they think of telemedicine, the broader definition offered by the Institute of Medicine is probably more appropriate. Clearly the use of telephone conversations, faxes, transmission of still images, and other varieties of electronic communication are all forms of telemedicine or telehealth. They simply represent different aspects of the technological base of telemedicine. These modalities are considered in more detail in the next section of this chapter.

It should also be noted that the Institute of Medicine's definition of telemedicine includes both clinical and nonclinical applications of telemedicine. Thus, both patient care and areas such as continuing medical education, administration, and management are all contained within the umbrella definition of telemedicine (often referred to as *telehealth* when used in this broader context).

It is also important to note that the Institute of Medicine feels that geographic separation or distance between the participants is a defining characteristic of telemedicine. One of the older terms for telemedicine was *distance medicine*, and this name is still sometimes used.

Since the defining characteristics of rural areas include the concepts of distance and sparse population, it is clear that telemedicine can play a significant role in the health care of rural citizens.

A CONDENSED HISTORY OF TELEMEDICINE

Electronic distance communication has been used for over 150 years. The first intercity public telegraph services were used between Washington and Baltimore in 1844. Twenty years later, during the Civil War, military physicians used the telegraph to order medical supplies and transmit casualty lists.[2] In 1876, Alexander Graham Bell patented the telephone and pioneered its use as a device for electronic speech transmission. Long-distance telephone links and companies offering telephone services began to appear in the 1880s. Based on several textbooks on the history of medicine, it is apparent that the usage of the telephone in medical practice began shortly thereafter. In 1948 the first transmission of radiologic images by telephone between two sites in Pennsylvania separated by a distance of 24 miles was described.[3] In 1959 the University of Nebraska used a two-way closed-circuit interactive telemedicine linkage to transmit neurologic examinations and other information across campuses to medical students. Subsequently, the Nebraska psychiatrists used the system for group therapy consultations and treatment. This telemedicine link, with the hospital over 100 miles distant, was also used to provide neurologic examinations, diagnoses of difficult psychiatric cases, case consultations, and education and training.[4] In 1959, a report also appeared describing a Canadian radiologist who did fluoroscopic diagnostic consultations using a telemedicine linkage.[5] During the early 1960s, telemedicine usages expanded to include radiotelemetry for monitoring anesthetized patients, and ship-to-shore and transoceanic transmission of electrocardiograms (ECGs). In the late 1960s, radio signals were used to transmit ECG rhythms from on-site fire department "first responders" to hospital emergency departments.[6] In the late 1960s, Massachusetts General Hospital expanded its prior telephone link with Boston's Logan Airport by adding an interactive television microwave link that provided ECG, stethescopic, microscopic, voice, and other capabilities. In this same time period, Massachusetts General Hospital was also developing telepsychiatry linkages with nearby veterans' hospitals.[7] During the 1960s and 1970s many other telemedicine applications were initiated, often supported by federal grants. Several of these were supported by the National Aeronautics and Space Administration (NASA) and demonstrated the efficacy of satellite transmission of telemedicine signals. Most telemedicine projects did not continue functioning after their grant funding was expended.

MODALITIES OF TELEMEDICINE

Table 16-1 lists the various types of telemedicine.

Telephone (Other than Telegraphy)

The use of the telephone probably represents the oldest and broadest application of telemedicine. Examples of the use of the telephone for support of medical practices abound. One example is found at the University of Washington School of Medicine, where the MEDCON system has been in use for over 25 years. This system pro-

TABLE 16-1   MODALITIES OF TELEMEDICINE

Telephone
Fax
Computer/modem-based modalities
Discipline-specific (teleradiology and telepathology) modalities
Video: real-time interactive and store-and-forward "Telepresence"

vides a toll-free access line that allows health care providers from the states of Washington, Wyoming, Alaska, Montana, and Idaho to contact, free of charge, clinical specialists practicing at the University of Washington School of Medicine. These contacts are free and often allow rural physicians to have access to most specialties for the purpose of discussing the medical care of specific patients. The advantages of the telephone system are manifold. Telephones are, at least in the United States, ubiquitous. They operate on an infrastructure that is already very widely distributed. It is difficult to find anyone who does not already know how to operate a telephone. Finally, the usage of the telephone, even for long-distance transmission, is relatively inexpensive. Unfortunately, there are also several disadvantages to the use of the telephone. These include the fact that, at this time, the standard telephone transmits only audio signals. Text and images are not transmitted by the standard telephone. Furthermore, both parties need to be present at a telephone receiver at the same time. This is often a significant disadvantage, as it is quite common for health care providers to participate in several rounds of "phone tag" before actually making contact with each other.

Fax

The next most common modality used for telemedicine is probably the fax machine. Examples of the use of fax machines in the practice of medicine are widespread. Transmissions of ECGs and fetal monitoring strips for interpretation and consultation are common. Additionally, most regional medical libraries fax medical articles to rural health care providers. The advantages of fax machines are similar to those of telephones. Over the last few years fax machines have become very common and are available in most rural practices in the United States. These units operate on the same electronic infrastructure used for the telephone system—an ever-present infrastructure that provides a great advantage for the fax machines. The cost of fax machines has diminished markedly from their high initial levels. Additionally, fax machines

have become quite easy to use and require little operator training. These systems handle text very well and are improving in their capabilities with "still" graphic images. Furthermore, the use of fax machines is not dependent upon the synchronous presence of both parties. Instead, a fax machine can transmit its images to the other party without regard to his or her presence at the receiving end. There are several disadvantages to fax machines. Unless there are two lines present, it is not possible to talk with the other party on the telephone about the faxed message while it is being sent. Furthermore, although faxes handle still images reasonably well, they cannot display motion.

Computer/Modem-Based Modalities

The next major area involved in telemedicine actually includes several modalities. The unifying factor is that each usage relies on a computer with a modem (a device for transmitting digital signals to or from a computer electronically, often via telephone lines). Specific applications of this modality include E-mail-based telemedicine, Internet-based telemedicine, and World Wide Web–based telemedicine. Many examples can be found in each of these areas. It is common for health care providers to use E-mail to consult with other health care providers about clinical situations. Concern has been raised about the security of these transmissions; often, specific patient identifiers are not used or encryption of the transmission is utilized. This remains, however, a popular mode of clinical discourse.

The use of the Internet and the World Wide Web presents another group of applications through which much telemedicine is accomplished. For example, the Communicable Disease Center sponsors multiple Web sites to send current information to providers around the world on topics involving communicable diseases. The National Library of Medicine has long sponsored Internet access programs to access the medical literature, including their MEDLINE and Grateful Med applications. This telemedicine modality, with its multiple applications, has a number of advantages. Computers and modems are both very common. Indeed, it is difficult to purchase a personal computer without a modem at this time. Most modems operate on the telephone system infrastructure, although some use other transmission systems (Ethernet, cable TV cables, etc.). Most do not require special digital or broad-bandwidth connections. This versatility makes the systems highly transportable. Once the system is set up and the user is trained, these systems provide significant convenience. The cost of the systems is relatively low, and the prices have been dropping dramatically over the past few years. These systems currently handle text and still images extremely well. Additionally, software advances promise that motion-oriented images will be handled more easily and satisfactorily in the future.

There are several disadvantages to the computer/modem-based systems. These include the need for user training, the need for equipment setup, and concerns about security. Security has been a significant concern with these systems, especially with those where the communication is Internet-based. The concern has been that hackers could intercept sensitive medical information that is associated with discrete patient identification.

Discipline-Specific Telemedicine

The next sets of telemedicine modalities are essentially discipline-based approaches to telemedicine. Probably the best example of these is teleradiology. As indicated in the earlier comments on the history of telemedicine, protocols to transmit radiographic images were first introduced in 1948, followed by protocols to transmit real-time fluoroscopy in 1959. Today, multiple examples of teleradiology exist in all parts of the United States, with some worldwide applications being developed. The general approach is for a radiographic image to be taken. The image may be recorded on standard x-ray film, or its signal may be directly digitized. If the image is recorded on standard film, it is then passed through a digitizer which, in a fashion conceptually similar to the way a fax machine

works, changes the image into a digital electronic format that can be transmitted. If film is not used, then the directly digitized image can be transmitted. The digital image signal is transmitted to a radiologist, who is usually stationed at a computer-based workstation. The radiologist interprets the image on the monitor and sends the interpretation back to the site where the image was originally obtained, often transmitting the interpretation electronically. This system is fundamentally a specialized subset of the computer/modem systems discussed above. As such, it has most of the same advantages as the computer/modem. Several specific additions are necessary, including special software and larger, higher-resolution monitors. The disadvantages are also similar to those of the computer/modem. Depending on the software being used, the system may transmit only images and not text. Otherwise, this has proven to be a highly popular and very practical use of telemedicine technology.

Another "discipline-based" approach to telemedicine is telepathology. In the telepathology systems, an electronic image of the microscopic field involved is transmitted from the site where the specimen is being processed to the site where a pathologist can provide interpretation for the specimen. In many ways, this process is similar to teleradiology in that the specialist is distant from the site of image processing. Because of the nature of interpretation of microscopic images and the normal need to vary the focal lengths of the image on a slide to allow "depth" to be present, there are some technical differences. Telepathology systems allowing interpretation of Pap smears and surgical pathology images are in wide use in some parts of the United States. The advantages and disadvantages of the telepathology systems are quite similar to those of the teleradiology systems.

Interactive Video and "Store and Forward" Video

When most people think of telemedicine, they visualize a real-time, interactive, two-way video transmission. This type of transmission has been widely used in telemedicine linkages. The early telepsychiatry programs at the University of Nebraska fall into this category. More recently, many of the rural projects funded by the Federal Office of Rural Health Policy have supported the creation of real-time, two-way interactive video linkages between rural practice sites and either regional "hub sites" or academic medical center hubs. These systems have many advantages. They handle both audio and motion-oriented video transmissions very well. They allow a real-time interaction between physicians or between physicians and patients. They are also quite easy to use, and both patient and provider acceptance has been very good. Among the disadvantages of these systems has been their cost. It is noted, however, that the cost of the systems is decreasing rapidly. Additionally, the systems have typically required a broad-band digital transmission infrastructure (other than standard telephone systems) to support them. Often, this broad-band transmission infrastructure is not available in rural sites. As the WWAMI Rural Telemedicine Network (the rural telemedicine program used by the University of Washington in Wyoming, Alaska, Montana, and Idaho) was installed, the broad-bandwidth digital transmission infrastructure had to be specially installed into several rural sites; it was not already present in these small towns. These systems, depending on their software, tend to handle audio and motion well but sometimes do not handle text well. Additionally, these systems require the synchronous presence of all parties and are thus time-bound. This last requirement has led many telemedicine developers to work toward store-and-forward video capabilities. These systems, variants of the real-time interactive video systems, are now in use at many sites. The store-and-forward systems allow the transmission of one-way video communication to another site (as opposed to two-way). The image and audio are recorded for playback at a later date in much the same way that an answering machine might recall a caller's comments for playback when the intended recipient can accept the message. Equipment of this type, using both still and video transmissions, is becoming much more common. The advantages include less expensive equipment, especially with still digital photography, than that required by the interactive systems. Because this is not real-time transmission, narrow (cheaper) bandwidths can be used. Additionally, these systems are not time-bound. The disadvantages are the lack of a real-time interactivity. It is noted, however, that the convenience often outweighs this disadvantage.

"Telepresence"

Much has been written about the use of *telepresence,* in which telemedicine is taken past communications to an active "physical" involvement with the environment at a distance from the site from which the signal originated. At the present time, all of the telepresence activities are experimental. It is, however, anticipated that, in the future, telemedicine will develop in this direction. Whether this direction of telemedicine development will be useful to rural patients and rural providers remains to be seen. The disadvantages are many, including an extreme broad-band infrastructure, high cost, and the experimental nature of the equipment. The potential advantages are uncertain at this point, but the systems may find early applications in microsurgical settings.

ACTUAL AND POTENTIAL APPLICATIONS OF TELEMEDICINE/ TELEHEALTH IN RURAL HEALTH CARE

Excellent studies have been done reviewing the potential applications of telemedicine. Some of these were discussed in the examples presented at the beginning of this chapter, and others have been mentioned in the discussion of the modalities of telemedicine. Commonly accepted telemedicine applications include the following[8]:

• Initial evaluations of patients, triage decisions, and pretransfer arrangement development

- Medical and surgical follow-up and medication checks
- Supervision and consultation for primary care encounters in sites where a physician is not available
- Routine consultations and second opinions based on history, physical examination findings, and available test data
- Transmission of diagnostic images
- Extended diagnostic workups or short-term management of self-limited conditions
- Management of chronic diseases and conditions requiring a specialist who is not readily available locally
- Transmission of medical data
- Public health, preventative medicine, and patient education applications

As the reader can clearly see, almost all of these applications have even more utility in the rural than in the urban setting. In areas where population densities are low, where distances are long, and where a majority of the health care providers (if there are any) are generalists, access to specialty care and consultations are common uses of telemedicine. Additionally, the other applications that Grigsby and colleagues mention are all appropriate for rural utilization. Telemedicine is a tool that can be applied to a large variety of problems. Table 16-2 lists the most

TABLE 16-2   APPLICATIONS OF TELEMEDICINE

Emergency medicine
Primary care
Cardiology
Orthopedics
General surgery
General medicine
Pulmonary care
Psychiatry
Pediatrics
Oncology
Dermatology
Radiology

SOURCE: From Allen and Wheeler,[14] with permission.

used applications at the time of this writing. The innovative rural provider is probably in the best position to define problems that telemedicine might play a role in solving.

CURRENT ISSUES IN TELEMEDICINE

A number of issues exist in telemedicine at this time. These are briefly considered in order to clarify some of the limitations of this modality.

Infrastructure and equipment represent areas of significant issues in telemedicine. In a situation analogous to that seen during the early days of personal computers, there is less than universal intercompatibility of telemedicine systems at this time. Current significant efforts are under way to create standards that will allow reliable interconnections between telemedicine equipment developed by different manufacturers. It is hoped that in the future, telemedicine systems will all be developed in compliance with these standards and will therefore be able to connect easily with each other. Until this is done, it is suggested that the consumer of telemedicine equipment carefully ascertain that it will be possible to create connections between the equipment being purchased and the equipment that it will link to. With regard to infrastructure, especially in rural areas, there have been ongoing problems due to *lack of a broad-bandwidth data transmission capability*. In most urban areas and between most urban areas, broad-bandwidth data transmission capabilities can be purchased from telephone companies, cable television companies, and other vendors. This is not universally the case in rural settings, and this lack of infrastructure has somewhat limited widespread rural applications of telemedicine.

It is important to mention costs with regard to both equipment and infrastructure. The cost of telemedicine equipment has declined rapidly over the past few years. It had been hoped, with recent federal legislation, that the cost of broad-bandwidth data and telemedicine image transmission would also decline. It remains to be seen, however, whether these changes will actually occur.

One significant point that must be considered regarding equipment and infrastructure decisions is the nature of the information being transmitted, along with the nature of the clinical situation involved. These two factors should determine the technological application that will be used. Too often, technology has been a tool looking for a problem to solve. For example, it is both inappropriate and much more expensive to use real-time interactive video telemedicine when a store-and-forward approach with still photographs will accomplish the task. It is hoped that the rural provider will identify a problem and select the appropriate technology to solve it.

Lack of reimbursement for services has been a major impediment to the development of telemedicine services. Most of the financially successful uses of telemedicine and telehealth services in the United States to date have occurred using telemedicine to assist with radiographic image interpretation or to assist with management of "contracted" health care services. The reason for the widespread success in these two areas has been the presence of reimbursement for these specific telemedicine services. Medicare and most health insurance plans will pay a radiologist for interpretation of a film in which telemedicine is utilized to transmit the image. Similarly, in settings where health care is "contracted," such as prison or correction system health care, the use of telemedicine could be included in the contract. Unfortunately, most health insurance programs so far have not included telemedicine services in the "covered services" for their insured patients. Concern has been expressed by health insurers that telemedicine might actually increase the utilization of specialty services or cause billing by two physicians for services occurring simultaneously. For this reason, there has been reluctance to include these services within the plans' coverage. Recently, the U.S. Congress instructed the Health Care Financing Administration to begin including rural tele-

medicine services among the services covered by Medicare. Unfortunately, the implementation of this payment, at least as of this writing, is such that it is doubtful that many rural telemedicine services will actually be covered. One of the essential requirements for future development of telemedicine/telehealth services will be reimbursement for these modalities of care.

Credentialing has been a minor issue in the development of telemedicine and telehealth services. In disciplines where image interpretation is the critical part of the telemedicine application (radiology, pathology, dermatology), discussions have occurred about the possible need for special credentialing of providers involved in the interpretation of these images. This may be an area for future development.

Licensure has been a significant issue as telemedicine has spread throughout the United States. Concern has been expressed by many state licensing boards that out of state providers would utilize telemedicine systems to provide care for patients in states where the providers were not licensed. This concern has led to new and more restrictive licensure laws in some states. Because of this issue, discussion has occurred about the possible need for a national licensure within the United States. If telemedicine is being used within a single state, this issue does not arise. However, if the telemedicine application involves several states, it may be necessary for the providers to be licensed in all of them.

Liability concerns have been expressed by many providers involved in telemedicine. Specifically, these providers wonder if the use of telemedicine within their practices will actually increase their exposure to professional liability litigation. As of this writing, no landmark cases have arisen and it does not appear that professional liability insurers are charging higher rates for physicians utilizing telemedicine in their practices. It is suggested, however, that physicians consult their professional liability carriers about this question prior to the adoption of telemedicine for their practices.

A number of *user issues* have been studied over the life of telemedicine. Patient and provider acceptance has been considered rather extensively. Generally, patients have been accepting of the use of telemedicine systems in provision of their health care. It has also been noted that both primary and specialty care physicians have shown a general acceptance of this technology. An interesting pattern has been reported by Grigsby and Sanders[9] and others with regard to the utilization of telemedicine systems. Specifically, they have noted that, when a telemedicine system is installed, there is often a sudden and significant high rate of usage among both providers and patients. As time goes by, instead of increasing, the usage usually drops to a far lower baseline. Indeed, sometimes the systems are eventually not used at all. It is unclear why this pattern is repeatedly observed. Possible explanations have been that the systems are not "user-friendly" enough to be convenient for providers and patients, that the providers have learned how to manage the problems for which they had been obtaining telemedicine consultations, or perhaps other reasons.

Patient confidentiality and security of information have been important issues in the development of telemedicine. As long as telemedicine is being conducted on dedicated telephone lines or broad-bandwidth data transmission lines, the information is relatively secure. Much concern has been voiced, however, that extra parties present at both ends of a telemedicine transmission might increase the chance of violating patient confidentiality. Furthermore, if data are sent on the Internet, the possibility that these data will be accessed by outside parties creates significant concerns. Before telemedicine is widely adopted and before Internet-based telemedicine achieves its ultimate potential, these areas will have to be adequately addressed. Current efforts are under way to develop encryption systems that would increase the security of telemedicine transmissions. This or other approaches may relieve this concern.

The last major telemedicine/telehealth issue is that of the development of "telemedicine etiquette" or "telemedicine protocols." For aspects of telemedicine that involve direct clinical interaction between a health care provider and a patient, the issue of etiquette and protocols is a significant one. For those of us who have been providing health care for a long time, the expected behaviors of a health care provider and a patient in an examining room are fairly standardized. These have been developed over many years, and both provider and patient have achieved a comfort level with these standards. Health care interactions based on a video system fall outside these comfortable protocols. Both patient and physician will have to become comfortable with this new form of interaction. Discussions will have to be held regarding who may or should be in the telemedicine "studio" (exam room), whether the interaction will take place in real time or whether a store-and-forward method will be used, what sort of chaperone will be required for sensitive examinations, and so on. Development of widely accepted protocols in these areas will render telemedicine and telehealth services more useful and more comfortable to both the patient and the health care provider.

EDUCATION AND TRAINING

At the present time there is a paucity of training programs that include preparation for telemedicine or telehealth services in their curricula. In the future, as this form of health care interaction becomes more common, it is anticipated that training programs will have to develop at the level of professional or medical schools, postgraduate training, and continuing education training. The technical skills required to use these complex systems must be learned, and the clinical skills required to optimally apply these systems to clinical situations will also need to be learned. It is hoped that educational material on these two topics will be included in programs designed to educate rural health care providers

TABLE 16-3   RESOURCES FOR TELEMEDICINE

Federal Telemedicine Gateway—compilation of hands-on telemedicine health care projects funded by the federal government	http://www.tmgateway.org
Telemedicine and Telehealth Networks—a magazine for professionals in the field of telemedicine	http://www.telemedmag.com/
Association of Telemedicine Service Providers (ATSP)—information on the ATSP annual conference, advocacy, the *Dispatch* newletter, databases, useful links, how to join the ATSP, and more	http://www.atsp.org 7276 SW Beaverton-Hillsdale Hwy. Suite 400 Portland, OR 97225 Telephone: 503-222-2406 http://208.129.211.51/
Telemedicine Information Exchange	2121 SW Broadway Suite 130 Portland, OR 97201 Telephone: 503-221-1620 http://www.telemedprimer.com
Telemedicine Primer: Understanding the Issues—a reference manual for telemedicine program implementation	1013 Ridgewood Ct. West Des Moines, IA 50265 Telephone: 515-223-9389

and ancillary personnel. This type of training will be especially important for those preparing for rural practice. It would also be beneficial if programs were developed to provide patient education regarding telemedicine and telehealth services. Indeed, if patients knew what to expect from these services, they would probably be more accepting of them. Resources to assist the provider wishing to learn about telemedicine are listed in Table 16-3.

FUTURE DIRECTIONS

In spite of the significant progress that has been made in telemedicine over the past decade, the volume of patients receiving clinical services utilizing the technology remains relatively low, with less than 25,000 patients receiving direct telemedicine services in 1996.[10] It is, however, anticipated that the number of patients utilizing telemedicine and telehealth services will continue to increase steadily. In 1996 a survey of 2400 nonfederal rural hospitals found that 17 percent were participating in a telemedicine network, while another 13 percent had plans to use telemedicine.[11] In another study, which analyzed rural hospital use of telemedicine technology, 68 percent of the rural hospitals using telemedicine technology were using it for the transfer of radiologic images. Many nonclinical applications, including educational and administrative meetings via telemedicine, were also being used. Smaller hospitals were the most likely to utilize telemedicine, and the highest interest in telemedicine was in the rural hospitals of the intermountain region.[12] At the present time, cost is the major limiting factor for rural hospitals interested in adopting telemedicine. The Federal Office of Rural Health

Policy reported that the average equipment purchase ranged from $134,378 for "spoke" sites (peripheral hospital sites) to $287,503 for "hub" sites (central regional centers). Transmission costs ranged from an average of $18,573 for spokes to $80,068 for hubs. Federal and state grants were the most common sources of funding for the telemedicine programs studied, and the majority of sites also received hospital financial support.[12] Clearly costs will have to be controlled and reimbursement developed if rural sites are to continue their increased usage of telemedicine. Thus, it is likely that the first trend in telemedicine will be a continued increase in its usage. It is anticipated that the very wide diversity of clinical applications of telemedicine will continue and that each medical discipline will find ways to optimize the usage of these technologies.

Changes are occurring with regard to trends in telemedicine technology. In the early 1990s, the trend was toward more real-time interactive video technology. This focus is now shifting toward more personal computer–based and store-and-forward applications. The desktop systems will probably be more convenient and more cost-effective than the larger "studio-based" systems. The store-and-forward approach will likely relieve health care professionals of the need to try to achieve synchronous transmission. Additionally, more sophisticated software products, including multimedia email, may broaden the existing applications and may solve some of the complexities regarding security of telemedicine transmissions on the Internet.[13]

A major question concerning the success of the future development of telemedicine will be dependent on government telemedicine policies. These policies, at the state and federal levels, will determine the answers to the issues of licensure, liability, reimbursement, and many other current areas of controversy. The move by the United States government to include, albeit in a very limited way, reimbursement for telemedicine in the services covered for Medicare patients will likely herald a new era in which more telemedicine services qualify for reimbursement.

CONCLUSION

Telemedicine and *telehealth services* are very general terms that refer to a wide range of technologies and applications. Rural patients and rural health care providers have benefited markedly from the use of these technologies. It is anticipated that the application of electronic communications and computing tools to rural health care will continue to be aggressively pursued. It is also anticipated that these tools will continue to provide additional methods through which the rural challenges of distance and sparse population can be managed.

REFERENCES

1. Institute of Medicine: *Telemedicine: A Guide to Assessing Telecommunications in Health Care.* Washington, DC, National Academy Press, 1996.
2. Zundel KM: Telemedicine: history, application, and impact on librarianship. *Bull Med Library Assoc* 84(1):71–79, 1996.
3. Zundel KM: Telemedicine: History, application, and impact on librarianship. *Bull Med Library Assoc* 84(1):71–79, 1996.
4. Perednia A: Telemedicine technology and clinical applications. *JAMA* 273(6):483–487, 1995.
5. Jutra A: Teleroentgen diagnosis by means of videotape recording. *AJR* 82:1099–1102, 1959.
6. Nagel EL, Hirschman JC, Mayer PW, et al: Telemedicine of physiologic data and aid to fire rescue personnel in a metropolitan area. *South Med J* 61:598–601, 1968.
7. Crump WJ, Pfeil TA: Telemedicine primer: an introduction to the technology and an overview of the literature. *Arch Fam Med* 4:796–803, 1995.
8. Grigsby J, et al: *Analysis of Expansion of Access to Care through Telemedicine.* Report 4: *Study Summary and Recommendations for Further Research.* Denver, Center for Health Research Policy, December 3–4, 1994.
9. Grigsby J, Sanders JH: Telemedicine: where it

is and where it's going. *Ann Intern Med* 129:123–127, 1998.

10. Grigsby B, Allen A: Fourth annual telemedicine program review: Part 2. United States. *Telemed Today* 5:30–38, 42, 1997.

11. Hassol A, Gaumer G, Grigsby J, et al: Brunswick, Maine: rural telemedicine—a national snapshot. *Telemed J* 2:43–48, 1996.

12. Federal Office of Rural Health Policy, Health Resources and Services Administration, US De-partment of Health and Human Services: *Exploratory Evaluation of Rural Applications of Telemedicine: Final report.* Washington, DC, US Government Printing Office, February 1997.

13. Grigsby J, Sanders JH: Telemedicine: where it is and where it's going. *Ann Intern Med* 129:123–127, 1998.

14. Allen A, Wheeler T: The leaders: US programs doing more than 500 interactive consults in 1997. *Telemed Today,* 6(3):36–37, 1998.

Rural Health Networks: An Organizational Strategy for Collaboration

IRA MOSCOVICE   ANTHONY WELLEVER

R ural health networks continue to capture the attention of providers and health care policymakers.[1] Variously viewed as tools for increasing the effectiveness of members and as vehicles for aiding the diffusion of managed care in rural areas, rural health care networks differ widely in their purpose, structure, and operating characteristics.

One example of a mature rural health network is the Rural Wisconsin Health Cooperative (RWHC).[2] RWHC is owned and operated by 24 rural hospitals and one urban hospital. It was started as a shared service corporation in 1979 and provides services to its members in areas such as multihospital benchmarking and other quality improvement initiatives, physical therapy, physician credentialing, emergency room physician staffing, and ongoing rural-specific continuing education opportunities. Recent RWHC initiatives include joint efforts with HMOs and insurers in the region to increase the effectiveness of a regional physician credentialing service and a strategic alliance with a regional independent practice association to support community-based primary care practice through the development of a pool of administrative specialists who will work with rural physician practices.

The success of RWHC points out the value to rural health providers of membership in an organization that can directly provide necessary services, negotiate group discount rates for members for services that need to be provided by other entities, and help members to adapt to changing environmental conditions such as the entry of managed care in rural areas.

To one degree or another, all rural health care providers participate in networking relationships. Rural providers, for example, refer patients to other providers according to custom and convention, share information routinely in a variety of public and private meetings, and occasionally join together to solve specific problems. Both the number of these relationships and their transitory and variable nature make them difficult to study on a large scale. Accordingly, this chapter focuses on only one kind of network—formal rural health networks. The chapter summarizes the results of the only available national survey of rural health networks and discusses lessons learned from recent site visits to rural health network demonstration programs.

A NATIONAL PERSPECTIVE ON RURAL HEALTH NETWORKS

We define a rural health network as a formal organizational arrangement among rural health care providers (and possibly insurers and social service providers) that uses the resources of more than one existing organization and specifies the objectives and methods by which various collaborative functions are achieved.[3]

Formal rural health networks share the following attributes:

Written Agreement: A written agreement specifies the purpose of the network, identifies who is a member of the network, and outlines the duties and responsibilities of membership.

Individual Autonomy: The members of the network retain their individual autonomy, but they may choose to delegate an explicitly limited portion of their autonomy to the network to foster greater coordination and/or integration.

Joint Action: The members of the network perform collaborative activities according to an explicit plan of action. Activities include the provision or coordination of management functions and clinical services.

This section presents a snapshot of rural health networks in the United States as of the beginning of 1996. These networks shared two common traits:

- They exhibited the attributes of formal rural health networks.
- They had at least one rural hospital member.

We gathered information on rural health networks via a national telephone survey conducted in the fall and winter of 1996. The survey response rate was 95 percent. The data depicted in this chapter's figures and tables are a result of this survey.

This information can be used in various ways:

- Providers who do not currently belong to rural health networks may learn more about the structure and functions of networks. This knowledge may help them decide whether to participate in rural health networks in the future.
- Providers who do participate in rural health networks may be able to gauge their progress compared to other networks and possibly to plan future steps.
- Policymakers who view the current status of

network development may be able to provide incentives for wider development of networks, remove barriers to network creation and expansion, and design programs that more directly influence the course of rural health network structure and functions.

Members and Relationships: The Structure of the Network

Of the 180 rural health networks identified, five main categories of network composition emerged:

- Rural hospitals only
- Rural and urban hospitals only
- Hospitals and physicians
- Hospitals, physicians, and others
- Hospitals and others (not physicians)

The most common type of rural health network is one composed exclusively of hospitals. Rural-hospitals-only networks account for 29 percent of all rural health networks, and urban-and-rural-hospitals-only networks account for 18 percent. Forty-two percent of networks contained physicians as members (Fig. 17-1). Participation of other health and social service providers or insurers in networks is much less common (Table 17-1).

New rural health networks are more likely than older networks to be composed of hospitals and physicians. Approximately one-half of rural health networks 3 years old or younger include both hospitals and physicians (and possibly others). In contrast, hospital-and-physician networks account for less than one-quarter of networks over 3 years old.

A popular form of organization, the rural health network existed in 44 states in 1996. Although the distribution of rural health networks is broad, it is not particularly deep. Only two states—Iowa and Nebraska—boast more than 10 networks; 10 additional states have between 6 and 10 networks. But the vast majority of states (32 of 50) have between 1 and 5 rural health networks.

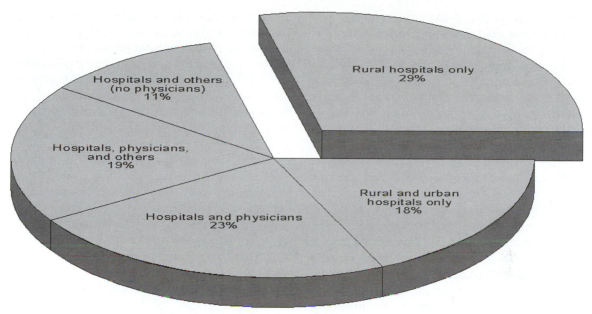

FIGURE 17-1 Types of rural health networks (n = 180).

This seems to indicate that, within most states, the creation of new networks is not attributable to a "bandwagon effect," whereby rural providers form networks to mimic the strategies of successful or apparently successful neighboring providers. To date, network participants appear to be motivated by their own strategic concerns and seem to have formed their networks without great reliance on established local or national models. To the extent that these rural health networks are successful, however, they themselves may provide models and stimulate a bandwagon effect within states in the future.

Although some rural health networks are over 20 years old, they are exceptions. Approximately 70 percent of rural health networks are 3 years old or newer. The older networks are more likely to be composed entirely of hospitals. These networks were formed primarily to share costly or difficult-to-supply services and to reduce costs. The newer rural health networks, which are more likely to include physicians and other providers, were formed to reduce duplication across providers, improve the continuity of care, and position providers to prosper in a managed care environment.

Governance and Management: Organizing the Network

Most rural health networks are incorporated, have a governing board, and are administered

TABLE 17-1   RURAL HEALTH NETWORK MEMBERSHIP

Member Type	Number (%) of Networks with This Type of Member
Rural hospitals	180 (100%)
Physicians	76 (42%)
Urban hospitals	71 (39%)
Mental health	19 (11%)
Home health	18 (10%)
Public health	18 (10%)
Nursing home	17 (9%)
Ambulance services	11 (6%)
Social services	11 (6%)
HMO/insurance	9 (5%)

according to written bylaws. Eight of ten networks are organized as either for-profit or not-for-profit corporations (Fig. 17-2).

The governing boards of rural health networks are composed primarily of health care providers. Approximately two-thirds of rural health network boards are composed exclusively of health care providers. The remaining network boards include some community members not involved in health services delivery.

The prevalence of formal incorporation and bylaws may be interpreted in several ways. The adoption of a formal structure may be indicative of the members' belief in the permanence of the network. Rather than a forum for solving a fleeting problem, members view the network as a "going concern" where various issues may be considered. On the other hand, incorporation and the writing of bylaws, potentially time-consuming activities, may be an unconscious substitute for taking substantive action. Overly rigid bylaws and mission statements created early in the network's development may also serve to throttle flexibility and innovation down the road.

Member dues, sale of network services, and government grants are the primary sources of income for rural health networks. Over one-half of all rural health networks rely on member dues for a portion of their operating income. Approximately 44 percent use the sale of network services to help finance operations; 31 percent have government grants (Fig. 17-3). Only one in five rural health networks relies exclusively on member dues to finance operations.

As networks mature, they are likely to concentrate on two primary sources of income: dues and sales of network services. Networks can be sustained by dues only if the members believe that they derive net benefits from membership. Furthermore, the budget of a network based on dues will always be constrained by the ability and willingness of members to contribute dues. The long-term survival of rural health networks, therefore, likely will be determined by networks' ability to sell services to members and others.

Forty percent of rural health networks employ a full-time director. Newer and smaller

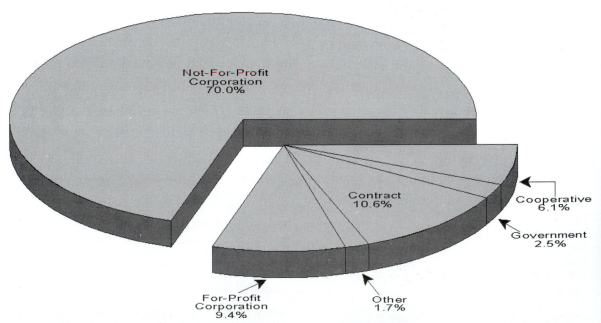

FIGURE 17-2 *Legal status of rural health networks.*

Chapter 17   Rural Health Networks: An Organizational Strategy for Collaboration

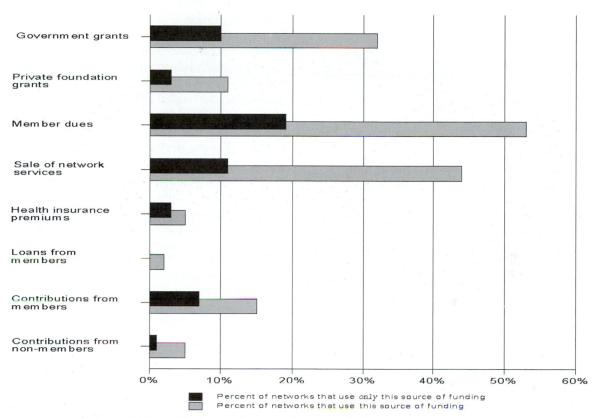

FIGURE 17-3 Sources of network funding and reliance on those sources.

rural health networks are less inclined to employ full-time staff. The employment of an executive director, however, is associated with a higher probability of network survival.[4] Qualified network directors can plan and implement network functions and services more expeditiously than a board of directors.

In the past, rural health networks developed slowly over a number of years. They moved through various stages, growing in complexity as members became more comfortable with one another and as the network produced desirable results. Many networks that form in today's rural health environment perceive that they do not have the same luxury of time. Yet, it is difficult to accelerate the development of a network because so little is known about the determinants of rural health network success.

The lack of models and the scarcity of "boil-

erplate" organizational tools has forced many networks to be created on their own. This act of self-creation consumes valuable time. It may be possible for policymakers and rural health networks themselves to take certain steps to accelerate the network development process, such as:

- Developing rural health network organizational and administrative procedure models for use by emerging networks.
- Providing targeted technical assistance to emerging rural health networks to help them overcome temporary problems in their development.
- Hiring qualified network administrators and endowing them with the authority for network development.

Functions and Services: The Business of the Network

Rural health networks form to accomplish certain objectives. Chief among these objectives is the production of collaborative functions that enable the members to fulfill their individual missions more fully and the development of clinical and insurance services to be offered to the public. Functional collaboration among members may lead to greater levels of integration, and more highly integrated networks may be associated with a greater probability of success in managed care environments. To measure integration of rural health networks, we developed an integration scale. This section reviews key trends in the business of networks, dividing findings between collaboration and integration and managed care linkages.

COLLABORATION AND INTEGRATION

The collaborative activities that members of rural health networks participate in most frequently are: (a) contributing capital to joint ventures, (b) establishing legislative and regulatory advocacy programs, (c) participating in continuing education programs, and (d) sharing staff. Almost one-half (46 percent) of rural health network administrators report that at least two of their members contribute capital to joint ventures, and almost one-third (30 percent) report that all of the members of their rural health networks contribute capital to joint ventures (Table 17-2).

Forty-three percent of network administrators report that at least two members participate in joint advocacy efforts. Thirty-seven percent report that at least two members "shared" continuing education programs, and 33 percent say that at least two members share staff.

Rural health networks exhibit only a modest amount of clinical and functional integration, but they do display a moderate amount of financial integration. On a scale of 0 to 100 (see Appendix 1 for calculation of scale), rural health networks averaged scores of 13.1 and 13.2, respectively, for clinical integration and func-

tional integration and averaged a score of 30.1 for financial integration.*

The great majority of rural health network members have not integrated their core functions with other members. Instead, rural health networks have tended to focus on support functions, such as legislative and regulatory advocacy and shared continuing education and staffing, that are peripheral to the core.

The creation of joint ventures is a special case. When the members of a network participate in a joint venture, they create a new organization—an organization that is not a member of the network—to provide a function or service that did not previously exist. Although this sort of collaboration is highly integrative, it is not an example of the coordination or combining of existing services of members. Members participating in a joint venture simply contribute capital and possibly their clinical or business acumen to the project.

Why have rural health network members not combined their core functions and key support services to a greater degree? Reasons may include lack of trust (which may be a function of network age), unwillingness to surrender autonomy, and ignorance of the purported benefits of integration.

MANAGED CARE LINKAGES

Overall, relatively few rural health networks contract with health maintenance organizations (HMOs) or self-insured employers. Twenty percent of rural health networks contract with HMOs and 21 percent contract directly with self-insured employers (Fig. 17-4).

Rural health networks composed of hospitals,

---

* *Integration* means the bringing together of previously separate and independent functions, resources, and organizations into a new unified structure.[4] *Clinical integration* denotes the coordination or combination of patient care services across members of the network.[5] *Functional integration* describes the coordination or combination of key support or administrative functions and activities across members of the network.[6] *Financial integration* indicates the sharing of capital, risks, and profits across members of the network.

TABLE 17-2   MEMBER PARTICIPATION IN RURAL HEALTH NETWORK FUNCTIONS[a]

Function	Percent Who Say at Least Two Members Participate	Percent Who Say All Members Participate
Use the same personnel policy manual	6.7	1.7
Use the same salary and wage system	6.7	1.7
Use the same chart of accounts	9.2	2.5
Use a consolidated network office for payroll and/or accounts payable	6.7	2.5
Use a consolidated network office for patient billing and collections	9.2	5.0
Use the same health professional recruitment program	25.2	13.4
Use the same networkwide management information system	21.0	8.4
Use the same networkwide materials management system	17.6	5.9
Use the same physician credentialing system	27.7	16.0
Use the same quality measurement and improvement program	16.0	8.4
Use the same clinical protocols	10.9	4.2
Use a system for sharing medical records among network members	11.8	6.7
Accept a portion of the risk of operating loss on network ventures	30.3	21.8
Accept a portion of the risk of business failure on network ventures	26.1	17.6
Contribute capital to network ventures	46.2	30.3
Use the same continuing education programs	37.0	25.2
Use shared staff	32.8	14.3
Participate in common legislative and regulatory advocacy efforts	42.9	31.9
Use a consolidated network office for marketing and community relations	16.8	10.0
Use a consolidated network office for planning	20.2	16.8
Use a consolidated network office or service for grant writing	25.2	17.6

[a]Networks with 20 or fewer members only, $n = 119$.

physicians, and others are significantly more likely to contract with HMOs and with self-insured employers on behalf of their members. Seventy percent of all rural health networks that contract with HMOs and 70 percent of health networks that contract with self-insured employers include physicians in their networks.

A slim majority (54 percent) of rural health networks that contract with HMOs receive a capitated payment from the HMO and distribute it to their members. The rural health networks contracting with HMOs tend to capitate

their primary care physician and hospital members and to pay their specialists on a fee-for-service basis. A total of 63 percent of primary care physicians and 43 percent of hospitals in rural health networks that contract with HMOs receive capitated payments from the network for providing services to HMO enrollees, while 58 percent of specialists in rural health networks that contract with HMOs receive fee-for-service payments from the network for providing services to HMO enrollees.

In the future, more rural health networks

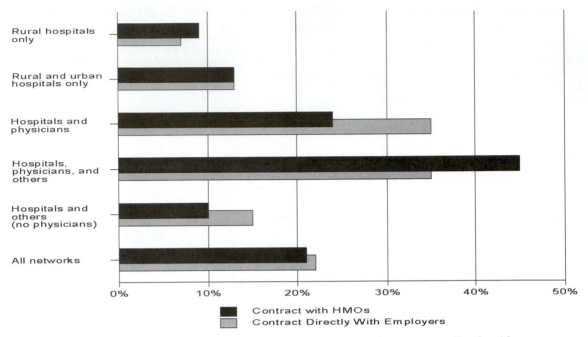

FIGURE 17-4 *Rural health networks that contract with HMOs or contract directly with employers, by network type.*

may be expected to contract with HMOs. More rural health networks also are likely to contract directly with employers and government programs to provide a range of services to covered enrollees to the extent they are permitted to do so by state insurance commissioners and Medicaid plans and by the Medicare program.

So few networks currently contract to provide services because the networks do not contain the range of services required by plans (for example, only four of ten rural health networks contain physicians) and because so few HMOs actually enroll rural residents. Expansions of Medicaid managed care programs under Section 1115 waivers and the Medicare risk program under the Balanced Budget Act of 1997 will likely encourage managed care development in rural areas.

If rural health networks are to be more useful to their members and the residents they serve, they will need to increase their integration of core activities and key support functions. Rural health networks need to develop the type of

coordination that will enable rural providers to thrive in a managed care environment. Many of the newer networks appear to be structurally prepared for integration in that they contain a variety of different kinds of provider members and include community representatives in network governance. Whether they will be able to transcend the barriers to integration remains to be seen.

LESSONS LEARNED FROM RECENT RURAL HEALTH NETWORK DEMONSTRATION PROGRAMS

During the past decade, a range of public and private programs have been implemented to support the development of rural health networks.[7] Some states—notably New York, West Virginia, and Florida—have implemented grant programs to support the development of rural health networks. The federal government has assisted and shaped rural health networks through the Essential Access Community Hospital (EACH) Program, the Medicare Rural Hospital Flexibility Program, and the Rural Network Development Grant Program of the Federal Office of Rural Health Policy. Private foundations also have provided resources for rural health network development, including efforts by the Robert Wood Johnson Foundation, the W. K. Kellogg Foundation, the Kansas Health Foundation, the Colorado Trust, the James Irvine Foundation, and the Claude Worthington Benedum Foundation. These grant programs have offered support to rural providers to develop collaborative solutions to their communities' health care problems.

We have had the opportunity to complete site visits to approximately 40 networks participating in the above initiatives. Although the site visits have not suggested the optimal path to assure success for rural health networks, they have provided some important insights into network development and operations. We believe the lessons presented here are central to the overall progress of rural health networks.

1.   Networks progress at their own speed. The formation and operation of rural health networks is an incremental process that requires a substantial amount of time. Rural health networks cannot be developed quickly and may require up to a decade to mature. Networks progress at their own speed. Network progress is influenced by many factors, including the quality of site leadership, the organization and commitment of local providers, the perception of environmental threats particularly as they relate to the regional managed care environment, the level and diversity of community involvement, and the historical relationships and current level of trust among the key participants at each site.

Service area definition also may influence network progress. Rural health networks frequently have designated the county as their service area for lack of a compelling reason for another choice. Caution should be used when selecting a larger service area that involves multiple counties because of the geopolitical issues

inevitably raised in such an endeavor as well as the practical limitations of meeting the needs of a diverse set of constituents. Defining a smaller service area at the subcounty level may seem conducive to the development of rural health networks. However, one needs carefully to consider the types of activities that are feasible with a limited population base and the level of trust among local health professionals before embarking on a subcounty project. Decisions on a relevant service area need to be based on more than just geopolitical boundaries. Other factors that should be considered include trade patterns, resource distribution, competition with and among communities, geographic barriers, and cultural barriers.

In sum, there are several reasons why networks develop and mature over extended periods of time. Rural health professionals, institutions, and policymakers need a long-term commitment to and investment strategy for networks if they want those networks to generate benefits for the rural populace.

2.   Integrated rural health networks need product lines that provide ongoing sources of revenue. The prestige associated with membership in a rural health network may diminish rather quickly if the network does not develop activities that provide benefits to its members and to the communities it serves. This is not a trivial point, as indicated by the difficulty that many networks have experienced in their search for a network mission that yields financial advantages for all members. Networks need to be able to differentiate their product lines from those of individual network members and also from those of other groups in which network members participate. Equally important, networks need to be able to develop new products that are clearly understood by providers, managers, and local communities.

At present, networks are more likely to be involved in the coordination of administrative functions (e.g., marketing, management information systems) and sharing of services provided by their members (e.g., health promotion) than in the direct provision and financing of health services. This may lead to identity problems for networks and confusion surrounding the issue of what the network does.

3.   Rural health networks are not well integrated. The rural physician group practice, rather than the rural hospital, may be the more appropriate foundation for network integration. Many of the networks we studied proved to be in the initial stages of development with regard to integration. Most of the sites have integrated some administrative functions (e.g., strategic planning, human resource administration), but few sites had made major strides toward integrating their members from either a financial or a clinical perspective. The reasons for the lack of progress along these dimensions include diverse network membership with different levels of stability and commitment, lack of organizational complexity and changing missions, inability to create a stable funding base for the network, and the nascent stage of information system development.

As networks develop and mature, an important issue will be what organization, or which individual, will provide the leadership for integration among network members. If the major purpose of network activity is service integration, the rural physician group practice, rather than the hospital, may be the key coordinating element. Networks need physician involvement to accomplish either clinical or financial integration. It is very difficult to stimulate strategies for the integration of health service delivery and financing if physicians are committed to maintaining the status quo. Physicians are essential to network efforts to improve quality and control costs.

Organization of the primary care medical community into a single group, independent practice association (IPA), or horizontal network can expedite integrated networking. Rural group practices are usually small and likely to be run as democracies. Typically less bureaucratic than hospitals, they have more flexible decision-making styles. However, most rural group practices do not yet have the sophisticated information systems now possessed by many rural hospitals. Rural physicians will need the support of hospitals or else may require more time to develop collaborative activities that lead to increased financial and clinical integration among rural health network members.

4.   The roles of external entities in network development vary and evolve over time. The value of participation of external entities should be measured by their effect on network accomplishments and the eventual transfer of control to local entities. The appropriate role for external entities (e.g., private foundations, consultants, government, nonlocal health care organizations) in developing rural health networks is not always obvious. Potential roles include educator, data collector and analyst, neutral convener, mutual arbitrator, provider of technical assistance, funding source for capital expenses, etc. These roles may change over time, with initial emphasis on community capacity building and later emphasis on technical consulting on specific projects. The benefits of the above roles may be large as long as local stakeholders are open to receiving support from nonlocal entities.

However, there are potential drawbacks to the use of external catalysts in motivating network development. External support for network development may allow network members to avoid making difficult choices between operating joint programs or maintaining autonomy. This may impede network maturation by delaying both the development of strong bonds of commitment between network members and the eventual local ownership of the networking process. Local entities need to define and accept meaningful roles for external entities that support their vision of an integrated delivery and financing system.

The issue of whether the benefits of network development and operations remain in rural communities is very important. Do community residents benefit from increased access to services, reduced costs, and enhanced quality of care? And do local health providers benefit from the stability created by increased use of their services and / or an enhanced ability to offer services relevant to the needs of community residents? The use of external catalysts may lead to a scenario in which the amount of resources allocated to network members expands due to the cooperative efforts of a nonlocal entity. The value of external catalysts' participation should be measured by their effect on network accomplishments (e.g., increased local retention of health expenditures, improved coordination of referrals, increased efficiencies due to shared staff, programs, or services).

5.   Although the recent popularity of rural health networks may have increased due to the anticipated expansion of managed care in rural areas, network members have little interest in increasing their financial risk. There is primary interest in developing services of the type provided by an administrative services organization (ASO) [e.g., claims administration, quality assurance/utilization management (QA/UM), credentialing, marketing, case management, information system linkages] that involve limited provider risk. Change is difficult to accomplish in many rural environments because of financial, technical, political, and leadership constraints; relative isolation and limited linkages to nonlocal entities; and the comfort associated with maintaining the status quo. The extent to which network development, supported by external expert facilitation and market-driven pressures, can provide leverage for changing the delivery and financing of health care in rural environments is not clear.

At this point in time, many of the networks that have interest in managed care activities are concentrating on developing ASO-type services (e.g., claims administration, QA/UM, credentialing, marketing, case management, information system linkages) that involve limited provider risk. Networks view this as a logical next step in their preparation for managed care and suggest that a successful ASO could be an important step toward the development of a locally based community health plan in the future.

The majority of rural health providers in networks do not feel the urgency of increasing their financial risk. They are, in many ways, still iso-lated from the constraints imposed by managed care. Consequently, they prefer to be involved with limited-risk managed care functions. In a similar vein, rural employers are interested in capping the financial risks associated with their employee health costs. They face constraints (e.g., union issues, multiple-site-employer issues, employee reluctance to change) in changing their health benefits packages or administration. This suggests that the implementation of managed care functions with greater financial risk by rural health networks may require a nonlocal partner as well as a well-designed plan for how risk will be shared among the key actors.

For those interested in ASO activities, financial feasibility analyses need to be completed. These analyses should view the ASO as a new business and examine issues such as the relevant scale of ASO activity, the potential volume of business based on service area population, and the required start-up and development costs. This information will help the key stakeholders to address the "make or buy" decision for ASO functions.

CONCLUSION

Rural health networks cannot address all of the challenges health professionals face in meeting local community needs. However, networks have the potential to maintain local access to health care services and support the implementation of managed care in rural areas. We make the following two recommendations to support rural health network development in the future:

• **Incorporate physicians into rural health networks to a greater degree than currently.** It is important for managed care contracting that physicians be part of a rural health network. Physicians are the primary provider group with which managed care organizations will want to contract. Managed care contracting may facilitate integration as network members strive to reduce duplication and improve efficiency. Physician participation in networks may be facilitated by organizing the physicians first, as with an independent practice association or a clinic without walls.

- **Increase community participation in rural health network planning and operations.** Community participation in rural health networks will help keep the focus of network activities on the community. Community members may also serve the network by mediating disputes between provider members, should they arise. Although community residents may be included in the planning and operations of networks by virtue of governing board seats, they may also contribute by participation in advisory committees and by the holding of board meetings that are open to the public.

REFERENCES

1. Casey M, Wellever A, Moscovice I: Rural health network development: public policy issues and state initiatives. *J Health Politics Policy Law* 22:23–47, 1997.
2. Rural Wisconsin Health Cooperative: RWHC Overview, http://www.rwhc.com, 1999.
3. Moscovice I, Wellever A, Krein S: *Rural Health Networks: Forms and Functions.* Minneapolis, MN, Rural Health Research Center, University of Minnesota, 1997.
4. Moscovice I, Christianson J, Johnson J, et al: *Building Rural Hospital Networks.* Ann Arbor, MI, Health Administration Press, 1995.
5. Morris R, Lescohier I: Service integration: real versus illusory solutions to welfare dilemmas, in Sari R, Hansenfeld Y (eds): *The Management of Human Resources.* New York, Columbia University Press, 1978.
6. Shortell S, Gillies R, Anderson D: The new world of managed care: creating organized delivery systems. *Health Affairs* 13:46–64, 1994.
7. Wellever A: Rural health networks, in T. Ricketts (ed): *Rural Health in the United States.* Oxford, England, Oxford University Press, 1999.

APPENDIX 1: NETWORK INTEGRATION SCALE

CALCULATION OF SCALE

For all networks with 20 or fewer members, we collected data on the number of members who participated in each of the 19 functions listed below. For each function, we calculated the percentage of network members who participate in the function. For each subgroup identified below, we calculated the average of the percentage participation scores. The functional integration scale is the average of the overall scores for human resources, accounting, planning and marketing, and management information systems. Integration scores range from 0 to 100. A score represents the percent of members who use, participate in, or contribute to a network function.

COMPONENTS OF INTEGRATION

1. Clinical Integration

- Use the same physician credentialing system
- Use the same quality measurement and improvement program
- Use the same clinical protocols developed or approved by network practitioners
- Use a system for sharing medical records among network members

2. Functional Integration

HUMAN RESOURCES
- Use the same personnel policy manual
- Use the same salary and wage system
- Use the same health professional recruitment program
- Use the same continuing education programs (e.g., for doctors and nurses)
- Use shared staff (e.g., nurses, physical therapists)

ACCOUNTING
- Use the same chart of accounts
- Use a consolidated network office for payroll and/or accounts payable
- Use a consolidated network office for patient billing and collections

- Use the same networkwide material management program

PLANNING AND MARKETING
- Use a consolidated network office for marketing and community relations
- Use a consolidated network office for planning

MANAGEMENT INFORMATION SYSTEMS
- Use the same networkwide management information system

3. Financial Integration
- Accept a portion of the risk of operating loss on network ventures
- Accept a portion of the risk of business failure on network ventures (i.e., responsible for paying creditors after business fails)
- Contribute capital to network ventures

APPENDIX 2: RESOURCES

Additional sources of information on rural health networks include:

- Rural Network Development Grant Program of the Federal Office of Rural Health Policy
    Contact: Jack Culp
    Office of Rural Health Policy
    Room 9A-55
    5600 Fishers Lane
    Rockville, MD 20857
    Phone: (301) 443-6894

- Networking for Rural Health, a project directed by the Alpha Center

Contact: Dan Campion
Alpha Center
1350 Connecticut Avenue, N.W.
Suite 1100
Washington, DC 20036
Phone: (202) 296-1818
Web site: www.ac.org

- Rural Information Center Health Service, a joint project of the Federal Office of Rural Health Policy and the National Agricultural Library
    Contact: Phone: 1-800-633-7701
    Web site: www.nal.usda.gov/ric/richs

CHAPTER 18

The Economics of Rural Practice

GEORGE E. WRIGHT

The hospital in Littletown, Mississippi (not its actual name), is the center for health care for two very low income rural counties that suffer from high rates of teenage pregnancy, low-birth-weight infants, and unmet pediatric needs. The service area has 20,000 people, and the nearest neighboring hospital is 45 miles away. The two senior physicians in town therefore recruited a pediatrician, who turned out to be capable and well liked by the community and her colleagues. But after 2 years, she reluctantly left town, unable to develop a financially viable practice. What went wrong? Building a full practice often takes 3 years, and salary guarantees did not last long enough. Young families are often the least able to pay and have the poorest insurance coverage. Medicaid paid poorly. Those families with insurance commuted long distances to work, and their health plans did not include local physicians. Finally, the three family physicians in town were reluctant to refer patients to the new pediatrician, particularly those with insurance coverage. The town needed a pediatrician but lacked the economic capacity to support one.

*T*his chapter is about the economic characteristics particular to rural practice. As the entire U.S. health system is being reorganized, are there factors that still differentiate the financial aspects of service delivery in nonmetropolitan settings? I will argue that this is indeed the case and that an enduring trend in the experience of hospitals, physicians, and other health providers is the economic pressure imposed by the very nature of the rural communities they seek to serve. Small markets, often with a restricted economic base, large fixed costs relative to a limited scale of operations, and systematic lower reimbursements combine to restrict rural income opportunities relative to urban practices. As illustrated in the actual example above, all too frequently these factors combine to undermine the economic viability of practices in just those communities most at risk of underservice. The issues presented are thus relevant to both individual practitioners and broader public policy concerns.

Although all health professionals confront the issues raised in this chapter, our discussion focuses on rural primary care physicians—a profession for which data and previous analyses exist. Given the wide spectrum of possible economic issues, the chapter is oriented around a single central theme: Why do rural physicians tend to earn less than their urban colleagues for comparable full-time practices? Answering that question will take the reader on a wide excursion into rural living standards, insurance coverage, third-party rate setting policies, and the level of competition. After reviewing these pressures, the chapter concludes with a discussion of the winds of change being introduced by managed care and the development of provider networks.

TRENDS IN RURAL PHYSICIAN INCOME

On average, physicians in nonmetropolitan areas have net practice incomes approximately 25 percent below those of their urban colleagues. Moreover, this $40,000 income differential has been increasing during the last 10 years.[1] However, this crude comparison ignores the differing mix of specialties; indeed, virtually all of the overall income gap is due to the comparative predominance of primary care physicians in nonmetropolitan areas. To illustrate this point, Table 18-1 controls for differences in specialty mix by summarizing a decade of change in the net practice incomes for the combined specialties of family medicine and general practice. The data are drawn from the American Medical Association's annual surveys, and the urban-rural categorization is according to the common official definition of Metropolitan Statistical Areas (MSAs). A central conclusion is that there appears to be little significant difference between rural areas and large metropolitan areas in either the level or growth of pretax income net of practice expenses (unadjusted for inflation).

When we look in more detail at these numbers, it is clear that rural family physicians (FPs) and remaining general practitioners (GPs) have to work harder for their income than their urban colleagues. In 1986, rural FPs worked 16 percent more hours than those in large MSAs. Over the next 10 years, while the average work week of rural FPs increased by 5 percent, that for urban FPs actually fell, expanding the work-hour differential to 24 percent. Rural FPs not only work longer hours but also report a consistent pattern of seeing more patients per hour and making three times as many hospital visits per week.

Compared to family physicians in large met-

TABLE 18-1   CHANGES IN REAL INCOME OF FAMILY PHYSICIANS IN URBAN AND RURAL AREAS, 1986–1996

Income Factor	1986	1996	Percent Change
Mean income per week			
Non-MSA[a]	$1,538	$2,496	62.3%
Large MSA	$1,456	$2,517	72.9%
Patient care hours per week			
Non-MSA	57.5	60.6	5.4%
Large MSA	49.5	48.9	−1.2%
Mean fee for follow-up visit			
Non-MSA	$19.30	$41.52	115.1%
Large MSA	$27.70	$50.93	83.9%
Visits per office hour			
Non-MSA	3.26	3.23	−1.2%
Large MSA	3.07	2.98	−3.0%
Hospital visits per week			
Non-MSA	22.3	14.5	−35.0%
Large MSA	14.0	5.6	−60.0%
Real income per hour			
Non-MSA	$26.76	$29.08	8.7%
Large MSA	$29.41	$36.34	23.6%

[a]Non-MSAs are rural areas excluded from the Bureau of Census definition of Metropolitan Statistical Areas. Large MSAs are those with more than 1 million population.

SOURCE: American Medical Association: *Socioeconomic Characteristics of Medical Practice.* Chicago, AMA, 1996 and previous annual editions.

ropolitan areas, whose inflation-adjusted income per hour increased by 23.6 percent, that of rural FPs increased by less than 9 percent over the period of a decade (see the last row of Table 18-1). This is clearly not the pattern of financial incentives appropriate to attracting more physicians to underserved rural communities. By 1995, rural family physicians earned $29 an hour, 25 percent less than the $36 an hour averaged by their counterparts in large MSAs.

An obvious question is the degree to which lower living costs in nonmetropolitan areas compensate for gaps in nominal take home pay. Although housing costs are typically lower, other expenses such as food, energy, and many consumer goods are higher, and others (e.g., travel, professional expenses, books) tend not to vary geographically. As a result, the urban-rural cost-of-living differential may not be as large as commonly supposed. According to one commercial source of geographic differences in cost-of-living estimates, the average cost of living for 30 small cities with less than 55,000 residents was only 3.3 percent below the national average, a small proportion of the income per hour differential illustrated at the bottom of Table 18-1.[2]

To compound the problem, national averages mask significant variations within the grand diversity of rural America. For example, the net income of all family physicians in the Mountain States averages over 20 percent less than that reported in the South.[3] Large variations exist even within rural areas of a single state. According to a 1997 survey from Washington State, the highest-earning quartile of full-time rural family physicians averaged twice the annual net income of the lowest-earning quartile.[4]

DOES PHYSICIAN INCOME MATTER?

How important are systematic rural income gaps for physicians and public policy? Although the case of the Mississippi pediatrician is perhaps extreme, systematic income deficits exacerbate any disadvantages a small rural commu-

nity faces in attracting and retaining primary care physicians. More to the point, the evidence shows that income does appear to matter to physicians. For example, a widely quoted study of the retention of physicians locating in low-income and isolated rural towns found poor income to be one of the primary factors associated with elevated exit rates.[5] Physicians leaving a practice location after less than 4 years on site had incomes substantially below those choosing to remain. In general, although current or potential income is seldom explicitly mentioned in surveys of medical students or physicians as a key consideration in career decisions, a long series of empirical studies has demonstrated the link between income incentives and specialty and location choices.[6] More importantly, physician income stands out as a factor that can be substantially affected by public policy. Compared to structural issues—such as lack of community amenities, challenging practice conditions, or unavailable spousal employment opportunities—government policy can enhance reimbursement rates, subsidize income through loan repayment, or offer location inducements. For individual physicians, understanding the forces that shape rural income potentials are important for evaluating alternative practice settings and developing strategies to strengthen rural practices.

WHY ARE RURAL PRACTICE INCOMES LOWER?

The question before us then is: Why? Why do we see persistent and apparently increasing earnings gaps associated with rural practice? The following sections examine four factors—the restricted income base of many rural communities, poor health insurance coverage of rural residents, a tradition of reduced reimbursement rates for nonmetropolitan areas, and spatial competition with other locations over market share.

TABLE 18-2   SUMMARY OF CHANGES IN CHARACTERISTICS OF METROPOLITAN AND NONMETROPOLITAN COUNTIES, 1980–1997

Socioeconomic Characteristics	Metropolitan Counties	Nonmetropolitan Counties	Ratio of Nonmetro/ Metro Counties
Population Characteristics			
Population Growth			
1980–90	12.7%	3.0%	0.236
1990–97	7.8%	6.6%	0.846
Net migration rate[a]			
1980–90	3.8%	−2.8%	0.132[b]
1990–97	2.1%	4.0%	1.905
Growth of population >65			
1980–90	10.3%	15.2%	1.475
1990–97	11.1%	5.4%	0.486
Income Characteristics			
Percent below poverty			
1980–90	12.2%	18.3%	1.500
1990–97	13.2%	15.9%	1.204
Per capita income[c]			
1989	$24,151	$17,091	0.708
1996	$25,944	$18,527	0.714
Per capita income growth			
1980–90			
1989–96	7.4%	8.4%	1.135

[a]Net migration rate equals the percent of the population lost or gained through migration.

[b]For negative percentage change, the ratio of Nonmetro to Metro counties is approximated by scaling the difference to a rural rate of 1.0% (e.g., −2.8/3.8 = 1/7.6 = 0.132).

[c]Income per capita adjusted to constant 1996 prices.

SOURCE: US Department of Agriculture, Economic Research Service: *Rural Conditions and Trends.* 8(2), 1999 and previous annual editions.

Fundamentals of Financially Viable Practices—Population and Economic Base

An obvious first place to look for an explanation of lower real incomes for rural physicians is the nature of the market they serve. Small, isolated communities with low incomes, high unemployment, and poor insurance coverage will have a limited pool of patients able to pay according to established fee schedules. Table 18-2 illustrates some of the key changes in the profile of rural versus urban America. In sum, rural households have, on average, lower incomes and higher poverty rates. But rural-urban differentials in the growth of income and population have witnessed a remarkable series of turnarounds, with a wave of growth followed by collapse followed once more by rapid progress. Rural population—after decades of falling because of long-term changes in labor requirements for farming and minerals extraction—rebounded during the 1970s, when there was a net migration from urban back to rural communities. This positive trend was reversed in the 1980s, owing in large measure to an extended rural recession. The population growth, at only 3 percent over 10 years, was only one-fourth that of metropolitan counties and reflected a strong outmigration (negative values denote net outmigration) from rural areas.

Table 18-2 also illustrates a subsequent remarkable turnaround back to the positive trends of the 1970s. In the 1990s, net migration into rural communities shifts from negative to positive, and at 4.0 percent is now twice the rate for MSAs. In other words, we are now witnessing a net population flow from urban to rural areas. Nevertheless, the total population growth of 6.6 percent still lags slightly behind that of urban areas. Although this turnabout in population growth is most pronounced in those rural counties adjacent to large MSAs, fully 75 percent of all rural counties now have growing populations—quite a turnaround from the previous decade, where the majority of counties lost population.[7]

This new dynamic trend has been accompanied by a shifting trend in age composition. Rural communities have for the last half century been home to a steadily increasing above-average proportion of elderly—20 percent were over 65, compared to an urban elderly proportion of 15 percent by 1990. Since then, however, the rate of growth of those over age 65 has dropped to one-third that of the previous decade. In contrast to the stereotype of graying farming communities abandoned by younger families in search of jobs, the proportion of rural Americans over age 65 is actually dropping, and the phenomenon is shared across a broad majority of counties.[8] This important development should not mask the fact that many rural communities still have high proportions of elderly, and thus their physicians are unusually dependent on the whims of Medicare payment policy. In Minnesota, for example, the proportion of people over age 65 in farming counties such as Lincoln or Cottonwood is double that of Minneapolis (22.6 compared to 11.3 percent). Starting in 2010, both rural and urban areas are projected to witness a pronounced growth in the proportion of the aged.[9] In sum, despite a legacy of exodus and continuing pockets of stagnation, overall population trends at the beginning of the new millennium do not systematically work against the vitality of rural practice.

Accompanying its rebounding population, rural America has also witnessed a general economic resurgence. During the 1980s, per capita income expanded at only two-thirds the rate of MSAs, so that by 1989, MSAs had per capita incomes over 40 percent greater than those generated in rural areas (incomes unadjusted for geographic cost-of-living differences and figures not shown in Table 18-2). However, during the economic expansion in the 1990s, rural per capita income expanded even faster than that of urban areas—and, in contrast to large cities, the proportion of inhabitants below the poverty line decreased. In sum, the change in relative population and average income growth is a pronounced turnaround in the trend of total purchasing power (the product of population and per capita income) in rural America. Whereas in the 1980s total income for rural areas grew only 3.4 percent, compared to 24.4 percent in MSAs, rural incomes expanded at the urban rate during the following decade.

Although this trend strengthens the economic base underlying rural practice, the improvement has occurred from a disadvantaged baseline. The rural-urban per capita income differential is still 40 percent; rural poverty rates are still above the urban average. Moreover, the rebound of the 1990s is fragile, and the positive trends illustrated in Table 18-2 were, at the turn of the century, slowing down. The worldwide general deflationary trend in raw material prices has lowered real incomes in farming, mining, and forestry. Economic crises in Asia and elsewhere have eroded export demand for rural products. Almost as many rural counties are dependent on manufacturing as on farming, and international competition has hit many of these areas hard. In sum, the majority of rural communities have witnessed an economic upturn, but one that is now under increasing stress. Long-term projections forecast a return to the pattern of income growth whereby rural residents lag behind their urban compatriots.[9]

Problems with Insurance Coverage

Even when rural families have the same income as urban residents, they are more likely to lack adequate health insurance. According to the 1996 National Medical Expenditure Survey, rural residents were more than one-quarter more likely to be uninsured (23.0 percent uninsured compared to 18.3 percent for MSA residents).[10] Within nonmetropolitan areas, those residents living outside of larger towns were notably more likely to depend on out-of-pocket payment rather than health insurance.[11] Although most rural communities are not as poor as the area served by the Mississippi pediatrician described at the opening of this chapter, the large and growing gaps in insurance coverage are a common phenomenon.

Why is this? The answer appears to involve the dependence of rural economies on small businesses. Nationwide, less than half of firms with less than 10 employees offer health insurance and one-quarter of the employees in such firms offering a plan decline enrollment.[12] When individuals are interviewed, virtually all of the urban-rural gap in employer-based insurance coverage can be explained by the disproportionate share of such small business in most rural employment.[13] To make matters more difficult for rural providers, rural small businesses are significantly less likely to offer health insurance as a benefit to their employees than firms of similar size in large MSAs.[14] Newly available data indicate that these problems are becoming worse. The percentage of employers offering health insurance in small firms is falling, the proportion of employees enrolling is eroding, and the plans they do enroll in have ever more restrictive coverage, higher deductibles, and increased copays.[15]

Accompanying the structural problems is the fact that many rural areas' experience with employer-based insurance has been a collapse in more and more states of its major alternative—the individual health insurance market. For self-employed farmers and others without employer-based coverage, the alternative of an individual policy is increasingly unaffordable or even unavailable.[16] Although this is a nationwide problem, the burden falls heavily on farming-oriented communities, where for too many residents the only affordable coverage has such high copays and deductibles that it basically constitutes a catastrophic policy (i.e., relevant primarily for high-cost episodes involving a hospitalization). In such circumstances physicians are for all practical purposes caring for patients making 100 percent out-of-pocket payments.

Exacerbating these structural problems with employment-based and individual health insurance, state Medicaid programs exclude higher proportions of rural than of urban low-income families because the former are more likely to be the working poor—employed, but in low-wage jobs generating incomes at or below the poverty line. Moreover, predominantly rural states tend to impose more stringent eligibility standards.[17] In addition to higher rates of uninsurance at any point in time, recent research has found that the median number of months without health insurance was three times longer among rural than among urban residents.[18] Nonexistent or inadequate health insurance both lowers patients' ability to pay and places a greater demand on office-based physicians for charity care. For example, rural family physicians in Washington State reported 25 percent more hours a week devoted to uncompensated care than their urban colleagues.[19]

Discounting Rural Fees

The lower incomes and higher rates of uninsurance typical of many rural communities undergird perhaps the principal cause of the lower real incomes of rural providers—lower fees. Compared to their urban colleagues, rural physicians have tended to ask for notably lower fees. Third-party payers traditionally offered a percentage of physicians' "usual and customary" fees, thereby locking a rural discount into payment policy. The resulting vicious cycle has affected all types of rural providers: lower fees meant lower incomes, which meant lower pay for assistants and less resources for equipment and office space. With the advent of cost-based prospective payment, the traditional lower costs froze the cycle into place, with low costs begetting low reimbursements, which in turn beget low costs.

The most notable examples of this phenomenon have been Medicare payment policies for HMOs and for rural hospitals, in particular the geographic differentials in the diagnosis-related group (DRG) prospective payment system. Capitation rates for Medicare HMOs are set as a discount from the average cost of treating all residents in each county in the United States. Since the average cost to Medicare for its rural beneficiaries is 15 percent less than that for urban areas, the HMO capitation rates are set commensurably lower.[20] Widely criticized as inequitable and responsible for the slow rural expansion of Medicare HMOs, a minimum payment was introduced in 1997, with no discernible effect on HMO expansion into rural areas.[21,22]

Medicare's inpatient hospital payment system was introduced in 1983 offering a flat rate for all patients within a particular diagnostic category. However, the payments were subject to two geographic adjusters: an area wage index, which shifted payments downward for areas with low average hospital wages, and a separate (lower) base rate for rural hospitals to capture other sources of lower costs. A long "antidiscrimination" campaign by rural advocates led to the removal of the lower rural base rate and the ability of rural hospitals to have their wage adjustment raised to that prevailing in nearby metropolitan areas. However, the basic downward wage adjustment remains in place for most hospitals, is widely viewed as flawed, but has nevertheless been applied to Medicare outpatient department payments as of the year 2000.[23]

Physician payments are influenced by the same lower-cost-requires-lower-reimbursement cycle. During the early 1990s Medicare phased in a shift from paying on the basis of "usual and customary" fees to a national, standardized resource-based relative value scale (RBRVS). Since the new methodology set out to increase the valuation of primary care services relative to surgical and diagnostic procedures, it promised an advantage to rural practice both by favoring primary care and shifting away from the urban bias of traditional fee schedules. In practice, the RBRVS has offered advantages, but modest ones. Table 18-3 summarizes the annual changes in Medicare physician payments for 2 years, 1991–92 and 1994–95. The first two columns show rates of change in average Medicare payment per service—a coefficient analogous to a change in average physician fees. Nationwide, the new system reduced payments per unit of service, with urban physicians earning 1.8 percent less and rural physicians gaining 2.2 percent more per billed service. As the system evolved, this initial rural advantage has been generally maintained, with physicians in the smallest places (those more likely to focus on primary care services) benefiting the most. An important characteristic of the system is its lack of stability over time. Payment rate increases and their differential effects among specialties and geographic areas shift substantially. Analyses are not yet available on the effect of the marked decreases in payment rates at the end of the 1990s.

Not shown in Table 18-3 is the fact that the 1994–95 increase in average payment rates of 6 percent for physicians in lightly populated counties lagged behind an overall 9 percent increase for primary care services. One reason for this reduced rural effect is an adjustment similar to the wage index for hospitals. Using an index of physician practice costs, physicians in high-cost areas have their payment rates increased, while the rates of those in low-cost areas are reduced. In practice, this is a highly unstandardized web of adjustments that differs markedly across states. In some, all physicians are subject to a common adjustment; in others, markedly different practice cost calculations are applied to different areas. Table 18-4 illustrates the degree to which the Medicare program uses these adjustments to discount rural doctors' payments. The coefficients compare physicians' practice costs to the national average. Thus physicians in California's large metropolitan areas have estimated costs 6.9 percent above the na-

TABLE 18-3   CHANGES IN THE RATE OF GROWTH OF MEDICARE PHYSICIAN PAYMENTS

Geographic Area	Medicare Payment per Service[a]		Service Volume per Physician		Total Medicare Revenue per Physician[b]	
	1991–92	1994–95	1991–92	1994–95	1991–92	1994–95
National average	−0.9%	3.8%	3.0%	4.1%	2.0%	8.0%
Metropolitan	−1.8	3.6	3.8	3.9	2.0	7.7
Rural counties	2.2	5.2	2.2	6.0	2.2	11.4
>25,000		4.8		7.1		12.2
<25,000		6.0		1.4		8.1

[a]Payment per service is the net effect of several payment policy decisions, including the shift from usual and customary fees to the prospective payment fee schedule, changes in the relative value of different services in the fee schedule, the annual increase in the base payment rate, and the geographic adjustments for differences in practice costs.

[b]The increase in total Medicare revenue per physician is the net result of changes in the payment rates per service (column 1) and the number of services per physician (column 2). It is measured as allowed charges, which includes patient deductibles and copayments not in excess of charge limits.

SOURCE: Physician Payment Review Commission: *Annual Report to Congress 1995*, table 2.2, and *Annual Report to Congress 1996*, table 9.1.

TABLE 18-4   MEDICARE ADJUSTMENTS FOR GEOGRAPHIC DIFFERENCES IN PHYSICIAN PRACTICE COSTS BY METROPOLITAN AND RURAL AREAS WITHIN SELECTED STATES (U.S. AVERAGE = 1.000[a])

State	Metropolitan Areas, 1–3 million	Nonmetropolitan Areas	Percent Nonmetro Discount[b]
California	1.068	0.956	−10.6%
Florida	1.053	0.955	−9.3
Georgia	1.010	0.912	−9.7
Illinois	0.986	0.889	−9.8
Kansas	0.982	0.896	−8.8
Louisiana	0.977	0.893	−8.6
Maryland	1.032	0.960	−7.0
Massachusetts	1.084[c]	1.012	−6.6
Michigan	1.137[c]	0.975	−14.2
Missouri	0.984	0.891	−9.4
New York	1.116	0.952	−14.7
Pennsylvania	0.963	0.918	−4.7
Texas	0.978	0.895	−8.5
Virginia	0.951	0.900	−5.4

[a]All values set relative to the national average practice cost, which hence has a value of 1.0.

[b]The discounts are not the actual ones generated by the current payment system but simulations by Health Economics Research Inc. using a standardized definition of payment areas recommended by the commission. For states not included, the commission recommends a single statewide area for calculating practice costs.

[c]Values for metropolitan areas above 3 million population since the state had none in the 1 to 3 million range.

SOURCE: Physician Payment Review Commission: *Annual Report to Congress 1996*, table 9.5.

tional average, and those practicing in its rural areas run 4 percent below (1.0 less 0.956). The within-state rural discounts calculated in the last column of Table 18-4 tend to run in the 9 percent range. The accuracy of the practice cost discounts has been widely questioned. For example, among rural physicians, those in Illinois receive 10 percent less in Medicare payments than those in Michigan because of their differential in practice cost index scores (the percentage difference between 0.975 and 0.889).

A focus on Medicare payment policy is relevant because of its dominant role in many rural practices and because other payers tend to copy Medicare's innovations. Medicaid, Blue Cross, and managed care entities are all using the RBRVS fee schedule. It is to the advantage of rural physicians that these other payers tend to find the practice cost adjustment too complex and apply a single fee schedule to all physicians within a state. We conclude this section by noting that Congress has introduced enhanced Medicare reimbursements for rural physicians located in a designated Health Professions Shortage Area (HPSA). The "HPSA Bonus" program offers a 10 percent add-on to the fees for such practices. As applied to rural areas, this bonus, which has been sharply criticized as an ineffective subsidy, appears in many cases to merely counterbalance the discounts affected by the Medicare Practice Cost adjustments.[24]

The Medicare incentive payments for HPSA physicians is one of several federal financial incentive programs designed to compensate for less desirable locations and the lack of adequate population and income bases. Hidden in the extreme diversity of rural communities are numerous stagnant, isolated, and/or impoverished communities with poor access to care and limited ability to adequately support private sector health care. These continue to present a fundamental challenge to health policy. To give but one example, there are 333 nonmetropolitan counties where one-third or more of the population are either African Americans, Native Americans, or Hispanics.[25] Most of these counties have been for decades among the poorest in America. Combining this with Appalachian mining towns, logged-out timber communities, failed manufacturing sites, and former transportation centers, we face an entrenched catalogue of high-need communities that remain persistently "underdoctored." However, such communities are not the rural norm. The U.S. Public Health Service estimates that strategically relocating only 2300 physicians would fill all the gaps in designated rural primary care shortage areas.[26] The issues for most rural physicians are thus less dramatic. Indeed, rather than shortages, many rural physicians find themselves in distinctly competitive situations—a topic to which we now turn.

Workloads and the Competition for Patients

Although we have previously documented the expanded workload of most rural physicians, the stereotype of the overworked rural physician laboring without respite defies the substantial variation in experience. For example, among rural family physicians in Washington State under age 65 and with an active clinical practice, 25 percent reported hours in excess of 50 per week. However, another 25 percent worked less than 36 hours.[4] Thus, although some rural physicians have difficulty coping with the demands for care, others increasingly find themselves concerned with the loss of patients to competition from dominant urban or rural commercial and referral centers. The case of the Mississippi pediatrician presented at the opening of this chapter vividly illustrates the phenomenon of competition even in very underserved areas.

The national data on Medicare workloads presented in Table 18-3 suggest a possible important split between physicians working in small rural counties with less than 25,000 population and those in larger rural counties. The service volume per physician in larger places increased far faster than the national average (7.1 versus 4.1 percent annual increases, respectively), while the growth experienced in small counties was only 1.4 percent. This low number is consistent with two contradictory hypotheses: (1) overworked physicians whose already filled practices cannot be further expanded or (2) small-town physicians struggling with declining market share. Whichever the case, the low rate of growth in volume per physician means that despite the relative improvements in Medicare fees, the share of small-town physicians in Medicare physician payments is not increasing. (That is, the rate of increase in total Medicare payments per physician in counties under 25,000 is no greater than the national average.)

Although hard data are lacking, rural physicians report that they are increasingly caught up in the dominant paradigm of American health care—competition. In rural settings, the small scale and distances among towns make competition among providers obvious and personal. Although the competitive reach of rural commercial centers or more distant cities is increasing, primary care physicians, as opposed to those in specialty care, are insulated by the reluctance of patients to travel extensively for primary services—a core fact that leaves physicians in geographically isolated towns with substantial shares of the market. However, this advantage depends on a host of factors, including the town's population, its vitality as a commercial center, and distances to alternative sources of care. Thus the share for physicians is less than 50 percent for places in the 2000-to-3000 range. Surprisingly, primary care physicians in the smallest rural places with under 2000 inhabitants have larger market shares than physicians in larger rural places. This phenomenon is perhaps related to the self-selective and unusual nature of small places that are able to attract and retain physicians.

The pull of competing towns, particularly from larger rural centers or metropolitan areas, can substantially lower the expected share for a community physician. For example, Table 18-5 compares the market shares for communities that are adjacent and nonadjacent to a metropolitan area. In all size categories save one, the market share of the local primary care physi-

TABLE 18-5   MARKET SHARE FOR RURAL PRIMARY CARE PHYSICIANS OF VISITS BY MEDICARE PATIENTS: WASHINGTON STATE, 1994 (STANDARD DEVIATION)[a]

Town Population Size	Market Share to Primary Care[b]	
	Nonadjacent to Urban Area	Adjacent to Urban Area
10,000+	78.9%	72.8%
	(21.5)	(32.0)
5000–10,000	59.0	50.3
	(15.4)	(20.3)
3000–5000	50.1	59.9
	(28.8)	(17.7)
2000–3000	48.9	42.1
	(35.2)	(28.5)
1000–2000	60.1	52.4
	(21.3)	(23.7)
Less than 1000	53.9	43.6
	(28.8)	(28.4)

[a]Rural towns were classified as adjacent or nonadjacent to urban areas according to their health service areas as defined by the Washington State Health Department.

[b]Market share is based on all visits by Medicare beneficiaries in an area to primary care physicians.

SOURCE: Unpublished tabulations by the author drawn from all Medicare Part B physician claims for calendar year 1994 for all beneficiaries over 65 living in Washington and receiving all of their care from physicians within the state.

cian is reduced for places overshadowed by urban concentrations. Does this mean that when local physicians lose patients, they are competing with urban areas? Recent work with the same Medicare data for Washington State by Hart and colleagues track the different geographic sources of physician visits.[27] For small towns not adjacent to metropolitan areas, the primary competition is not from urban but rather from other rural providers. For such places, 49 percent of patient visits to primary care physicians leave the local market; 17 percent are shifted to urban physicians, 21 percent to larger rural places with over 100 hospital beds, and 11 percent to other small towns.

A key point in this analysis is that Medicare data overstate the local market share. That is, elderly patients are known to be much less willing to travel long distances. Indeed, it is not uncommon for small rural hospitals to serve almost exclusively geriatric populations, while younger residents drive past local providers to distant towns. Part of the difficulty is on the demand side—a local perception of quality and the advantages of specialists over primary care practitioners. Part is also due to supplier characteristics, in particular the unwillingness or inability of local family physicians to offer quality obstetric and prenatal care. Nevertheless, a central fact facing most rural practitioners is that the rapidly expanding and increasingly dominant commercial and referral centers will pose ever greater competitive challenges. As the following concluding discussion illustrates, the nature of these challenges is still evolving.

WINDS OF CHANGE—RURAL MANAGED CARE AND NETWORKS

The dominant paradigm of rural practice—solo or small group practices paid by fee for service—is clearly changing, but at a much slower rate than in urban areas. Although prepaid health care in the United States was originally a rural concept (the first HMO was started for Oklahoma farmers in 1929), rural providers have viewed the steady expansion of managed care with considerable misgiving. However, perceptions of the rural impact of managed care have changed with experience. In 1990, only 11 managed care organizations (MCOs) were rural-based, and less than half of urban-based plans even included a nonmetropolitan county in their declared service areas.[28,29] Responding to the prospect of a universal system of competitive managed care, a 1993 consensus conference in Little Rock, Arkansas, concluded that physicians and hospitals in remote or low-income rural areas were likely to be overwhelmed by massive urban-centered organizations and recommended that only "collar" counties immediately adjacent to MSAs be fully opened to reorganization by MCOs.[30] Subsequent experience

has shown the opposite to be true: managed care has found it expensive to organize and operate in small towns and their surrounding, lightly populated hinterlands. Although by 1997 over three-quarters of MCOs included a rural county in their service areas, the effects on physician practice have largely been limited to the MSA collar counties.

Difficulties MCOs face in more remote areas include the following: (1) absent large employers, the cost of marketing a health plan to numerous small businesses is high; (2) absent existing large provider networks, the cost of individually organizing numerous small-scale providers and introducing uniform statistical reporting is substantial; (3) absent a large health workforce, plans have limited choices in negotiating partners; and (4) absent a large initial enrollment, health plans are in a weak bargaining position with physicians and hospitals. In short, beyond the ring of counties surrounding MSAs, "health plans need physicians more than physicians need the health plans."[31] The reality of these constraints has recently been illustrated by the fate of the publicly mandated managed care purchased by Medicare, Medicaid, and state-funded safety-net plans. The pressure of falling capitation rates has occasioned a disproportionate exodus of plans from rural counties.

In this environment, the introduction of managed care has occasioned to date few major changes in the finances and operations of many rural practitioners. Managed care is delivered through contracts with loosely organized independent practice associations (IPAs), where member physicians are generally reimbursed according to a discounted fee schedule. In most cases, practitioners are asked to bear little risk; the proportion withheld for incentives and contingencies is limited and largely returned. Although there is a potential for intrusive utilization controls and disruption of established referral networks, the limited evidence to date from case studies and small surveys suggests that such developments are more the exception than the rule for more remote rural providers. A less benign experience may await providers in close-in collar counties, but evidence is so far lacking.

As always in describing rural America, generalizations mask an enormous diversity of experience with MCOs. For example, physicians serving communities with a single dominant employer are vulnerable to abrupt shifts in health plans and conditions of participation that they are powerless to influence. Moreover, the growth of managed care has spawned an even more pervasive development with a strong negative potential—highly competitive rural networks that pit physicians against each other and their local hospitals.

Although some MCOs are organizing their own provider networks, the fact that managed care entities prefer to work with established groupings places a premium on the development of integrated networks—the broader the geographic coverage of networks independent of any one MCO, the stronger the position in negotiating with third-party insurers. Moreover, a network based on a core of specialty care providers benefits from a far-flung stable of primary care physicians who will provide referrals.

There are a bewildering variety of ways in which expanding urban and rural-based physician networks are organized. For example, equity-based entities ask physicians to become partners in exchange for a share in future earnings. Physician-hospital organizations (PHOs) are hospital-based but can consist of open or closed membership and be centralized or decentralized.[32-34] Highly centralized versions of integrated networks may directly purchase rural primary care practices. In the latter phenomenon, physicians may find selling out highly advantageous, particularly given the uncertainty over the future value of small independent practices. The selling physician may be offered a guaranteed income substantially larger than current net income, an infusion of capital, better access to specialists, locum tenens coverage, and assistance with billing and practice management.

The question of why it would pay a network to guarantee a practice more than its current net income is addressed in Table 18-6, which uses survey data to illustrate the relationship between the income of a primary care practice for 2000 patients and their total health expenditures. Although the practice nets $112,000 after expenses, total billings from all sources of care have an expected value of over $3 million. A small-town physician indeed sits on a valuable franchise! The gross revenue from specialty physician referrals alone is estimated to be

TABLE 18-6   ILLUSTRATION OF A POTENTIAL VALUE OF A RURAL PRIMARY CARE PRACTICE SERVING A TOWN OF 2000 TO A MULTISPECIALTY NETWORK

Medical Expenditure Category	Estimated Spending Per Capita	Total Value for Population = 2000
Total medical expenditures per person, 1997	$2,375	$3,130,000
Total MD office visits, expenditures per person	444	928,000
Share of rural primary care physicians (@ 45%)	209	417,600
Market share of local primary care physician (@ 80%)	167	334,000
Less practice costs (including insurance and taxes totaling 2/3 gross income)	111	222,000
Net primary care physician income	56	112,000
Gross value of potential specialty referrals	235	470,000

SOURCES: Estimates by the author based on analysis of the National Medical Expenditure Survey updated to 1997 prices; 1994 Part B Medicare physician claims for Washington State; American Medical Association, Socioeconomic Characteristics of Medical Practice, 1997; and an unpublished survey for the Washington Academy of Family Physicians by LG Hart, 1998.

worth $470,000. For a multispecialty network or HMO, even a small increased share of the total through redirected referrals could be well worth underwriting a loss on the primary care practice.

Unfortunately, expanding networks can undermine the often fragile structure of a local community's health care—precisely the outcome feared by the Little Rock conference on rural managed care mentioned earlier. In adversarial situations where an external network has the single goal of enrolling physicians to support a centralized specialty hub, admissions are diverted from the local hospital, laboratory tests that were a traditional mainstay of the local hospital are shifted to newly equipped physicians' offices, previously hospital-based ambulatory procedures are conducted in distant or mobile specialty centers, and local home health agencies are confronted with a competitive network-supported agency. In such situations, expanding the scope of services comes at the expense of the economic viability of local hospitals and related facilities. Although such a trade-off may be a net benefit to the community, the restructuring is driven by the economic interests of some actors without wider public accountability.

The threat of external control of physician practices has led some local rural hospitals to purchase physician practices themselves. However, this has tended to prove financially disadvantageous, since new hospital admissions were not generated and the productivity of the now-salaried physicians often declined. Moreover, the decline of rural managed care has removed the financial advantages for highly integrated networks. By the end of the 1990s the practice of purchasing physician practices had declined.

The limited expansion of managed care into rural areas has to date spawned only occasional examples of destructive agglomerating networks, and strategies are available whereby physicians can work with local hospitals and their communities to direct the forces of change to mutual advantage.[35,36] Since the ultimate well-being of rural practice depends on a strong web of health facilities and providers, a major challenge for the future is managing the evolving reorganization of physician practices to both benefit physicians and maintain the long-term vitality of rural health systems.

REFERENCES

1. AMA: *Socioeconomic Characteristics of Medical Practice 1997*. Chicago, American Medical Association Center for Health Policy Research, 1997.
2. Economic Research Institute: *The 1997 Geographic Reference Report*, 11th ed. Redmond, WA, Economic Research Institute, 1997.
3. AMA: *Socioeconomic Characteristics of Medical Practice 1997*. Chicago, American Medical Association Center for Health Policy Research, 1997, table 43.
4. Hart LG: Unpublished results, Washington Academy of Family Physicians 1996–97 survey of family physicians. Seattle, WA, Department of Family Practice, March 1998.
5. Pathman DE, Konrad TR, Ricketts TC: The comparative retention of National Health Service Corps and other rural physicians: results of a nine-year follow-up study. *JAMA* 268(12):1552–1558, 1992.
6. Rizzo JA, Blumenthal D: Physician labor supply: do income effects matter? *J Health Econ* 13:433–453, 1994.
7. Bowers D, Hamrick K, eds: *Rural Conditions and Trends*. Socioeconomic conditions issue, 8(12). Washington, DC, Department of Agriculture, Food and Rural Economics Division, October 1997.
8. Personal communication, Calvin Beale, US Census Bureau.
9. Braschler C, Nelson G, Van der Sluis E: *1995 RUPRI Rural Baseline*. Report P95-1. Columbia, MO, Rural Policy Research Institute, April 1995.
10. *Health Insurance Status of the Civilian Noninstitutionalized Population: 1996*. MEPS research findings no. 1. AHCPR publication no. 97-0030. Rockville, MD, Agency for Health Care Policy and Research, 1997.
11. *Annual Expenses and Sources of Payment for Health Care Services*. National medical expenditure survey research findings 14. Rockville, MD, Agency for Health Care Policy and Research, 1992.

12. Cooper PF, Schone BS. More offers, fewer takers for employment-based health insurance 1987 and 1996. *Health Affairs,* Nov–Dec 1997, pp 103–110.

13. Coburn A, Kilbreth E: *Urban-Rural Differences in Employer-Based Health Insurance Coverage of Workers.* Working paper no. 13. Augusta, ME, Maine Rural Health Research Center, University of Maine, March 1998.

14. Rice T, Pourat N, Levan R, et al: *Trends in Job-Based Health Insurance Coverage.* Policy report. Los Angeles, CA, UCLA Center for Health Policy Research, July 1998.

15. Rice T, Desmond K, Purant N. *Dark Clouds in Pleasantville: Trends in Job-Based Health Insurance, 1996–98.* Los Angeles, CA, UCLA Center for Health Policy Research, July 1999.

16. Gabel J, Hunt K, Kim J: The financial burden of self-paid health insurance on the poor and near poor, in Custer G (ed): *Health Insurance Coverage and the Uninsured.* Report of the Commonwealth Fund, November 1997. Washington, DC, Health Insurance Association of America, December 1998.

17. Frenzen PJ: Health insurance coverage in U.S. urban and rural areas. *J Rural Health* 9(3):204–214, 1993.

18. Mueller KJ, Kashinath P, Ullrich F: Lengthening spells of uninsurance and their consequences. *J Rural Health* 13(1):29–37, 1997.

19. Unpublished results from Hart LG: Washington Academy of Family Physicians 1996–97 survey of family physicians. Seattle, WA, The University of Washington, Department of Family Practice, March 1998.

20. Laschober MA, Olin GL: *Health and Health Care of the Medicare Population: Data from the 1992 Medicare Current Beneficiary Survey.* Rockville, MD, Westat Inc, November 1996.

21. Blumberg LJ, Evans A: Reform of the Medicare AAPCC: learning from previous proposals. *Inquiry* 35(10):62–77, 1998.

22. McBride TD, Penrod J, Mueller K: Volatility in Medicare AAPCC rates: 1990–1997. *Health Affairs* 16(5):172–180, 1997.

23. Wellever A: *Hospital Labor Market Area Definitions under PPS.* Working paper no. 7. Rural Health Research Center, University of Minnesota, 1994.

24. General Accounting Office: *Physician Shortage Areas: Medicare Incentive Payment Not an Effective Approach to Improve Access.* HEHS-99-55. Washington, DC, GAO, March 1999.

25. *Rural Conditions and Trends* 8(2). Washington, DC, Economic Research Service, Department of Agriculture, February 1999.

26. Council on Graduate Medical Education Tenth Report: *Physician Distribution and Health Care Challenges in Rural and Inner-City Areas.* Rockville, MD, Health Resources and Services Administration, Department of Health and Human Services, February 1998.

27. Hart LG, Rosenblatt RA, Lishner DM, et al: *Where Do Elderly Rural Residents Obtain Their Physician Care? A Study of Medicare Patients in Washington State.* Rural health working paper series. University of Washington WWAMI Rural Health Research Center, 1999.

28. Krein S, Casey M: Research on managed care organizations in rural communities. *J Rural Health* 14(3):180–199, 1998.

29. Casey M: Serving rural Medicare risk enrollees: HMOs' decisions, experiences, and future plans. *Health Care Fin Rev* 20(1):73–81, 1998.

30. *Health Care Reform in Rural Areas.* Report of an invitational conference sponsored by the Robert Wood Johnson Foundation, March 1993. Washington, DC, Alpha Center, 1993.

31. Christianson J: Potential effects of managed care organizations in rural communities: a framework. *J Rural Health* 14(3):169–179, 1998.

32. Alexander JA, Vaugn T, Burns R, et al: Organizational approaches to integrated health care delivery: a taxonomic analysis of physician-organization arrangements. *Med Care Res Rev* 53(1):71–93, 1996.

33. Burns LR, Thorpe DP: Physician-hospital organizations: strategy, structure and conduct, in Connors R (ed): *The Organization and Management of Physician Services: Evolving Trends.* Chicago, American Hospital Publishing Company, 1997.

34. Dynan L, Bazzoli GJ, Burns LR: Assessing the extent of integration achieved through physician-hospital arrangements. *J Health Care Mgt* 43(3): 242–262, 1997.

35. *Rural Prescriptions for Managed Care: A Roundtable.* Rockville, MD, Office of Rural Health Policy, Department of Health and Human Services, 1995.

36. Silbaugh B: The rural health care enterprise: keeping up with the city slickers. *Phys Exec* 22(5):19–23, 1996.

CHAPTER 19

Practice Management in a Rural Setting

WALTER L. LARIMORE   SUSAN REHM

There are too many "dry" business education textbooks! We wanted to try a new approach and present our rural practice management advice in a new venue—an ongoing ficticious case study. The examples, while occasionally exaggerated, are based on actual experience in either practicing in or working with practices in rural settings. Our hope is that you enjoy this method of instruction and find the information useful, entertaining, and occasionally amusing. Rural practice management is not a matter to take lightly. There are significant differences from managing a suburban or urban practice. While this chapter could not begin to address all of the nuances, we tried to cover the "basics." Good luck with your rural medical practice career.

A DAY IN THE LIFE OF . . .

It is an unseasonably cold day in November in a small town in mid-central Iowa. Frost dusts the fields, recently shorn of their crops, and glistens on the tops of the silos, barns, and rooftops. The autumn leaves—crimson, gold, and orange—still cling to the trees, reflecting the sunlight on their frosty surfaces.

At the curbside of a narrow road, in front of the family's mailbox, three elementary school children wait for the bus. Corn shocks and pumpkins are positioned against the farmhouse's porch. On down the road, a crow perches on a fence post, its head cocked and its bright eyes seeking out an intriguing object on the ground. The Black Angus cattle are milling about the pasture, their breath frosty in the morning air. Chickens scurry about, scrambling to be first for their feed, which distracts them while the eggs are being gathered from their nests.

It is Friday and the town is preparing for the high school football team's annual homecoming. The team is undefeated and is playing its cross-state rival that evening. The civic leaders of the town are meeting for breakfast at the local cafe, finalizing plans, over coffee, for the festivities that will follow: the morning parade and football game. The town square is decorated for the occasion with festive posters and banners decorating the windows of the local merchants, which include a pharmacy (complete with soda fountain), hardware store, antique shops, and farm insurance agency, to name a few. The clock on the majestic red brick courthouse that graces the town square chimes 7:00 a.m. Most of the buildings date back to the late 1800s and house family businesses of many generations.

Meet Dr. Simpson

Dr. Frank Simpson, a family physician, rises from the table in the cafe and waves a cordial farewell to his colleagues, saying "See you tonight!" He makes his way to the cashier. He has approximately 90 minutes to drive to the hospital, which is 25 miles away, check on his patients, and be back at his clinic in time to see patients beginning at 8:30 a.m. The town in which Dr. Simpson resides has a population of 800. However, the service area averages 9000; the majority of the patients are on Medicare or working and uninsured. A few local major employers provide health insurance. There are very few physicians in the area, and Dr. Simpson shares call with a group of three other primary care physicians in neighboring communities. There is little industry in the area; most of the commerce is agricultural. There are a few medium-sized manufacturing operations; these have insurance plans for their employees.

As Dr. Simpson makes his way to the front of the cafe, one of his patients approaches him. The patient, a new mother whose baby Dr. Simpson recently delivered, describes symptoms of colic. Dr. Simpson reassures her that the condition is probably nothing serious but encourages her to make an appointment if the symptoms worsen or she continues to be concerned.

Dr. Simpson heads to the hospital, which has 35 beds. While driving to and from the hospital, he listens to continuing medical education (CME) tapes. The closest tertiary hospitals are 2 1/2 to 3 hours away. His patients are doing well, so he is able to leave a bit ahead of schedule. He arrives back at the clinic around 8:15 a.m.

Dr. Simpson is in his mid-forties. He and his wife, Meredith, met in college and have lived in the community for the past 9 years. Dr. Simpson's father had been a physician but practiced in a larger community. After a brief stint in a metropolitan area, the Simpsons relocated, seeking a simpler, more relaxed lifestyle. They have two daughters, Melody and Stacey, aged 16 and 13.

Flu Bug Arrives Early

Influenza had hit the community early this season, and hard. Unfortunately, one of its victims is Dr. Simpson's nurse. So one of the receptionists, who is cross-trained as a medical assistant, will substitute today. This means, however, that Dr. Simpson's wife, who serves as office manager, will cover for the receptionist. Typically this is not a problem, but it is time for Medicare and Medicaid claims to be filed, and Mrs. Simpson had planned to spend the day testing the new electronic billing system the clinic had recently implemented. Their insurance clerk had requested the day off well in advance, as her son was playing in the football

game that evening and she was having pregame dinner guests. In the meantime, the clinic's cash flow would suffer.

Fortunately, many of the patients simply wanted flu shots. The morning was progressing fairly uneventfully when a patient with an emergency entered the office, having suffered a severe laceration from operating a chain saw. Dr. Simpson was able to suture it successfully and the patient was expected to recover fully, but the unexpected surgery took nearly 45 minutes to perform.

A patient suffering from bronchitis walked in. Dr. Simpson suggested that if she'd quit smoking, she would be healthier. After numerous attempts at motivation, what seemed to finally make an impact was the ever-increasing price of cigarettes. Lunchtime was spent hurriedly eating fare from the local Pizza Hut while a pharmaceutical saleswoman from 200 miles away touted the latest hypertension medication.

A middle-aged man showed up after lunch. He handed Dr. Simpson's wife $25. That spring, a rattlesnake had bitten the man. As he had no insurance, he could only afford to pay for his treatment by the month. Dr. Simpson's wife greeted him with warmth and familiarity. She accepted his cash without querying him about future payments on the unpaid balance of his bill.

The Community "Family"

The day was winding down. Around 4:30 p.m., a group of young women from the high school pep club burst through the door, bearing a balloon/floral bouquet in the high school's colors. It was a gesture of gratitude to Dr. Simpson for providing medical care for the high school athletic teams and to Mrs. Simpson for helping organize a bake sale to help send the high school band to music camp. The Simpsons brimmed with pride and gratitude.

Later that evening, at the high school football stadium, the crisp starlit air was scented with smoke from the earlier pep rally bonfire. Hot dogs roasted on the concession stand grill and the fragrance of hot chocolate wafted through the bleachers. Remnants of crepe paper from the day's events stirred in the breeze. The parade floats were parked along the track surrounding the football field. A wrought iron settee and chairs were positioned for the crowning of the homecoming queen and her court during the half-time ceremonies.

The hometown team was ahead by a field goal. During a time-out, the cheerleaders performed. Posing in a pyramid on the soft asphalt track, one of the anchor cheerleaders lost her footing and the cheerleader on the top of the pyramid fell to the ground. She lay motionless, surrounded by the other cheerleaders, who were alternately trying to comfort her and fight back tears. Dr. Simpson was summoned, and he raced to her aid.

SPECIAL CONSIDERATIONS OF RURAL PRACTICE

The intention of this chapter is to not paint a picture portraying rural practice as a laid-back, bucolic lifestyle. Granted, there are distinct benefits, such as a sense of community and family, the opportunity to serve in a role of civic leadership, and a simpler lifestyle. In addition, rural physicians frequently have the opportunity to have an enhanced scope of practice by performing maternity care and more procedures. There also is less competition for patients.

On the other hand, rural practice has a number of potential drawbacks. As there may be few colleagues to share coverage with, rural physicians spend more time on call and find it difficult to be able to take time off for vacation, for relaxation, or to pursue CME opportunities. The void in access to peers and advanced technology can also create a sense of isolation. Lack of local enterprise means little or no employer insurance coverage, so the practice is dependent on private pay, Medicare, and Medicaid. An average rural practice consists of 32.9 percent Medicare patients, compared to 24.6 percent for urban physicians. Managed care is rapidly encroaching in the rural marketplace. (See Appendix 19-1.)

There are many trade-offs when one is considering rural practice. For starters, rural physicians provide more patient care than their urban counterparts. Table 19-1 provides a breakdown of hours worked per week in various settings.

TABLE 19-1   BREAKDOWN OF HOURS WORKED PER WEEK IN VARIOUS SETTINGS

Patient Encounters Per Week	Rural	Urban
Office visits	110.0	98.3
Hospital visits	10.0	16.0
Nursing home visits	6.2	2.3
Home health supervision	12.3	7.4
Total hours in direct patient care	46.4	41.0
Total hours practiced	55.2	51.8

SOURCE: *Facts about Family Practice.* Leawood, KS, American Academy of Family Physicians, 1998.

Rural physicians also receive less reimbursement from Medicare and Medicaid than do urban physicians. This adds up to less take-home pay, reduced annual net income (versus urban physicians), and greater professional expenses.

WHAT TYPE OF PRACTICE IS BEST FOR YOU?

It was well after midnight when Dr. Simpson returned home. Fortunately, Ashley, the injured cheerleader, was not seriously hurt. She was taken to the hospital as a precaution. She was going to have a nasty headache for the next day or so, and numerous bumps and bruises. After several hours of observation, she was sent home under her parents' care.

While Dr. Simpson was at the hospital, he dropped in on one of his elderly patients, Mrs. Morris, a 65-year-old widow, who was suffering from pneumonia as a complication of terminal cancer. Her discomfort had worsened. Dr. Simpson adjusted her medications and spent 20 minutes sitting at her bedside, holding her hand, talking to her, and then saying a prayer with her. The patient was prepared for "her transition" and deeply appreciated Dr. Simpson's care for her physically, emotionally, and spiritually. Her family members had gone home for the day, and she hadn't felt comfortable talking in such terms with them, as she "didn't want to burden them." As she drifted off to sleep, Dr. Simpson quietly disengaged his hand and left.

In addition to feeling frustration about the limitations on treatment options, Dr. Simpson had to admit that he felt like he might be burning out. Between his hospitalized patients, clinic patients, nursing home and homebound patients, and limited call sharing, he frequently put in an average of 60 hours a week, while making less money than his urban colleagues for his effort. That left little time to spend with his family, not to mention that he could barely squeeze in time to pursue CME and keep up on his professional reading. It had been years since he had been able to indulge in any of his favorite hobbies, such as fishing or photography. He rarely exercised, and meals frequently consisted of coffee or what he could grab and gulp down on the go. How could he counsel patients on the benefits of a healthy lifestyle if he himself didn't follow his own advice? If he were lucky, he could work in one or two 3- or 4-day weekends around selected holidays. The precious time he could devote to civic and church activities, which he found very fulfilling, was dwindling. It was time for a change.

Earlier in the month, Dr. Simpson had been approached by a large health system in a major metropolitan area 300 miles away. The system wanted to solidify its presence throughout the state and was in the process of acquiring the local hospital, with the promise of upgrading the facility, purchasing new technology, and providing a full range of outreach services locally. The health system was also interested in forming some type of collaborative relationship with Dr. Simpson, such as buying his practice and having him function in the role of employed physician.

The other local physicians had been approached as well. It did seem lucrative: a handsome salary, time off, and freedom from the administrative burdens of operating a practice. The health system also hinted at the possibility of recruiting an associate to the practice. It was a lot to contemplate. Would his patients and the community think he'd "sold out"? What were his colleagues going to do? He had finally fallen asleep when the phone rang.

Consider Your Options

The practice buyout option that our fictitious Dr. Simpson has been offered is not uncommon in today's rural practice. Gone are the days when the solo rural physician arrived in town, hung out the shingle, and saw patients flock in the door. However, for a physician starting or restarting a private practice, Appendix 19-2 includes a time line for starting a rural practice and Appendix 19-3 includes common tax, license, and privilege requirements to start a practice. However, there are many types of practice configurations to consider:

Solo practice. This would be ideal for the physician who values autonomy and a broad scope of practice.

Joining an established practice. Typically, this is a situation where a rural practice wants to recruit new providers to augment a group whose members are preparing for retirement or where the workload exceeds the available manpower.

Public Health Service student loan forgiveness. If a physician agrees to practice in an underserved area for a designated period of time, his or her student loans will be forgiven.

Income guarantee. In this contractual configuration, a hospital or health system will cover the physician's business expenses, including income, while the practice is being established in the community. The income guarantee will be established for a given amount spread over a specific time period. The objective is that once the physician is actively seeing patients, the amount advanced every month will eventually decrease and will be paid back.

Health system employee. As in our example, a health system, in an effort to establish and strengthen geographic presence, will approach a rural community. In exchange for more economic stability and updated technology, the health system will either acquire or take over management operations of hospitals and rural practices. Physicians and their personnel will become employees of the health system.

Community health center. Community health centers (CHCs) are federally supported clinics designed to provide health care to all patients regardless of ability to pay. Physicians are employees of the CHC.

Rural health clinic. See Appendix 19-4 for a discussion of rural health clinics (RHCs).

PENNY WISE VERSUS POUND FOOLISH

After thinking it over and discussing it at length with his family, Dr. Simpson decided to explore his options, including the offer from the metropolitan health system. He made an appointment with his accountant, Bill Markham, who advised him to engage a practice management consultant to perform a survey of the practice. The accountant and the consultant would work together to perform a valuation of the practice to ensure that the purchase offer made by the health system was equitable. Dr. Simpson also consulted with his attorney, who concurred with the accountant's advice and reiterated that Dr. Simpson should *not* sign any document without it first undergoing legal review.

During lunch, Dr. Simpson shared the accountant's advice with his wife. How would they go about finding a good consultant? How much would it cost? Would they be able to find somebody willing to travel to rural Iowa? Mrs. Simpson teasingly reminded her husband that she did have a degree in business and that it would not be difficult for her to find a qualified consultant.

In evaluating any type of practice opportunity, it is extremely important that you gather as much information as possible. Far too often, physicians trustingly sign contracts without having received the benefit of professional business advice. They suffer the consequences later.

True, it *is* expensive to hire a consultant and/or attorney, and for a newly graduated resident or physician in a rural practice, this can be a financial hardship. However, more often than not, you will save money in the long run. For example, assume you decided that paying $5000 for a practice valuation was too expensive and you accepted the health system's offer to purchase your practice. Down the road, you learn that your practice was undervalued by $17,000. There's nothing you can do about it then.

Working with Professional Business Advisers

A number of practice management resources are available through professional organizations (see Appendix 19-5). However, one may also obtain help from a practice management consultant. Tips for working with a consultant are given in Appendix 19-6. There are many resources to assist in locating consultants and attorneys who specialize in health care. One of the best options is word-of-mouth recommendations from trusted colleagues. Other reliable options include your state specialty academy, the state or local medical society, the National Association of Healthcare Consultants, or the American Bar Association.

In addition to appraising medical practices, consultants and attorneys provide a broad scope of services, including (1) starting a new practice; (2) evaluating a managed care contract; (3) evaluating an employment contract/practice opportunity; (4) preparing for a Medicare audit; (5) reviewing the practice's reimbursement systems; and (6) converting the practice to a rural health clinic (see Appendix 19-4).

How to Interview a Consultant or Attorney

Mrs. Simpson narrowed down her search for consultants to three firms. As she prepared to interview the consultants by phone, she made a list of specific questions to ask each candidate. There were three screening criteria that the firms had to meet before she proceeded with the interviews: (1) they had to have had experience with rural practices, (2) they had to have been in business for at least 2 years, and (3) they had to be willing to work with the Simpsons' local accountant and attorney. Once Mrs. Simpson was satisfied that a firm had met her screening criteria, she evaluated it based on the criteria in Appendix 19-7.

The Final Decision

The Simpsons decided on a consulting firm based in a neighboring state. Yes, it would be more costly in the area of travel expenses, but the consultant assured them that she could complete her initial duties in about a week. A benefit was that she was not from the same area as the health system whose offer she would be evaluating, so she could be objective.

Katherine James was with a health care consulting firm located in Nebraska. Her firm had been in business for 11 years and served health care providers exclusively: physicians, dentists, and veterinarians. Katherine had been with the firm for 3 years. Her previous experience had been with a large health firm in Minnesota. She had worked with rural providers in her former state and was perfectly willing to work with the Simpsons' attorney and accountant. In fact, her firm preferred that type of arrangement, since the local accountant and attorney would be more familiar with the rules and regulations in Iowa.

Katherine's first visit was in April. She flew to Iowa and rented a car to drive to the Simpsons' clinic. It was a gorgeous day, sunny and warm. The Simpsons' clinic grounds were landscaped with redbud, flowering plum, Bradford pear, and maple trees. The clinic itself was a simple red brick and white frame structure with dark green trim. However, it had been added onto numerous times throughout the years, which gave it a haphazard, puzzle-piece appearance. Still, the grounds were neat, the parking lot had been recently blacktopped, and the exterior paint was fresh and chip-free.

"How pretty," Katherine thought, as she entered the clinic. Patients occupied practically every chair in the reception area. To Katherine's practiced eye, the room was clean and tidy but sparse. Patients were either thumbing through months-old magazines, reading materials they had brought themselves, or sitting there looking anxious. One elderly lady occupied herself with her crocheting. Young children were running around, playing together and undoubtedly exposing one another to their various maladies. "Too bad they can't bring some of the beauty of the outdoors inside," Katherine thought, as she approached the receptionist.

The receptionist, who was busy with a phone call, ignored Katherine. Finally, she looked up and made eye contact. She placed her hand over the mouthpiece of the phone. "What do you want?" she asked, almost rudely.

Katherine smiled as she thought to herself, "Obviously this receptionist does not realize or appreciate the fact that if I were a patient, I would be paying her salary." She smiled at the receptionist. "Hello," Katherine replied pleasantly. "I am Katherine James and I have an appointment with Meredith Simpson."

The receptionist's eyes narrowed and Katherine could just sense the "Oh, it's *her*, the hatchet woman!" impression. "She'll be with you in just a moment," the receptionist replied curtly. "Please have a seat," and she returned to her phone call, which, from what Katherine overheard, appeared to be of a personal nature.

"Gladly," Katherine thought. "I'll just catch up on last year's *Field and Stream* fly-fishing advice."

She waited nearly an hour. Mrs. Simpson rushed out and apologized. She'd been detained at a meeting at the hospital.

Mrs. Simpson took Katherine on a tour of the clinic. There were eight exam rooms. "Before Frank took over the practice, this clinic originally had four physicians. For a while, we also had a physician assistant, but he found a better-paying job in the city and left." She shrugged. "What can you do?"

Both Dr. and Mrs. Simpson had private offices. Two other rooms (added-on space), which Katherine assumed had been offices for the long-since-departed physicians, served as a supply storage room and medical records overflow area. The clinic also had a small x-ray room and procedures room. There was another room, just behind the reception area, that was the business office. In that room was the single practice computer terminal, a 386.

Adjoining the business office was another room where all of the medical records files were stored. It was apparent that the business office/file room had also been added on to the facility. The odd configuration of space made it difficult to navigate efficiently between common work areas. Although this was not apparent from the outside, the clinic had a second floor and basement. The second floor was used for storing supplies and included an employee break room, complete with a kitchenette and television set. The basement was used to store old medical records and x-rays that had belonged to the previous physicians. Katherine's initial assessment of the clinic was that it was immaculate but definitely in need of a "face-lift."

THE PRACTICE SURVEY

Katherine met with Dr. and Mrs. Simpson and their local accountant, Bill Markham. The four of them decided that, first, the best course of action would be for Katherine to conduct a practice survey. *A practice survey is a comprehensive overview of all operating systems of the practice.* It was more expensive than the Simpsons had anticipated, but both Katherine and Bill convinced them of its importance. Once Katherine had a thorough understanding of how the practice functioned, she could point out the deficiencies that needed to be corrected before a practice valuation was conducted.

Step 1: First Impressions

Katherine had gotten a good first-hand perspective of a patient's experience in the reception room. Patients showed up late for their appointments or not at all, and there was considerable "walk-in" traffic. It was not uncommon for several family members to show up as a group for a single appointment. Dr. Simpson frequently ran late—based on his hospital census—and, since he performed obstetrics, that could throw the schedule off at any time. Frankly, Katherine was surprised that Dr. Simpson was able to see everybody. However, he did so at the expense of often not leaving the clinic until 8:00 or 9:00 in the evening. The atmosphere of the office was more like that of an emergency room at a hospital.

In addition to the scheduling problems, Katherine observed a lack of professionalism among the front office staff. For example, instead of putting callers on "hold," the receptionist would sometimes simply cover the mouthpiece of the phone so that she could talk to patients who approached the front desk. Other times, the phone rang so

incessantly that callers were immediately put on hold without so much as a word.

The front office staff were amazingly informal in their approach to patient communications. Katherine heard a billing clerk call out into the reception area, "Maggie Walters, is your date of birth November 21, 1963?" or, "Mr. Williams, are you now on Medicare?" Katherine knew that this would be a potentially difficult situation to address. Although the familiarity and collegiality between the office staff and patients was positive, the casual approach to professional communication bordered on violating confidentiality.

Katherine decided that the first order of business would be for the practice to revamp its scheduling system. For example, Dr. Simpson should plan a given number of time slots per week when he would see new patients or perform H&P's or well-woman checkups on established patients. He should also plan specific times for his obstetric patients to come in for their prenatal checkups. There should be a specified block of time each day for "walk-ins," and, of course, emergencies would be treated as such. If a patient wanted other family members to be seen, they would have to make individual appointments. Once the practice had gotten a handle on patient flow, other operating procedures could be addressed. Katherine also wanted the practice to eventually get to the point where patients would not have to wait more than 15 minutes beyond their appointed time before being seen.

Managing the Appointment Book

Emergencies can create disarray in even the most carefully planned schedule. However, there is much a practice can do to effectively manage routine appointments. One helpful hint is to make sure that whoever is scheduling appointments gets a clear idea from the patient about the nature of the office visit, so that adequate time can be allotted.

Telephone triage systems are being used more in physician practices. These systems guide personnel through a series of questions to ask the patient about symptoms, onset, duration, and so on. The patient's response will guide the receptionist in determining how quickly the patient needs to be seen. In some cases, the patient may need to be referred to the emergency room; sometimes, the problem can be managed with an over-the-counter remedy.

Our advice would be for the physician to thoroughly review any telephone triage system before implementing it and to be very careful in training the staff. In some practices it may be perfectly appropriate to allow an experienced receptionist who has no formal clinical training to make these types of decisions. In other offices, this responsibility is better delegated to a "triage nurse." Again, this decision will depend on available personnel and practice resources.

Remodeling and Redecorating the Reception Area and Exam Rooms

Second, Katherine recommended that the reception area be made more "cozy." She suggested bringing some of the beautiful outdoor landscaping of the clinic inside, in the form of green plants, such as pothos, airplane plants, and philodendrons, which required little maintenance. "Plants," she pointed out, "are supposed to help keep the air cleaner." (To which Dr. Simpson raised a skeptical eyebrow!) She also recommended subscribing to one of the national magazine services that provide popular magazines at a discounted rate.

Katherine was also going to look into ordering colorful health information posters that could liven up the walls after a fresh coat of paint was applied.

The exam rooms didn't need a lot of work; again, some fresh paint and current educational reading materials would suffice. The Simpsons wanted to hold off on making major investments in capital improvements until they'd decided whether or not to become affiliated with the metropolitan health system.

Appearance Does Matter

It is not expensive to improve the appearance of your reception area and exam rooms. There are many simple decorating techniques that can be implemented, even on the leanest of budgets. Patients waiting in the reception and exam rooms, who are ill or in pain, are already anxious. Making their wait as comfortable and relaxing as possible increases patient satisfaction.

Your decorating efforts can double as patient education opportunities. There are health promotion companies that provide posters, pamphlets, and many other resource materials that are attractive as well as informative. Some practices have television sets in their reception areas that feature educational programming on health topics. Another reception area decorating trend is to have an aquarium; it is relaxing to watch exotic tropical fish. Again, this is a matter of personal choice and availability of resources.

Step 2: Taming the Telephones

Katherine contacted the local phone company to run a "busy study." This is a service in which the phone company monitors accessibility at various times during a day. The practice received a report detailing hourly utilization and how many calls placed to the practice were "lost"—in other words, how many patients tried to call the practice and gave up because they received a busy signal or got frustrated with being on hold.

As expected, Monday morning between 8:00 and 10:00 a.m. had the highest percentage of lost calls. Another time period that had a high number of lost calls was between 3:30 and 4:30 p.m. The receptionist explained that during that time period, patients usually called in for prescription refills and laboratory results. There were also specific days of the month when the volume of lost calls was high all day. Mrs. Simpson and Katherine finally deduced that those days coincided with the times when the clinic sent out patient account statements. The clinic would then receive calls from patients who had questions about their bills.

Is Your Telephone Technique Driving Away Patients?

The Simpsons' telephone company performed a busy study for the practice free of charge. In addition to restricted access, how were the patients treated when they called the office? Dr. Simpson's receptionist, Martha, had a rather curt manner because she was always so overwhelmed with calls and walk-in traffic. "Simpson Clinic," she'd snap. "Hold please!" Without giving the patient an opportunity to respond, she immediately placed the call on hold. A good customer service practice is to answer the phone with a cordial greeting such as "Good morning; Simpson Clinic. This is Martha speaking. How may I help you?" Yes, it would take a few more seconds to deliver the extended message, but it would make a better impression on the clinic's patients.

What? More Phones?

The clinic had four phone lines. There were two for the front desk, a private line for Dr. Simpson, and the fourth line primarily for Mrs. Simpson. This line, however, was often used by the back-office staff. It was also used when the clinic was filing electronic claims.

Katherine's immediate suggestion was to increase the number of phone lines by a minimum of two. She recommended having a direct line for the clinical staff for calling back patients with test results and for patients to call with prescription refill requests. The second new line would be dedicated to billing/insurance use. That line would also be used for the modem.

The next suggestion from Katherine was to establish specific times when patients could call the clinic for routine information. For example, requests for prescription refills would be handled between 10:00 and 11:00 a.m. and 3:00 and 4:00 p.m., which would still allow adequate time for the prescription to be filled the same day. Katherine would then work with the clinical staff to determine when would be a convenient time for them to call patients with test results.

It was suggested that there be one designated time period during the week to call patients who had normal test results. Obviously, patients who had questionable test results would be called immediately. The new phone number for the billing/insurance department would be publicized the next time that patient statements were mailed.

Last, Katherine suggested that time be taken each day for staff to call patients to remind them of their next day appointments. The staff, including

Mrs. Simpson, immediately balked at the idea, arguing that there simply was not enough time. Katherine did agree with them that it would be time-consuming—at first. She reminded them of the high number of "no-shows" and how much time was spent trying to follow up. It not only caused unexpected openings in the schedule but also obliged Dr. Simpson to spend extra time documenting the failed appointments in the patients' charts. Once patients got used to being reminded of their appointments, they would be in the habit of keeping them.

The Telephone—Friend or Foe?

The telephone "hold button" is one of the hardest-working members of your medical support team! There is no effective way to avoid having to put patients on hold. However, you can reduce the amount of time patients have to wait by employing some of the strategies discussed above. Having enough phone lines and establishing specific times for addressing routine calls can help make phone traffic flow much more smoothly.

Step 3: Personnel and Professionalism

Dealing with employees can be challenging. The supervisor-employee relationship is one of the most difficult to manage. The problem in the Simpson Clinic was even more complicated.

For starters, some of the employees were "inherited" from the previous physicians and became employees of the Simpsons. Second, Mrs. Simpson, because she was a gregarious and nonconfrontational person, frequently blurred the lines between manager-subordinate and personal friendship. In a large city, it is easier to draw lines of demarcation between management and staff because there is less likelihood of crossing paths after hours. In a small community, it is a very different case. Several of the Simpsons' employees attended the same church as the Simpsons. Husbands of employees served on the same civic committees as Dr. Simpson. The Simpson girls attended school with the sons and daughters of the Simpsons' employees and were friends with them.

A community event would bring everyone together.

Katherine knew what a difficult situation she faced. How could she tell Mrs. Simpson that her management style was possibly contributing to some of the clinic's personnel problems? With Mrs. Simpson's permission, Katherine interviewed all of the clinic employees and asked them the same set of questions: (1) How long have you been in your present job? (2) What do you like best about your job? (3) What do you like least about your job? (4) Do you have any suggestions as to how to serve patients better?

These were the clinic's employees:

Martha. Martha, the receptionist, had worked for 11 years for the previous physicians. The Simpsons had employed her for 9 years. Martha also provided back-up support in billing and insurance filing.

Janice. Janice had been hired by the Simpsons. She had completed a medical assistant program and worked with Dr. Simpson and his nurse. Janice also provided back-up assistance to Martha in the front office. She had also been cross-trained to work in the laboratory. Janice had worked for the Simpsons for 3 years.

Donna. Donna had worked for the previous physicians but had quit to go work at the community hospital in the radiology department. The Simpsons hired her back shortly after they'd taken over the practice. Donna was an x-ray technician and could also perform medical assisting duties. Donna had worked for the Simpsons for 8 years.

Lori. Lori, a medical technologist, managed the Simpsons' in-house laboratory and performed phlebotomy. She came from a neighboring community. She and her husband had lived in another state for several years but then decided to "return home" to raise their family. The Simpsons had hired her 4 years earlier.

Denise. Denise, the insurance/billing clerk, had worked for the Simpsons for 8 years. The previous billing clerk, who had worked for the former physicians, had retired. Denise also served as an administrative assistant to Mrs. Simpson.

Nancy. Nancy was newly hired as transcriptionist because Dr. Simpson had decided that it would be more efficient if he dictated his progress notes.

Nancy was also to perform back-up receptionist and administrative duties. She had previously worked out of her home performing transcription services for a medical group in a neighboring community but lost her job when the group decided to implement an electronic medical records (EMR) system. She had been with the Simpsons less than a year.

Gail. Gail worked part time in the insurance/billing department. As she had children in high school and middle school, she was not interested in working full time. Gail had worked part time for the Simpsons for a year. Previously, Gail had worked for an insurance agency in town.

Mary. Mary was Dr. Simpson's nurse. She had a BSN and, prior to working for Dr. Simpson, had worked in a community of similar size in Kansas. Her husband had been transferred to Iowa. Gail had been employed by the Simpsons for 9 years.

The Survey Results

As Katherine sat down with each employee, she tried hard to alleviate their anxiety but did not make any promises about job security. She was surprised by the responses she received from the employees. They all reported a high level of job satisfaction and especially enjoyed the interaction with patients. They reported that the Simpsons were generous in granting requested time off and that they were rewarded each year with a handsome Christmas bonus and a lavish luncheon at the local country club. The employees also remarked that they felt "part of the family." Their main complaints involved the long hours they frequently were required to work and the lack of new equipment. They also expressed some confusion as to their job duties. There were, however, specific references to one employee who abused the system with her frequent absenteeism. She also allegedly often came in late. This caused ill will among the other staff, who would "retaliate" by taking extra long lunch breaks and leaving early. There were also complaints that two employees, who were smokers, appeared to be entitled to more breaks (outdoors) during the day than the nonsmokers.

The employees had few suggestions as to how to improve patient care beyond hiring additional staff and upgrading equipment. Katherine then realized that these employees were "satisfied" because they had little or no alternative employment opportunities. The employees were not doing a poor job, but Katherine knew that the Simpsons' number of FTEs (full-time-equivalent employees) far exceeded the national average for family physicians of 3.5 FTEs per physician. Plus, in order to attract and keep their employees, the Simpsons provided a higher-than-average salary *and* benefits. Katherine knew that several of the positions could be combined or eliminated. Cost centers, such as radiology, could be shifted elsewhere—for example, to the hospital's outpatient clinic.

Full-Time Equivalent

The term FTE refers to the number of full-time employees required to support one full-time family physician. The average number of FTEs for a family practice is 3.5; however, practices that are extremely busy, performing a wide variety of procedures and services, can have 4.5 to 5 FTEs per family physician.

How to Approach This Hornet's Nest?

Katherine decided that she had to have a heart-to-heart talk with Mrs. Simpson. The two arranged to go out to dinner one evening and talk about Katherine's findings. First, Katherine brought up the employee who was frequently absent and late, Nancy.

"This is a real problem," Mrs. Simpson admitted. "She is a single mother with a young child. Frequently, her absences are due to the child's being ill with asthma. She recently went through a nasty divorce and her husband left the area. I know for a fact that he does not pay child support, so it is a real struggle for her. Family support is very limited. Her mother has died and her father is disabled and unable to provide child care. It goes on and on. I don't know what to do. I try to be accommodating, but it does become challenging. Still, it would be devastating to her if she lost her job."

Katherine then asked Mrs. Simpson if she knew that Nancy's "work ethic" was eroding morale among the other employees.

Mrs. Simpson said she had some awareness that something was amiss with the staff but couldn't pinpoint exactly what. No one had brought the problem to her attention. Katherine said that while it would be very difficult, Mrs. Simpson had to discuss the problem with Nancy. Perhaps there were community resources that Nancy was unaware of that could help her in times of crisis.

Katherine brought up the problem of the smokers taking frequent breaks. Mrs. Simpson said she didn't know what to do. If she had her preference, *none* of the clinic's employees would smoke. Katherine said that the way to curtail the problem was to establish a new office policy allowing only two breaks a day (for an established amount of time) for *all* employees.

Then Katherine broached the subject of Mrs. Simpson's treating her employees as friends instead of subordinates. Expecting a defensive response, Katherine was surprised when Mrs. Simpson acknowledged the error of her ways. "You would think I'd know better," she admitted. "What can I do? I'm going to see many of them tomorrow night at a church social. I can't suddenly go back to work Monday and act like the boss."

Katherine agreed. It would be disastrous to implement such dramatic change immediately, so she recommended the gradual approach. The first thing they'd do would be to review job descriptions. Mrs. Simpson admitted that the practice didn't have formal job descriptions. The two agreed that the next order of business would be to draft job descriptions for all staff.

Clearly defined job descriptions are your best strategy in establishing employee job expectations, giving you a standard against which to compare employee performance. Your staff will appreciate the clarification and structure job descriptions provide.

Step 4: Job Descriptions, Personnel Policies and Procedures, and Performance Appraisals

The next morning, Katherine and Mrs. Simpson sat down and discussed formal employee job descriptions. They worked together for some time until Mrs. Simpson completed her first job description—for a billing/insurance clerk (Appendix 19-

8). Once the first one was completed, the rest followed in fairly rapid order. It is often assumed in many medical practices that trained professionals inherently "know what to do." However, it is essential that performance expectations be documented in writing.

Next, Katherine asked whether the practice had a performance appraisal process in place. Mrs. Simpson said that she had a form she'd created a few years ago. However, she did not feel qualified to assess the performance of the clinical personnel fairly. She didn't want to burden her husband with yet another administrative duty, so she more or less let the entire process fall by the wayside. If Dr. Simpson experienced any problems, which he apparently didn't, he was supposed to discuss them with his wife. However, he had never expressed any dissatisfaction, so Mrs. Simpson assumed all was well. If there were problems with the administrative staff, Mrs. Simpson addressed them, even though it was difficult for her, because many of the problems, from her perspective, were "petty and trivial" and seemed to stem from a "long-timer" versus "short-timer" attitude.

"Why can't people just come to work and do their job?" she lamented.

Job descriptions were drafted for all employees, even though Katherine knew that eventually some of the positions would be combined and eliminated. However, she was sensitive enough to realize that she could only implement so many changes at a time.

Components of a Job Description

A job description should include the title of the position, name and title of the immediate supervisor, and work hours. It should list, as bullet points, the position's primary daily responsibilities. Last, it should summarize other secondary responsibilities in paragraph form. This paragraph should end with the stock phrase, "Other duties as assigned." The job description concludes with a list of qualifications for the position. See Appendix 19-8 for a sample.

Conducting a Performance Appraisal

Katherine reviewed the performance appraisal form Mrs. Simpson had developed; it was very comprehensive. Katherine made a few minor suggestions, such as adding an area to the bottom of the form for the employee to write her comments about the appraisal of her performance. She recommended that each employee receive a performance appraisal on the anniversary of her initial employment date and every 6 months thereafter. Dr. Simpson agreed to participate in evaluating the performance of the clinical personnel. Examples of performance appraisal criteria are shown in Table 19-2.

It is helpful to use as simple and as objective evaluation measures as possible. For example, you might have ratings of "Does Not Meet Expectations," "Meets Expectations," and "Exceeds Expectations" or "Less Than Satisfactory," "Satisfactory," and "Highly Satisfactory."

You may wish to reiterate your ratings with explanations, either written or verbal, so that employees thoroughly understand exactly why you assessed their performance as you did. It is also helpful to have examples of specific performances that led to the particular rating.

We suggest that there be an area at the end of the form where the supervisor can write a summary of the employee's performance within the evaluation period. The employee should also be allowed "equal space" to write his or her reaction to the appraisal, as well. Some appraisal forms also include space to write performance goals for the next evaluation period, strategies

---

TABLE 19-2   EXAMPLES OF PERFORMANCE APPRAISAL CRITERIA[a]

Attendance and punctuality
Knowledge of job duties
Productivity
Professionalism
Commitment to continuing education
Problem solving
Patient relations
Teamwork

---

[a]This will vary depending on the employee's duties and status (e.g., clinical, administrative, supervisory, etc.)

for improvement, and so on. That is totally up to you.

Last and most important, both the supervisor and the employee must sign and date the performance appraisal form, whether or not the employee agrees with the assessment. This is your practice's evidence that the employee received the appraisal. We are reluctant to mention the "L" word, but this is to your advantage in the event of potential litigation, such as a wrongful discharge suit.

In conclusion, the performance appraisal is *not* the time to drop "performance bombshells." Nothing should come as a surprise to the recipient. Keep the tone objective, impersonal, and professional. Avoid using the words *you* and *I* in conducting the discussion. Allow the employee enough time to absorb and process your message. Be willing to hear the employee's point of view, particularly if he or she is in disagreement, and to answer any questions. Act in the role of a coach who is willing to work with the employee to either improve or enhance performance. Some supervisors give the employee a copy of the completed evaluation form prior to the one-on-one discussion. Again, that depends on your personal management style. However, we do not recommend simply handing the employee a copy of a completed performance appraisal form in lieu of actual discussion.

Personnel Policies and Procedures

In addition to job descriptions, a personnel policy and procedures manual is the foundation on which you can base your assessments of your employees' job performance. For example, had the Simpsons been more conscientious in this area, many of the morale problems they were now dealing with, such as abuse of work hours, would have been avoided.

A topic that needs to be very clearly stated in the personnel policy and procedures manual is the disciplinary process. Today's society is highly litigious in the area of employer-employee relations. Therefore it is to the practice's benefit to implement a formal disciplinary pro-

cess. There should be a systematic approach to corrective action. For example, in dealing with the employee who shouted questions at patients in the reception area, Mrs. Simpson should, first, address the problem with the employee, in private. If the behavior continues, the employee should receive a written warning, which would clearly spell out the consequences should the problem behavior not cease.

Should that fail, the practice could either place the employee on probation or terminate her. This would depend on the seriousness of the infraction. When a corrective action process is going on, carefully document all communication with the employee. A suggested personnel policies and procedures manual that would be appropriate for a practice such as the Simpson Clinic is outlined in Table 19-3. These are just some suggestions of what to include in a personnel policies and procedures manual. The content will vary by individual practice.

Job Applicants

Although Katherine was not anticipating that the Simpsons would be hiring any additional staff in

---

TABLE 19-3 TOPICS TO BE CONSIDERED IN A PERSONNEL POLICY AND PROCEDURE MANUAL

Work hours (including scheduled breaks)
Salary and benefits
Drug screening
Patient confidentiality
Time off (vacation, sick leave, holidays, etc.)
Performance appraisals
On-the-job injuries
Disciplinary action
Emergency procedures[a] (although the clinic has emergency escape route maps strategically posted)
Employee health and safety (e.g., needlestick, hepatitis B vaccinations, etc.)

---

[a]This addresses emergencies such as fire, inclement weather, etc. The clinic had well-established procedures on patient emergencies.

TABLE 19-4 DOS AND DON'TS FOR INTERVIEWING JOB APPLICANTS[a]

DO ask them to describe their prior work experience.

DO call previous employers and references.

DO ask them to describe what they liked about a previous job.

DO ask them to describe how their qualifications meet the needs of your job.

DON'T ask them how old they are.

DON'T ask them about daytime child-care arrangements if they have children.

DON'T ask them if they are married.

DON'T ask them about religion, religious holidays, etc.

DON'T ask them how they plan to get to work.

[a]This is not a comprehensive listing but offers a few examples. The point we are addressing is that it is illegal for an employer to discriminate on the grounds of age, gender, race, and religion.

the near future, she did review the clinic's job application, which had been ordered from a commercial supplier of printed forms. It was appropriate and contained language such as "Equal Opportunity Employer."

In the past, the rule had been for Mrs. Simpson to interview all job applicants and for Dr. Simpson to talk to those who were invited back for a second interview. "Do's and don'ts" for interviewing job applicants are seen in Table 19-4. This is not a comprehensive listing but gives a few examples. The point we are addressing is that it is illegal for an employer to discriminate on the grounds of age, gender, race, or religion. Once again, going back to the halls of justice, job applicants have filed lawsuits, based on the above criteria, against potential employers for not hiring them.

Don't Keep Them Hanging

A frustration often voiced by job seekers is the failure of potential employers to follow up after an interview. Busy as you are, call back when you said you would, even if the hiring deliberations are taking longer than you had anticipated. To applicants who were disqualified after the first interview, send a form letter thanking them

for their interest but explaining that you have selected a candidate whose qualifications met the requirements of the position. Keep the letter brief and objective. Do not go into specific detail as to why the particular applicant was not considered. Follow the same procedures if a former employment candidate calls you to inquire as to why he or she was not hired. You are under no obligation to provide an explanation.

A quick note about employment references. This is another potential legal minefield. If an employer calls you for a reference on a job applicant, the prudent response is only to verify the term of employment and the salary. In a small community where you know other employers, this can be uncomfortable, because you want to "play straight" with your colleagues. Just keep in mind that whatever you say could possibly be held against you. Employees have successfully sued former employers on the grounds that the former employer's less than favorable reference precluded the employee from getting a job.

Step 5: Reimbursement

The next area Katherine looked into was the practice's payer or reimbursement mix. Some of the coding resources that Katherine and her staff used for reimbursement are listed in Table 19-5. Sixty percent of the practice's income came from the federal government through Medicare and Medicaid. Approximately 30 percent came from private payments, and the rest came from insurance and managed care plans. The accounts receivable (AR) age was approximately 130 days. The average age of AR for a rural family practice is 75 to 90 days.

Accounts Receivable

Accounts receivable represents the amount of money owed to a practice from billable charges, as from Medicare, Medicaid, managed care plans, individual insurers, and private payers. *AR age* is the amount of time (in days) it takes for the payer(s) to reimburse the practice. Typically,

TABLE 19-5   PHYSICIAN CODING RESOURCES[a]

A wide selection of coding resource products can help physicians report their services. The following are available from the American Medical Association:

AMA CPT products (various formats for CPT (floppy disk; magnetic tape); also specialty minibooks, Hospital Outpatient CPT

Health insurance claim forms

Medicode Insurance Directory—information on more than 5000 third-party payers and self-administered corporations; includes MediGap insurers, 800 and fax numbers, HCFA 1500 guidelines.

St. Anthony's ICD-9-CM Code Books for Physician Payment

AMA Color Coded ICD-9-CM

ICD-9-CM on Disk

St. Anthony's HCPCS Level II Code Book

Medicare RBRVS: The Physician's Guide

Medicode Code It Right

Medicode Coders' Desk Reference

AMA HCPCS Level II Code Book

[a]To order or for a complete catalogue with a description of each product listed, call 1-800-621-8335.

the older the account balance, the more difficult it will be to collect payment.

> Katherine evaluated the practice's fee schedule, which hadn't been updated in 3 years. Her analysis revealed that Dr. Simpson was being underreimbursed for evaluation and management (E&M) services. It was apparent that Dr. Simpson, fearing an audit from his local Medicare carriers, was undercoding his procedures. Katherine was able to help Dr. Simpson improve both his documentation and his coding, thereby increasing his fees in accordance with local Medicare and insurance reimbursement allowances. Katherine knew that there were billing software packages which would analyze the charges and suggest the appropriate E&M code for the visit.

Evaluation and Management

E&M and preventive medicine services are the primary groups of numeric codes used to communicate to a third party the medical service or the amount of time spent providing a medically related service. Physicians obtain these numbers from the American Medical Association's (AMA's) *Current Procedural Terminology* (CPT) book. These services are reimbursed based upon the resource-based relative value system (RBRVS).

In order to be adequately reimbursed, the physician must document correctly either the time spent with the patient (if counseling takes up more than 50 percent of the face-to-face time with the patient) or the patient's history and exam and the type of medical decision making used. The AMA's CPT book discusses this process in detail. In addition, any procedures performed or resources used (such as supplies) must be charged separately. In addition, the physician's staff must correctly provide the diagnosis codes for each service rendered using the numeric codes listed in the *International Classification of Diseases*, 9th ed., with clinical modifications (more commonly called the ICD-9-CM code book). The details of proper CPT and ICD-9-CM coding are beyond the scope of this chapter but are crucial to adequate and fair reimbursement for physician services.

Usually a practice management consultant is helpful in improving this area of practice economics. In addition, coding seminars are available from a variety of professional associations [including the AMA, the American Academy of Family Physicians (AAFP), and the Medical Group Management Association (MGMA)] for physicians and their staffs.

> At this point Katherine met with the billing personnel, which included Denise, Gail, Martha, and Mrs. Simpson [2.75 full-time equivalents (FTEs) were dedicated to this particular job function]. First she asked them how frequently they updated each patient's insurance information. Although this process was tedious for the patients, they did so at every office visit simply because coverage was so frequently subject to change.
>
> "Excellent," Katherine replied. She then queried them about their collection practices. Were they

collecting the patients' copayments (where applicable)? How were they handling private payment accounts? Did any of the local patients have secondary Medicare payer plans? If not, was there a possibility of introducing them into the community? How often were statements sent out? Did the practice file electronic claims? Did they use a collection agency?

Mrs. Simpson recoiled at the mention of a collection agency, but admitted that they were not as diligent as they should be about collecting private payments and insurance copayments. It was very difficult, since everyone who worked at the clinic seemed to be aware of the individual patients' financial situations. For example, there was the man who was making monthly payments on his treatment for the rattlesnake bite. Everyone in the clinic knew that the man was a farmer and that the past year had been very difficult for him. How could they, in good faith, ask him to increase his monthly payments to the clinic?

This is a difficult philosophical dilemma in rural practice. The easy answer would be to increase fees, hoping that the differential would be covered by the Health Care Financing Administration (HCFA). Unfortunately, rural providers are reimbursed at a lesser rate than their suburban and urban counterparts. Federal legislation to lessen the differential should become effective during the year 2000.

Katherine next suggested an equally difficult change to consider: being more assertive about collecting insurance copayments, deductibles, and private payment amounts. The usual approach was that whoever was manning the reception desk would ask for the copayment or payment. If the person didn't have the cash or a check, the receptionist would simply wave it off and say, "We'll bill you" or "Just bring it in next time."

Katherine empathized with the situation of the patients but encouraged the receptionist to collect any copays at the time the patient signed in. First of all, she explained, it was in direct violation of the particular plan's contract to waive copays. Second, the patients, in order to uphold *their* end of the bargain, *expect* to pay the deductible, copay, etc. Katherine produced a quick example. Suppose

that one patient per hour did not pay his or her copay, using an average of a $10-per-visit copay. Right there, that would be a loss in cash flow to the practice of $80 to $100 per day (depending on how long the clinic was open that day). Multiply that times the number of days a month, and it adds up—fast!

Your Personal Philosophy

For a change of pace, instead of giving you advice for discussion, how do you personally feel about this?

REGULATORY COMPLIANCE

In addition to adhering to HCFA guidelines, medical practices have other regulatory guidelines to meet. The three we will address here are those of the Occupational Safety and Health Administration (OSHA), the Clinical Laboratory Improvement Act (CLIA), and the Americans with Disabilities Act (ADA).

The OSHA guidelines most applicable to medical practices are the existence of policies and procedures regarding blood-borne pathogens and exposure to hazardous chemicals. The Simpsons had purchased a commercial OSHA compliance program that could be customized to the practice. The clinic offered hepatitis B vaccinations to all employees, and all exam rooms as well as the laboratory were equipped with wall-mounted sharps boxes. The employees also wore gloves during patient encounters where there was the risk of being exposed to body fluids. The hospital offered, as a perk to its referring clinics, a hazardous waste transporter. [For more information about OSHA compliance, call 1-800-221-2469.]

Physician office laboratories (POLs) must comply with the regulations of the CLIA. CLIA was implemented to uphold the quality of laboratory testing, not only in hospitals but also in private practices. The Commission on Laboratory Accreditation (COLA) can accredit POLs. Many medical specialty societies offer proficiency testing (PT) programs, in which POLs can enroll to make sure their practices meet CLIA guidelines. Because the

Simpsons' clinic provided more extensive laboratory testing than the minimum exempt from CLIA regulation, it was enrolled in a national PT program. For more information about COLA, call 1-800-298-8044.

The Americans with Disabilities Act (ADA) was implemented to provide equal access to persons with disabilities to employment opportunities and public facilities. The level of compliance with ADA laws is contingent upon the size of the facility and how many are employed. In the Simpson Clinic, the doors and hallways were wide enough— barely—to accommodate wheelchairs and one of the rest rooms had been reconfigured to be handicapped-accessible. [For more information about ADA, call the U.S. Department of Justice ADA Hotline at 1-800-514-0301.]

FOUR MONTHS LATER

It was late summer when Katherine returned to work with the Simpsons. It was a hot day, around 89 degrees, and humid. The sky was a dark greenish-gray with a low bank of dense dark clouds forming a wall.

"This doesn't look good," Katherine thought, as she pressed the accelerator. Finally, as she proceeded along the sparsely traveled highway, the sky began to look lighter but still ominous. The wind was picking up and she saw a flash of lightning off to the west. About 5 miles from town, the lightning became more frequent and she heard thunder.

"Any time now!" Sure enough, as soon as Katherine parked the car in the driveway of the Simpsons' clinic, the storm broke full force, so she decided to remain in her car and wait it out.

The wind was blowing so hard that the trees were almost parallel to the ground. It was raining so torrentially that she could barely see. Then she heard the familiar ping-ping of hailstones on the rental car's exterior. She saw an extremely intense bolt of lightning and heard what sounded like an explosion. The storm lasted another 10 minutes or so and then quickly subsided. The clouds were breaking up and the air was about 20 degrees cooler.

Katherine walked toward the clinic door, then she noticed huge billows of smoke in the sky. Suddenly she was nearly knocked to the ground by a mass exodus of people leaving the clinic, with Mrs. Simpson in pursuit.

"Meredith," Katherine gasped. "What happened?"

"There's a fire downtown," Mrs. Simpson replied. "Lightning. Two of our patients who were in the waiting room are members of the volunteer fire department and that's why they ran out. The others left to go see how they could help. Come on."

The two jumped into Mrs. Simpson's car and they sped off.

When Katherine saw the historic downtown square, she nearly burst into tears. Mrs. Simpson did. An entire block was engulfed in flames. Gone were the pharmacy, a beauty shop, a video rental store, a Chinese restaurant, a shoe repair store, and a laundromat.

"Melody's best friend's mother owns the beauty salon," Mrs. Simpson told Katherine.

Firefighters from neighboring communities arrived, but their efforts were futile. "Just let it burn itself out," the fire chief proclaimed. "Everybody's out and there's nothing more we can do." As a precaution, the firefighters worked to prevent the fire from spreading to other buildings. Business owners and citizens, in total despair, watched the blaze.

Dr. Simpson and Mary, his nurse, arrived. "Is anybody hurt?" he asked.

Without waiting for an answer, he made his way to the waiting ambulance to help the emergency medical technicians (EMTs). One firefighter was suffering from smoke inhalation. Another had minor burns caused by falling debris.

Blankets and beverages appeared to comfort the shocked and drenched business owners and patrons who had fled the burning structures.

"It looks like things are under control here," Mrs. Simpson said to Katherine. "Let's go back to the clinic."

As they drove back to the clinic, Mrs. Simpson told Katherine about the various people who had owned the businesses destroyed by the lightning fire. She doubted that most of them were adequately insured. Although the buildings were brick, their age and proximity, plus the false fronts of the structures, had caused the fire to spread rapidly. She was already thinking of what kind of community relief efforts could be organized to help the business owners get back on their feet.

"Those buildings were part of the national historic register, so there might be some type of federal relief they can apply for," she said, as she parked the car in the clinic's driveway.

As Katherine followed Mrs. Simpson into the clinic, she noticed that many of the suggestions she had offered during her previous visit had been implemented. The reception room looked much more inviting, and prominent signage announced the clinic's new policies about the collection of fees at the time of service; it also listed the new phone numbers for prescription refills, test results, and billing inquiries. Katherine also noticed that she wasn't greeted by Martha's familiar scowl. "Where's Martha?" she asked.

"Quit," Mrs. Simpson replied. "She apparently didn't like the new way of doing things around here, so she left. The last I heard, she and her husband were taking some time to travel. So we moved Janice into that position. It's working out quite well."

As they settled into Mrs. Simpson's office, Mrs. Simpson told Katherine of another personnel change. Nancy was gone as well. As it turned out, Nancy was also doing the transcription for a practice in another town. As there were more physicians in that group, the volume and therefore the pay was higher. Frequently, on the days when she called in sick or with a sick child, she was actually working at home for the other practice. So she was collecting sick pay from the Simpsons while also being paid by the other practice.

"Did I feel taken for a ride," Mrs. Simpson confessed. "Here I felt so sorry for her, when all along she was taking advantage of us. We haven't replaced her yet. We're still trying to decide what to do. If we join the health system, we might get electronic medical records (EMR), so we eventually may not need a transcriptionist."

While they were talking, Mrs. Simpson was interrupted by an important phone call.

"Good news," she mouthed to Katherine.

"OK, OK," she said, as she made notes. "We'll make sure you have all the necessary information. Thank you so very much. Goodbye."

A pharmacy in the neighboring town had called the clinic to offer its services to patients because of the fire. It would be considerable work for the office staff to transfer information, but it had to be done. Katherine made a mental note to bring in pastries, from the bakery that had survived the fire, the next morning.

PREPARING THE PRACTICE FOR MANAGED CARE

The purpose of Katherine's visit was to see how things were going and to move into the second phase of her practice survey. In the few short months since her last visit, two managed care plans had been introduced in the area and four area employers had signed on. In order to be competitive, the Simpsons had to demonstrate that they were able to provide quality care in a cost-effective manner. Katherine introduced three new components that would help prepare the practice for managed care:

1. *Patient satisfaction.* The managed care plans and their clients, local employers, would want to know how satisfied patients are with the care the clinic provided. The best way to measure this would be by administering patient satisfaction surveys. The patients would be asked to rate the services performed: for example, how long they had to wait beyond their appointed time, courtesy and professionalism of the front office staff, and communication with Dr. Simpson. The feedback would provide a wealth of information as to how the practice could be improved. Patients should then be surveyed again after a predetermined time period and the results compared.
2. *Medical records documentation.* Although Dr. Simpson was very good about completing his charting on a timely basis, there were other specific documentation requirements of managed care plans, such as using a problem list and medication flow

sheet. Fortunately, Dr. Simpson used both, so this was not another new procedure to be implemented. Katherine advised him to keep in mind that each plan might have its own documentation requirements, so he might still be required to make adjustments.

3. *Preventive services.* Managed care plans abide by the preventive services guidelines set out in the Health Employer Data and Information Set (HEDIS). HEDIS cites specific preventive services and indicates how frequently they need to be provided, based on patient age, gender, risk factors, etc. For example, HEDIS recommends that diabetic patients be referred on an annual basis to an ophthalmologist for an eye exam. Dr. Simpson felt that he did a fairly good job in this area but admitted that he could improve. The problem was that traditionally, many of the local employer insurance plans did not cover preventive services, and patients were reluctant to pay out of pocket for medical care when "they weren't sick."

Dr. Simpson said that many of his patients, as well as the community in general, received some preventive services at the annual health fair sponsored by the hospital. Participants would have their height, weight, and body mass index (BMI) calculated, as well as body fat percentage, via calipers. Other services provided were blood pressure checks, cholesterol testing, and skin cancer screening. On hand were Hemoccult tests for people to take home, and information about screening for breast, prostate, and colon cancer. Now that the hospital was under the management of the suburban health system, there was talk that the health system would bring its mobile mammography unit to the next year's health fair.

Dr. Simpson also promoted annual immunizations for children and conducted a back-to-school clinic each autumn, where children could receive their required shots and physicals. He also promoted influenza and pneumococcal vaccines each winter.

Katherine realized that he was doing the best he could, and the problem was with educating the patients about the importance of preventive care. She found a preventive services provision system that included prompts for both the physician and the patient. Brightly colored stickers, sticky notes, patient handouts, and educational posters re-

minded Dr. Simpson when patients were due for preventive services.

He and Mary worked out a system where she would prompt the patient during a visit about the procedures that were needed. For example, when a woman came in for her annual Pap smear, Mary would remind her, when appropriate, that she needed to schedule a mammogram. The patient still had the option to decline the services, but at least Dr. Simpson now had documentation that the patient had been counseled.

THINGS ARE LOOKING UP

Although it was too soon to see long-term results, Katherine was quite pleased to see that many of her suggestions had been implemented and were working successfully. In addition to the physical improvements, she noticed that the reception area was not quite as congested. The phone did not ring quite so frequently. The front-office staff spoke to one another quietly, and when the phone rang, Katherine discovered that callers were treated in a much more courteous and professional manner.

Katherine approached the front-office staff, and, to her surprise, she received a friendly greeting. Feedback from the staff indicated that the changes she had suggested were working, particularly in the telephone situation. The additional lines took a great deal of pressure off the front-office staff. Patients were slowly beginning to follow the procedures about calling the new numbers with their routine questions.

The staff still grumbled about the amount of time it took to place appointment reminder calls to patients, since there were few results to show for their efforts. However, everyone seemed happier and morale had improved. The smokers still managed to steal an occasional break here and there, but the abusive patterns of the past were gone.

Gail, who worked part time, was quite good at working with patients about their financial arrangements. She had come up with installment payment plans that, although Katherine didn't quite agree with them, seemed to work, and they fell within the guidelines of legally acceptable collection practices. The clinic's AR record had improved somewhat but still fell short of national averages.

THE PRACTICE VALUATION

Katherine met with the Simpsons, their accountant, and their attorney. The health system had sent out an appraiser to perform a practice evaluation and had made an offer. Dr. Simpson wanted to have an independent appraisal conducted for comparison. Bill, the accountant, recommended an appraiser to work with him.

Entire books have been published on the subject of medical practice valuations. A very simple definition of a practice valuation is that if determines the financial value of the practice (assets minus liabilities). A common measure of the value of tangible assets is their *book value,* which is the original purchase price minus depreciation. *Modified book value* is the purchase price of something depreciated over its estimated useful life. *Goodwill* describes intangible assets. A partial listing of the tangible and intangible assets and liabilities of a medical practice is given in Table 19-6.

Pretend that you have been approached by an outside entity to purchase your practice. Using the listing of liabilities, tangible assets, and goodwill and the book value method, come up with an approximation of what your practice is worth today.

THE OUTCOME

While the health system's valuation was slightly less than the Simpsons' appraisal, the difference was not great. After considerable contemplation, Dr. Simpson decided to forgo the offer, at least at that time. It was a very difficult decision. Had he accepted the offer, he as well as the rest of the clinic's personnel would have become salaried employees of the health system and eligible for benefits. Although he would get a good deal financially, the employees would not. In fact, many of them would have to take pay cuts, consistent with the health system's "rural differential." The continuing medical education (CME) reimbursement package was not that generous either.

Then there were all of the details about contracts, withholds, incentive/production bonuses, etc.—not to mention the lecture they'd been given on their AR status.

However, in processing it all, Dr. Simpson kept coming back to the bottom line—that he would no longer be in control of his practice—and he admitted that he was just not ready to hand over the authority to an outsider.

NOT SUCH A GREAT DEAL

Although he was disappointed, Dr. Simpson was also relieved that things didn't work out with the health system. However, the clinic forfeited many capital benefits, such as a new facility and computer system and the promise of a new associate. Dr. Simpson would have dearly loved a new, modern facility, but he did not want to have to leave the existing location. Katherine said that structural rehabilitation was not her forte, so she offered the services of an architectural firm that her organiza-

---

TABLE 19-6 PARTIAL LISTING OF THE TANGIBLE AND INTANGIBLE ASSETS AND LIABILITIES OF A MEDICAL PRACTICE

Tangible assets
  Furniture
  Equipment
  Supplies
  Accounts receivable
  Leasehold improvements
Intangible assets or goodwill
  Medical specialty
  Practice location
  Growth potential
  Collection ratio
  Financial status
Liabilities
  Mortgage
  Accounts payable
  Taxes
  Salaries and benefits
  Insurance

tion subcontracted with. At this point, Dr. Simpson was getting really nervous. Did he do the right thing? Only one physician in the area had accepted the health system's offer, and he seemed fairly content with the arrangement so far.

Katherine asked the Simpsons to prioritize the needs of the clinic. They rated an improved computer system first, followed by a remodeling of the clinic. Logically, if the first two objectives were fulfilled, it would make the clinic more attractive to a prospective associate for Dr. Simpson.

HOW TO SELECT A COMPUTER SYSTEM FOR A PHYSICIAN'S OFFICE

Katherine was quick to move ahead on this because she knew that a system upgrade would make clinic operations more efficient. For example, the practice could generate bills and file claims electronically, but another advantage would be that the software could be used to schedule appointments. Dr. Simpson was ambivalent about implementing electronic medical records but did condone the option of adding an application that would prompt patients to schedule appointments for preventive services. Katherine suggested that the practice purchase a fully integrated system that included both administrative and clinical functions. The EMR application could be implemented when Dr. Simpson felt comfortable in doing so.

The first step was determining what operating procedures could be automated. The clinic was already filing its HCFA claims electronically because the regional Medicare carrier had provided them with a point-of-service (POS) system. However, the existing operating system and modem capabilities made this process extremely slow and frustrating for the billing/insurance staff.

The clinic also had a billing system that was several years old. Although it functioned adequately, the large volume of patient information on file was rapidly consuming memory, which meant frequent system crashes. Both Dr. and Mrs. Simpson were quick to agree on dumping the old system and going with something new. The front-office staff was also excited about the prospect of having an electronic scheduling system. However, it was also quite apparent that some anxiety existed about whether the computer would replace them in their jobs.

High-Tech versus High-Touch

Should employees be worried that they might be replaced by a computer? This would depend. In some practices, that outcome would clearly be part of the objective, to reduce overhead, and if a computer could eliminate some FTEs, fine. In other practices, the goal is to have the computer system perform some of the more routine tasks so that the employees can spend their time doing other work. For example, if your receptionist is using the computer to schedule appointments, she might have time available to distribute and analyze patient satisfaction surveys. If the billing clerk is not struggling to post payments and charges and file claims, she may be able to work with your patients to collect past-due accounts. The bottom line is that health care is still a highly personal "high-touch" industry that not even the most sophisticated technology can replicate.

Katherine and Mrs. Simpson spent considerable time reviewing trade journals and visiting medical software vendors' Web sites. They also talked to the staff at another practice that was using an Electronic Medical Records (EMR) system and were invited to conduct a site visit. It was decided that Janice, Denise, Katherine, and Mrs. Simpson would go. It was going to be difficult to have that many staff out of the office for an afternoon, but it was important that those people who would be using the computer system the most have an opportunity to provide feedback. Table 19-7 lists resources from the AAFP for computerizing a practice.

The Site Visit

Mid-Central Iowa Family Practice was a 90-minute drive from the clinic, and there were five physicians on staff. It was a warm Indian summer day and the leaves were just beginning to turn. The sky was clear blue, and red sumacs along the roadside were accented by black-eyed susans. Monarch but-

TABLE 19-7   OFFICE COMPUTER RESOURCES FROM THE AMERICAN ACADEMY OF FAMILY PHYSICIANS

FP Net, the American Academy of Family Physicians' clearinghouse for computerization resources (*http://www.aafp.org/fpnet/*) has the following resources:

AAFP monograph, *Family Physicians and the Year 2000: Preventive Medicine for the Millennium Bug*

AAFP monograph, *How to Select a Computer System for a Family Physician's Office*

Software product information with direct links to vendors' web sites and software reviews

Computer tutorials and basic web-site resources

Information and links to hardware vendors and specialty hardware

Information on medical computing education

Information on CME and non-CME courses and meetings

Information on and links to medical computing organizations

Information on and links to family practice management articles, medical computing journals and books, and AAFP resources on computerization

"How To. . ." Computer system selection guidelines, resources on selection and implementation of software

---

terflies floated in the breeze. Mid-Central had been using a billing system for several years and had recently implemented an EMR system. A Tuesday afternoon was purposely selected for the site visit because it would be a busy day—though not as overwhelming busy as a Monday—and it would be beneficial to see the staff using the computer during a peak time.

Mid-Central's reception area was full. Patients checked in and the receptionist pulled up their records on the computer screen to verify insurance coverage. Another receptionist had the telephone cradled against her shoulder as she searched the system for an open appointment slot. Like a typical busy medical office, there were stacks of correspondence and patient charts covering the work areas. Even though the staff had computers, there seemed to be more than enough work to do. "Why

are there patient records in there?" Janice whispered. "I thought they were on EMR?"

"Good question. Let's ask," Katherine replied.

Mrs. Simpson, Katherine, and Janice were shown into the manager's office; there was also a computer terminal on her desk. Everyone crowded around the desk while the manager demonstrated the patient registration and scheduling processes. After all the questions were answered, the next stop was the billing office, where a staff of three was busily entering charges and payments and going through a thick computer printout of insurance claims reports.

One of the clerks demonstrated how to enter charges and payments and how the EMR system would suggest the appropriate E&M code after the physician completed the visit note.

"That reminds me," Janice interrupted. "If your practice is using EMR, why are all of these paper records still sitting around?"

"Because we are still in the implementation process," the clerk explained. "For a while, we'll use the EMR to print out progress notes and so on and file that information in the patient's folder. Once everyone gets used to the new system, we'll go paperless. We are transferring information from the paper charts into the EMR. Anyone who has any spare time does this. We're about one-third of the way finished."

"But how do you know what information to put into the EMR?" Janice asked.

"We left that up to the doctors," the clerk replied. "Our vendor developed a chart summary form for us to use, so all of the information is consistent from record to record. There should be a blank one lying around here somewhere that I can show you." She rummaged around and pulled a form out of a stack of papers and handed it to Janice.

"Unfortunately, the physician who was to demonstrate the EMR for you has been called away on an obstetric emergency, so we've asked his nurse to show you," the manager explained.

After a quick demonstration at the nurses' station, the group returned to the manager's office before departing. "How did this process work out for you?" Mrs. Simpson asked.

"I would be lying if I told you it was a piece of cake and went very smoothly," the manager answered. "There still are bugs to be worked out, but we're getting there. The worst hangup we had was trying to get the vendors to work together to integrate the products."

"What do you mean?"

"Well, when we started the process, we decided to get just the billing/scheduling system, but the physicians wanted the whole works, the EMR, too, at once. We picked out a billing system and, as it turned out, the vendor had recently developed an EMR system. We thought that we'd hit pay dirt, but the physicians didn't like that particular vendor's EMR and wanted to go with a different product. The hassle—not to mention cost—involved the billing software vendor, who was extremely reluctant to create an interface from his end to work with the EMR product. Obviously, he wanted us to buy his EMR product. However, we persevered, and it is now working out."

"That's very interesting," Katherine noted. "So would you recommend that we just look at those software products that offer *both* billing and EMR applications?"

"Not necessarily," the manager replied. "You need to get the products that work best for your physicians and office staff. I am just cautioning you that you may run into potential problems if you buy software products from many different vendors. I would make it perfectly clear up front that you want a flexible system."

"Did you end up laying off any of your staff?" Janice asked.

"We did get to the point where we no longer needed our second transcriptionist," the manager replied. "We'd had a contract employee in another town who was doing some of our transcription electronically. Now, we can get by just fine with one. When we go paperless, there is plenty of other work for her to do, such as scanning information into the system."

"How did you get the office staff and the physicians to use the new system?" Mrs. Simpson asked.

"It wasn't difficult. Our practice had been using a billing and scheduling system for several years, so upgrading that particular component was not difficult and was very much welcomed by the staff because the other system was obsolete and was creating more problems than support. We are probably in a better position than a lot of practices about the EMR issue. The doctors here *wanted* it. Well, let's say three out of five were gung-ho; the other two eventually came along, but rather reluctantly. It took a lot of patience, support, and peer pressure, but the other two doctors finally began using it, and now they're used to it. That is why we took a two-step implementation approach. At first, we used parts of the EMR applications with the paper charts. Once the doctors were comfortable with that, we began getting ready to go totally paperless. We just now bought a new scanner, so I have the support staff entering information from the paper charts into the EMR and scanning reports and correspondence."

After a few more minutes of questions, Mrs. Simpson and her staff thanked the personnel of Mid-Central Family Practice and headed home. During the drive, they thought of more questions they wished they'd asked. They agreed that the visit probably would have been more useful if they'd gone to a smaller practice, but they didn't know of any other practices locally that had a sophisticated system.

"I can see the practicality of using an EMR in a five-doctor practice," Mrs. Simpson said. "I just don't know if it would work in a solo or, if we're really lucky in the future, two-doctor practice. It looked to me like using an EMR would take even more time than documenting by hand or transcription, having to go through all of those screens and checking off stuff. Then who has time to sit down and enter all of that data, even if it *isn't* the entire chart?"

Back at the clinic, Dr. Simpson remained uninspired by EMR. "I have heard all about what happened at Mid-Central," he said. "One of their doctors kept us all quite entertained at the hospital telling us about the latest disaster. I also know that it cost considerably more than they'd planned for because they had to get some kind of 'black box,' or whatever you call it, so that everything would work together properly. I don't know," he shook his head. "I'm afraid I'm going to have to veto this one. I've stayed out of much of this reengineering process, but this is one area where I say no. For one thing, we can't afford it, though I'm fully in support of getting new equipment, Internet, and a billing / scheduling system. Second, I simply do not have time to learn how to use it. So for now, no EMR!"

Softening a bit, he added, "I'll tell you what. I'll make an effort to learn what I can about EMR, and when the day comes that we get a second physician, we can make that decision together."

Change is a scary process, even if it eventually will be for the better. It is especially difficult for individuals who are used to being in control, such as physicians. Throwing too much at them at once can be overwhelming. Be diligent in introducing major changes gradually.

When going on a site visit to see a demonstration of a computer system, select a practice (if at all possible) similar to yours, so the comparison will be more meaningful. Second, prepare a list of questions in advance. Obviously, you will think of more things you'll wish you'd asked after the fact.

WORKING WITH VENDORS

Mrs. Simpson and Katherine narrowed the search to three practice management software vendors. Two of them also had an EMR system. The next

TABLE 19-8   SOME KEY POINTS A REQUEST FOR PROPOSAL FOR COMPUTERIZING A PRACTICE SHOULD ADDRESS

Hardware and software requirements
Training
Technical support (on-site, by phone, modem, tutorial, etc.)
Warranty
Ownership of source code
Replacement of defective equipment
Ability to integrate with products from other vendors
ALL Costs

step was to have the vendors submit a request for proposal (RFP). Some key points an RFP should address are outlined in Table 19-8.

The source code is the documentation used by the programmer to create the software. Licensees of the software should request that the source code be placed in an escrow account so it is accessible. It is not unheard of for vendors to go out of business or quit supporting some of their products. The source code will allow you to correct your software in the event that something goes wrong.

SIGNING THE CONTRACT

The Simpsons made their final selection and went with one of the products that also included an EMR component. The vendor tried to convince them that it was less expensive to purchase the "package deal," but the Simpsons held firm and said it was a strong consideration for the future. The vendor pulled a contract out of his briefcase and slid it across the table to Dr. Simpson.

"Just sign on the dotted line, Doc," he said with a smile, offering Dr. Simpson a pen. Dr. Simpson returned the smile, saying, "Not until after my attorney looks it over."

Software purchase contracts must be carefully reviewed by your attorney. Don't be pressured into signing anything on the spot. The contract must address the issues covered in the RFP. This advice bears repeating. There have been too many cases of physicians being left in the lurch by software vendors because they were not protected contractually. And if the contract did not spell out the vendor's responsibilities, the vendor is legally in the clear.

RECRUITING A NEW PHYSICIAN

Without the benefit of the health system's resources, the Simpsons knew that recruiting a new physician to the area would be difficult or impossible.

The new computer system had been successfully implemented and the practice's cash flow had improved significantly, which was also partly attributed to signing up with the new managed care plans in the area. Although they could not afford to make major renovations, the Simpsons had been able to make several leasehold improvements to the clinic. New furniture had been purchased for the reception area (for both patients and personnel). The maze-like layout of the business office had been reconfigured, providing more space and a logical traffic flow. Dr. Simpson's and Mrs. Simpson's offices had been modestly remodeled, as well as one of the empty physician offices. The employee break room had also received a face-lift, and the upstairs supply area had been cleaned out and reorganized so that the supplies stored in one of the physician offices could be relocated.

After consulting with the state medical society about how long to keep old medical records and x-rays, Mrs. Simpson hired Melody, Stacey, and some of their friends for after-school work a few hours each day to go through the thousands of records to determine which ones needed to be retained and which ones could legally be discarded. Once the basement was cleared out, shelves were installed to store the medical records overflow.

Katherine had given Mrs. Simpson the names of several physician recruitment firms. And, before she went back to Nebraska, she worked with Mrs. Simpson to develop a "practice opportunity profile," which incorporated a fact sheet about the practice, including approximate service area, annual gross billings, square footage of the clinic, number of employees, equipment, and hospital affiliation. It also included information about the community and surrounding areas. There was an interesting brochure about the historic town square and information about local lakes, fishing, camping, and hunting. They also included copies of the new practice information brochure, which mentioned the new phone numbers and office procedures for patients. Last, they included a 5 × 7 color photo of the clinic, taken during the spring when all of the trees and flowers were in full bloom. The previous year, the Simpsons' place had been chosen for one of the local newspaper's "Beautiful Yard of the Month" awards and a photo had been taken.

Mrs. Simpson began making phone calls. The prognosis for finding a good match for Dr. Simpson and the community, plus the fees the recruitment firms charged, was discouraging. However, one firm did agree to come to meet the Simpsons and size up the potential.

Warren Andrews arrived at the clinic on a Thursday, late afternoon. It was a blustery February day, bitterly cold and gray, and snow threatened with an occasional burst of flurries.

Upon meeting Mrs. Simpson, Warren immediately complained about the weather.

"Yes, I'm sure this climate is quite a shock compared to Dallas," Mrs. Simpson replied nonchalantly.

Warren seemed unimpressed with the clinic and barely spoke to the employees when introduced.

"Are you hungry?" Mrs. Simpson asked. "I thought I'd take you for a drive around town, then we are having dinner at the country club with the hospital administrator and his wife."

"You're kidding? There's a country club *here*?" he replied.

Mrs. Simpson did not respond and drove him around town, pointing out the schools, neighborhoods, churches, and community recreation center.

"So everybody around here's just a farmer?" he asked.

"No. There is quite a bit of private industry. A company that manufactures wheels for railroad cars is in the process of relocating here, which means a lot of new jobs. There are also many family-owned businesses." She headed into the town square.

"What happened here?" he asked. "There's nothing here. Don't tell me—a tornado passed through." He chuckled at his own "humor."

"No," Mrs. Simpson replied lightly. "This is Iowa, not Kansas, and the brick color scheme is red, not yellow. There was a lightning strike during a thunderstorm last summer. It was devastating. Many people lost everything. The town's in the process of rebuilding, but there have been some delays because of the weather."

Warren remained silent for the remainder of the tour.

Dinner at the country club was uncomfortable. It was apparent that Warren was not interested in the Simpsons and the community as clientele.

As they dropped Warren off at his motel, Dr. Simpson politely informed him that he felt that potential for a professional relationship was lacking, and Warren was free to return to Dallas.

"Now what?" he asked his wife.

PLAN B

Mrs. Simpson called Katherine, who was appalled at Warren's patronizing behavior, as her firm had worked with his firm on numerous occasions.

"Luck of the draw," Mrs. Simpson replied. "He apparently has no use for 'farmers' and 'country bumpkins.'"

The next plan of action was to place ads in the recruitment classified ads sections of national medical journals. This was very expensive but essential. Mrs. Simpson also contacted physician placement programs at hospitals, residency programs, and medical associations. The clinic received a few calls now and then, and Mrs. Simpson had a practice opportunity profile sent to each caller, but there was little follow-up.

"What are we doing wrong?" Mrs. Simpson asked Katherine. "I have even had Melody's boyfriend create a web site for us, thinking that would be a good way to reach residents."

"Nothing," Katherine reassured her. "I think the web site is a great idea. Just keep in mind that primary care residents begin to get inundated with employment offers as early as their intern year. And health systems are making a major play for rural practices. You must just be patient and persistent."

"Do you think we made the wrong decision in not going with the health system?" Mrs. Simpson asked. "It's not too late to reconsider, is it?"

"You can only do what is best for your practice, your patients, and, most importantly, you and your family. Let's ride it out a bit longer and see what happens. Did the health system give you a final deadline for reconsideration?"

"No. But we're sure the door won't remain open forever."

At the conclusion of the conversation, Katherine knew better. The Simpsons now had a highly lucrative practice, which would be a tremendous benefit to the health system. Actually, the Simpsons held the trump card. However, Katherine did not want to influence them or falsely raise their hopes.

When It Rains . . .

In the early summer, the Simpsons began to get many serious inquiries, not only through the web site but also via letters and phone calls. After their resumes were reviewed, several candidates were invited to visit the clinic for personal interviews. Each successive candidate was more disappointing than the last. One physician had a spotty work history and had jumped around among rural communities in several states. As it turned out, he had repeatedly lost his license to practice because of suspected abuse of controlled substances, and he was only one step ahead of the law.

One candidate had excellent skills but had lived in the United States for a very short period of time. He was personable and eager to work and had a good command of the English language, but in talking with Dr. Simpson, it was apparent that he would need extensive clinical training to be able to provide the scope of practice in a rural setting.

Dr. Simpson needed someone who could "hit the ground running." Another physician was interested, but his wife freaked out during the site visit.

"What do you people do around here for fun?" she whined.

Both Simpsons were growing discouraged.

The Right Place at the Right Time?

It was a balmy summer evening. The temperature was in the nineties and cicadas buzzed in the background. The Simpsons' small vegetable garden was in full yield. Dinner had included a tomato/zucchini casserole and fresh cucumbers. The flower beds around the house boasted red, pink, and orange zinnias; blue Victorian salvia; white begonias; red, pink, and yellow-gold roses; hostas; and yellow and orange day lilies. The lawn was sadly in need of a good mowing, which would have to wait until the weekend.

Now accustomed to having a bit more free time in the evenings, Dr. Simpson finished dinner, helped the girls clear the table, and left for a meeting.

Dr. Simpson was a member of the advisory council of the local community college. He listened to a long presentation of potential candidates for faculty appointments. "I'd rather be mowing," he thought. "I'm so bored, I sound like a bumper sticker!"

Suddenly, his interest was piqued. The college wanted to expand the faculty of its new information technology department. It had an exceptional candidate that it was considering for the department chairmanship. The glitch was that there were "no opportunities" for his wife, a family physician who had recently completed her residency. Dr. Simpson nearly leapt from his seat to respond to the discussion.

After the meeting, he approached the community college faculty coordinator and informed her of the situation at his clinic. Could she please speak to the wife of the faculty candidate and see if she would be interested?

YET ANOTHER INTERVIEW

Dr. Simpson received a call from Dale Morris, the candidate that the community college was considering for the position of chair of its information technology program. Dr. Simpson explained the situation and asked whether Mr. Morris's wife would be interested. To Dr. Simpson's dismay, Mr. Morris was very deliberate in his response.

"Well, I'll have to talk to her," he replied. "Can you send her some information about your practice?"

"We can do even better," Dr. Simpson replied. "We have our own web site." He gave Mr. Morris the address.

"Cool," Mr. Morris replied, now much more interested in the opportunity with the Simpsons. He

asked Dr. Simpson several questions about information technology at the clinic.

Although Dr. Simpson was still a computer novice, he was able to answer the younger man's questions. Dr. Baines (who had retained her maiden name) and her husband were from small towns in Iowa and had met in college. A site visit and interview was arranged.

Dale Morris and his wife arrived promptly. They seemed quite nervous as they talked with the Simpsons. Once Dr. Baines felt more at ease, she seemed very comfortable in the clinic. She was friendly to the employees, and Dr. Simpson was impressed with her resume and track record in her residency program. She also had highly positive references.

Dr. Baines had a list of questions for the Simpsons. These are listed in Table 19-9.

Table 19-9 provides just a partial listing of potential questions. If you were evaluating a practice opportunity in a rural community, what additional questions would you ask?

As she was originally from a small community, Dr. Baines did not have a lot of questions about the region beyond local industry, employment, and insurance coverage. She thought the town square was charming and lamented the fire. The reconstruction process was halfway completed. She liked the practice's computer system and asked Dr. Simpson about implementing EMR.

He threw up his hands. "Three against one," he laughed, referring to his wife, Katherine, and Dr. Baines. "Uncle! Seriously, I am contemplating it."

The Simpsons decided to make Dr. Baines an offer. It was clear that her husband was very interested in the position at the community college. It seemed too good to be true. Dr. Baines had the Simpsons' offer evaluated by her attorney and, after a few minor revisions, accepted.

Prior to Dr. Baines officially coming to work, there was much to be done. They showed her the new office and asked her for suggestions on how to decorate it. The next step was to hire a nurse for Dr. Baines, which took a month but was accomplished. Then, the clinic held an open house to

TABLE 19-9   SOME KEY QUESTIONS TO ASK BEFORE JOINING A PRACTICE

What is the daily patient volume?

How many patients per day will the new doctor be expected to see? How many of these will be new patients? Will more appointment time be allotted for new patients?

How many new patients did the practice acquire annually? (The Simpsons had to turn new patients away!)

What is the payer mix? Will the new doctor see all of one type of payer (managed care, Medicaid, Medicare)?

What is the accounts receivable balance?

How will the new doctor be paid (salary, percentage of billing, percentage of production)?

Will there be any bonus for performance?

Is partnership or ownership of the practice an option? When? Under what specific terms?

What is the practice's philosophy about managed care?

What is the practice's philosophy about preventive services?

What type of equipment is available? If newer or additional equipment is needed, how will it be paid for?

Will the new doctor have a dedicated staff?

What are the call arrangements?

How financially viable is the hospital?

What subspecialty services are available?

What benefits are available, such as a CME allowance?

Who covers the cost of malpractice insurance? Is tail coverage included?

introduce the community to its newest physician. The community welcomed Dr. Baines, and she had a full schedule awaiting her on her first day of practice.

ONE FINE DAY. . .

Katherine and her husband, Mark, were changing planes at the airport in Kansas City en route to San Francisco. They decided to get a bite to eat during the layover. As they strode through the terminal, someone called out, "Katherine. Katherine!"

Katherine turned around and saw Meredith Simpson. The two embraced. Then Katherine introduced Meredith and Mark. "I must get a new magazine for the long flight, so I'll meet you at the gate," Mark said, tactfully departing the scene.

"So how are things going?" Katherine asked Meredith.

"Well, see for yourself," Meredith said, stepping aside.

Katherine saw Dr. Simpson approaching with Melody and Stacey. All three carried soft drink cups and carry-on bags.

"We're on our way to Phoenix. We're also going to the Grand Canyon," Meredith said.

"So I take it that Dr. Baines is working out OK?" Katherine asked.

"She's going great," Meredith replied. "The patients and staff love her. This is the first vacation we've taken since the girls we're this big" (she gestured with her hand).

"We're so excited for you!"

Dr. Simpson came forward and shook Katherine's hand. Katherine noticed that he had a sophisticated 35-mm camera slung around his neck.

"I can't thank you enough," he said. "Lots of good things have happened. The town square is almost entirely reconstructed. It looks just like it did 200 years ago—except nobody has lived long enough to know the difference. Ha! Ha! The official dedication is on May 17. Can you make it?"

"Wouldn't miss it for the world," Katherine replied. She turned away.

"Well, our flight is about to board. I'll see you soon." Meredith squeezed Katherine's hand, then turned her attention back to her family.

CONCLUSION

As we stated at the start of this chapter, there are too many "dry" business education textbooks! Our hope is that you found this method of instruction interesting and entertaining and that you found the information useful. Rural practice management is not a matter to take lightly. It is significantly different from suburban or urban practice management. Although this chapter could not begin to address all of the nuances, we have tried to cover the "basics." Good luck with your rural medical practice career. Additional Internet resources are shown in Appendix 19-9.

APPENDIX 19-1   RURAL PRACTICE AND MANAGED CARE

Managed care is now a reality for the vast majority of rural physicians. More than 80 percent of rural physicians have at least one managed care contract (compared to a national average of 85 percent) and more than one-half of all rural counties have at least two competing health maintenance organizations (HMOs).[a] The percentage of rural medical practices with managed care contracts varies from a low of 62 percent in Michigan to a high of 98 percent in Colorado. On average, rural practices generated 30 percent of their income from managed care contracts in 1997, with discounted fee for service being the primary payment method (as opposed to capitation, fee withholds, or bonus incentive payments.)

In most current rural managed medical systems (as opposed to urban), the physicians share little or no financial risk. In addition, some managed care plans (even Medicaid) result in increased revenues for rural physicians (which primarily happens by reducing the number of uninsured patients seen by the rural physician.)[b] Many rural physicians are finding ways to gain leverage with the health care payer systems via managed care and are finding increased potions to increase income, increase satisfaction and increase services provided.[c,d]

Managed Care Resources for Rural Physicians

- AMA Doctors' Advisory Network: This resource is for AMA members only and is a network of select physicians, lawyers, and business consultants who are experts in managed care. First you talk to a member of AMA's legal department, who will as-

sess your needs and refer you to qualified individuals from their database of managed care experts. Call 1-800-AMA-1066.

- Strategies-for-Change Workshops: Interactive managed care and health system reform workshops for physicians. Workshop faculty are experienced experts in managed care and they know the local and regional issues that will directly affect rural practices. Workshops are hosted locally by medical societies, hospital medical staffs, specialty societies, and other groups. Contact 1-800-AMA-1066.

- AAFP monograph, *Principles of Interaction between Family Physicians and Health Plans.* (http://www.aafp.org/socioeconomics/rep 203.html).

- AAFP monograph, *FPs and Managed Care: A View to the 90s.* A comprehensive publication written for the AAFP by a managed care expert. Included are a comprehensive glossary of terms and bibliography of MHC literature. Cost $15.00. Call 1-800-944-0000.

- AAFP monograph, *Requirements Related to Managed Care Plans, Utilization Review—Programs and Point of Service Plans.* (http://www.aafp.org/managed/require.html).

[a]Guardino JR: Managed care comes to rural America. *Fam Pract News,* July 1, 1998, p 52.
[b]"Medicaid managed care good for rural docs." *Fam Pract News,* July 1, 1998, p 52.
[c]Ranney RJ: Rural practice and managed care: a success story. *Fam Pract Mgt,* May 1998, pp 37–44.
[d]Christianson JB, Hamer R, Knutson D: HMO financial arrangements with rural physicians. *J Rural Health* 13(3):240–252, 1997.

Family Practice Management Resources to Read

Flanagan L: Keys to success in medicaid managed care. *Fam Pract Mgt,* February 1997. (http://www.aafp.org/fpm/970200fm/cover.html).

Fields MA: Re-engineering for managed care: a practice in transition. *Fam Pract Mgt,* May 1997. (http:// www.aafp.org/ fpm/ 970600fm/ cash.html).

Spicer J: Making patient care easier under multiple managed care plans. *Fam Pract Mgt,* February 1998. (http://www.aafp.org/fpm/980200fm/spicer.html).

Spicer J: Coping with managed care's administrative hassles. *Fam Pract Mgt,* March 1998.

(http://www.aafp.org/fpm/980300fm/cover.html).

Ranney RJ: Rural practice and managed care: a success story. *Fam Pract Mgt,* May 1998. (http://www.aafp.org/fpm/980500fm/rural.html).

Davis KG: The managed care transition: touching all the bases. *Fam Pract Mgt,* May 1998 (http://www.aafp.org/fpm/980500fm/transit.html).

APPENDIX 19-2   TIME LINE FOR STARTING TO PRACTICE MEDICINE— A YEAR BEFORE STARTING PRACTICE[a]

1. Make final decision on practice location. (E, GP, SP)
2. Check on membership for: (E, GP, SP)
   County medical society
   State medical society
   National medical societies
   Specialty societies
3. For comparison purposes, get in writing details of contracts from groups or corporations you are considering joining. (E, GP)
4. Begin to examine net worth in terms of capital available for start-up costs. (SP)
5. If possible, reserve office phone number. (SP)
6. Find out the date when telephone books are printed. Have your name listed in both the white and yellow pages. (SP)
7. Visit banks and begin shopping for a loan. Pick up loan applications and meet loan officers. Determine what information the bank needs to evaluate your loan application. (SP)
8. Open:
   Checking account, personal (E, GP, SP)
   Checking account, business (SP)
   Savings account, personal (E, GP, SP)
   Savings account, business (SP)
9. Draw up an income/expenditure projection for first year of practice. Talk with several bankers regarding borrowing money; submit applications. (SP)

Key: E, employed physician; GP, group practice physician; SP, starting a solo practice.

SOURCE: From *Starting a Medical Practice: The Physician's Handbook for Successful Practice Start-up.* Chicago, American Medical Association, 1996, with permission.

APPENDIX 19-3   TAX, LICENSE, AND PRIVILEGE REQUIREMENTS TO PRACTICE MEDICINE

State medical license	Call the State Board of Medical Examiners. The process can take 6 to 9 months.
Medical staff privileges	You will need to apply for privileges with each hospital or outpatient center and with each insurance company (PPO, HMO) with or in which you will practice. The process can take 6 to 9 months.
Drug Enforcement Agency (DEA)	You must notify the DEA of your change of address (1-800-882-9539).
State narcotics license	Most states require you to have a state narcotics license. Check with the state board of medical examiners or the state chapter of the AAFP.
Universal provider number (UPN)	The UPN is assigned by the Health Care Financing Administration (HCFA). This number will be assigned when you apply for a Medicare provider number.
Business license	This may include city, county, and/or state licenses. Usually the state board of medical examiners can give you this information.
Laboratory license	If you plan to do any laboratory work at your office, you will need a Clinical Laboratories Improvement Act (CLIA) number. The AAFP can assist you with information on obtaining a number and obtaining ongoing proficiency testing.
Employer identification number (EIN)	The EIN is needed by all employers. An accountant, business consultant, or CPA can assist with this.
State tax identification number	An accountant, business consultant, or CPA can assist with this.

U.S. Medical Licensure Statistics and Current Licensure Requirements, 2000 ed. Chicago, American Medical Association, 2000 (to order call 1-800-621-8335; order OP399099BCG).

If you're planning to start or move your practice, you'll find this book an invaluable aid. The only single source containing current statistics and information on medical licensure requirements for every state in the United States. Includes the following information:

State board licensing policies as of January 1996

The most current information on the U.S. Medical Licensing Examination (USMLE)

Requirements for Federation Licensing Examination (FLEX) and Foreign Medical Graduate Examination in Medical Sciences (FMGEMS) examinations

Reciprocity/endorsement policies

Fees, renewal intervals, and CME requirement

National board and Educational Commission for Foreign Medical Graduates (ECFMG) requirements

Details on the Special Purpose Examination (SPEX)

Current guidance for Department of Defense licensure

An Immigration overview of international medical graduates

For up-to-date information on the DEA's Controlled Substances Registration Program, call 1-800-882-9539.

SOURCE: *Starting a Medical Practice: The Physician's Handbook for Successful Practice Start-up.* Chicago, American Medical Association, 1996.

APPENDIX 19-4   PLANNING AND MANAGING A RURAL HEALTH CLINIC

In 1977, the U.S. Congress passed legislation, Public Law 95-210, that established criteria for the establishment of federally certified Rural Health Clinics (RHCs.) The law was designed to support and encourage access to health care by rural residents. Congress noted that because of economic conditions, the rural population was becoming poorer and more elderly and that rural physicians were becoming older and not being replaced upon retirement by younger physicians. It also was noted that provision of health care to the rural poor and elderly was more costly to them than to those populations in urban areas.

The number of Rural Health Clinics (RHCs) has proliferated in the past 10 years due to decreasing reimbursements from the standard fee-for-service system. Because RHCs receive cost-based reimbursement, rural physicians are turning to this program to be able to continue providing service to the rural poor and elderly. Rural Health Clinic status has helped maintain health care in areas that otherwise have not historically been able to recruit or maintain providers.

Health care provision to rural populations through Rural Health Clinic certification does the following: (1) it allows access in areas that otherwise would not have sustainable health care; (2) it encourages midlevel providers to be an integral part of the health care delivery system; (3) it gives rural citizens the opportunity to learn and accept the skills of midlevel providers; and (4) it allows the potential for other services to be brought to the rural area that otherwise would not be available in a private practitioner's office, such as dietetic, social work, and physical therapy services.

The Rural Health Clinics program eligibility requires that the practice be in a medically underserved area (MUA) or a health professional shortage area (HPSA). Midlevel providers are required by the enabling federal law to be key Rural Health Clinic components in the delivery of primary health care services. The program clearly has the potential for enhancing Medicare and Medicaid revenues for rural primary care practices in underserved areas. However, although the opportunity for enhanced reimbursement is attractive, the financial and operational impact that a conversion to this cost-based reimbursement program can have on a practice must be studied in detail and understood. A number of resources can help physicians study this option.

To find out if your community qualifies as a MUA or HPSA, contact the Department of Health and Human Services' Health Professional Shortage Area Web site at http://www.bphc.hrsa.dhhs.gov/databases/hpsa.cfm

APPENDIX 19-5   PRACTICE MANAGEMENT RESOURCES

- The Practice Success Series is a series of eight excellent books available at reasonable prices. The titles are as follows: (1) *Starting a Medical Practice;* (2) *Managing the Medical Practice;* (3) *Financial Management of the Medical Practice;* (4) *Personnel Management in the Medical Practice;* (5) *Managing Managed Care in the Medical Practice;* (6) *Integration Strategies for the Medical Practice;* (7) *Buying, Selling, and Owning the Medical Practice;* and (8) *Assessing the Value of the Medical Practice.* Call 1-800-621-8335 to order.
- Practice Management Workshops
  The AMA has workshops on a variety of topics for physicians and medical office staff, offered in conjunction with other groups. Topics available include the following: (1) starting to practice smart; (2) joining a partnership or group; (3) financial control of your practice in 30 minutes a day; (4) the competitive edge: tips and tools for a medical practice; (5) billing and collecting in a medical practice; (6) personnel principles: building a practice team; (7) quality service; (8) positive relationships for patients and staff; (9) electronic billing; (10) CPT coding; (11) ICD-9 coding. Call 1-800-366-6968 to enroll.
- Practice Management Helpline
  Direct access to a health specialist at the AMA. Call 1-800-AMA-1066.
- Practice Tips
  AMA Financing and Practice Services, Inc., offers a variety of tips from the pros in a free booklet, the *Physician's Financing/Management Source Book.* Tips are offered on topics such as unsecured lines of credit, lease versus purchase of office equipment, phone smarts, and collection tips. Call 1-800-366-6968.
- Practice Management Tutorial
  A personal practice management instructor can give you an introduction to the business aspects of medical practice and what to look for before you join a group or partnership. You can team up with a few of your colleagues and arrange for this personalized, interactive learning experience to be conducted at your site. The tutorial combines highlights from several popular practice management workshops. Spouses are encouraged to attend. Time and travel costs can be reduced by bringing the AMA instructor to your site. Call 1-800-366-6968.
- AMA'S *Physicians Socioeconomic Statistics*
  The information you need for success in hospital marketing and staffing and determining compensation levels and hours for hospital medical staff. This resource offers reliable, accurate data and analysis of physician fees, hours, patient visits, income, expenses, and weeks worked. Call 1-800-621-8335; order #OP193100. Also available on CD-ROM.
- AMA's *Medical Groups in the U.S.*
  The ideal reference for anyone interested in current trends or involved with planning for the ongoing success of any existing group. The only source of comprehensive information on medical groups. It summarizes and analyzes the latest survey data and census information for more than 16,000 medical groups throughout the country. Call 1-800-621-8335; order #OP390398.
- MGMA's *The Development and Management of Medical Groups*
  For those interested in forming a group practice or learning about the group practice model and how it works, this is the book! This text provides a solid understanding of what group practice is, how it originated, and what market forces are making group practice attractive to physicians. Practical information on forming a group practice, implementing a group practice model, developing physician compensation plans, understanding governance issues, physician-administrator relations, and group practice economics is given. 1996. Call 303-397-7877; order #OLC-4856.
- *Code of Medical Ethics: Current Opinions with Annotations*
  This collection of ethical opinions provides you and your patients with guidance on today's issues and problems: genetic testing, rationing of health care, withdrawal of life-sustaining medical treatment, reproductive issues, and economic conflicts of interests. It also includes: principles of medical ethics (core ethical principles), fundamental elements of the patient-physician relationship (basic rights to which patients are entitled from their physicians), and patient responsibilities. Call 1-800-621-8335; order #OP632398.

APPENDIX 19-6   TIPS FOR WORKING WITH A MANAGEMENT CONSULTANT OR ATTORNEY

1. When you are formally engaging the services of a management consultant or attorney, you will

need to have some type of contract or letter prepared that defines the terms agreed to.

2. Prepare the staff and other physicians for the arrival of the consultant if the project involves working on site. The presence of a consultant may be an imposition on staff members, especially if they were unaware that problems existed in the practice.

3. Cooperate with the attorney or consultant. If relevant practice information is requested, comply. For example, a consultant may want to review many years' history of insurance payments while conducting a reimbursement audit. Or it might be necessary to pull medical records to review documentation. Assign a key staff person to be the consultant's on-site contact.

4. Request ongoing progress reports. The consultant or attorney should be keeping you posted about how things are going.

5. Listen to the consultant's or attorney's recommendations with an open mind. If you don't agree with something being suggested, speak up. However, be willing to compromise. The advantages a consultant or attorney brings to the situation are expertise and objectivity.

6. Implement the consultant's or attorney's recommendations with a positive attitude. Impending change is daunting.

7. If you are unhappy with the way the consultant or attorney performs, speak up. Poor communication is the most frequently cited cause of a deteriorating relationship and unfavorable results.

SOURCE: Adapted from the American Academy of Family Physicians, 2000, with permission. FP Assist: Tips for working with a management consultant or attorney. Leawood, KS, AAFP, 2000 (http://www.aafp.org/fpassist).

APPENDIX 19-7   CRITERIA FOR SELECTING A PRACTICE MANAGEMENT CONSULTANT OR ATTORNEY

1. **Availability.** How quickly are you able to speak to a consultant? Did the consultant call you back? If so, how quickly? Was the consultant you talked with the one who would be assigned to work with the practice? Was the initial phone consultation free?
   Why? The responsiveness of a consulting or law firm to your initial inquiry is a significant indicator of how interested it is in engaging you as a client. If the firm is overly subscribed, it may not have the time to give your situation the attention it deserves. In some instances, the consultant with whom you initially speak will not be the consultant who works with you. Your project may be assigned to another consultant/attorney in the firm. That is not necessarily a drawback, but you will need to consider that individual's qualifications. Last, find out whether the initial inquiry is billable. You don't want to be surprised down the road by a statement. Typically, most firms will not charge a prospective client for an initial inquiry.

2. **Situation analysis.** Describe your practice problem to the consultant or attorney. It is a good sign if he or she asks questions that indicate experience with the problem(s) at hand.
   Why? A consultant or attorney who either asks nothing or reflects a "been there, done that" attitude either knows little about your particular situation or may be acting in a dismissive or patronizing manner and may not be prepared to devote the necessary attention to your account should you hire him or her.

3. **Fees.** How does the firm bill for its services?
   Why? Some firms bill on an hourly basis. Others will have a flat rate for performing a specific service, such as contract evaluation or a practice survey. Travel expenses—such as transportation, lodging, meals, and incidentals such as long-distance phone calls—for the consultant or attorney are always billable to the client. Get the specifics in writing. Does air fare mean coach or first class? What follow-up services will the practice be billed for (such as additional training, phone support, or reports)?

4. **Conflict of interest.** Does the firm have a vested interest in a particular product, such as a software package?
   Why? If a firm is supporting a particular product, regardless of what it is, there is an incentive for its clients to use that product. Therefore, the consultant or attorney may try hard to get your practice to use it. Is he or she really trying to sell you something?

5. **References.** Have the firm provide you with references, particularly from practices that are similar to you own. Contact them!
   Why? You'll want to talk to other physician practices that have used the firm's services to assess

their level of satisfaction. Granted, a firm is not going to give you the names of clients who were not happy. Nonetheless, it is essential that you check this out on your own. If a firm will not provide you with appropriate references, that is a huge red flag!

6. **Formalize the offer.** If it looks like a "go," ask the consulting firm to provide your practice with a written request for proposal (RFP) or request for quote (RFQ). For a law firm, request a letter of engagement.

    Why? Having the consulting or law firm spell out up front the services it will provide and an estimate of the cost will let you know up front what you can expect to result from the professional relationship. Appendix 19-6 outlines tips for working successfully with a consultant or attorney.

7. **Inform your staff.** Let them know that an attorney or consultant will be visiting the practice and most likely will enlist their assistance.

    Why? To lessen the anxiety of your employees. It is perfectly natural that they will deem the presence of an "outsider" as the end of their employment, which more often than not is a total misconception. In addition, the consultant or attorney will need access to crucial data, such as medical charts or billing information. Therefore the cooperation of the staff is needed to make the encounter successful.

APPENDIX 19-8   SAMPLE JOB DESCRIPTION

Title: Billing/Insurance Clerk
Supervisor: Meredith Simpson, Office Manager
Hours: 8:00 a.m. to 5:00 p.m., Monday to Friday, occasional weekends.
Responsibilities
  Accurately posts all daily charges and payments into the computer system.
  Prints the daily activity and audit reports.
  Files claims electronically.
  Prepares and mails patient statements on a monthly basis.
  Reviews remittance reports from insurance companies.
  Responds to patient requests regarding statements and payments.

Additional responsibilities include providing back-up assistance and phone coverage to the receptionist and other duties as assigned. The position requires good verbal communication skills and a customer service attitude. Working knowledge of medical billing software and Medicare regulations is preferable.
Qualifications
  High school graduate
  Minimum of 2 years' employment experience, preferably within a health care environment.
  Typing speed of 60 wpm.
  Familiarity with basic principles of accounting.
  Familiarity with ICD-9 and CPT coding.
  Familiarity with medical terminology.
  10-key by touch.
The Simpson Clinic is an Equal Opportunity Employer.

APPENDIX 19-9   INTERNET RESOURCES[a]

- Bureau of Primary Health Care Programs: http://www.bphc.hrsa.dhhs.gov/bphc/index 1.htm
  The BPHC is the largest bureau within the Health Resources and Services Administration and provides support for high-quality community-based preventive and primary care.

- *Family Practice Management:* http://www.aafp.org/fpm/
  The official practice management journal of the American Academy of Family Physicians helps family physicians adapt their practices to the changing health care system.

- Federal Office of Rural Health Policy: http://www.nal.usda.gov/orhp/
  The ORHP operates out of the U.S. Health Resources and Services Administration.

- FP Assist: http://www.aafp.org/fpassist/
  FP Assist is available on the AAFP's Web site and is a clearinghouse to find consultants or attorneys to assist in rural practice management. Consultants can assist you in the following areas: practice overview, office operations, practice start-up, billing/collections/reimbursement, patient relations/marketing, financial issues, practice valuations, medical practice planning, personnel issues, computerization, medical records, personal financial management and retirement planning, partnership

issues/physician relations, managed care issues, physician office laboratory issues, office planning and new building design, practice consolidation, physician-hospital issues, practice management instruction, rural health issues and/or rural health clinic (RHC) conversion. The Web site is divided into two sections, ConsultLink and LawLink.

- FP Net: http://www.aafp.org/fpnet/
  FP Net is the American Academy of Family Physicians' clearinghouse for computerization resources.
- Medical Group Management Association: http://www.mgma.com/
  MGMA is the leading organization for group medical practice professionals.
- The National Organization of State Offices of Rural Health: http://www.ruralcenter.org/nosorh/
  NOSORH is an influential voice for state rural health concerns. The members of NOSORH strive to develop increased communication and involvement with the 50 State Offices of Rural Health, build strong relationships with other health care groups, and find the sources of revenue to improve its effectiveness and can help physicians locate resources necessary for successful practice.
- National Rural Health Association: http://www.nrharural.org/
  A national membership organization whose mission is to improve the health and health care of rural Americans and to provide leadership on rural issues through advocacy, communications, education, and research.
- National Rural Health Resource Center: http://ruralcenter.org/nrhrc/
- National Rural Health Services Research Database: http://www.muskie.usm.maine.edu/rhsr/default.asp
  The Federal Office of Rural Health Policy's database of funded rural health services research projects under way in the United States.
- Practicing in Underserved Areas: Funding resources: http://www.aafp.org/special/resource/index.html
  This directory has been prepared to identify and describe financial aid programs, scholarships, fellowships, grants, awards, and other incentives to attract and retain health care personnel in scarcity areas.
- Quality Clearinghouse: http://www.aafp.org/quality/
  This AAFP site is devoted to helping family physi-

cians with resources to improve the quality of care they provide and links to national guidelines for care.

- Rural Health Information: http://www.scan.org/ruralhealth.html
  Provides resources relating to rural health care issues including health care access, health care financing, health care professions education for rural practice, and rural research funding, to name a few.
- Rural Health Resources: http://ahec.msu.montana.edu/ruralhealth/resources.html
  Federal Office of Rural Health Policy (ORHP) links to other federal, national, and state resources.
- Rural Information Center Health Service: http://www.nal.usda.gov/ric/richs/richs.htm
  RICHS is a joint project of the Office of Rural Health Policy, the Department of Health and Human Services, the National Agricultural Library (NAL), and the U.S. Department of Agriculture.
- Rural Information Center Publications: http://www.nal.usda.gov/ric/ricpubs/abtricpb.html
  The RIC publications cover a broad range of topics. Publications are divided into two categories in this menu. The first is Rural publications, and the second is Rural Health publications.
- Rural Family Medicine: http://www.ruralfamilymedicine.org/
  The Official Site of STFM Rural Interest Group, which has information for family practice residents and practicing physicians about rural America; it presents sites giving an overview of the sociocultural factors of rural life.
- Rural Health Web-Ring: http://www.ruralhealth.org.au/
  This ring comprises sites dedicated to rural health issues. It includes government, educational, and hospital sites that contain information relevant to rural health.
- Rural Health Grants—HRSA: http://www.nnlm.nlm.nih.gov/scr/scnn/9701/Hrsgrant.html
  A list of rural health grants from the Health Resources and Services Administration's (HRSA) Office of Rural Health Policy for Rural Health Outreach, Network Development, and Telemedicine Grant programs.
- Rural Recruitment and Retention Network: http://www.3rnet.org/
  The Triple R Net is made up of 45 state-based organizations such as State Offices of Rural Health, Area Health Education Cooperatives (AHECs), Coopera-

tive Agreement Agencies, and State Primary Care Associations.

[a]Although these Internet sites were active at the time of publication, the Internet is a fluid medium and some or many of the site addresses given above may have changed. However, in general, the organization names should still be accurate and may be found with an Internet search engine.

Resources to Read

Medical Group Management Association's (MGMA) *Group Practice Personnel Policies Manual* discusses such standard personnel issues as selection, compensation, and evaluation but also adds policies related to legislation such as the Americans with Disabilities Act (ADA) and the Family and Medical Leave Act (FMLA). It also highlights policies related to issues of workplace violence and electronic communications. It includes a disk of generic policies that can be used or modified as appropriate. The 1997 price was $150.

Would your practice do better as a certified Rural Health Clinic? *Fam Pract Mgt*, November/December 1995, p 58.

Wade TL, Brooks EF: *Planning and Managing Rural Health Centers*. Cambridge, MA, Ballinger, 1979.

1. Carlson RP: The art of choosing the right practice consultant. *Fam Pract Mgt*, April 1997. http://www.aafp.org/fpm/970400fm/cover.html.

CHAPTER 20

Quality of Care in Rural Settings: Bringing the "New Quality" to Rural Practice

JOHN B. COOMBS

A CASE FOR QUALITY

You have recently been elected to the board of your local hospital district. During the election, your platform was based on returning the local health care delivery system to the level of trust and quality it had been known for in the past. Now—along with your fellow four commissioners, the hospital administrator and her staff, and the local physicians—you are anxious to begin addressing local concerns that the quality of care has been slipping and your once respected hospital is now thought to be second rate. Despite the rumors and concerns, in the recent election, the community passed a bond issue focused on infusing capital into the hospital to bolster its worsening financial condition and the threat posed by less Medicare money, given the Balanced Budget Act now being put in place. You had interpreted this action as a tangible show of support for local health care and a vote of confidence that solutions to the emergency concerns could be found. Several pieces of information are available to you beyond the financial information:

• A recent survey of district residents commissioned by the hospital administrator confirmed local concerns on quality: poor service in the emergency room, nurses who did not seem to care, and poor condition of home health care when patients were "pushed out the door" before they were ready to go home.
• The local general surgeon had retired after 35 years of practice, and there was a lack of confidence in his newly recruited partner—this coupled with rumors of bad outcomes after surgery at your hospital.
• A recent newspaper article (with an accompanying op-ed piece) indicated that hospitals not accredited by the Joint Commission (JC) provided poorer care than those that were accredited, and that they lacked public scrutiny. The op-ed piece pointed out the decision of your hospital 8 years ago to give up seeking JC accreditation because it cost too much.
• Following a publicly covered local lawsuit, two of the community's most popular family physicians decided to drop obstetrics from their practice, forcing many residents to seek care 30 miles away.

As a new board member, where might you start to address these concerns and begin to return the hospital to its once trusted position and perceived quality? You decide to start by learning more about what makes up quality in rural settings and to discover some of the things that are known about the composition of quality in rural hospitals.

Access, Quality, and Cost— The Rural Environment

Over the course of the last decade, driven by the continued, dramatic rise in the cost of health care, the states and the federal government have attempted to create sweeping changes in health care through public policy initiatives. During these years, cost reduction, insurance reform, and universal coverage were at the center of the debate. For the most part, access—centering around universal sponsorship, service, and quality—seldom was the primary focus of change.

Quality was taken as a given. There appeared to be no crisis in quality, and—for most of those involved in health care reform—issues of cost were addressed as if we had quality to spare.

In rural America, access has been and remains the central issue in health care delivery. Many rural communities do not have access to basic health services—primary care, specialty consultation, health promotion and disease prevention, emergency care, substance abuse treatment, mental health, and occupational health. Access to care in underserved areas is even more difficult for the uninsured and elderly, who make up a greater proportion of the rural population compared to their urban counterparts.

The public debate on lowering cost has not been focused on rural areas. Although approximately 25 percent of the U.S. population lives in rural areas with proportionally more elderly residents than in urban areas, less than 5 percent of the Medicare budget and 6 percent of overall hospital expenditures[1] are actually spent in rural communities. The shortage of primary care and the dearth of tertiary centers in rural communities has limited the number of costly procedures and hospital services delivered. Geographic barriers and their associated problems have also limited access to such specialized care for rural residents.

Managed Care and Rural Communities

In an effort to reduce the burden for the federal budget created by the rising cost of Medicare and an aging U.S. population, managed Medicare (also known as Medicare part C/Medicare HMO) has been developed. This product capitates providers and attempts to make costs more predictable for the federal government. The penetration of managed Medicare, like other managed care programs, into rural areas has been slower than in most urban areas. Data from

TABLE 20-1   PERCENT OF (ELIGIBLE) POPULATION ENROLLED IN COMMERCIAL, MEDICAID, AND MEDICARE HMOs AND PREPAID HEALTH PLANS

	Rural	Urban
Commercial HMOs (8 states)	7.8%	25.7%
Medicaid (all states)	10.5%	27.1%
Medicare (all states)	0.7%	10.8%

SOURCE: From Moscovice et al.,[3] with permission.

1995 presented in Table 20-1 demonstrate these differences. The percentage of rural capitated managed care for Medicare is approximately one-tenth of that seen in urban areas; for commercial and Medicaid, it is one-third.

Reasons most frequently cited for this lag in HMO growth in rural communities are the lack of provider networks; low per capita cost indices, which limit reimbursement; and the low population density of Medicare recipients found in many rural communities.[4] The perception by many plans that adverse selection (sicker and more complex patients) is more prevalent in rural communities has not been confirmed by a recent study focused on four chronic conditions.[5]

No objectively gathered information about the quality of care provided under managed care in rural communities has been published to date.

Attempts to reduce costs so far have primarily depended on "managed competition" between multiple providers within a given locale. As a consequence, the introduction of managed care has been more rapid in urban settings. Given the lag in rural communities, these new directions in the methods under which care is provided run the risk of decreasing access to care, especially for Medicare, in rural settings.

Through all of this public debate, interest in cost containment, and movement toward managed care, how has quality been judged? The recently published Institute of Medicine's Roundtable on Health Care Quality[6] concludes that the answer to this question is, "not well." Noting that the quality of health care can now be "precisely defined and measured with a degree of scientific accuracy comparable to that of most measures used in clinical medicine," the report concludes that serious and widespread problems exist throughout American medicine, in both small and large communities, and it calls for a systematic effort to overhaul how we deliver health care services.

Perception of Quality in Rural Health

The quality of medical care provided in rural communities has generally been perceived to be inferior to that available in urban settings. In 1992, Keeler and colleagues from the Rand Corporation[7] published a study that examined five diseases in the Medicare population derived from random samples of 297 hospitals taken from 1981 to 1982 and 1985 to 1986. The study concluded that "quality varies from state to state, but teaching, larger and more urban hospitals have better quality in general than nonteaching, small and rural hospitals." The study acknowledges that outcomes and explicitly measured criteria significantly improved in rural hospitals between the two time periods, although the study considered only medical diseases (as opposed to surgical, obstetric, or pediatric diseases). Nevertheless, a media blitz was ignited, noting poor quality in rural communities and strengthening the call for closure of "unnecessary" rural facilities. Other reports, not accorded similar media interest, have shown that the quality of care in rural facilities is equal to or better than that provided in larger urban facilities. Two examples include Welch et al.,[8] who considered a variety of quality indicators and found that the surgical care provided in rural hospitals had better overall outcomes when compared with urban controls. Measuring the frequency of adverse events (injuries caused by medical intervention) in New York hospitals, Brennan and colleagues[9] found that these rates were lower in rural facilities.

Over the course of the last 15 years, nearly 10 percent of the approximately 2800 U.S. rural hospitals have closed. From 1980 to 1990, a total of 558 acute care facilities closed, 60 percent of which were rural. By 1995, following a variety of mergers and a continued annual closure rate on average of 2.5 percent, only 2236 rural hospitals remained open, with approximately 183,000 beds.[10] These closures, forced largely by failing finances and the inability to attract adequate providers into small communities, contributed to the perception that many rural facilities were unnecessary. Furthermore, they gave credibility to the feeling that such closures would not adversely affect the quality of care available to local residents. Adding to this widely accepted view was the fact that 75 percent of the approximately 50 rural hospitals that closed in 1988 were within 20 miles of the next hospital.[11] What appeared on the surface to have a minimal effect on access and quality actually carried significant consequences for reduced quality of care within the rural communities affected. Nesbitt and colleagues,[12] focusing on obstetric cases, noted a significant increase in morbidity and cost to local residents when their hospital closed. Contrary to Keeler's statement that "despite their generally lower quality, rural hospitals symbolize a small town's identity, provide means to attract physicians that will make medical care more convenient, and provide jobs for the community,"[7] rural hospitals appear to contribute to better outcomes and quality of care for the population as a whole. One expects that these improved outcomes are particularly significant to those low-income residents without the means to travel, given the generally poor availability of public transportation in rural communities. This sequence of information again underscores the key role that access plays in the overall quality and outcomes of care in rural settings.

Rural and Urban—The Evolution of Assuring Quality

In 1982, Congress introduced a new method for monitoring the performance of physicians and hospitals providing care to Medicare beneficiaries. The earlier system utilizing approximately 200 Professional Standards Review Organizations (PSROs) designed to introduce peer review was replaced by a smaller number of statewide utilization and quality-control peer review organizations (PROs). Whereas PSROs could only recommend that payment be denied when poor quality was discovered, PROs could actually deny Medicare reimbursement and recommend a range of other sanctions, including exclusion from the program. In the first years of the program, a disproportionate number of rural providers were sanctioned. Several sanctions occurred in Texas, creating several cases where the only hospital and physician in a rural community were threatened with exclusion. A review of these procedures led to the requirement that groups responsible for rural peer review would include practicing rural physicians and brought about a change in due process in order to protect providers from any bias introduced by reviewers during the review proceedings.

A key principle emerging from this debate was that the standard of care in both rural and urban settings should be considered to be the same, though access and geographic distances might substantially modify how care was provided. Two examples of this difference in delivery included a greater utilization of rural facilities "for social reasons" and the use of "itinerant surgeons," the latter being surgeons who periodically provided surgical care in a rural community but primarily practiced elsewhere. In 1988, with less than full support of the American College of Surgery, the American Hospital Association recognized the importance of itinerant surgery to access to care for rural citizens and went on to develop a set of parameters to guide rural hospitals in the quality oversight of outreach surgeons. These were the American Hospital Association's *Guidelines for Credentialing Outreach Surgeons*, published in 1988.

Challenges to Providing Quality Medical Care in Rural Settings

Several key factors influence medicine's ability to provide quality medical care and the oversight of quality in rural communities:

1. *Inadequate providers: incomplete services across the full continuum of care.* As mentioned above, many rural communities are underserved and most suffer from a lack of services involving such areas as mental health, substance abuse, specialty consultation, and occupational health.

2. *Inadequate financial resources.* Most rural hospitals are either losing money or operating with thin margins. They are disadvantaged by differential payments for government programs that favor urban reimbursement, and inadequate financial resources are the unfortunate norm among rural hospitals. The commonly evoked phrase "No margin, no mission, and lower quality" seems especially applicable to rural facilities and providers. Lack of adequate capital reduces the ability of the rural provider to invest in new technology, including information systems.

3. *Volume-outcome relationship.* Certain surgical procedures exhibit a volume-outcome relationship in which a higher volume of patients undergoing a procedure at a hospital is associated with better outcomes.[13] However, this relationship, using mortality as a measure, does not seem to exist in all diagnoses, especially those conditions commonly cared for in small rural hospitals.[14]

4. *Bypass of rural providers by rural patients.* Patients frequently perceive that "bigger is better"—that smaller providers do not have the latest technology and that rural physicians are less qualified.[15] The choice by patients to bypass local providers may substantially reduce the volume of patients served, select for the cases seen, and reduce the base upon which providers can sustain services, potentially undermining the viability of a physician's practice.

5. *The lack of a system.* Most rural providers are independent and frequently compete for sparse resources. The absence of a cooperative system to bring small rural providers together often does not allow for the sharing of resources to address quality issues or benchmark outcomes. Two examples of successful efforts to create a system to support

quality have been published. Both describe cooperative efforts to link providers for the purpose of instituting a quality improvement program.[16] One demonstrated the cooperative collection of data to support change in the care of patients with myocardial infarction.[17]

6. *Distance and geographic barriers.* The often wide distribution of providers and seasonal change in the nature of geographic barriers to transportation create the need for unique approaches to care that are absent in urban settings.

7. *Constraints on quality assurance.* Within hospitals, smaller numbers of patients, fewer clinical departments, a smaller number of patients per disease category, and limited dedicated support staff all make conducting quality review more challenging. The small number of physicians on a rural medical staff, peer relationships, and limited numbers within a given specialty also make peer review difficult. Confidentiality and the lack of technical support require innovative approaches and careful attention to the process of review.

8. *Limited automated information management support.* Although, overall, the availability of automated clinical information is increasing for hospitals in general, the American Hospital Association (AHA) reports that fewer than 20 percent of all hospitals (both urban and rural) are set up to regularly provide profiles of quality measures routinely collected. Again, the relative paucity of capital, coupled with other more pressing needs for precious dollars, limits the availability of information systems to track clinical indicators, utilization statistics, and other outcome measures. Though lagging behind urban areas, the increased presence of managed care plans accredited by the National Committee on Quality Assurance (NCQA) should increase the availability of periodic reports in rural communities through the use of Health Plan Employer Data and Information Set (HEDIS) measures discussed below.

9. *Appropriateness of accreditation standards for rural hospitals.* Since 1988, the Joint Commission on Accreditation of Healthcare Organizations (JCAHO), responding to the fact that the majority of rural facilities are not accredited, has changed the composition of site-visit teams to include visitors familiar with small rural facilities. In addition, changes made in 1998 in the accreditation standards and performance measures to better reflect rural quality care and accommodate rural facilities and attempts to keep the cost of accreditation reasonable have been made. These efforts focused on encouraging more rural hospitals to seek accreditation.

To date, the NCQA has not initiated a similar look at the potential need to modify the HEDIS data set in order to clearly reflect quality in rural communities. Failure to do so has limited the usefulness of HEDIS measures to rural providers.

The remainder of this chapter further explores what is currently known about the practice and measurement of quality in rural communities. The evolution of the "new quality" embodied in evidence-based medicine is examined and explored from a rural perspective. Finally, challenges and future directions for quality measurement in rural communities are examined.

WHAT WE KNOW ABOUT QUALITY IN RURAL PRACTICE

Perception of Quality and Satisfaction of Service

From 1985 through 1988, the WWAMI* Rural Hospital Project (RHP) (supported by the W. K. Kellogg Foundation) assisted selected communities in improving the financial stability and quality of their local health care systems.[18] In

---

* *WWAMI* stands for the Washington, Wyoming, Alaska, Montana, and Idaho regional medical education program based at the University of Washington School of Medicine.

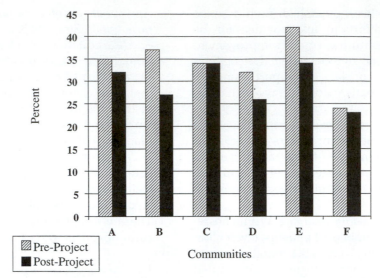

FIGURE 20-1 *Percent of respondents with nonlocal hospitalizations that indicated they did not use the local hospital because of concern about the quality of care—1985 and 1989.*

most of the project communities, substantial improvements were recognized, including better organizational performance, increased surgical volume (2- to 10-fold increase), enhanced hospital market share (increased by as much as 6 percent), higher operating margin (up to 9.1 per-

cent), and favorable public satisfaction with hospital services (up to a 13 percent increase). Within the six communities studied, the RHP surveyed the opinions of rural residents regarding the quality of care provided by local hospitals and providers. Figures 20-1 and 20-2, taken

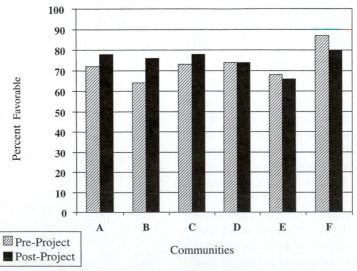

FIGURE 20-2 *Evaluation of overall quality of local hospital care—1985 and 1989.*

from results of the project, demonstrate, among project communities, both baseline opinions of perceived quality and any changes following implementation of the project objectives.

If perception is reality (or at least a reflection of reality), patient and community levels of satisfaction for services are also a reflection of the overall value that is placed on available health care. Looking beyond inpatient services, the project also measured satisfaction with services across the full continuum of care. Results presented in Fig. 20-3 are the averages in 22 rural communities.[18]

These results reflect both access to and satisfaction with specific services within a rural community. During the early 1990s, fueled by health care reform, a dramatic increase in many of the services depicted in Fig. 20-3 occurred. Most of the new services were developed by rural hospitals. Table 20-2 summarizes the highlights of this growth, which occurred from 1991 to 1995.[7] A substantial percentage of increased outpatient (OP) visits came from outreach specialty visits from neighboring urban communities, enhancing access to specialty consultation within the community.

Quality of Specific Programs and Disease Management

A review of the literature reveals a limited number of studies that specifically examine the quality of care provided in rural communities. Table 20-3 summarizes the area and number of studies found in the literature. In the following, these studies and their findings are briefly reviewed.

The greatest number of entries in the literature were in the management and prevention of trauma in rural communities. All studies noted a higher mortality rate for vehicular accidents in rural areas.[19] Reports centered on direct trauma center transfer versus local hospital use and reduction of preventable deaths. A study done in Virginia[20] concluded that direct transfer to trauma centers brought improved outcomes, whereas in Washington State,[21] the authors concluded that the primary use of rural hospitals

did not result in increased mortality rates and did appear to reduce unnecessary transfers and their associated costs and family burden. A carefully done study in Florida[22] found that the situations involved in producing injury (high posted speed and dark road environment, more prevalent in rural settings) was primarily responsible for the greater mortality rates in rural areas—more so than the availability and accessibility of medical care.

Whereas one study did not find obvious preventable deaths in rural areas,[21] most reported overall preventable death rates of approximately 13 percent.[23,24] In comparing rural with urban outcomes, preventable deaths were found to be twofold higher in rural, prehospital time (trauma scene to hospital transport time), first physician contact (sixfold higher), and crude death rate (threefold higher) when compared with urban settings.[25] In looking across studies, one concludes that a consistently higher rate of adverse outcomes from trauma occurs in rural areas. In addition, given variation by state in reported outcomes, the organization of trauma care and protocol followed for such care in a given rural locale is best determined either locally or by region. In many settings, especially where distances are greatest, the role of the rural hospital improves trauma care and contributes to better outcomes. Efforts to decrease emergency medical service (EMS) response time and to provide continuing education and training in trauma care for rural hospital-based emergency care providers are the recommendations most frequently made by researchers. However, as underscored in the Florida study,[22] the factors relevant to rural areas of high posted speed and dark road environment represent ongoing challenges to reducing the carnage created in rural communities by motor vehicle accidents.

In the area of children's health, Bronstein et al.[26] reported substantial differences in the care provided to rural and urban Medicaid recipients with the diagnosis of urinary tract infection (UTI) and otitis media (OM). The study showed that, when compared with that in similar urban settings, care provided in rural communities

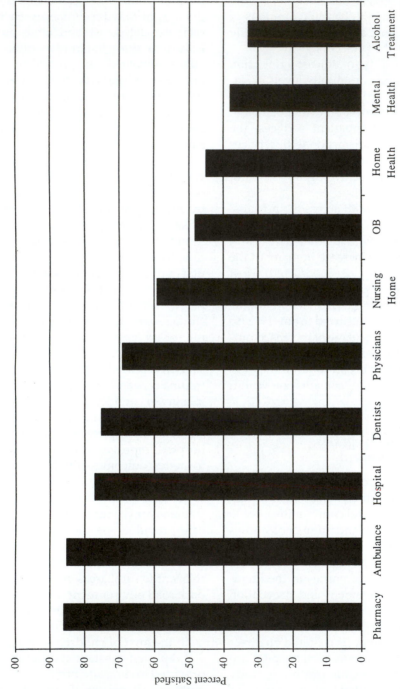

FIGURE 20-3 *Average satisfaction rates for various medical services within 22 rural communities.*

TABLE 20-2   GROWTH OF CONTINUUM OF CARE SERVICES SPONSORED BY RURAL HOSPITALS 1991–1995

	1991	1995	% Change
Skilled nursing care	678	811	+19.6%
Hospice	285	498	+74.7%
Home health service	828	1138	+37.4%
Nonemergency outpatient service			+88.3%

was less expensive, with fewer ancillary services and facility charges. However, in considering quality indicators, rural providers used fewer urine cultures (UTI) and were less likely to see the child back after the acute illness (OM). This lower utilization was judged by the authors as being below standard. Carcillo et al.[27] reported that, over a 3-year period, the introduction of consistent preventive services and comprehensive care to an underserved rural community reduced hospitalizations and emergency department visits and also decreased the number of low-birth-weight infants as well as the risk of congenital syphilis, childhood tuberculosis, and child mortality. While not disparaging the quality of rural services, this study again underscores the important role of improved access within underserved rural areas in benefiting the overall health status of the community.

The nature and quality of perinatal services

TABLE 20-3   RURAL QUALITY OF CARE LITERATURE BY TOPIC AND NUMBER OF STUDIES

Area of Study	Number of Studies
Myocardial infarction	1
Childhood illness prevention	2
Health promotion in the elderly	2
Surgery	1
Perinatal care	3
Diabetes	1
Mental health	3
Trauma care	7

in rural areas are described in several published studies.[12,28,29] Hart et al.[29] observed that rural providers use fewer overall resources (fewer intrapartum days, less epidural anesthesia) than their urban counterparts while noting no difference in outcomes between the two groups. Nesbitt and coworkers[12] noted that when local care is not available and women are required to leave their community for obstetric care, a greater proportion of complicated deliveries as well as higher rates of prematurity and higher costs of neonatal care are seen as compared with care in a local rural hospital. These studies indicate comparable quality of rural care to urban care but again underscore the critical role that access plays in determining optimal outcomes in rural communities.

Myocardial infarction (MI) and diabetes care in rural areas have also been studied from a quality perspective. Hand[30] studied the outcomes of MI when no facility for cardiac catheterization existed in rural hospitals. When compared with suburban and urban sites where cardiac catheterization was most often immediately available, comparable rates of transfers, admissions, and complications were found. The mean in-hospital mortality rates for rural hospitals did not significantly differ from those at the other sites despite the absence of immediate access to cardiac catheterization. Catheterization rates in the suburban and urban facilities ranged from 8 to 20 percent. The authors concluded that the absence of high-technology mechanical methods for reperfusion (as is the case in most rural facilities) may not increase mortality from MI. Zoorob and colleagues[31] studied the practice patterns of rural family physicians in the management of non-insulin-dependent diabetes mellitus. Using a retrospective record review and comparing documented indicators with American Diabetes Association standards, rural areas were considered to be below standard in the use of dietary counseling (66 percent), exercise counseling (33 percent), and performance of glycosolated hemoglobin (15 percent) and annual funduscopic (66 percent) and foot (64 percent) examinations. However, the study failed to use appropriate controls, thus limiting its usefulness.

In the area of mental health, three studies reviewed the availability of mental health services and the treatment of depression in rural communities. Looking at the perceptions of rural Wisconsin residents of the availability and quality of mental health services, Tarnan and Menz[32] reported that the availability and quality of both inpatient and outpatient services are better overall for adults and that children, adolescents, and minority and geriatric populations have limited access to needed services. Rost and colleagues[33] studied 21 rural primary care practices and reported that findings demonstrated lower depression detection rates at the initial visit as well as lower 5-month remission rates (32 versus 70 percent) when compared with findings in other studies in urban sites. However, no urban controls were directly provided in this study. The authors noted, among rural practitioners, a low compliance with Agency for Health Care Policy and Research (AHCPR) published guidelines for depression management as to the regimen of antidepressant medications prescribed. The authors concluded that "outcomes for major depression may be worse in rural family practice settings than in urban settings." In another study by the same authors focusing on the management of depression in rural areas,[34] despite fewer per capita providers trained to provide mental health services in the rural study areas, no rural-urban differences were noted in the rate, type, or quality of outpatient treatment for depression. However, significantly fewer specialty care visits for depression were recorded, and depressed rural individuals had a threefold increase in hospitalization for physical and mental health problems. In addition, rural subjects reported significantly more ($p = 0.05$) suicide attempts during the 1-year period. The authors, noting the key influence of access to care, conclude that "additional work is warranted to determine how to alter barriers to outpatient specialty care if the rural health care delivery system is to provide cost-effective depression care."

One concludes from these studies that access to mental health diagnostic and treatment services is the primary component to the provision of quality mental health care within rural communities.

Implementing Quality in Rural Communities

Some literature exists on implementing quality-focused efforts in rural settings.[35-37] Each study carefully tracks the factors that support and the pitfalls encountered when applying continuous quality improvement,[16,38-40] administrative change,[41] audit and feedback,[42] reengineering,[43] and case management to clinical care delivery.[44,45] Reports have also indicated that competition between proximate rural hospitals and their medical staffs often enhances access and the quality of available programs.[46] The use of innovative health promotion programs using waivered services from Medicare and mobile outreach for seniors have also been described,[47,48] though no difference in health outcomes has been reported from these trial programs. However, improved health screening rates, higher immunization rates, and decreased utilization of emergency services have been realized from these efforts.

In each of these process improvement efforts, authors note a similar list of barriers to overcome in implementing quality improvement.

1. *Time constraints.* When implementing a new process improvement, work-load and time constraints of providers are not adequately taken into account and recognized.
2. *Physician autonomy.* Medical staff leadership and support are often lacking.
3. *Technical support.* Rural providers often lack technical support, specifically access to data and outcomes measures.
4. *Limited participation.* Nursing and physician staff are often resistant to change.
5. *Resource constraints.* Small budgets and thin margins challenge planning processes.
6. *Small departments.* It can be difficult to initiate

improvement initiatives in single-person or very small departments.

7. *Lack of benchmarks.* It can be difficult to obtain comparative benchmark data (see Gates[17] for Vermont's approach to this issue).
8. *Volume.* There are challenges in improving low-volume processes.

Many of these issues are the same as those faced in urban settings, though a low volume of processes and a small work-force size are issues unique to rural areas. Some of these barriers have been addressed by rural hospitals affiliating with other rural and/or urban facilities to deal with quality, access, and financial issues. Between 1991 and 1995, there was a substantial increase in the number of rural hospitals joining systems (8.5 percent increase), alliances (4.7 percent increase) and networks (greater than a 30 percent increase).[10] Reports of the successful use of these affiliations for the purpose of quality improvement either do not exist or have not been documented in the literature.

MOVING TOWARD THE "NEW QUALITY"— EVIDENCE-BASED MEDICINE

In the past, quality has been defined and based on the structure or organization of health care delivery systems, the processes by which care is delivered and overseen, and, to a lesser degree, the outcomes of care. Examples of each of these three categories include optimal organization of hospitals (a board, medical staff structure, intensive care units, etc.), processes to support quality (including a delineated credentialing process and quality plan), and tracking of outcome indicators such as mortality and nosocomial infection rates. Similarly, quality assurance was the centerpiece of providing oversight for quality, focusing on adherence to the institutional quality plan, providing peer review, and emphasizing risk-management services. Several reviews on the evolution of quality have recently been written.[49–54]

Over the past decade, quality has evolved toward a substantial if not fundamental change. While the previous focus on "implied quality" was derived from defined structures, processes, and a limited number of reported outcomes, the "new quality" draws its definition from explicit dimensions found in a much wider array of outcome measurements, clinical practice guidelines, and the principles of continuous quality improvement. Quality assurance is being supported by quality assessment and improvement, while retrospective utilization review has given way to concurrent, explicitly defined processes of care (care maps, critical paths) reviewed through periodically reported indicators of process compliance.

With this shift from the "old" quality to the "new," evidence-based medicine (EBM) has emerged.[55,56] EBM embraces four components: scientific and clinical evidence appraisal, explicit process-of-care definition, decision-making support, and outcomes measurement. Figure 20-4 outlines these essential elements and provides examples of components frequently used to build an evidence-based approach to the provision of care.[57]

Successful evidence-based approaches depend on the ability of an organization to generate or obtain data that support outcomes measurement. Linking patient-specific information traditionally found in the medical record with defined "best practice" gleaned from a rapidly evolving base of knowledge and process of care is critical to the optimal application of EBM. The measurement and monitoring of outcomes depend heavily on the availability of timely, accurate data derived from the clinical provider-patient interaction. [58–60]

In addition to the move toward EBM, accreditation of health care institutions and health plans has undergone substantial change in the last decade. The Joint Commission (JC), the traditional accrediting agency for hospitals, initiated its "Agenda for Change," a program designed to identify specific indicators of quality across a broad span of clinical areas. From this initial effort has emerged the IM System and

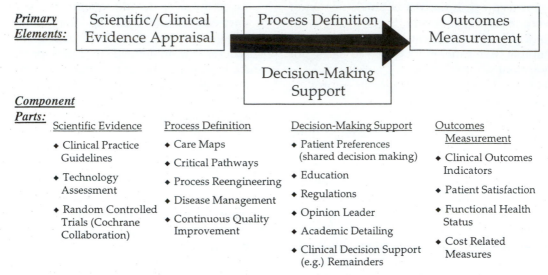

FIGURE 20-4 The primary elements and component parts of evidence-based medicine. (From Coombs J, Norris T: The electronic record: linking patient care and the management of quality in clinical practice. New Med 2:215–222, 1998, with permission.)

National Library of Healthcare Indicators, which provides hospitals and health systems with a base of indicators upon which to measure outcomes of care and monitor processes. These indicators have been integrated into the JC's accreditation process. In 1997, JC began ORYX, which allows hospitals to choose a performance measurement system from among 60 systems contracted with JC. Hospitals and health systems accredited by JC are now required to choose a minimum of 10 separate measurements from one or more of five specified consensus-based measure sets (www.jcaho.org).

In 1988, the National Committee for Quality Assurance (NCQA) was founded to accredit health plans (payers, HMOs, etc.) and develop a standardized data set which would allow industry (as purchasers of health care), providers, and the general public to have access to and compare outcomes of various plans. The Health Plan Employer Data and Information Set (HEDIS) is now being utilized by many groups to rate quality and compare plans (www.ncqa.org). Both the changes made by JC and the emergence of NCQA have provided

further support for the introduction of EBM. To date, no separate rural set of performance measures or quality indicators has been delimitated by either JC or NCQA.

Evidence-Based Medicine in Rural Settings

During this early period of EBM, few differences stand out between EBM as it applies to rural and urban areas. Clinical practice guidelines (CPG) are written for the most part without reference to application in urban or rural settings. This may not always make practical sense. When time frames for various interventions are established (such as the 30-minute decision-to-incision guideline for cesarean section when unrelenting fetal distress is diagnosed), there has not been a rural and an urban guideline but rather just one standard. The assumption that this "one standard fits all" may not be practical.

CPGs have assumed equivalent access to new technology upon which to execute best practice. Though reports of dissemination of new technology in obstetric care reveal near equivalency in rural when compared to urban hospitals,[61,62] the assumption that this is also the case across a vast scope of all health care delivery is unlikely.

Decision support strategies and explicitly defined processes of care (e.g., disease-management critical pathways and case management) appear to show few differences at present between urban and rural settings, though the challenges to be overcome during implementation appear to be somewhat different between the two settings.[14,35,37–42]

However, there appears to be some urban advantage in the ability to measure outcomes. One might expect that, given the substantial financial outlay to create better information systems, rural would lag behind. Likewise, several other factors, such as less detailed claims data (given slower penetration of rural by managed care and systems and the absence of accreditation performance measures and benchmarks specific to rural communities), heighten concern that this gap might widen rather than close. One potential result of this inability of rural areas to keep up with explicit measurement is reinforcement of the still widely held perception that rural medical care delivery is of poor or undetermined quality.

Future Directions and Challenges

The application of the "new quality" embodied in the addition of performance-based measures to the accreditation process and EBM is just beginning throughout the American health care delivery system. In the face of this evolving change, the future of quality in rural health care faces challenges that are different from those in most urban settings.

1. *Access to care remains the single most important element for improving quality in rural communities.* Many rural areas continue to lack easy access to basic physician and hospital services. Most rural communities lack access to basic services across the continuum of care, such as mental health, substance abuse care, hospice, and accessible specialty services. As

mentioned throughout this chapter, once access is addressed, outcomes of care improve in many instances.

2. *Vertical integration of services continues to be the exception rather than the rule in most rural settings.* As mentioned above, horizontal integration across the continuum of care within rural communities continues to have many gaps. Likewise, attempts to create vertical integration between urban-based and rural providers have been traditionally based on simply increased market share for the urban system rather than improvement of access and quality for rural cities.

3. *Information management and system support will be critical to the successful implementation of evidence-based medicine and the "new quality."* This is true in both urban and rural areas, though the scarcity of investment capital for information systems (IS) in rural communities will make this task more challenging and most likely an unattainable goal in the near future. In the absence of adequate IS, rural communities will continue to struggle to demonstrate quality. Some fear that in the long run the failure of IS development in rural areas to keep pace with the rest of the health care industry will make rural practice less viable.

4. *The evidence-based approach should carefully focus on clinical practice guidelines that take into account special challenges presented by the rural setting (implementation barriers, access to technology, etc.) as well as strategies to support definition and implementation of low-volume processes in an explicitly defined fashion.* Given the paucity of rural integrated networks and the relatively slow penetration of managed care into rural settings, dissemination strategies for clinical practice guidelines must also be innovatively crafted so as to assist rural providers in implementing "best practice."

5. *Accreditation bodies must continue to acknowledge the different needs of rural providers and institutions for accreditation standards and performance indicators that specifically reflect quality in rural settings.* Both HEDIS and ORYX

performance measures and indicators of quality must separately address the question of rural care and adjust, as appropriate, the constellation of indicators which truly reflect quality in the rural setting.

WHAT ABOUT THE CASE STUDY?

Having learned something about quality in health care in rural areas, as the new board member you have decided that the following principles of approaching quality concerns in your hospital include:

1. *No margin, no quality.* It is essential that a plan be developed to make sure resources given to the hospital are put to good use—to improve access to services, enhance customer service and a caring attitude among staff, and reinstitute lost or diminished services (such as obstetrics and surgery of high quality) to the point of meeting community needs.
2. *Access to care in rural areas remains the principal component of quality.* This includes adequate services beyond the walls of the hospital (such as home health, long-term care, and hospice) and proper attention to coordination of services for patients.
3. *You cannot manage what you cannot measure.* When you were able to objectively look at outcomes of surgical care, you found that, in fact, outcomes have improved since the introduction of the new surgeon, including patient satisfaction. Now all you need to do is get the work out. You are also convinced that the hospital would be wise to start investing in better information systems that can not only help keep track of business considerations but also measure clinical outcomes.
4. *A fresh look should be taken at seeking accreditation by the JC.*

The quality of health care in rural areas continues to be perceived as being lower than that in urban areas. This is despite studies showing that the quality of rural care, though access-sensitive, is consistently equal to or better than that found in comparable urban settings. The quality of rural care, largely and ideally determined by the degree and scope of access to both basic and specialized services, can be determined only by taking local factors into account—a situation that makes sweeping conclusions difficult and most often inaccurate.

The introduction of evidence-based medicine and the move to create explicitly defined outcome measures upon which to judge quality will further place rural care at a disadvantage in seeking to judge quality. Despite the likelihood of a widening gap in attempts to demonstrate quality differences between rural and urban areas, continued efforts to enhance information sources of clinical measures from rural settings and to assist accreditation agencies to select rurally sensitive accreditation standards and performance measures must be pursued. Only through efforts such as these can the American public be assured of equal access to the abundance of quality medical care available in the United States regardless of where they reside.

REFERENCES

1. Hart LG, Amundson B, Rosenblatt RA: Is there a role for the small rural hospital? *J Rural Health* 6:101–118, 1990.
2. Casey M: *Serving Rural Medicare Risk Enrollees: HMOs' Decisions, Experiences and Future Plans.* Working paper no. 119. Minneapolis, MN, University of Minnesota Rural Health Research Center, November 1997.
3. Moscovice J, Casey M, Krein S: *Rural Managed Care: Patterns and Prospects.* Minneapolis, MN, University of Minnesota Rural Health Research Center, April 1997. www.hsr.unm.edu/centers/rhrc/vhvc.html:
4. Serrato C, Brown RS, Bergeron J: Why do so few HMO's offer Medicare risk plans in rural areas? *Health Care Fin Rev* 17(1):85, 1995.
5. Call KT: Rural beneficiaries with chronic conditions: assessing the risk to Medicare managed care. Working paper no. 23. Minneapolis, MN,

University of Minnesota Rural Health Research Center, May 1998.

6. Chassin MR, Galvin RW, and the National Roundtable on Health Care Quality: The urgent need to improve health care quality. *JAMA* 280(11):1000, 1998.

7. Keeler EB, Rubenstein LV, Kahn KL, et al: Hospital characteristics and quality of care. *JAMA* 268(13):1709, 1992.

8. Welch HG, Larson EH, Hart LG, Rosenblatt RA: Readmission after surgery in Washington state rural hospitals. *Am J Public Health* 82:707, 1992.

9. Brennan TA, Hebert LE, Laird NM, et al: Hospital characteristics associated with adverse events and substandard care. *JAMA* 265:3265, 1991.

10. *A Profile of Non-metropolitan Hospitals 1991–1995*. Chicago, American Hospital Association, AHA Center for Healthcare Leadership, Section for Small or Rural Hospitals, 1997.

11. *MedHealth.* May 14, 1990; 44(19):2.

12. Nesbitt TS, Connell FA, Hart LG, Rosenblatt RA: Access to obstetric care in rural areas: effect on birth outcomes. *Am J Public Health* 80(7):814, 1990.

13. Hughes RG, Hunt SS, Luft HS: Effects of surgeon volume and hospital volume on quality of care in hospitals. *Med Care* 25(6):489, 1987.

14. Schlenker RE, Hittle DF, Hrincevich CA, Kaehny MM: Volume/outcome relationships in small, rural hospitals. *J Rural Health* 12(5):395, 1996.

15. Rieber GM, Benzie D, McMahon S: Why patients bypass rural health care centers. *Minn Med* 79:46, 1996.

16. Busteed S, Barwick S, Grubb L: The challenges of implementing quality improvement in small rural hospitals. *Quality Lett* 25, July–Aug 1994.

17. Gates PE: Think globally, act locally: an approach to the implementation of clinical practice guidelines. *J Qual Improv* 21(2):71, 1995.

18. Rosenblatt R: The WAMI rural hospital project (6 parts). *J Rural Health* 7(5):473, 1991.

19. Mueller BA, Rivara FP, Bergman AB: Urban-rural location and the risk of dying in a pedestrian-vehicle collision. *J Trauma* 28(1):91, 1988.

20. Young JS, Bassam D, Cephas GA, et al: Interhospital versus direct scene transfer of major trauma patients in a rural trauma system. *Am Surg* 64(1):88, 1998.

21. Grossman DC, Hart LG, Rivara F, et al: From roadside to bedside: the regionalization of motor vehicle trauma care in a remote rural county. *J Trauma* 38:14–21, 1995.

22. Miles-Doan R, Kelly S: Inequities in health care and survival after injury among pedestrians: explaining the urban/rural differential. *J Rural Health* 11(3):177, 1995.

23. Maio RF, Burney RE, Gregor MA, Baranski MG: A study of preventable trauma mortality in rural Michigan. *J Trauma* 41(1):83, 1996.

24. Esposito TJ, Sanddal ND, Hansen JD, Reynolds S: Analysis of preventable trauma deaths and inappropriate trauma care in rural state. *J Trauma* 39(5):955, 1995.

25. Esposito TJ, Maier RV, Rivara FP, et al: The impact of variation in trauma care times: urban versus rural. *Prehosp Disaster Med* 10(3):161, 1995.

26. Bronstein JM, Johnson VA, Gargason CA: How rural physicians compare on cost and quality measures for Medicaid ambulatory care episodes. *J Rural Health* 13(2):126, 1997.

27. Carcillo JA, Diegel JE, Bartman BA, et al: Improved maternal and child health care access in a rural community. *J Health Care Poor Underserved* 6(1):23, 1995.

28. Thompson M, Curry MA, Burton D. The effects of nursing case management in the utilization of prenatal care by Mexican-Americans in rural Oregon. *Public Health Nurs* 15(2):82, 1998.

29. Hart LG, Dobie SA, Baldwin LM, et al: Rural and urban differences in physician resource use for low-risk obstetrics. *HSR: Health Services Res* 31(4):429, 1996.

30. Hand R: Rural hospital mortality for myocardial infarction in Medicare patients in Illinois (abstr). *AHSR FHSR Annu Mtg* 12:58, 1995.

31. Zoorob RJ, Mainous A: Practice patterns of rural family physicians based on the American Diabetes Association standards of care. *J Commun Health* 21(3):175, 1996.

32. Tarnan MS, Menz FE: Professional perceptions of availability and quality of mental health services in Wisconsin. *Wisconsin Med J,* January 1997.

33. Rost K, William SC, Wherry J, Smith ER: The process and outcomes of care for major depression in rural family practice settings. *J Rural Health* 11(2):114, 1995.

34. Rost K, Zhang M, Fortney J, et al: Rural-urban differences in depression treatment and suicidally. *Med Care* 36(7):1098, 1998.

35. O'Shaughnessy J, Clark L, Dye N, et al: Success factors for the future survival of rural hospitals. *Best Pract Benchmark Healthcare* 2(1):1, 1997.

36. Merkens B, Spencer JS: A successful and neces-

sary evolution to shared leadership: a hospital's story. *Int J Health Care QA* 11(1):i–iv, 1998.

37. Yasin MM, Green RF: A strategic approach to service quality: a field study in a rural health care setting. *Health Mktg Q* 13(1):75, 1995.

38. Gates PE: Clinical quality improvement: getting physicians involved. *Qual Rev Bull* 19(2):56–61, 1993.

39. Kabcenell AI, Cohen AB, Merrill JC: Importing a model of hospital quality from the Netherlands. *Health Aff (Millwood)* 10(3):240–245, 1991.

40. Dugar B: Implementing CQI on a budget: a small hospital's story. *J Qual Improv* 21(2):57, 1995.

41. Dwore RB, Murray BP, Parsons RI, et al: Revenue enhancement through total quality management / continuous quality improvement (TQM / CQI) in outpatient coding and billing. *J Hosp Mktg* 9(2): 63, 1995.

42. Newell SD, Englert I, Box-Taylor A, et al: Clinical efficiency tools improve stroke management in a rural southern health system. *Stroke* 29:1092, 1998.

43. Furch G, Linderbery J: A rural hospital's zero-based redesign of discharge planning. *Continuum* 16(2):1, 1996.

44. Bertram DA, Thompson MC, Giordano D, et al: Implementation of an inpatient case management program in rural hospitals. *J Rural Health* 12:54, 1996.

45. Bushy A: Case management: considerations for coordinating quality services in rural communities. *J Nurs Care Qual* 12(1):26, 1997.

46. Krein SL, Christianson JB, Chen MM: The composition of rural hospital medical staffs: the influence of hospital neighbors. *J Rural Health* 13(4): 306, 1997.

47. Lave JR, Ives DG, Traven ND, Kuller LH: Evaluation of a health promotion demonstration program for the rural elderly. *HSR: Health Serv Res* 31(3):261, 1996.

48. Alexy BB, Elnitsky C: Rural mobile health unit: outcomes. *Public Health Nurs* 15(1):3, 1998.

49. Blumenthal D: Quality of healthcare: Part I. Quality of care—what is it? *N Engl J Med* 335:891–894, 1996.

50. Brooks R, McGlynn E, Cleary P: Quality of health care: Part 2. Measuring quality of care. *N Engl J Med* 335:966–970, 1996.

51. Chassin M: Quality of health care: Part 3. Improving the quality of care. *N Engl J Med* 335:1060–1062, 1996.

52. Blumenthal D: Quality of health care: Part 4. The origins of the quality-of-care debate. *N Engl J Med* 335:1146–1149, 1996.

53. Berwick D: Quality of health care: Part 5. Payment by capitation and the quality of care. *N Engl J Med* 335:1227–1231, 1996.

54. Brooks R, Karnberg C, McGlynn E: Health system reform and quality. *JAMA* 276:476–480, 1996.

55. Evidence-Based Medicine Working Group: Evidence-based medicine—a new approach to teaching the practice of medicine. *JAMA* 268:2420–2425, 1992.

56. Sackett D, Rosenberg W, Gray J: Evidence-based medicine: what it is and what it isn't. *BMJ* 312:71–72, 1996.

57. Coombs J, Norris T: The electronic record: linking patient care and the management of quality in clinical practice. *New Med* 2:215–222, 1998.

58. Grandia L, Pryor T, Willson D: Building a computer-based record in an evolving integrated health system, in Steen EB (ed): *Proceedings of the First Annual Nicholas E Davies CPR Recognition Symposium*, Schaumburg, IL, Computer-based Patient Record Institute Incorporated, February 1995, pp 5–33.

59. Schoenbaum S, Barnett G: Automated ambulatory medical records systems: an orphan technology. *Int J Technol Assess Health Care* 8:598–609, 1992.

60. Evans R, Burke J, Classen D: Computerized identification of patients and high risk for hospital-acquired infections. *Am J Infect Control* 20:4–10, 1992.

61. Rosenblatt RA, Sanders GR, Tressler CJ, et al: The diffusion of obstetric technology into rural US hospitals. *Int J Technol Assess Health Care* 10(3): 479–489, 1994.

62. Rosenblatt RA, Dawson AJ, Larson EH, et al: A comparison of the investment in hospital-based ultra sound in Wales and Washington state. *Int J Technol Assess Health Care* 11(3):571–584, 1995.

Community-Oriented Primary Care and Rural Health Services Development

ROBERT L. WILLIAMS   PETER J. HOUSE

A young father rushed into the rural clinic cradling his limp toddler. While running on to the clinic's resuscitation room, he gave the history that the child had been well. Earlier that brisk winter day, the family had traveled from their home in an impoverished rural area to a small neighboring city to do some shopping. The child had been well when he was put in the back seat of the car for the 40-mile trip home, and he slept for most of the ride. When the family arrived home, though, they could not wake him and they immediately drove to the clinic.

On arrival in the resuscitation area, the 14-month-old child was unresponsive, with absent vital signs and sluggish pupils. Cardiopulmonary resuscitation was immediately started by the clinic team as diagnostic efforts began. Cardiovascular resuscitation was successful, but there were no spontaneous respirations and the child remained comatose. A screening test for carbon monoxide by the clinic staff suggested a toxic level. The child was airlifted to the regional pediatric intensive care unit on 100% oxygen. Unfortunately the child's condition failed to improve. When brain death was confirmed, the child was taken off life support and died. Definitive tests for carboxyhemoglobin initially drawn at the rural clinic confirmed the cause of death as carbon monoxide poisoning.

A month later, a second infant was brought in to the same clinic unresponsive, with absent vital signs and unreactive pupils. Again, the child had been well until driven from his rural home to a small convenience store, where he had been left in the pickup truck's cab with the engine and heater running while his mother picked up a few grocer-

ies. This time, resuscitation was unsuccessful, and tests again confirmed the cause of death as carbon monoxide poisoning. Subsequent tests performed on the passenger compartment of the vehicles involved in these two cases demonstrated toxic levels of carbon monoxide caused by faulty exhaust systems coupled with car body damage.

In a quiet moment after the second infant's death, one of the clinic physicians reflected on the diagnostic and treatment efforts with the two children. Although both children had received rapid, up-to-date care with maximal technological support, in neither case did it make any difference to the ultimate outcome. For these children, advanced care delivered when the children presented for care was useless. The limits of office- or clinic-based primary care were made strikingly clear by the circumstances of these two children.

In response to the deaths of these children, the clinic launched a program reaching beyond its confines in order to prevent similar deaths in the future. Forming a partnership with public health officials and with small community governing councils in the area, the clinic led a multifaceted program to reduce exposure to vehicular carbon monoxide. Community education was initiated in the clinic, in community meeting houses, and through the radio and newspapers. Screening for toxic carbon monoxide levels in vehicle interiors was carried out by public health officials at area post offices and community meetinghouses. Drivers whose vehicles demonstrated toxic levels were educated about the problem—its mitigation and correction. Data from this program demonstrated that one of every six local vehicles screened exceeded the Environmental Protection Agency's standards for exposure to carbon monoxide. However, over the next 5 years, no further cases of carbon monoxide poisoning were seen at the clinic.

OVERVIEW OF COMMUNITY-ORIENTED PRIMARY CARE

Physicians everywhere fill important roles in their communities, but this is especially true of rural physicians. In small communities, physicians are often called upon for advice or assistance in a variety of community matters, many of which are beyond the scope of clinical practice. Pathman et al.[1] have outlined four ways in which physicians are involved in their communities:

1. By identifying and intervening in the community's health problems.
2. By being aware of local cultural groups' health problems when treating patients.
3. By coordinating the community's health resources in the care of patients.
4. By assimilating into the community and participating in its organizations.

Given their important position in small communities, rural physicians are often active in all four of these areas. The first area, identifying and intervening in the community's health problems, is one in particular in which rural physicians tend to be more active than their urban counterparts. The relative shortage of public health personnel in rural areas coupled with geographically distinct patient populations means that rural primary care physicians are often led to adopt a community or population-based perspective on problems seen in their clinical practice. Community-oriented primary care (COPC) is one way of putting that perspective into practice.

What Is Community-Oriented Primary Care?

COPC is a set of processes that merge the care of individuals with the care of communities. It arises from a recognition that health and illness in the person are influenced by the family and by the community. Although illness may occur in the individual, the factors that cause it are often complex and multifactorial. Some of those factors originate from close personal relationships, while others stem from the broader community a person resides in. Prevention or treatment of the disease in the individual may require attention to those family or community-based factors as much as it requires attention to the individual. All the care given to the two children in the rural clinic after they arrived with carbon monoxide poisoning did nothing to affect their illness outcome. The solution to the problem causing their deaths required looking beyond the children.

At its most basic, COPC simply requires an awareness of the importance to health of this link between individuals and their families and community, together with an effort to influence that link at both the personal and community levels.

Community-Oriented Primary Care and Rural Health

COPC has deep roots in rural health. Almost all of the earliest descriptions of what later came to be called COPC came from rural areas. Rural practitioners are often presented with views that make clear the links between the person and the community. Pickles, a rural British general practitioner, used observations about his patients to elucidate some of the principles of transmission of hepatitis A in the 1920s.[2] Sidney and Emily Kark, who later articulated many of the concepts of COPC and developed models of its application, began by developing communitywide programs to decrease nutritional and infectious diseases among their Zulu patients in rural South Africa in the 1930s.[3] In the United States, work on the rural Navajo reservation in the 1950s along with later work in several areas of the Indian Health Service all demonstrated the concepts of COPC even before the term was coined.[4,5] In fact, it is likely that many more examples of the type of practice now called COPC have existed in rural areas for years.

What is the place of COPC in the practice of medicine in rural areas now? In those rural areas where resources are limited and health care providers are few, a population-based approach like COPC is a natural fit. Under these circumstances, providers have a de facto monopoly over health care for a geographic area. From this position, it is much easier for providers to see the links between the individual and the community, and it becomes even more important for the provider to act on those links.

Even where such "monopoly" conditions do not exist, both rural and urban providers must begin to take the population perspective if they wish to further improve the health of their individual patients. Increasingly, the major causes of ill health are behavioral. Dietary habits, risk-taking behaviors, substance abuse, and exercise habits are primary determinants of cardiovascular disease, trauma, and certain infectious and neoplastic diseases that are the major causes of morbidity and mortality today. Our ability to influence these determinants while focusing only on the individual is very limited. It is only through taking both individual and population-based approaches that improved results can be expected.

COPC potentially gives communities a greater voice in the way their health care is delivered. Especially in medically underserved areas, where both health care resources and health care consumer options are limited, community input can be an important means of feedback to the provider. In keeping with this view, some proponents of COPC emphasize a community empowerment aspect of the concept. However, taking a COPC view does not inherently require a major participatory role for the community. The process can conceivably (if unwisely) be conducted entirely by a physician without direct input from the community.

Community-Oriented Primary Care and Managed Care

Beyond these theoretical reasons why COPC is a good fit in rural environments, there are grow-

ing pragmatic reasons linked to managed care to support COPC in rural areas. Initially, when managed care organizations enter an area, they compete with each other for patients first on the costs of care, then on the quality of care they deliver. Once costs and quality begin to equilibrate, plans compete with each other based on the health of the populations they cover.[6,7]

It is clear from those areas where managed care has become more established that the population-based approach is becoming important. It is also becoming clear that the plans will not assume all of the risk for maximizing the health of their covered lives. Rather, they will act to pass some of the risk on to the providers with whom they are affiliated. An example of how plans will pass this risk on to providers is shown by the fact that providers in some areas are being held accountable for immunization rates among their enrollees. To respond to such demands for accountability, providers will need to be familiar with a population-based approach like COPC and follow it.

One further pragmatic reason for adopting a COPC approach relates to resource utilization. Managed care has created pressure for increased efficiency of resource utilization. Improved outcomes are expected with diminished resources. Where resources are limited to begin with, it becomes imperative to utilize them most efficiently. COPC offers the potential to target scarce resources most efficiently by identifying practice and community risk or disease patterns so they can then be acted on and by linking practice-based preventive care with community-based efforts.

GETTING STARTED

The most important aspect of getting started with COPC is to begin to consider the community aspects of ill health as it is seen in the practice. What are the patterns of ill health being seen in the practice? How are these conditions influenced by the family and community circumstances of the patients? Are there actions that could be taken in the practice or in the community to either prevent or improve these conditions? A willingness to broaden the view from the individual patient to the "community" of patients and then on to the larger community is the most important first step.

Although this appears to suggest that the COPC process must be started by a clinician, this is not necessarily so. The process can be initiated by any interested person or group. Managed care plans, community organizations, hospitals, public health departments, health educators, and community leaders all have an interest in this relationship, and from this interest could start the COPC process. Regardless of who initiates or leads the process, clearly the best way to carry it out is as a collaboration of interested parties. COPC should be seen as a team process. In situations where resources are limited, as is often the case in rural areas, assistance can be essential for following through on ideas. Additional perspectives, expertise, and information that team members can bring are often invaluable in the problem solving that is at the heart of the COPC process.

Although the composition of a team to work on COPC would be heavily dependent on the situation in each rural site, people from any of the groups listed above could be considered. Representatives from Area Health Education Centers, universities, cooperative extension services, offices of rural health, foundations, or statewide professional organizations may also be helpful as team members. A team could be assembled either informally or through a more formal process [Community Health Services Development (CHSD), Community Decision Making (CDM), Planned Approach to Community Health (PATCH), etc.] to be described later in this chapter. The nature of the problems and the community itself should guide who is brought into the team.

What Is It Exactly?

Figure 21-1 displays an idealized diagram of the COPC process. The diagram should not be seen as prescriptive. In real life, activities shown as

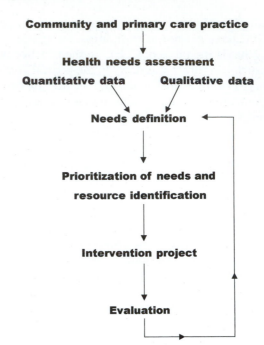

FIGURE 21-1 *The community-oriented primary care process.*

sequential may take place out of order, may occur at the same time, or may not be done at all. The COPC process is highly situational: what works well in one setting may be irrelevant in another. Nevertheless, the diagram provides a useful structure for considering the types of activities that can be part of the COPC process.

What Is the Problem?

The driving force for the COPC process is the perception of a health-related need or problem existing in the community. Often this problem is identified through the personal experience of a health care worker, as was the case with the children with carbon monoxide poisoning. Although this has the advantage of energizing the work involved, it may lead to overlooking equally important areas for intervention. A more systematic approach to identifying the health needs of a community can help with this.

Traditionally, health needs have usually been

identified through review of available statistical data describing the population of interest. This remains an essential part of the COPC process. Review of these quantitative data is important to clarify and prioritize causes of morbidity and mortality. However, many problems will require knowledge about how people in the community view their problems. Qualitative data of this type from the community are an important complement to quantitative data in understanding the community's health needs.

"Community"

Before beginning to gather these data, it is important to consider first how to define one's community. Many rural practitioners would find it easy to describe their communities geographically. However, some practices may define their communities using socioeconomic, cultural, age, or other criteria. For example, a clinic serving Native Americans in a rural area of mixed ethnicity may not consider a geographic definition of community appropriate for their purposes.

The advantage of defining the community as something extending beyond the group of people who seek health care is that it begins to include people who may have health needs but have not sought care. Since one of the goals of COPC is to extend preventive care to those within and beyond the practice who have not yet received it, this is a desirable way of defining community. However, for practical reasons, it is often easiest to start by simply considering those people who have sought care through a practice to be a community.

GETTING THE DATA—QUANTITATIVE

Regardless of how the community is defined, the next step is to begin to gather and review data about the health of the community. Dramatic advances in information technology over the last 5 to 10 years have made the task of reviewing quantitative data about the health

status of a community more realistic than it previously was.

It is important to consider what the goals of reviewing the data are. Is there a specific topic or problem in mind, or is the interest more in understanding the broad picture of health in a community? Regardless of what the specific data needs are, the emphasis must be on realistic methods of gathering, processing, and using the data. This means that despite advances in information technology, the ideal must often still be exchanged for the attainable.

Most practices collect clinical data only as part of the billing process. In many instances, summaries of clinical data gathered from billing records will be a rich source of information for the COPC process. When clinical information is collected solely for billing, though, limits on the range and type of data are inevitable. Given the expense and difficulty of parallel collection of data for clinical purposes, however, these limitations are usually accepted. With further development and adoption of electronic medical records, the quality and access to summary clinical data should improve.

Some other potential sources of quantitative data on health measures of a community are listed in Table 21-1. Census data—which not only provide important health information but are also important for calculating rates of other health indicators—are now available, often in electronic form, from a variety of sources, including many public libraries. Vital statistics, reportable diseases, and summary hospital dis-

TABLE 21-1   COMMON SOURCES OF QUANTITATIVE HEALTH DATA ABOUT COMMUNITIES

Census data
Hospital discharge data
Vital statistics
Cancer registry data
Reportable disease data
Disease-specific data
Managed care organization preventive service data

charge data are other types of quantitative data that should be available electronically to most rural practitioners through state and local agencies (e.g., state and county health departments, offices of rural health, rural health associations, and hospital associations). In some areas, community or market surveys may be available and offer useful data.

There are several common obstacles that might be encountered in collecting and organizing quantitative data. One of these is the proprietary nature of some of these data. Organizations engaged in competition in the health care marketplace might not be willing to share proprietary data about the community. A practical solution to this problem can be to develop mutually beneficial "partnerships."

Information overload can present a different type of problem when the goal is to view a broad picture of the health status of the community. Many sources of community health data present that information in an overwhelming array of measures. However, Zyzanski et al. have shown that it is possible to select relatively few indicators without loss of information.[8] Although one may want to add additional indicators for specific clinical questions, they have shown that one measure of the distribution of age across the community and one measure of income can constitute an acceptable minimum.

Mapping of health measures is often very useful, as visual images of data distributions provide compelling presentations. Although mapping software is rapidly developing, a decision to include mapping capabilities in the quantitative community assessment carries with it some limitations. Relatively few types of data are available on a communitywide basis and "geocoded" (address or geographic area markers attached to each case) in order to map. Mapping packages vary in their data-handling capabilities and their corresponding prices and can be quite time consuming to utilize.

Regardless of how the data are reviewed, it is important to recall some limitations. Secondary data, because they are collected for other purposes, may vary in reliability, validity, and rele-

TABLE 21-2   PRACTICAL APPROACH TO COMMUNITY ASSESSMENT USING QUANTITATIVE DATA

Be realistic; set goals that make sense given the many competing demands on your time and the resources available.

Decide whether your interest is in a specific problem (with focused data needs) or a broader understanding of the practice or community's health.

Get data on the part of the community seeking care—those seen in the practice: age, sex, diagnoses, preventive care status.

Find partners who both have an interest in the same question and may have access to data you need—e.g., public health departments, hospitals, managed care organizations.

If the interest is in the broad view of the community's health, start with getting census data (useful for viewing distribution of risk factors as well as for calculating disease rates).

Consider using mapping software only if there is a specific interest in viewing the distribution or clustering of a health indicator.

vance when applied to COPC purposes. Furthermore, the relatively small amount of data available from any practice or community, particularly if a condition of interest is uncommon, means that any variation in those data over time or over a geographic area may be the result of random variation rather than true differences.

What should one do then? Table 21-2 provides some suggestions about a practical approach to the review of quantitative data as part of a community assessment for COPC. The most important first step is to set realistic goals and avoid the time commitment and frustration that might come from efforts to set up elaborate databases.

Two examples demonstrate how these data can be used in COPC. DeGolia, in unpublished work, was concerned about the problem of untreated hypertension in the community where his practice was located. After first determining the number of residents being seen at the practice with this diagnosis and their age, sex, and racial distribution, he derived an estimate of the overall portion of community residents being seen in the practice. By matching these data with national data on the prevalence of hypertension by age, sex, and racial group, he was able to estimate the number of untreated hypertensives in the community. By carrying out this analysis at the level of a census tract in the community, he was able to target a specific area for plans to increase outreach and education about hypertension. When resources are limited, such targeting can increase their effectiveness.

In another example, concerns were raised in a semirural area about an apparently rising incidence of cancer and whether, if this increase were confirmed, it might be due to industrial groundwater contamination.[9] Data were compiled on all cases of cancer seen in the practice and on all cases of cancer recorded in the county through a regional cancer registry. Tying these data to age-sex profiles for the practice and for the county (defined as the community), maps of the county were generated, which located incident cases and projected incidence rates for both the practice and the county, by census tract, of the most common cancers. Viewing these maps and the lack of clustering of cases pro-

vided some reassurance to those concerned about cancer incidence.

GETTING THE DATA—QUALITATIVE

Although review of quantitative data about a practice's or community's health status can be very informative, a fuller understanding of the community's health needs often requires qualitative data as well. Data of this type can supply answers to three questions that are relevant to COPC: (1) Why does this problem exist? (2) How can this problem be best solved? (3) What are the priorities among a group of needs? Answers to these questions will not always be found in quantitative data—they require ideas and opinions.

There are a number of methods of collecting qualitative data. Here again, the emphasis must be on feasibility in a busy setting. The method chosen should be rapid, inexpensive, productive of useful information, and easily used by clinical staff. Table 21-3 lists some possible methods, each of which has its own advantages and disadvantages. For instance, focus groups are relatively expensive yet appear to have greater ability to provide emotional or personal

TABLE 21-3   SELECTED METHODS FOR GATHERING QUALITATIVE DATA FROM A COMMUNITY

Method	Key Advantages	Key Disadvantages[a]
Key informants/key informant trees	Good for identifying local resources for assistance	May give "accepted" responses
Focus groups	Provides emotive content	Requires group facilitation skills; greater cost
Long interviews	In-depth exploration of questions	Limited range of responses
Telephone surveys	Does not require respondent to come to a meeting	Misses those without phones; limited depth of responses
Mail surveys	Wide range of responses; flexible timing	Requires literacy; limited depth of responses
Nominal groups	Useful in prioritizing among choices	Requires greater time investment by respondents

[a]All methods are subject to selection and response biases. Careful attention must be given to minimizing and recognizing the effects of these biases.

content than the others listed. Phone surveys seem to provide a wider range of responses and are useful for contacting less mobile persons, but they do not appear to elicit volunteers to help with implementing COPC plans, as some of the other methods do.

The type of nondirective interviewing that these methods require is a natural fit for many trained in clinical interviewing. It is important to remember, however, that the validity of qualitative data very much depends on the way they are collected. Sampling should assure that a full range of information is supplied; the interview must be truly nondirective; and the analysis must be open-minded so as to minimize the potential for biased data.

Here again, an appropriate balance between methodologic rigor and feasibility must be struck. Most clinicians have neither the experience nor the resources to carry out in-depth qualitative research as part of a community assessment. Table 21-4 presents some suggestions for practical approaches to gathering this information in a clinical setting. The key is to use care in the data collection and analysis while maintaining healthy skepticism about the information gathered.

An example can show how qualitative data can be useful in COPC. Staff at a clinic were concerned about poor attendance in follow-up for abnormal Pap smears. Their reminder letters mentioning the possibility of progression of the cervical lesions were failing to improve attendance. Through use of three qualitative data-collection methods (focus groups as well as mail and phone surveys), the staff found that community members' fatalism about cancer was a major factor in missed appointments. The reminder letter, by aggravating the fatalistic view, was worsening the problem. In light of this finding, the practice chose to revise the letter to emphasize personal control over health. Information of this sort could not have been obtained from quantitative data.

GETTING THE JOB DONE

So Much to Do, So Little Time

A common problem is that health needs quickly exceed the available time and resources, making prioritization essential. Although priorities may be "preselected," as in the case of vehicular carbon monoxide poisonings or when outside agencies such as managed care organizations impose population-based performance standards, in other circumstances several important needs may be identified. Systematic approaches to setting priorities among competing needs, such as cost-benefit analysis, are not useful in the COPC setting because of the difficulty in applying general data to the local setting or in obtaining valid local data.

Priorities are usually chosen based on a combination of participant interest and skills, available resources (time, personnel, funding), and the availability of interventions that are thought likely to be effective. It is important, however, to be sure that interest, resources, and interven-

---

TABLE 21-4   PRACTICAL APPROACH TO COMMUNITY ASSESSMENT USING QUALITATIVE DATA

Be realistic; set goals that make sense given the many competing demands on your time and the resources available.

Clarify whether the interest is in a specific problem (with focused data needs) or a broader understanding of the practice or community's health.

Clarify whether the interest is in getting explanatory information, new ideas, or a sense of priorities.

Select at least two methods of data gathering to enhance data validity; choose the methods most likely to get the information needed from the portion of the community of interest.

Balance the need for care in gathering qualitative data with what is feasible in practice; pay most attention to how the people to be interviewed are selected, to nondirective interviewing, and to keeping an open mind while reviewing the data.

tions are well matched so that failure or frustration are not the result. It is important, as well, that the intervention is acceptable to the community. This is best assured by continuing communications between those leading the COPC process and those in the community who will be affected by the decisions. Such continuing communication helps to guide not only the selection of priorities but also the subsequent intervention.

Successfully carrying out COPC work is dependent on this match between interest, resources, and interventions. How much of each of these is required depends on the nature of the problem, the community, and the approaches followed. As mentioned previously, it is important to develop partners in the process. Teams of interested people are much more likely to succeed than one individual, particularly where resources are limited. Realistic objectives must be established. Avoid the disappointment trap caused by setting goals that are unrealistically high or so low that interest is lost.

So What? Has It Made a Difference?

It is useful to evaluate whether the results of COPC work have been worth the effort. Has the targeted health problem been improved in the hoped for way? Though evaluation of an intervention is rarely a principal objective, it is important to consider early in the process so that there is a means in place to clarify successes and areas for improvement in subsequent efforts.

Although the specific health indicator that is the focus of a COPC intervention is a natural measure for evaluation of the intervention, it is important not to overlook other equally useful outcomes. Some examples of other worthwhile outcomes of the COPC process could include establishing the partnerships that drive the COPC plan; increased involvement of community members in their health care; improved professional satisfaction of the health care providers; spinoff effects on nontargeted health conditions; and increased community awareness of the targeted health problem.

WHAT CAN BE EXPECTED?

Published Studies of Outcomes

There are relatively few published studies of the effects of COPC on health outcomes. The Institute of Medicine, in its study of COPC, studied several practices following the COPC process.[10] It found "examples of improved health outcomes," particularly in rural practices. Reductions in complications from streptococcal infection, gastroenteritis and dehydration, hearing loss, and tooth decay were some of the examples cited. Another study in paired rural communities found a reduction in blood pressures in the community where cardiovascular disease was a target of COPC interventions.[11] In a rural North Carolina community, residents who received care at a practice described as following the COPC model had improved control of hypertension compared with residents who sought care elsewhere.[12] Another publication reported the results of a private foundation effort in the late 1980s to establish model rural COPC practices in several sites across the country.[13] Mixed results were obtained over the 3 years of funding, as health practitioner turnover and competing time demands were problems. The most important problem, however, appeared to be a lack of methods and skills for putting the model into effect.

Costs

There is little information about the marginal costs or financial benefits of the COPC model. A few case studies have reported cost estimates of elements of the process, and one study attempted to give rough estimates of overall marginal costs.[13,14] However, it is difficult to know how well the specific cost estimates given in these few studies represent the true costs of COPC work. Given the highly situational nature of COPC and the range of activities that could be considered COPC, much more work is needed for a full understanding of its costs or financial benefits. The true costs or benefits of

COPC will be known only once the process is studied from start to finish, including any reduction in overall costs due to health gains from the interventions. Reflecting how highly dependent the COPC process is on the circumstances of each location, funding for COPC work published in the literature has come from a variety of sources. In general, it is likely that future resources for COPC will come from the interested partners in the process, each of which will contribute some measure of personnel, time, or money.

Secondary Benefits

Conceptually, the COPC process could have a number of benefits beyond the specifically targeted health condition. Some of these have been mentioned previously (community empowerment, improved provider satisfaction, improved efficiency of health care resources, etc.). Only limited anecdotal data are available to assess whether these benefits are achieved.

Obstacles

Although managed care—with its emphases on prevention, cost-efficiency, and population-based care—has begun to remove the financial disincentives that were a major barrier to COPC in previous years, there are still obstacles to overcome. The methods and outcomes of COPC are not yet well enough understood for clear recommendations on the best paths to follow to be made. The transition from identifying health needs to designing and carrying out effective interventions may also be difficult. Most importantly, COPC requires a major change in perspective for clinicians, whose focus is otherwise entirely on the well-being of the individual. For rural practitioners, this perspective may come into view more easily through their role in the community.

The COPC process may take longer than expected and involve negotiating a variety of topics with COPC partners. Sustaining interest through to completion may become an obstacle. The fruits of all these labors may take some time to appear.

In some areas, competition between health care providers or between managed care organizations may make it difficult to build effective COPC partnerships. Indeed, when managed care organizations enter a community, the changes they drive may be disruptive to existing community health efforts.

THE FUTURE

Certifying and funding agencies, including Medicare and Medicaid, are beginning to hold managed care organizations accountable for the health of the populations they serve. Recent versions of the Health Plan Employer Data Information Set (HEDIS), quality measures developed by the National Committee for Quality Assurance (NCQA), place increasing importance on measures of the enrolled population rather than simply on service provided to those who present for care. The result of this is that providers will be increasingly supplied with population-based data from the managed care organizations with which they affiliate. Although these data will likely be restricted to the population of "covered lives" of the managed care organization, they will increase the motivation to look at the health of communities as part of personal health services. Regardless of whether it is called COPC, there will be a growing interest in the linkage of personal health services and community health.

It is likely that this linkage will take many forms. There is no single model of COPC, and there is no one way for putting in place the concepts of population-based health care. The future will hold a variety of models for making this linkage.

No matter what the form of the model, a central characteristic will be a collaborative service partnership. Managed care organizations, providers, health departments, and community

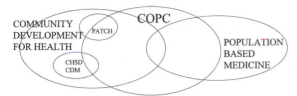

FIGURE 21-2 Diagrammatic relationships between approaches to community health.

organizations are finding common ground in the need to look at both personal and community health services. Each brings unique strengths to the table yet needs the assistance of others to influence the health of communities and individuals.

Recognition of the importance of a collaborative approach to improving the health of the community has led to the development of integrated programs aimed at building community capacity for health improvement. These programs, which closely resemble the COPC process in many ways (see Fig. 21-2), focus on community development as the key to success in health-improvement efforts.

CHSD, CDM, AND PATCH

Two approaches of this type that have been broadly applied to health systems are Community Health Services Development (CHSD) and Community Decision Making (CDM). Both of these approaches are based on the premise that the most important determinant of the strength of a health system is its linkages to the community it serves.[15] The two approaches also share the strategy of using outsiders to launch projects while relying on locals to take action and keep things going. A third approach, PATCH, is similar but does not rely on outside consultants.

The Community Health Services Development (CHSD) approach grew out of the work done in the rural Northwest in the late 1980s under the Rural Hospital Project (RHP), sponsored by the Kellogg Foundation.[16] Although the RHP started with a research focus, it con-cluded with community development. Under the RHP, researchers gathered information about communities with a hope of understanding how the local health systems worked. CHSD was initially developed as an approach for using research findings to help communities strengthen their health systems. Since then, over 50 rural communities in the Pacific Northwest have participated in a CHSD project.

CHSD starts with a commitment on behalf of local decision makers (e.g., the board of the local hospital or the county commissioners) to go through a planned approach to improving the local health care system. There is agreement to participate in the design, implementation, and analyses of a series of assessments. Further, they agree to share with the broader community the results of the assessments. Finally, they agree to participate in a planning process that develops strategies for working on issues that come from the assessments.

Figure 21-3 shows the flow of the CHSD process. A key concept is that most of the work of the assessments is done by outsiders. Although the overall process is managed by a single entity (in the Pacific Northwest, this has been the University of Washington in conjunction with the state-based Area Health Education Centers), those assigned to the assessment team are a mix of academicians and private consultants. Needs assessments, the communitywide goal-setting meeting, the community survey, and the organization review can be planned and carried out by health administration professionals. The financial review requires specific expertise that can come from private consultants. A physician typically leads the scope-of-services review, a process that depends on clinician-to-clinician interaction. Each of these assessments is described in more detail elsewhere.[17]

Assessments done in this fashion, using outside consultants, can be costly. If outsiders are retained, the community or its agencies may have to provide the funding for the outside assistance. The community could raise this money itself or get help from granting agencies such as foundations or government programs. Con-

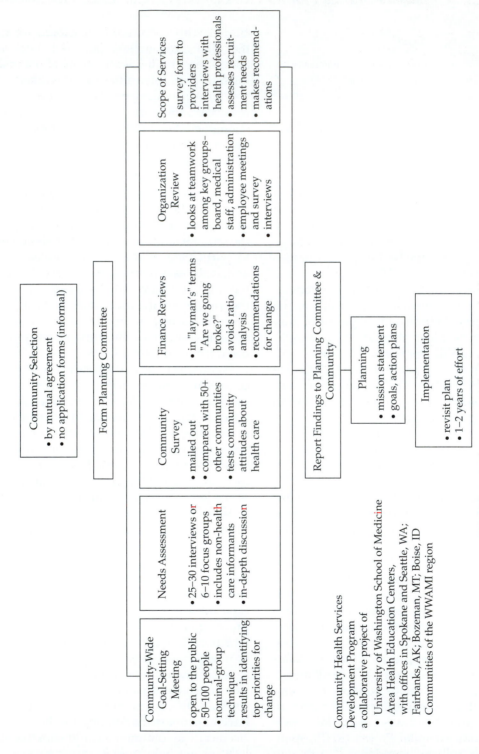

FIGURE 21-3 *The community health services development process.*

ducted in this way, the cost can be as low as $1000 for a single assessment (such as an organizational review) or as high as $20,000 for a community survey. A complete CHSD-type project, with all assessments and a planning process, could cost $40,000 to $60,000.

Although outsiders take prime responsibility for the assessment phase and they facilitate the planning phase, the decisions are solely the responsibility of the community. The local planning committee considers the assessments and agrees upon a set of strategies for making things better. Optimally, the plan undergoes continual review and refinement, thereby increasing the likelihood that tasks will be completed.

Community Decision Making (CDM) focuses most closely on the assessments and relies on the community's wisdom to make decisions about future directions for the health system. In the information gathering stage, CDM focuses on the needs assessments and the community goal-setting meeting. CDM places the highest importance on the process of gathering information and building local community development capacity. To move the process along at the local level, the community appoints a "community encourager" who is charged with scheduling meetings, compiling information, and organizing the community goal-setting meeting. Before starting the project, the community encourager attends an intensive weeklong training camp led by professional community developers.

While both CHSD and CDM use a community goal-setting meeting, CDM was the first to make this a central part of the assessment. The meeting is a broadly publicized, all-comers meeting with very careful facilitation. Under the guidance of encourager-trained local facilitators, the community discusses its likes and dislikes concerning the local health system. The meeting culminates with the full group voting on the top priorities for changes to the health system.

A manual for developing and carrying out a CDM project can be purchased from the Moun-

tain States Group [1607 West Jefferson, Boise, ID 83702 (208-336-5533)]. CDM is particularly attractive as a way to get started on community-based planning because the project has a great workbook and the encourager does the bulk of the work.

CHSD and CDM are two examples of ways communities can partner with outsiders to strengthen their health systems. Although well over 100 communities have applied these two methodologies, there are many other approaches that may work as well or better in any given community. The Centers for Disease Control and Prevention has a similar program entitled Planned Approach To Community Health (PATCH). It differs from those programs just described primarily in its reliance on community members for the entire process, including the assessments and facilitation. Community members are provided with packets of materials that supply guidance for the whole process along with visual aids for use in meetings. This packet has been successfully used in many areas of the country over the last decade. Most state health departments have a state coordinator for PATCH. Readers unable to identify their state coordinator may wish to contact the Centers for Disease Control and Prevention directly. Contact information is given at the end of the chapter.

Experience in fields outside of health is relevant for many of the community development activities involved in these programs. For example, Cooperative Extension has been working with communities for decades. The National Rural Resource Center in Duluth, Minnesota (218-720-0700), can provide more information on other approaches.

SUMMARY

COPC provides a conceptual structure for applying population-based health care to meet the needs both of individuals and their communities and of the managed care delivery system.

Advances in the last decade have led to the development of programs for helping communities to put the concept in place, and to develop specific methods for feasibly carrying out the COPC process.

REFERENCES

1. Pathman DE, Steiner BD, Williams E, et al: The four community dimensions of primary care practice. *J Fam Pract* 46:293, 1998.

2. Pickles WN: *Epidemiology in a Country Practice.* Baltimore, Williams & Wilkins, 1939.

3. Kark SL, Cassel J: The Pholela Health Centre: a progress report. *S Afr Med J* 26:101–104, 131–136, 1952.

4. Deuschle KW: Community-oriented primary care: lessons learned in three decades. *J Commun Health* 8:13, 1982.

5. Nutting PA, Strotz CR, Shorr GI, et al: Reduction of gastroenteritis morbidity in high-risk infants. *Pediatrics* 55:354, 1975.

6. Goldsmith JC, Goran MJ, Nackel JG: Managed care comes of age. *Healthcare Forum J* Sept/Oct:15, 1995.

7. Randall TG, Schauffler HH: Health promotion and disease prevention in integrated delivery systems: the role of market forces. *Am J Prev Med* 13:244, 1997.

8. Zyzanski SJ, Williams RL, Flocke SA: Selection of key community descriptors for community-oriented primary care. *Fam Pract* 13:280, 1996.

9. Mettee TM, Martin KB, Williams RL: Tools for community-oriented primary care: a process for linking practice and community data. *J Am Board Fam Pract* 11:28, 1998.

10. Institute of Medicine: *Community-Oriented Primary Care: A Practical Assessment, I: The Committee Report.* Washington, DC, National Academy Press, 1984.

11. Gold MR, Franks P: A community oriented primary care project in a rural population: reducing cardiovascular risk. *J Fam Pract* 30:639, 1990.

12. O'Connor PJ, Wagner EH, Strogatz DS: Hypertension control in a rural community: an assessment of community-oriented primary care. *J Fam Pract* 30:420, 1990.

13. Kukulka G, Christianson JB, Moscovice IS, et al: Community-oriented primary care: implementation of a national rural demonstration. *Arch Fam Med* 3:495, 1994.

14. Williams RL, Flocke SA, Zyzanski SJ, et al: A practical tool for community-oriented primary care community diagnosis using a personal computer. *Fam Med* 27:39, 1995.

15. Starkweather DB, Cook KS: Organization-environment relations, in Shortell SM, Kaluzny AD (eds): *Health Care Management: A Text in Organizational Theory and Behavior,* 2nd ed. New York, Wiley, 1988, p 334.

16. Amundson BA, Rosenblatt RA: The rural hospital project: conceptual background and current status. *J Rural Health* 4:119, 1988.

17. House PJ, Hagopian A: Community health services development program, in McSwan D, McShane M (eds): *Issues Affecting Rural Communities: Proceedings of the Conference.* Townsville, Queensland, Australia, James Cook University of North Queensland, 1994, p 66.

ADDITIONAL READING ON COMMUNITY-ORIENTED PRIMARY CARE

Connor E, Mullan F (eds): *Community-Oriented Primary Care: New Directions for Health Services Delivery.* Washington, DC, National Academy Press, 1983.

Nutting PA (ed): *Community-Oriented Primary Care: From Principle to Practice.* Albuquerque, NM, University of New Mexico Press, 1990.

Rhyne R, Bogue R, Kukulka G, et al: *Community-Oriented Primary Care: Health Care for the 21st Century.* Washington, DC, American Public Health Association, 1998.

USEFUL RESOURCES/ADDRESSES

American Academy of Family Physicians, 8880 Ward Parkway, Kansas City, MO 64114; Phone: 816-333-9700; email: fp@aafp.org; http://www.aafp.org/

Cooperative Extension of the U.S. Department of Agriculture—a source of help for community level activities: http://www.reeusda.gov/

Federal Office of Rural Health Policy, Health Resources and Services Administration, 5600 Fishers Lane, Room 9-05, Rockville, MD 20857; Phone: 301-443-0835; a source of ideas for funding and a means to link with resources to help with projects: http://www.nal.usda.gov/orhp/

National Center for Chronic Disease Prevention and Health Promotion, CDCP, Mailstop K30, 4770 Buford Highway NE, Atlanta, GA 30341; Phone: 770-488-5426; email: zwc6@cdc.gov

National Rural Health Resource Center, Suite 404, 600 East Superior Street, Duluth, MN 55802; Phone: 218-720-0700; email: nrhrc@ruralcenter.org; www.ruralcenter.org/nrhrc; provides technical assistance, information, and tools to build healthy communities.

PART FOUR

Education for Rural Practice

T he shortage of physicians in rural America is a long-standing problem that has persisted, as physicians have continued to preferentially settle in metropolitan, suburban, and other nonrural areas. The last 20 years have seen a variety of strategies introduced by governments and by medical education programs in an effort to ameliorate this problem and promote the choice of rural practice by physician graduates.

The goal of this section is to describe recent developments in education for rural practice along a continuum including medical school, residency training, and continuing education of clinicians practicing in rural areas. As in earlier sections of this book, our particular focus is directed to the special problems of educational preparation for practice in small rural communities with populations of less than 10,000 people. The educational needs of clinicians in such settings are different in scope and depth from their counterparts in metropolitan areas. Rural health care providers are frequently challenged with minimal resources as well as by urgent and emergent clinical problems across the full spectrum of primary care; they must call upon a wide range of cognitive and procedural skills to care for these patients. Rural physicians tend to work longer hours and see more patients per week than their colleagues in urban or suburban practice. Close teamwork with a small number of colleagues is essential in order to survive and prosper in rural practice over years.

The selection, recruitment, and retention of rural clinicians is a perennial challenge and is addressed at each step along the educational "pipeline" to rural practice. Special curricular needs are also addressed, including advanced obstetrics, emergency care, and other procedural competencies. Special educational strategies, such as rural training tracks, are described and assessed. Where appropriate and possible, future directions are also projected as they relate to the changing nature of rural practice in the twenty-first century, as the organizational changes described in the last section take hold and medical informatics are more broadly applied.

John P. Geyman

CHAPTER 22

Predoctoral Education for Rural Practice

JAMES R. BLACKMAN

I n order to meet the continued demand for rural practitioners, medical schools with primary care missions and those that desire to increase their output of rural health care providers must continue to review policies and programs that could increase their output of generalist physicians. Although family physicians make up the largest component of the rural-based health professional work force, other primary care providers such as general internists, general pediatricians, physician assistants, and nurse practitioners as well as other specialties (surgery) also contribute significantly toward meeting our rural health care needs.

The academic medical literature is replete with studies suggesting ways for medical schools to improve their output of primary care physicians. However, the interplay between admission policies, curriculum, and the institutional environment is complex and extremely difficult to study. Often programs with a strong curricular emphasis on primary care are also the same ones that attract or preferentially admit students with a stated interest in primary care. There have been several attempts to improve the validity and usefulness of conclusions drawn from literature review.[1-3] Multiple confounders and lack of randomized trials make it difficult to develop substantiated recommendations for strategies to increase the production of rural physicians. This makes it difficult for medical schools to react responsibly to recommendations. This chapter does not attempt to continue the debate about what policies or pro-

grams are most effective but rather brings together those elements that seem most successful in identifying and training students for rural practice. A continuous educational pipeline is proposed, designed and organized to stimulate or continue to foster student interest in rural practice. A case study is presented to illustrate the importance of combining multiple program initiatives in an effort to increase students' interest in primary care. Important factors that may assist in this process are reviewed, such as the culture of the institution, admission policies, and curricular elements.

Gretchen Johnson was born and raised in a small northern Minnesota community located on the Iron Range. Her father was a minister and the family was heavily involved in community activities. She was delivered by her family physician, who provided care for her parents and brothers and sisters. Following graduation from high school, she attended a small private college and actively participated in its premedical club. She had a good college premedical adviser and participated in an externship program with area family physicians.

Following graduation from college, she was accepted into the University of Minnesota-Duluth School of Medicine. She was impressed with the school's mission to increase the number of well-trained family physicians for rural and nonurban areas of the state of Minnesota. The school's admission's committee was impressed with Gretchen, not only because of her excellent scholastic record but also because of her background in humanitarian activities, including spending time in a third-world country during college. They were also impressed with her stated desire to become a rural family physician.

As part of her training in Duluth, she participated in the first-year family practice preceptorship, where she had the opportunity to spend 12 half days learning about the practice of medicine directly. During the second year of her training, she participated in additional preceptorships in family practice in a rural community. Following completion of her first 2 years of medical school, Gretchen chose to enter the University of Minnesota's Rural Physician Associate Program (RPAP), which was developed to diminish the shortage of rural primary care physicians throughout the state. Following completion of two 6-week rotations (internal medicine and obstetrics/gynecology), she spent 9 months in a rural training site. While on RPAP, she experienced the personal and professional lifestyle of a rural physician. She was able to evaluate and treat patients in clinic, hospital, emergency room, and nursing home settings. She assisted in surgery, consulted with other health care professionals, and served as a resource to the community. After completion of her RPAP experience, she completed her fourth year at the University of Minnesota campus in Minneapolis and then entered a northern Minnesota family practice residency program that was committed to training physicians for rural areas.

After completion of her residency training program, she joined the group of family practice physicians that provided her RPAP experience. She now functions as an RPAP preceptor.

This case study demonstrates the importance of exposing students to a continuous educational pipeline designed to stimulate and/or foster interest in rural practice. Although the student is fictional, the Minnesota programs are now and remain highly successful. The University of Minnesota medical education programs are described further later in this chapter.[4,5]

INSTITUTIONAL CHARACTERISTICS FAVORING PRIMARY CARE

Most organizations develop a culture that significantly influences the behavior, values, productivity, and satisfaction of its members.[1,6–9] In academic institutions, the primary institution (with which the medical school is affiliated) influences medical school policies (promotion, tenure), which is influential in determining the type of faculty and students who are attracted to and succeed in the academic setting. The primary forces forming the culture of an academic institution are its faculty, admission policies, and students. The type of medical school (public or private) influences the mission, which in turn influences faculty composition. The presence of primary care faculty, the number of full-time versus part-time faculty, and the number of academic versus clinical faculty are all important. To be successful in producing a significant proportion of primary care graduates, a medical school should have a large proportion of academically credible primary care faculty. This faculty influences the culture of the institution through committee activities (admissions, human subjects, curriculum) and by occupying leadership positions. The expanded primary care base now necessary to support medical schools can provide increased primary care faculty and student teaching opportunities.

The average age of all faculty in higher education by the year 2000 will be 55.[1] If medical school faculty are representative, most physician faculty completed their training in schools that had no departments, clerkships, or rotations in primary care. These same faculty may have done their residency training at sites with no primary care residents. As a result, they are bound to have misunderstandings and misconceptions about the skills of primary care physicians. When a large proportion of full-time primary care faculty are present within the medical school, they not only interact with and continue to foster students' interest in primary care but also have increased interaction with other faculty members, which may help to promote an understanding of primary care within the institution.

Public schools, when compared with private schools, provide significantly greater proportions of primary care graduates.[10,11] High-producing schools have departments of family medicine, the majority of which are affiliated with three or more family practice residency sites. They also have a sponsored Area Health Education Center (AHEC) and are less research-intensive. Institutions that produce significantly smaller numbers of primary care graduates tend to be private institutions of large class size and are often heavily research-intensive. However, it is not inconsistent to be both a large provider of primary care graduates while at the same time being research-intensive. Those institutions that do both have a strong institutional commitment to primary care coupled with a dedication to help relieve the shortage of rural health care providers.

ADMISSION POLICIES FAVORING PRIMARY CARE

When all other admission criteria are equal [the Medical College Admission Test (MCAT) scores and the grade point average (GPA)], it may be possible to increase the medical school's output of primary care providers by careful attention to admission criteria that favor primary care.[1,12–17] Students select specialties by trying to match the characteristics of a specialty with career needs, personal needs, and social needs.[1] Personal needs and student values are closely related and are influenced by life experiences, demographic factors, and personality characteristics. Student values are also influenced by medical school experiences, including the culture of the institutions in which the student receives medical training. Although personality characteristics have been difficult to study, student values may more visible. Students who expressed an interest in primary care at matriculation and who perceive long-term patient care as desirable are more likely to select primary care career pathways.[15] Medical student attitudes toward psychosocial aspects of treatment may also be important.[18]

Students who enter primary care fields tend to be older, female, have lower income expecta-

tions, value longitudinal relationships with patients, have an expanded background in social sciences, and may have had some international or human service experience prior to entering medical school.[19,20] Older students may have a clearer picture of their professional goals, are less influenced by the culture of the institution, and are more interested in a residency of shorter duration owing to accumulating debt load and responsibility for other family members. Although women are more likely than men to choose a primary care specialty, they are significantly less likely to enter practice in a rural setting.[21] Students that come from rural backgrounds (or have spouses that do) and who state an interest in primary care, particularly family medicine, at the time of matriculation are more likely to end up in primary care. However, even though significant numbers of students with a stated strong interest in primary care may be admitted to medical school, a significant percentage of those students will ultimately change their minds and move away from a primary care career.[1–4] This "leakage" away from primary care may in part be related to the student not having a solid understanding of what it means to be a primary care physician and also having had little or no experience with physicians in other specialties. As discussed, the culture of the institution can also significantly influence student career choices. More work needs to be done regarding changing values and attitudes as students progress through medical school.

THE PIPELINE TO RURAL PRACTICE

A student's interest in primary care may begin very early, perhaps even prior to entering high school. Early contact with examplary health care providers coupled with an opportunity to see or experience some form of medical practice could be valuable. Programs designed to capture the interest of high school students and assist in preparing them for health care careers have been developed by medical schools. Physicians can actively participate with high school students by being involved with athletic programs, providing seminars at local schools, and being strong positive role models within the community.

When students begin their liberal arts education, a high-quality premedical adviser program should be available to assist them regarding career opportunities in medicine. Often, premedical advisers are not physicians and may have had minimal contact with the medical profession. Regional medical schools should have a strong interest in working with premedical advisory programs and faculty should be willing to attend various premedical club gatherings or to participate in classroom discussions clarifying the roles and responsibilities of being a physician. Community physicians should also participate. They could offer students the opportunity to join them and see the practice of medicine at first hand. Premedical students should be encouraged to participate in these externship programs and should also be encouraged to seek out humanistic experiences such as international travel in underserved areas. In addition, students should be encouraged to take more social science and humanities courses. These courses help to foster humanistic values, which are needed for rural practice.

Many medical schools provide early exposure to local rural family practice experiences during the first and second years of medical school.[1-3,22] Although these early primary care experiences do not appear to directly influence primary care specialty choice, they reinforce already existing interests and provide a process by which students can clarify their values.

Many medical schools have developed special programs to increase their output of generalist physicians. Some examples follow:

At Jefferson Medical College in Philadelphia, a program entitled The Physician Shortage Area Program (PSAP) was started in 1974. Special medical school admissions policies combined with special education programs (faculty advising, required third-year family medicine clerkship, and fourth-year subinternship in family medicine) have produced a dramatic and sustained positive impact. PSAP graduates were about 10 times more likely to combine a career choice in family medicine with rural practice than non-PSAP graduates. Eighty-five percent of PSAP graduates either chose a primary care specialty or practiced in a rural or small metropolitan area or a physician shortage area. Their special admission policy gives preference to otherwise qualified applicants from rural backgrounds with stated intentions to practice family medicine in rural and/or underserved areas.[23,24] A 5.5-fold increase in the number of rural primary care physicians resulted from a special admissions process when compared with a regular admission's process without preference for rural background and interest in primary care.[25,26]

The University of Minnesota-Duluth School of Medicine has, for many years, had the highest proportion of graduates entering family practice of any medical school in the country. Our case study was written to emphasize the importance of their programs and to demonstrate how a series of educational experiences can continue to foster a student's interest in rural practice. The Duluth program is a classic example of what can result from a clear institutional commitment to rural health. Since the school's existence (1972), 53.4 percent of students have entered the specialty of family practice and an additional 15.8 percent have chosen another primary care specialty (Table 22-1).[4,5] During this time, the national rate of entry into family practice was approximately 13 percent. The Rural Physicians Associate Program (RPAP) was established in 1971 as one of the University of Minnesota's programmatic responses to diminish the shortage of rural primary care physicians throughout the state. This 9-month elective experience is open to 40 third-year medical students at either the University of Minnesota-Duluth or the University of Minnesota Twin Cities Campuses. RPAP replaces 24 weeks of elective time and 12 weeks of unscheduled time in the third- and fourth-year curriculum. Through careful documentation of community-based experiences, RPAP students may "opt out" of two or three required clerkships (surgery, pediatrics, and

TABLE 22-1 PROPORTION OF
UNIVERSITY OF MINNESOTA GRADUATES
SELECTING FAMILY MEDICINE
RESIDENCIES CATEGORIZED
BY EDUCATIONAL EXPERIENCES
IN MEDICAL SCHOOL; ALL UNIVERSITY
OF MINNESOTA MEDICAL SCHOOL
GRADUATES (1976–1998)

	Number of Family Physicians	Percent	Total
• 4 years Minneapolis • No RPAP	716	17.0	4211
• 2 years Duluth • 2 years Minneapolis	335	45.3	740
• 4 years Minneapolis • Plus RPAP	371	68.7	540
• 2 years Duluth • 2 years Minneapolis • Plus RPAP	171	75.3	227
Total graduates	1593	27.95	5718

SOURCE: From References 5 and 6, with permission.

primary care medicine). Participating students receive a scholarship of $13,000 ($9000 provided by the state of Minnesota and $4000 provided by the physician, preceptor, and/or clinic).

To date, 858 third-year medical students have participated in the RPAP program. Of these, 750 have completed their residency training and are now in practice. Sixty-one percent are in rural or small-town communities and 64.5 percent practice in Minnesota. Again referring to Table 22-1, a total of 68.7 percent of Minneapolis-based students who participated in RPAP entered family practice residency programs. Of the Duluth students who participated in RPAP, 75.3 percent chose family practice. These data do not include students who have chosen other primary care specialties since there is no information available regarding which students subspecialized after entering internal medicine and pediatric residency programs.

Rural primary care providers are important contributors to both programs and are largely responsible for the success that has been achieved. Their special efforts help to solve the problem of short supply rural health care providers.

Mercer University was founded with a mission to produce primary care physicians for rural and underserved areas of Georgia. This medical school adopted the McMaster model for problem-based learning in the basic science years and has promoted generalist values and practice throughout the 4 years of predoctoral education. Percentages of students choosing family practice residencies and other primary care programs remain very high.[27]

The University of Washington School of Medicine serves as the only medical school for the five-state area of Washington, Wyoming, Alaska, Montana, and Idaho (WWAMI). Medical students admitted from the respective WWAMI states take their first year at state universities within their home state. During their clinical years they have the opportunity to take community-based clerkships, most of which are in rural areas. The University of Washington School of Medicine also provides the WWAMI Rural Integrated Training Experience (WRITE) program for third-year medical students within the WWAMI states. During this experience, students spend 6 months in a rural community following 8 weeks of inpatient medicine, 3 weeks of inpatient pediatrics, 4 weeks of inpatient psychiatry, and 6 weeks each of inpatient surgery and obstetrics/gynecology. Students who complete the WRITE program obtain credit for 6 weeks of family medicine, 4 weeks of ambulatory internal medicine, 3 weeks of ambulatory pediatrics, and 2 weeks of ambulatory psychiatry in addition to elective credit. Although this is a new program, 12 of the 13 students admitted to date are women.

Prior to the institution of WWAMI (pre-1974), 31 percent of University of Washington School of Medicine graduates entered primary care. Since 1974, these numbers have exceeded 50 percent. Of those post-1974 students without WWAMI experience, 27 percent have entered primary care, whereas of those students who participated in the WWAMI remote site experiences, 61 percent have entered primary care. Although remote experiences may affect specialty selection, it may also be true that students who are already interested in primary care are most likely to take WWAMI clerkships.[28]

In late 1991, the Robert Wood Johnson Foundation announced a Generalist Physician Initiative (GPI) grant program designed to help medical schools increase the number of generalist physicians. A summary has recently been published.[29] Dartmouth Medical School, one of 16 U.S. medical schools to receive a GPI grant, made significant curricular changes. A first- and second-year course called Longitudinal Clinical Experience (LCE) was developed to place the students in the offices of practicing physicians one-half day each week. Students observe clinical practice and practice basic physical examination techniques. Small- and large-group activities reinforce and clarify clinical experiences. In addition, an interdisciplinary primary clerkship was developed in the third year. This clerkship groups outpatient experiences in pediatrics, family medicine, and internal medicine together in a required 16-week block. Dartmouth College has seen the number of its graduating medical students entering primary care programs increase from 38 percent in the year preceding the GPI to more than 50 percent with the graduating class of 1997.[30] Also as part of the GPI, Eastern Carolina University developed goals and objectives to undertake a comprehensive curriculum review, integrate primary care principles across the first year of medical school, develop a problem-based learning course, include primary care community experiences in medicine and pediatric clerkships, develop a partnership with the Area Health Education Center (AHEC) to increase the number and quality of community primary care faculty, and provide faculty development for generalist academic faculty.[31]

West Virginia School of Osteopathic Medicine has educated, placed, and retained more primary care physicians in Appalachia (1978–1999) than any other U.S. medical school. This school has a clear mission to serve Appalachia and continues to promote rural practice from admission to placement. West Virginia School of Osteopathic Medicine participates in the Southern Regional Education Board (SREB) with Georgia, Mississippi, Maryland, and Alabama. Students from these states may matriculate at West Virginia School of Osteopathic Medicine without paying out-of-state tuition and fees. As of 1999, 50 percent of the school's first 40 graduates had entered primary care in rural Appalachia.[27]

In Australia, government funds have been identified to support the Rural Health Support, Education and Training (RHSET) program. A Faculty of Rural Medicine has been organized within the Royal Australian College of General Practitioners and guidelines have been established for rural academic general practice units. These units are to be based in exemplary rural "demonstration" practices and will be involved in practice-based research as well as teaching of medical students, residents, practicing physicians, and allied health professionals.[32] A Rural Medical Curriculum Design Project has developed specific curricular goals and objectives in surgery, anesthesia, and obstetrics.[33,34] Both Canada and Australia see the need for further curricular design for more effective preparation for rural practice.[35] A Canadian Rural Medicine Network is being organized by the College of Family Physicians of Canada for these purposes.[36]

Factors that clearly influence primary care specialty choice during the third and fourth years include having an appropriate advising system readily available to students, having a required third-year family medicine clerkship, of at least 6 weeks duration, and the provision of other longitudinal training experiences for students.[1,16,27,32,37] The influence of the RPAP program was quite dramatic in this regard.

A strong advising program must be in place in the medical school to serve as a linkage with the various programs that are offered within the institution. Student advisers located within the medical school must have a strong interest in the students' professional development and should be an unbiased resource to help students sort out their professional lives.

One of the most significant components of predoctoral education for rural practice is the training received within the community.[1,14,37] Community-based training is highly significant in terms of fostering a student's interest in rural practice. More and more schools are recognizing the importance of exposing students to appropriate role models in primary care. Medical schools are allowing more community-based rural physicians to contribute to their academic programs. A better balance has been achieved between hospital-based subspecialty training and community-based primary care training. A greater proportion of medical training has been shifted to the outpatient and community-based sites where the majority of medical care is practiced. As medical schools continue to add more required family practice clerkships, more and more rural primary care settings have been recruited to provide important teaching activities. The characteristics of ideal clinical physicians have been identified (Table 22-2).

TABLE 22-2   CHARACTERISTICS OF IDEAL CLINICAL TEACHERS

Breadth of clinical knowledge
Enthusiastic
Energetic
Enjoys teaching
Friendly
Clinically competent and credible
Well organized
Accessible
Interested in students
Interested in patients
Sets good example
Models appropriate behavior
Provides feedback
Responds to questions
Communicates performance expectations

SOURCE: Modified from Sheets KJ, Harris DL: Questions asked by family physicians who want to serve as medical student preceptors. *J Fam Pract* 42:503–511, 1996.

TABLE 22-3   WHAT STUDENTS CAN LEARN FROM A PRECEPTOR

Real medicine outside the academic medical center
Doctor-patient relationship skills
Doctor-doctor relationship skills
Medical knowledge
Procedural skills
Negotiation skills
Application of basic science knowledge
Practice management
How to handle acute medical problems
How to handle chronic medical problems
How to work with specialists and subspecialists in consultation/referral situations
How to work with community resources/agencies

SOURCE: From Society of Teachers of Family Medicine. Preceptor Education Project: workshop materials and instructor's manual. Kansas City, MO: Society of Teachers of Family Medicine, 1992, and from Sheets KJ, Harris DL: Questions asked by family physicians who want to serve as medical student preceptors. *J Fam Pract* 42:503–511, 1996, with permission.

Students benefit significantly from clinical experiences based in a community outside the boundaries of the academic medical center. Rural preceptors have much to teach, find themselves continually challenged by the presence of students and residents, and stay connected to their regional medical school for social, educational, and clinical reasons (Table 22-3).

Serving as a preceptor takes time, not only in terms of teaching (an additional 45 to 60 minutes per day) but also regarding meeting the academic medical center's requirements for evaluation, feedback, and grading.[38] Working with patients while obtaining feedback on their skills helps build the students' confidence. Rural preceptorship experiences also offer the opportunity to examine community needs. Most medical schools provide appropriate clerkship handbooks and may provide regular preceptorship training workshops, particularly regarding teaching skills, evaluation, and feedback. Although it costs money and time to teach medical students in the office, serving as a preceptor is intellectually stimulating and an investment in the future of rural practice.

SUMMARY

To be successful in meeting the health care needs of our rural areas, medical schools must give serious consideration to the provision of a continuous educational pipeline throughout the 4 years of medical school that is designed to stimulate and foster students' interest in rural practice. These important educational opportunities must be linked by an appropriate and unbiased advising system located within the medical school. All things being equal (GPA, MCAT scores), special admission policies could be considered. Students from rural backgrounds and with a stated interest in primary care (particularly family practice) could be preferentially selected. Rural clinical experiences during the first and second years of medical school assist in reinforcing interest in primary care among students. Required 6-week family practice rotations should occur in the third year and at a community-based teaching site if possible. Longitudinal experiences such as RPAP or WRITE should be considered in those schools lacking longitudinal training opportunities. Other primary care experiences in the third and fourth years should be considered. Of major importance throughout all of these educational experiences is the development of community-based teaching faculty outside the academic institution who are willing to share their clinical expertise and practice with students. These clinical faculty should be appropriately recognized within the institution and should receive ongoing faculty development regarding teaching skills, evaluation, and feedback. Through this highly cooperative and highly integrated effort, we will move closer toward meeting the health care needs of our rural populations.

REFERENCES

1. Bland CJ, Meurer LN, Maldonado G: Determinants of primary care specialty choice: a non-statistical meta-analysis of the literature. *Acad Med* 70:620–641, 1995.

2. Meurer LN: Influence of medical school curriculum on primary care specialty choice: analysis and synthesis of the literature. *Acad Med* 70:388–397, 1995.

3. Geyman JP, Hart LG, Norris T, et al: Physician education and rural location: a critical review. In press.

4. Boulger JG, Beathick, Repesh L, et al: Reinforcing medical students' decisions to practice family medicine in a rural setting: the University of Minnesota, Duluth School of Medicine and the Rural Physician Associate Program (unpublished).

5. Boulger J: Family medicine education and rural health: a response to present and future needs. *J Rural Health* 7:105–115, 1992.

6. Lynch DC, Newton DA, Grayson MS, Whitley TW: Influence of medical school on medical students' opinions about primary care practice. *Acad Med* 73:433–435, 1993.

7. Campos-Outcalt D, Senf J, Watkins AJ, Bastacky S: The effects of medical school curricula, faculty role models, and biomedical research support on choice of generalist physician careers: a review and quality assessment of the literature. *Acad Med* 70:611–619, 1995.

8. Xu G, Veloski J, Barzanski B: Comparisons between older and usual-aged medical school graduates on the factors influencing their choices of primary care specialities. *Acad Med* 72:1003–1007, 1997.

9. Colwill JM, Perkoff GT, Blake RL, et al: Modifying the culture of medical education: the first three years of the RWJ generalist physician initiative. *Acad Med* 72:745–753, 1997.

10. Rosenblatt RA, Whitcomb ME, Cullen TJ, et al: Which medical schools produce rural physicians? *JAMA* 268:1559–1565, 1992.

11. Whitcomb ME, et al: Compiling the characteristics of schools that produce high percentages and low percentages of primary care physicians. *Acad Med* 67:589–591, 1992.

12. Hull AL, Glover PB, Acheson LS, et al: Medical school applicants' essays as predictors of primary care career choice. *Acad Med* 71:37–39, 1996.

13. Kassebaum DG, Szenas PL: Medical students' career indecision and specialty rejection: roads not taken. *Acad Med* 70:938–943, 1995.

14. Boulger J: Factors influencing primary care career choices (unpublished).

15. Senf JH, Campos-Outcalt D, Watkins AJ, et al: A systematic analysis of how medical school char-

acteristics relate to graduates' choices of primary care specialties. *Acad Med* 72:524–533, 1997.

16. Rubeck RF, Donnelly MB, Jarecky RM, et al: Demographic, educational, and psychosocial factors influencing the choices of primary care and academic medical careers. *Acad Med* 70:318–320, 1995.

17. Basco WT, Buchbinder SB, Duggan AK, Wilson MH: Associations between primary care-oriented practices in medical school admission and the practice intentions of matriculants. *Acad Med* 73:1207–1213, 1993.

18. Brock DM, Schaad DC, Guo J, et al: Development and psychometric properties of the Washington primary care interest inventory. *Acad Med* 73:1299–1304, 1993.

19. Kassebaum DG, Szenas PL, Schuchert MK: Determinants of the generalist career intentions of 1995 graduating medical students. *Acad Med* 71:1998–1209, 1996.

20. Xu G, Rattner SL, Veloski JJ, et al: A national study of the factors influencing men and women physicians' choices of primary care specialties. *Acad Med* 70:398–404, 1995.

21. Xu G, Rattner SL, Veloski JJ, et al: A national study of the factors influencing men and women physicians' choices of primary care specialties. *Acad Med* 70:398–404, 1995.

22. Dobie SA, Carline JD, Laskowski MB: An early preceptorship and medical students' beliefs, values, and career choices. *Adv Health Sci Educ* 2:35–47, 1997.

23. Rabinowitz HK: Recruitment, retention and follow-up of graduates of a program to increase the number of family physicians in rural and underserved areas. *N Engl J Med* 328:934–939, 1993.

24. Rabinowitz HK: A program to recruit and educate medical students to practice family medicine in underserved areas. *JAMA* 249:1038–1041, 1983.

25. Rabinowitz HK: Estimating the percentage of primary care rural physicians produced by regular and special admissions policies. *J Med Educ* 61(7):598–600, 1986.

26. Rabinowitz HK, Diamond JJ, Markham FW, et al: A program to increase the number of family physicians in rural and underserved areas: impact after 22 years. *JAMA* 281:255–260, 1999.

27. Ackermann RJ, Comeau RW: Mercer University School of Medicine: a successful approach to primary care medical education. *Fam Med* 28:395–402, 1996.

28. Atkins RJ, et al: Geographic and specialty distributions of WAMI program participants and nonparticipants. *J Med Educ* 62:810–817, 1987.

29. Blake RL: Increasing the production of generalist physicians. *Acad Med Suppl* 74:S1–S14, 1999.

30. Brooks WB, Orgren R, Wallace AG: Institutional change: embracing the initiative to train more generalists. *Acad Med Suppl* 74:S3–S8, 1999.

31. Grayson MS, Newton DA, Klein M, et al: Promoting institutional change to encourage primary care: experiences at New York Medical College and East Carolina University School of Medicine. *Acad Med Suppl* 74:S9–S15, 1999.

32. Hays RB, Bridges-Webb C, Harris M, Bushfield M: ARGPUs—academic rural general practice units. *Med J Aust* 157:473–474, 1992.

33. Craig M, Nichols A: training curricula in surgery, anaesthesia, and obstetrics for rural GPs. *Aust Fam Physician* 22:1218–1219, 1993.

34. Craig M, Nichols A, Price D: Education for the management of obstetric conditions in rural general practice: a curriculum statement for a major in obstetric studies in the Rural Training Programme of the Faculty of Rural Medicine, Royal Australian College of General Practitioners. *Aust NZ J Obstet Gynaecol* 33:230–239, 1993.

35. Rourke JT: Postgraduate training for rural family practice: goals and opportunities. *Can Fam Physician* 42:1133–1138, 1996.

36. Rourke JT, Rouke LL: Rural family medicine training in Canada. *Can Fam Physician* 41:993–1000, 1995.

37. Brazeau NK, Potts MJ, Hickner JM: The Upper Peninsula Program: a successful model for increasing primary care physicians in rural areas. *Fam Med* 22(5):350–355, 1990.

38. Sheets KJ, Harris DL: Questions asked by family physicians who want to serve as medical student preceptors. *J Fam Pract* 42:503–511, 1996.

CHAPTER 23

Graduate Education for Rural Practice

John P. Geyman

John Jones grew up in a small town in Ohio and decided in high school that he wanted to become a physician. Having enjoyed a rural background growing up, his goal was to become a generalist physician in a small town, probably out West. He attended a state medical school in his home state with a traditional predoctoral curriculum and no rural track or electives. After graduation, he entered a family practice residency program in a western state. He was attracted to the program by its location in a western state not too distant from wilderness areas, by the program's strong reputation (including other residency programs in internal medicine, surgery, and obstetrics/gynecology at the same institution), and by the opportunities for his wife to further her education and employment.

The 18-resident family practice residency was based in a family practice center adjacent to a 350-bed university-affiliated teaching hospital. Most inpatient rotations were in that hospital, while obstetrics/gynecology and pediatrics rotations were provided in other hospitals elsewhere in the city. The program director had spent 15 years in private family practice in a nearby suburb before entering full-time teaching. The other full-time faculty had similar practice experience in suburban settings. The program did not have a clear-cut mission in terms of goals for its graduates, almost all of whom had gone on to group family practice in metropolitan areas. The program valued diversity in its selection process, with a nearly equal distribution by gender and about 20 percent minorities. Since the program had to provide coverage on a regular basis to rotations in medicine, pediatrics, and obstetrics/gynecology, there was

a minimal amount of elective time over the 3 years of the program. There was no opportunity for advanced obstetric training; there were also no faculty role models with rural practice experience and no organized rural electives.

After 3 years in the program, Dr. Jones felt well trained in many areas of family practice but not well prepared in obstetrics or in procedural or emergency care for his anticipated needs in rural practice. He had experienced no reinforcement during his training for his original rural practice goals. Upon completion of his training, with some regret, he joined three other family physicians in a nearby suburban practice that appeared to best meet his family's needs, including his wife's new position in a local law firm.

T he above circumstances are played out time and again in graduate education programs, across both disciplines and borders. Most such programs are located in cities, owing in large part to the ready availability of the multidisciplinary teaching resources and plentiful hospital beds required by traditional residency programs. Very few have a mission of preparing graduates for rural medical practice. For those programs that do espouse that mission, there are many steps along the way that threaten to derail the trainee from his or her original goal to establish practice in a rural area of need.

The goal of this chapter is to explore the challenges of graduate education for rural practice, including such aspects as recruitment and selection, program organization and curriculum, types of rural experiences, and reasons for success or failure in preparing graduates for rural practice. Lessons, both positive and negative, are touched upon, together with comment concerning future directions.

BACKGROUND

The shortage of physicians in rural areas has been a long-standing problem that has persisted for generations in the United States and in many other countries around the world, as physicians preferentially settle in metropolitan, suburban, or other nonrural areas. Although many initiatives have been attempted by state and federal governments in the United States and abroad to address the problem of geographic maldistribution of physicians, the problem remains chronic, and many of these efforts have either failed or met with limited success. Some of the challenges to recruitment and long-term retention of physicians and other health care providers in rural practice involve the adequacy and relevance of educational preparation, while others involve the rural environment itself.

Before one can address this subject with any precision, the term *rural* must be clarified. There are many definitions and interpretations of this term. For the purpose of this chapter, our focus is on communities of less than 10,000 people not adjacent to metropolitan areas, or "small rural." This is where the real challenges of rural practice are seen—not in small communities immediately adjacent to a large metropolitan area.

As has been evident from the opening chapter of this book, rural health care is extremely complex, and there is no single profile fitting all rural areas. That the nature of rural life is being subjected to major change is well illustrated by the findings of Cordes in a 1990 paper exploring seven myths about rural America. He found that (1) rural populations in the United States are no longer declining but increasing, (2) farming has given way to manufacturing as the major source of employment in rural areas, (3) there are more similarities than differences in the economic structure of rural and urban America, (4) rural areas are no longer isolated from mainstream urban life, (5) rural people share much of the knowledge and many of the attitudes and beliefs of urban people, (6) rural people are *not* happier and healthier than their urban counterparts, and (7) rural America is much more diverse than previously thought.[1]

About 20 percent of the U.S. population, over 50 million people, live in rural areas, while only 9 percent of physicians practice there.[2] More than 22 million Americans live in Health Professions Shortage Areas (HPSAs), defined as areas with less than one primary care physician per 3500 people.[3] Despite big increases in the total number of physicians since World War II, most have settled in metropolitan areas, thereby worsening the chronic problem of geographic maldistribution of physicians.[2]

It is apparent from Chap. 22, on predoctoral education for rural practice, that selection, education, recruitment, and retention of physicians and other health professionals in rural practice involve a long "pipeline." This chapter deals mainly with educational programs themselves, but some attention is necessarily also paid to issues of selection, recruitment, and retention, including the changing environment of rural practice. Our focus is on family practice as a classic example of the problems being addressed and approaches being taken to preparing physicians for small rural practice. This is not to say that other specialties or types of health professionals are not involved in rural practice but that family physicians represent a core need in such areas and that most of the available literature bears on the family practice experience in training rural health providers. Small rural communities require generalists with a broad range of medical knowledge and skills who are capable of sharing after-hours call. Internists, pediatricians, and obstetrician/gynecologists typically need a catchment area large enough to support five or more physicians, not the usual small rural environment.[2]

GRADUATE MEDICAL EDUCATION

Example of Family Practice

Graduate training in family practice not only deals directly with the major generalist physician provider in rural practice but also illustrates well the challenges, problems, and progress in this area. We first examine the U.S. experience with graduate education for rural practice, including program orientation, requisites for training, and special educational strategies. Brief comparative commentary is then added concerning graduate training for rural generalists in several other countries.

United States

RURAL MISSION AND LOCATION

A recent national study of U.S. nonmilitary family practice residency programs revealed 151 programs claiming a rural mission. This number can be misleading, however, in both directions. The extent and quality of actual rural emphasis is often unclear from a program's claim. In addition, it is known that some programs with bona fide rural emphasis have not claimed a rural mission; there are 25 programs in the United States with either a rural training track (RTT), rural clinic, or rural fellowship that did not claim a rural mission.[4,5] There is considerable regional variation of rurally oriented programs, as shown in Fig. 23-1.[4]

In terms of program location, Saver and colleagues profiled the locations of all U.S. family practice residency programs by urban influence codes. They identified 96 programs listing some kind of rural descriptor (out of more than 480 programs). Among these, there were 31 RTT sites in 26 programs in clearly rural locations, with an additional 22 non-RTT programs in rural locations.[6]

NECESSARY REQUISITES FOR RURAL TRAINING

A recent national study by Norris et al. surveyed over 600 family physicians in current rural practice in order to identify their individual educa-

tional needs assessments. They found many particular educational needs beyond those required in many metropolitan settings, including emergency care, general trauma care, advanced obstetrics, pre- and postoperative care, and surgical assisting.[7] It is clear that curricula of family practice residency programs need to be strong in all of the above areas. In addition, residents in training for rural practice must have required rotations or elective experience in actual rural settings. They must have exposure to positive role models of physicians practicing in rural communities as well as an ongoing nurturing environment during their residency training for their future practice goals.

SPECIAL EDUCATIONAL STRATEGIES

RESIDENT SELECTION   It has become abundantly clear that family practice residency programs committed to preparing family physicians for rural practice must pay careful attention to selecting residents most likely to pursue that goal. Many factors have been shown to play an important role in the selection, recruitment, and retention of physicians in rural areas. These interrelate and play out before, during, and after a young physician's medical school and residency training years. Two factors have been demonstrated by Rabinowitz and colleagues to be especially influential in this regard. Based on a 22-year experience with the Physician Shortage Area Program (PSAP) at Jefferson Medical College in Philadelphia, they found that a *special medical school admission policy* (including rural background and stated goal for rural family practice) together with a *special educational program* (faculty, advising, required third-year family medicine clerkship, and fourth-year subinternship in family medicine) led to a sustained positive impact on the selection of future family physicians and their retention in rural practice. They found that PSAP graduates were four times more likely to practice family medicine (52 versus 13 percent) and ten times more likely than non-PSAP graduates to combine a career choice of family medicine with rural practice

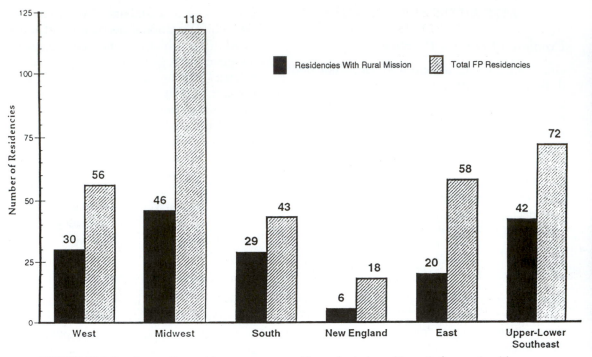

FIGURE 23-1 *Family practice residency programs with rural missions. (From Reference 4, with permission.)*

(21 versus 2 percent). In addition, they found that long-term retention in rural practice is high, with 87 percent of PSAP graduates who were practicing family medicine in rural areas between 5 and 10 years ago still so involved today.[8]

Another national study of 380 family practice residency programs (68 percent response rate) and over 1000 residents examined the choice by residents of their initial practice location. That choice is indeed complex, as shown in Table 23-1, which shows that the decisions of the graduating residents' significant others were the most important of many factors.[9]

The latest information from annual surveys of the Association of American Medical Colleges (AAMC) provides useful insights based upon 1995 graduates of U.S. medical schools. Only 294 senior medical students (out of 13,000 respondents and 16,000 total graduates) declared an interest in future practice in rural communities of less than 10,000 people. Compared to

their nonrural classmates, rurally oriented students were slightly older; more likely to be married and to have children; usually white; graduating from public medical schools; and more likely to prefer family practice. Twice as many took rural/international electives and did volunteer work in public health clinics or other programs for underserved areas.[10]

The gender of the medical graduate is also an important factor. For example, there are less than 7000 female physicians now practicing in rural America; the overall male/female ratio across all 50 states for practicing rural physicians is 5.4 to 1.[11] Although the future gender distribution of rural physicians needs to be closely monitored, experience so far calls for targeting male applicants for rurally oriented residency training. At the same time, consideration should be given to exploring whether and how rural practice can become more attractive to female physicians.

TABLE 23-1   MOST IMPORTANT FACTORS TO GRADUATING FAMILY PRACTICE RESIDENTS IN CHOOSING THEIR FIRST PRACTICE SITE[a]

Factor	Rank	Percent Responding Important[b]	Mean Likert Rating
Significant other's wishes	1	85.2	4.30
Medical community friendly to family physicians	2	76.3	4.02
Recreation/culture	3	60.7	3.64
Proximity to family/friends	4	60.1	3.64
Significant other's employment	5	59.0	3.55
Schools for children	6	58.2	3.44
Size of community	7	53.8	3.49
Initial income guarantee	8	52.8	3.45
Benefits plan	9	52.8	3.42
Proximity to spouse's family/friends	10	51.3	3.37
Weather/geography	11	50.6	3.45
Need for physicians	12	46.1	3.25
Significant other's school opportunities	13	45.6	3.04
Maximum potential income	14	45.4	3.24
Familiar with physicians in area	15	35.6	2.92
Community service commitment	16	35.2	2.86
Affordable housing	17	33.5	2.97
Opportunity to teach	18	31.5	2.86
Familiar with hospital	19	31.0	2.81
Loan payback plan	20	27.6	2.49
Signing bonus	21	26.3	2.61
Residency nearby	22	22.1	2.48
Medical school nearby	23	13.4	2.19
Military service commitment	24	13.3	1.74

[a]$n = 1012$

[b]4–5 on Likert scale on which 1 = not important and 5 = very important.

SOURCE: From Costa AJ, Schrop SL, McCord G, Gillanders WR: To stay or not to stay: factors influencing family practice residents' choice of initial practice location. *Fam Med* 28:214–219, 1996, with permission.

LOCATING RESIDENCY PROGRAMS IN OR NEAR RURAL AREAS   Two main approaches have been taken by U.S. family practice residencies in terms of program location: (1) the "one and two" program or rural training track (RTT) and (2) the Area Health Education Centers.

One and two programs were developed in the late 1970s, combining a first residency year in a large urban teaching center with the next two residency years in a small family practice group practice and associated community hos-

pital in a distant rural community.[12] Up to seven programs were established at that time, but the idea did not catch on and most such programs ended up as 3-year programs in the smaller community. In more recent years, the very similar rural training track (RTT) has emerged as a more successful approach. Rosenthal and colleagues recently completed an initial evaluation of RTTs based on a 1996 survey. They found that over half of the RTT sites are in HPSAs; that each family practice center has an average of three full-time faculty; that the average size of the associated rural hospital is 173 beds (range 14 to 308 beds); and that of the first 99 RTT graduates, 76 percent had entered rural practice.[13] Based on the early experience of these RTTs, Rosenthal et al. identified the following five major elements of successful RTTS: (1) academically sound urban component of program, (2) supportive urban medical center, (3) financially viable rural hospital, (4) modern rural practice unit, and (5) robust rural community.[13]

Although the experience of RTTs has so far been promising, there are several problems that go beyond the traditional residency program. Resident recruitment, of course, can be more difficult than usual, since a major move is required after the first year for the resident and his or her spouse if married. Many challenges are encountered in the organization and development of an RTT, including issues of accreditation, match numbers for resident selection, and new communication and collaborative arrangements between participating institutions. Funding is also a problem, since reimbursement for rural health services is less than for similar services in urban settings, and mechanisms for Medicare graduate medical education (GME) payments to rural hospitals and teaching units is either unavailable or problematic.

The National Area Health Education Center (AHEC) Program was established in 1970 with an overall goal to serve the health care needs of rural and other underserved populations. Many regional and statewide AHECs have been formed since then, emphasizing primary care education in community hospitals affiliated with academic health science centers. AHECs have provided the means for community-based medical education at predoctoral, graduate, and continuing medical education levels. Critics feel that this program is expensive and duplicative of other parts of the medical education establishment. Supporters point to the marginal experience that AHEC counties in North Carolina with less than 50,000 people averaged 3 to 5 percent higher primary care physician-to-population ratios than non-AHEC counties between 1975 and 1985.[14] Linkages between AHECs and family practice residencies are also a mixed story. Blondell and colleagues studied all AHEC projects around the country, reporting in 1989 that only about two-thirds of 38 AHEC projects had some interaction with family practice resident programs and that AHEC resources are underutilized by family practice residencies for rural education initiatives.[15]

CURRICULAR BREADTH   Much of what is known about the presence, extent, and content of rurally oriented curricula in U.S. family practice residency programs was revealed in a recent study by Bowman and Penrod of 100 rurally oriented family practice residencies. They found that two-thirds of these programs provide specific didactics on rural topics; that 80 percent emphasize computer skills, including Internet access; that 60 percent use telemedicine for teaching purposes or consultation; and that 45 percent have library holdings on rural health resources. On the other hand, they found that many other subjects were not yet presented, including rural hospital issues, rural health policy, networking, significant other's transition, and adaptation of the physician, as well as others. Responding programs listed a number of areas in which rural physicians may feel inadequately prepared, such as advanced obstetrics, medical specialties, geriatric home care and assessment, counseling, and community assessment.[4]

It is common wisdom today that family practice residents with future plans for rural practice need advanced training in emergency care and life support, including Advanced Cardiac Life Support (ACLS), Advanced Trauma Life Support (ATLS), and Pediatric Advanced Life Support (PALS). They need considerably more than a basic 2-month rotation in obstetrics. They need a more extensive array of procedural competencies than their urban counterparts. They also need leadership and communication skills in order to be effective in leading a sizable health care team in the care of both individual patients and community health problems. Further commentary on some of these areas is provided else-

TABLE 23-2   SELECTED CHARACTERISTICS AND RURAL PRACTICE CHOICE BY FAMILY PRACTICE RESIDENCY GRADUATES

Number of required rural months	0	1	2	3	4–6	22+
(Number of programs with rural months)	(212)	(82)	(29)	(15)	(4)	(11)
Graduates choosing rural practice	24.4%	36.5%	45.6%	52.3%	51.0%	68.5%
Number of obstetric months taken	0	1	2	3	4	>4
(Number of programs)			(141)	(111)	(71)	(30)
Graduates choosing rural			23.8%	31.2%	34.1%	42.1%
Number of other graduate programs used	0	1	2	3	4–6	
(Number of family practice programs)	(138)	(33)	(27)	(28)	(127)	
Graduates choosing rural (mean)	37.3%	26.4%	25.1%	27.4%	22.5%	

SOURCE: From Bowman RC, Penrod JD: Family practice residency programs and the graduation of rural family physicians. *Fam Med* 30:288–292, 1998, with permission.

where in this book, as in Chap. 7 (on emergency care) and Chap. 9 (on perinatal care). The positive influence on choice of rural practice exerted by extent of rural rotations and obstetric training is shown in Table 23-2.[4]

SPECIAL RURAL EXPERIENCES   Many family practice residencies offer 4- to 8-week community practice rotations or preceptorships in rural family practice settings. These experiences can be usefully employed by residencies that have not developed a coherent rural mission or curriculum. They can be helpful to residents who may be considering future careers in rural practice but clearly need to be supplemented by additional training in typical areas of need, as described above.

FELLOWSHIPS   Another educational approach taken by some family practice residency programs is the creation of various kinds of fellowships, typically 1 year in duration. Based on self-report of 353 responding programs, Bowman and Penrod identified 42 obstetric fellowships, 16 rural fellowships, and 70 programs with various kinds of procedural emphasis.[4] Most of these fellowship programs are too new to be fully evaluated or reported in the literature. An exception is the fellowship in rural family medicine at Tacoma Family Medicine, Washington. Norris and Acosta recently reported their first 5-year experience with this 1-year fellowship.

The curriculum included 6 months of advanced obstetrics (including cesarean section competency), a 1-month rural rotation in community medicine, and 5 months of electives. The most commonly chosen electives have been (in descending order of frequency): obstetric ultrasound, colposcopy, anesthesia, gynecology, sports medicine, minor surgery, orthopedics, neonatal intensive care, and exercise stress testing. There have been 40 to 60 applicants each year for the 8 fellow positions. Some 90 percent of fellows have felt that the fellowship met their needs, and 80 percent of its graduates are practicing in communities with less than 10,000 people, while the others are in academic practice, large community practice, or a surgical fellowship (the latter included one graduate preparing for missionary service overseas).[16]

Figure 23-2 summarizes various educational strategies that have been found useful in increasing the supply of rural physicians along a pipeline continuum from high school and college through the medical education years.[17]

Some Comparisons from Other Countries

Although each country has a unique set of circumstances relating to graduate education for rural practice, it is interesting to note many similarities as well as some unique differences in approaches to the worldwide problem of chronic geographic maldistribution of physi-

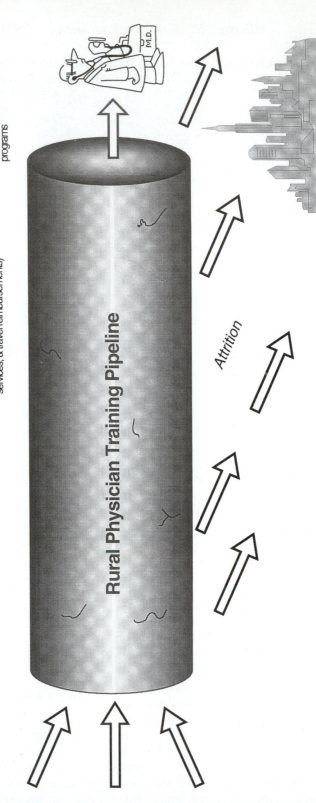

High School/College

- Rural and minority health professions programs (e.g., AHEC sponsored)
- Early admissions programs
- Primary care mentorship programs
- Rural observation experience
- Local high school encouragement & opportunity activities

Medical School

- Rural mission
- Admission policies
- Profiling of candidates
- Curricula for primary care
- Advisor and mentor programs
- Rural experience programs

Graduate Training

- Selection Process
- Location of residencies
- Rural goals of programs
- Rural curricula/experience, e.g.,
  - breadth of curriculum
  - rural rotations
  - rural training tracks (RTTs)
  - fellowships
- Rural training support (e.g., e-mail, telehealth teaching, library services, & travel reimbursements)

Rural Practice

- Continuing medical education (CME)
- National Health Service Corps (NHSC)
- Indian Health Service (IHS)
- Other approaches to sustain and nurture retention in rural practice, e.g.,
  - telehealth
  - reimbursement incentives
  - retention & clinical support programs

Rural Physician Training Pipeline

Attrition

FIGURE 23-2 Physician education and rural location: a pipeline continuum. (From Geyman JP, Hart LG, Norris TE, et al: Physician Education and Rural Location: A Critical Review. Rural health working paper no. 49. Seattle, WA, WWAMI Rural Health Research Center, University of Washington, 1999, with permission.)

cians. Rourke has compiled an excellent resource based on published work around the world on this subject—*Education for Rural Medical Practice: Goals and Opportunities: an Annotated Bibliography*.[18] Educational approaches to training physicians for rural practice are also included in the final chapters of this book, which deal with Canada, Australia, the United Kingdom, South Africa, and China, respectively. Of comparative interest here is the fact that *all* of Canada's 18 family practice residencies offer rural practice experience to their residents[19]—quite a contrast with the relatively limited proportion of U.S. family practice residencies that do so.

EXPERIENCE OF OTHER SPECIALTIES

The published literature contains scant reference to educational initiatives to prepare physicians in specialties other than family practice for rural practice. Saver and colleagues recently went beyond a literature search to conduct key informant interviews and E-mail postings to *listservc* for educators in other specialties, and their retrieval of relevant reports was still extremely limited.[6]

The few articles found from this search suggest that rural medical education in other specialties is not of high priority. There are a small number of internal medicine residencies located in rural counties, but these are in large multispecialty groups (e.g., the Geisinger Clinic) with more of a referral than primary care practice.[6] Two small pilot programs involving short rural clinic rotations for internal medicine residents at Harvard and in Florida were reported about 20 years ago, but no later follow-up reports were published.[20,21] In 1995, the University of Minnesota Internal Medicine Residency Program reported on a 1-month ambulatory care block rotation in community settings, but it is unclear how rural these sites are.[22]

In pediatrics, a rural primary care pediatrics residency program was established about 15 years ago at Dartmouth-Hitchcock Medical Center. Residents spent 1 day per week in their second and third residency years in selected practices in towns within 45 miles as well as 3- to 4-week rotations in all 3 years; no follow-up evaluations have been reported.[23]

In surgery, the University of Louisville established a third-year rural surgery rotation in the 1970s. After 10 years with this project, Asher and colleagues reported that the residents' experience was useful educationally, and that 44 percent of the 58 responding graduates subsequently entered rural surgical practice.[24] Although a rural surgery track is presently in a planning stage at the Oregon Health Sciences University, there is no available evidence today of a currently operational general surgery program in the United States with a rural orientation and mission.[25]

CURRENT STATUS OF GRADUATE MEDICAL EDUCATION FOR RURAL PRACTICE

As is apparent from the foregoing, the last 25 years have seen considerable growth of knowledge and experience concerning educational strategies to address the problem of geographic maldistribution of physicians in rural areas. Some excellent educational models have been developed, together with a sizable number of active family practice residencies with a rural mission. At least three main steps are required, however, if the number of rural physicians is to be increased and kept in line with the needs of a growing rural population: (1) identify candidates for rural generalist practice early in the educational pipeline (i.e., preferably before medical school admission), (2) establish and maintain excellent rural training opportunities for medical students and residents, and (3) minimize the barriers to long-term retention in rural practice by creating a nurturing environment for such practice.

Recruitment of Rural-Oriented Applicants

In the first instance, much has been learned concerning the most likely candidates to pursue future rural practice. At the University of North Carolina, Madison has found that a service orientation as revealed by medical school applicants on their application essay (i.e., volunteer activities, social need content, Peace Corps) was a strong predictor ($p = 0.0001$) of a generalist career 7 years later.[26] Based upon what is now known about generalist specialty choice and rural practice, Rosenthal has recommended the following approaches to increase the number of rural physicians[27]:

1. Determine medical school's mission (does it include rural?)
2. Profile applicants
    MCATs, GPA (threshold), community of origin, community service work, specialty intent
3. Admit students with plans consistent with school's mission
4. Require rural immersion experiences in curriculum
5. Follow up

The above recommendations are logical and on target, but much still remains to be done to increase the potential applicant pool of future rural physicians. It is now clear, for example, that the most likely candidates to become rural generalist physicians are white, usually male, have rural background/interests, favor primary care (especially family practice), and have demonstrated social concerns and interest in people. Yet admissions committees of many U.S. medical schools still do not include primary care physicians or have a special rural track, and the selection process of most family practice residencies does not explicitly target the above criteria.

Rural Training Opportunities

In the second instance, a number of educational approaches have already been demonstrated to be effective in preparing and placing graduates in rural practice. Rural physicians require a broader range of knowledge and skills than their counterparts in urban practice with close proximity to consultants in most specialties and the technology/resources of larger hospitals. Rural physicians must have excellent procedural skills in emergency medicine, obstetrics, minor surgery, orthopedics, and perhaps anesthesia. They must be skilled in community medicine, be attuned to team and group practice, and have computer and business skills. This broad spectrum of knowledge and skills can be acquired in a 3-year family practice residency, but only if the program has a strong rural mission and a carefully structured curriculum. Rural training tracks (RTTs) and rural fellowships have been shown to be promising toward this goal.

Although there is room for optimism from the progress described above, many barriers and concerns persist; these still threaten the further development of generalist education for rural practice. Accreditation requirements are one such barrier, as they still do not accommodate the needs of rurally oriented programs (e.g., one versus two residents in an RTT at any one time, or an overly narrow definition of the "Family Practice Center").[11] Another important barrier is the difficulty of funding rural GME programs. The North Carolina Rural Health Research and Policy Analysis Program, for example, has found that rural physicians are more dependent on Medicare and Medicaid than urban physicians, yet they are reimbursed at lower rates.[3] Still another potential concern is the recent trend towards hospital practice in many urban settings, which could lead to a decreased emphasis on inpatient training in some residency programs.

Retention in Rural Practice

It has become clear that rural residency training cannot enjoy long-term success if the rural practice environment is hostile or unappealing to program graduates. The trend toward small group practice and networking among rural physicians is one positive trend making rural practice much more attractive and viable than in the past. It has become almost impossible to sustain a rural solo practice over any length of time. Some of the newer approaches to continuing medical education, to be discussed in the next chapter, represent another means by which rural physicians can keep up. Telehealth is likely to see increased use for both continuing medical education (CME) and consultation, providing still another way of decreasing the isolation of rural physicians. Federal legislation in 1997 established reimbursement mechanisms for telehealth services for Medicare beneficiaries residing in HPSAs starting in January 1999. The National Library of Medicine has committed $42 million over the next few years to 19 demonstration projects in order to evaluate the effectiveness of telehealth services in various clinical and geographic settings.[28] There is also some recent progress toward dealing with reimbursement problems in rural practice. Starting in 1997, for example, Medicare reduced the urban/rural payment differential by consolidation of rural and urban areas in some states, while the Medicare Incentive Program provides a 10 percent supplement in some rural areas.[2]

In circumstances where a small rural hospital is either closed or on the brink of closure, Ambulatory Hospital Services Districts have been found effective in stabilizing local rural health services in Arizona and Washington State and have authorizing legislation in 33 other states.[29] In addition, federal legislation in 1997 established a Critical Access Hospital Program in an effort to stabilize threatened small hospitals as limited service facilities.

COMMENT AND FUTURE DIRECTIONS

Returning to the case vignette at the start of this chapter, it is likely that Dr. Jones would have realized his goal of becoming a rural generalist physician had he experienced rurally oriented exposure and training in his predoctoral and residency years. His original goal was to become a family physician in a small town, but he had no opportunity to reinforce that goal during his medical school years. He then entered an urban family practice residency program, albeit in a rural western state, without any rural emphasis or reinforcement of his rural goals. The end result of his selection of practice in a metropolitan area was only to be expected, as his educational needs for rural practice were not met and as he and his wife became enculturated to an urban lifestyle.

Based on the progress and increased knowledge gained over the last 25 years with medical education for rural practice, it seems certain that more rural physicians can be trained and retained in rural practice if the number of family practice teaching programs with explicit rural missions can be increased, accreditation restrictions relaxed, and fiscal problems addressed for rural teaching practices. Rural training tracks (RTTs) and rural fellowships are especially promising in this regard. Equally important, of course, is a selection process in both medical schools and residency programs favoring applicants with qualifications, traits, and interests consistent with the needs of future rural practice.

Finally, it will be important to closely monitor the progress and problems of rurally oriented medical education programs at all levels. The health care system is rapidly changing and the rural health care environment is still fragile. Federal and state health care policy will have to be sensitive to the special needs of rurally oriented medical education and the vital fabric of rural practice if the health care needs of the nations's growing rural population are to be met and well served.

REFERENCES

1. Cordes SM: Come on in, the water's just fine. *Acad Med* 65(12 suppl):S1–S9, 1990.
2. Council on Graduate Medical Education: *Physician Distribution and Health Care Challenges in Rural and Inner-City Areas.* Tenth Report. Washington, DC, U.S. Department of Health and Human Services, Public Health Service, Health Resources and Services Administration, 1998, February 11.

3. North Carolina Rural Health Research and Policy Analysis Program; Chapel Hill, NC. *Rural Health News* 413:3, 1998.

4. Bowman RC, Penrod JD: Family practice residency programs and the graduation of rural family physicians. *Fam Med* 30:288–292, 1998.

5. Acosta D: Medical education: current status of residency fellowships in rural health, in presentation at STFMs Working Group on Rural Health, Chicago, May 13, 1998, p 48.

6. Saver BG, Bowman R, Crittenden RA, et al: *Barriers to Residency Training of Physicians in Rural Areas.* Working paper no. 46. Seattle, WA, WWAMI Rural Health Research Center, 1998.

7. Norris TE, Coombs JB, Carline J: An educational needs assessment of rural family physicians. *J Am Board Fam Pract* 9:86–93, 1996.

8. Rabinowitz HK, Diamond JJ, Markham FW, Hazelwood CE: A program to increase the number of family physicians in rural and underserved areas: impact after 22 years. *JAMA* 281:255–260, 1999.

9. Costa AJ, Schrop SL, McCord G, Gillanders WR: To stay or not to stay: factors influencing family practice residents' choice of initial practice location. *Fam Med* 28:214–219, 1996.

10. STFM Group on Rural Health: *Rural Family Doctor.* Kansas City, MO, Spring, 1998.

11. Doescher MP, Ellsbury KE, Hart LG: The distribution of rural female generalist physicians in the United States. WWAMI RHRG. Working paper no. 44. Seattle, WA, University of Washington, February 1998.

12. Geyman JP: The "one and two" program: a new direction in family practice residency training. *J Med Educ* 52:999–1001, 1977.

13. Rosenthal TC, McGuigan MH, Osborne J, et al: One-two rural residency tracks in family practice: are they getting the job done? *Fam Med* 30:90–93, 1998.

14. Hynes K, Givner N: The effects of Area Health Education Centers on primary care physician-to-population ratios from 1975 to 1983. *J Rural Health* 6(1):9–17, 1990.

15. Blondell RD, Smith IJ, Byrne ME, Higgins CW: Rural health, family practice and area health education centers: a national study. *Fam Med* 21:183–186, 1989.

16. Norris TE, Acosta D: A fellowship in rural family medicine: program development and outcomes. *Fam Med* 29:414–420, 1997.

17. Geyman JP, Hart LG, Norris TE, et al: *Physician Education and Rural Location: A Critical Review.* Rural health working paper no. 49. Seattle, WA, WWAMI Rural Health Research Center, University of Washington, 1999.

18. Rourke J: *Education for Rural Medical Practice: Goals and Opportunities: An Annotated Bibliography.* Moe, Victoria, Australia, Australian Rural Health Research Institute, Monash University, 1996.

19. Rourke JT: Postgraduate training for rural family practice: goals and opportunities. *Can Fam Physician* 42:1133–1138, 1996.

20. Stern RS, Calkins D, Lawrence R, Delbanco T. Joining a rural practice: A pilot program in primary care education in internal medicine. *J Amb Care Mgt* February: 89–95, 1980.

21. Crandall LA, Reynolds RC, Coggins WJ: Evaluation of a rural clinical rotation for medical residents. *J Med Educ* 53:597–599, 1978.

22. Parenti CM, Maldow CF: Training internal medicine residents in the community: the Minnesota experience. *Acad Med* 70(5):366–369, 1995.

23. Kairys S, Newell P: A rural primary care residency program. *J Med Educ* 60:786–792, 1985.

24. Asher EF, Martin LF, Richardson JD, Polk HC: Rural rotations for senior surgical residents: influence on future practice location. *Arch Surg* 119:1120–1124, 1984.

25. Saver BG, Hart LG: Personal communication, September 8, 1998.

26. Madison DL: Medical school admission and generalist physicians: a study of the class of 1985. *Acad Med* 69:825–831, 1994.

27. Rosenthal TC: Factors influencing medical student selection of primary care careers. *Tex J Rural Health* Spring:28–37, 1994.

28. National Rural Health Association: *Issue Paper on the Role of Telemedicine in Rural Health Care.* Kansas City, MO, NRHA, February, 1998.

29. Taplin SE, Geyman JP, Gimlett D: The public hospital district for ambulatory care: an option to stabilize rural health services in crisis. *J Am Board Fam Pract* 7:493–502, 1994.

CHAPTER 24

Continuing Medical Education for Rural Practice

JEFFREY A. STEARNS

Continuing medical education (CME) is the overall process by which physicians acquire knowledge, skills, and attitudes after leaving residency (graduate medical education) and entering practice. It encompasses all of the learning experiences that physicians engage in with the conscious intent of continuously improving the performance of their professional duties (quality assurance and competence) and meeting their professional responsibilities. Optimal CME is relevant and highly self-directed. The physician should specifically select the appropriate content, learning methods, and learning resources to improve knowledge, skills, and attitudes required in his or her daily professional life.

The purpose of this chapter is to look at this overall process, especially as it applies to rural practitioners. CME, for a variety of reasons but particularly because of specialty board certification and state licensure requirements, has become a multimillion dollar industry. There is a growing literature on the process of CME and dozens of approaches, with variable efficacy, to attaining it. This chapter defines CME very broadly to encompass a variety of learning mechanisms in order to look at current CME; suggest an evidence-based approach for attaining our CME while focusing on individual relevancy; and examine how CME may be presented in the future, given the constantly expanding world of electronic communication.

BACKGROUND OF CONTINUING MEDICAL EDUCATION

Definition of Continuing Medical Education

CME is the lifelong process of education that physicians follow after leaving residency. It encompasses a broad range of formal and informal learning activities engaged in by physicians, with the goal of maintaining and improving professional competencies in relation to quality assurance. It must therefore be self-directed and highly specific to be relevant to the daily professional activities of the practitioner.

Increasingly, undergraduate medical education includes the goal of "lifelong" learning skills as an important competency for graduating students. The explicit process by which one pursues this competency is actually the objective of multiple courses. The entire problem-based learning approach to medical education teaches a process of problem definition and specific information gathering. Although the need to maintain competency for practice has long been accepted and remains the major objective of CME, the ability to pursue this goal has been greatly enhanced and facilitated by the "information superhighway" and advances in computer and communication technology. Although the CME requirements for state licensure and board certification may drive formal CME, a mechanism for information organization, access, and mastery assumes great importance for maintaining this competency as the twenty-first century begins. This is particularly significant for the situations of rural practitioners.

Traditionally, physicians, the CME "industry," and the accreditation process focus on CME in the form of a didactic process, most often consisting of lectures, conferences, and skill-acquisition practicums; in addition, journals and/or audiotapes, etc., play a role. It is important to look beyond this somewhat delimiting definition, as we are faced with the exponential growth of information, quality assurance/practice performance, and clinical outcomes. Consequently, continuing medical education for the future must be defined as any measure that attempts to get practitioners to modify their practice performance with the ultimate goal of improving the quality of outcomes for patients, practices, or the many other stakeholders in the process of health care delivery.[1] This broader definition allows many additional methodologies to be applied to the process of lifelong learning.

Motivation for Continuing Medical Education

The overarching reason for lifelong learning and engaging in the process of CME must be the assessment and maintenance of professional competence. The continuing quality of patient care (in all its definitions) is contingent on professional competence. The desire to be up to date and to provide quality care is a deep-rooted, highly ingrained characteristic of physicians, but the scrutiny of external entities also provides increasing motivation to pursue continued professional improvement. Beyond this broad goal are more specific motivators:

- Seeking information to address an individual patient's problem or an unusual diagnosis
- Needing CME as a requirement for membership in professional organizations or maintenance of licensure

- Meeting the challenge of teaching medical students and residents
- Changing scope of practice or taking on new responsibilities
- Satisfying curiosity about new approaches to diagnosis and therapy

It is important to understand that the specific reasons to seek new information should actually drive the choice of methodology to achieve the continuing education.

Literature on Continuing Medical Education

An important question to ask in the process of reviewing CME is "Does it work?" There is a growing literature on this subject, and it has become a legitimate area of academic inquiry. Davis and colleagues at the University of Toronto have a series of articles[1-3] that scrutinize this question. Both the increasing commercialization of the CME process and the quality-assurance movement demand an answer to this question. Davis and colleagues define CME from a broad prospective to include all educational interventions that seek to change physician behavior or patient outcomes. They have categorized a number of interventions, many of them "classic" CME, others less traditional, for examination through a rigorous evaluation process. The categories examined include:

- Educational materials (noninteractive printed materials, audiotapes, videotapes, computer-generated materials)
- Formal CME programs (courses, seminars, rounds, meetings, lectures, conferences, workshops, small group discussions, traineeships, teleconferences)
- Local, community-identified opinion leaders or educational specialists
- Outreach visits ("academic detailing" by doctors of pharmacy or other education professionals)
- Patient-linked interventions, like audit with

feedback, including chart review with peers or supervisors or chart reminders
• Combinations of these activities

Of the 160 interventions, 62 percent showed an improvement in at least one outcome. Of significant concern was that the more traditional methods of CME showed little or no change in physician behavior or patient outcomes. The community-based strategies, such as outreach visits, or the patient-linked strategies, such as audits, were more successful.

Davis and colleagues apply a strict quantitative methodology to evaluate outcomes of CME, eliminating the studies using more qualitative methods of evaluation. If one accepts that the ultimate goal of CME is to change physician behavior and to affect patient outcomes, the process of current CME must also be reexamined. A more important conclusion to be drawn may be that CME must be focused on specific individual needs or patient problems rather than on the acquisition of more generalized information.

Another study in 1992 by Kwee[4] of rural providers in Oregon asked a number of important questions about CME. This study examined CME in relation to a specific topic (geriatrics) and involved a variety of types of rural providers. The investigators found general interest in CME on this topic, for the full range of motivational reasons. They also identified a number of barriers to CME, such as location, timing, and distance to travel. Therefore, as one looks at CME of all types for rural providers, it is important to ask three key questions:

• Is it relevant to the situation?
• Is the information valid?
• What is the work required to attain it?

The next section examines various types of traditional and newer CME opportunities, attempting to apply an "evidence-based" approach to CME.

AN EVIDENCE-BASED APPROACH TO CONTINUING MEDICAL EDUCATION LEARNING OPPORTUNITIES

A new approach to evaluating the constantly expanding world of medical information utilizes the concept of evidence-based medicine (EBM),[5] which has been defined as an approach to practicing medicine in which the clinician is aware of the evidence in support of clinical practice and the strength of that evidence. This process involves a rigorous methodology of scrutinizing information from the medical literature regarding diagnosis and treatment. It evaluates the strength of the evidence presented and acknowledges areas of uncertainty or unclear direction. It asks what has actually been proven and differentiates this from inference or consensus-based conclusions. In this sense, EBM "deemphasizes intuition, unsystematic clinical experience, and pathophysiologic rationale as sufficient grounds for clinical decision making and stresses the examination of evidence from clinical research."[5] Although it is true that medical students are now being taught this methodology, few practicing clinicians have either the expertise or the time to spend on this process.

In this regard, Slawson et al.[6] have taken this process to a more user-friendly level in their conceptualization of disease-oriented evidence (DOE) and patient-oriented evidence that matters (POEM). DOE addresses information aimed at increasing the understanding of disease, its etiology, prevalence, pathophysiology, pharmacology, prognosis, etc. Unfortunately, DOE comprises the majority of the medical literature and textbooks as well as a significant amount of CME. Although this information is critical to the understanding of disease, it is less helpful in focusing clinical decision making on a particular patient's situation.

POEMs, on the other hand, deal with evidence that matters in patient care. For example, an article about the prostate-specific antigen (PSA) assay may report the sensitivity, specificity, and predictive value for identifying men with prostate cancer. This may inform the reader about how good this test is at identifying men at an early stage of the disease. This is a DOE. It, then, might be assumed that an earlier diagnosis of the disease would allow it to be cured. A randomized trial evaluating the overall effect of this early detection on the mortality of men with prostate cancer would provide this additional information and this would be a POEM. An even better POEM would be the study showing that early detection by use of the PSA test would lead to improved quality and length of life.

Articles are increasingly being written using an EBM methodology to derive POEMS. For several years the *Journal of Family Practice* has had a series on POEMs, and many of its articles are formatted to help physicians derive information that directly informs them about patient management. These series are now actually available on the Internet at http://jfp.msu.edu/ebp.htm. Utilization of POEMs draws the physician closer to a form of CME that directs specific changes in physician behavior and leads to better patient outcomes.

Another way to look at medical information obtained through any process of CME is to use Curley's[7] usefulness equation

$$U = R \times V/W$$

where

    U = usefulness of medical information
    R = relevance to everyday practice
    V = validity of information
    W = work done to obtain information

Thus, the focus is on relevance of information to the specific situation, the validity of the information obtained, and the work required to obtain it.

The next section takes an EBM approach to looking at the various forms of CME. Given the barriers to CME for rural providers, it is important to maximize relevance and validity and minimize the work required to attain it. This process will maximize the usefulness of CME for rural physicians.

Educational Materials

Among the more commonly accepted forms of continuing education are a variety of educational materials. These are largely noninteractive and printed materials, like journals/articles, books, newsletters, practice guidelines, audio and videotapes, and computer-based learning mechanisms (CD-ROM). They are basically static and dated, with little or no flexibility or interaction. Official CME credit can be obtained using many of these educational materials, often for very little cost. Unfortunately, the literature on CME has not shown these to be greatly effective in either changing provider behavior or improving patient outcomes.

Journals

Medical journals, such as the *New England Journal of Medicine* and *Journal of the American Medical Association,* are examples of "knowledge creation" journals.[8] These largely contain new data and periodically offer reviews that synthesize knowledge. Using the usefulness equation, there is often little of immediate utility, offering many more DOEs than POEMs. A large amount of time is required to assess validity, making this process very work intensive.

Another form of journals are the "translation" or "throwaway" journals. These offer summaries of expert reviews on various topics. They are often short (little work) and may deal with relevant topics but generally fail to provide the information needed to properly assess validity.

In the past few years, among the journals published specifically for family and general internal medicine, some have appeared that are practice-based, with research support. Several contain clinically based research formatted for EBM evaluation, with many DOEs, some POEMs, and primary-care oriented reviews. In the *Journal of Family Practice* (JFP), for instance, there is a specific column on POEMs that are available on line on the Internet and catalogued. These journals are attempting to address components of the usefulness equation delineated above. A variety of primary care newsletters are also available that summarize the recent literature for providers. They are often relevant and require very little work, yet they pose the same problem of assessing validity (expert opinions), and they are expensive. A new newsletter that addresses these concerns is *Evidence Based Practice*, published by the *Journal of Family Practice*.

Academic Reviews

Another type of educational material is the "academic review," the most common being the textbook. These are potentially a good source of POEMs, especially in that they are very relevant on a specific topic and generally accessible. However, textbooks often lack the ability to assess validity and are often out of date. Reviews from journals and audio or videotapes have similar strengths and weaknesses. For rural providers, audiotapes have significant convenience, and the *AudioDigest* has been available for many years, providing CME at moderate cost. Unfortunately, they cover general topics and may not prove relevant. Another emerging resource is the CD-ROM, for the computer. Some of these are actually interactive, but again they tend to cover broad areas, which may not provide the necessary level of relevance. CD-ROMs require little work but are expensive and can quickly become dated.

"Medical Cookbooks"

Another type of educational information is the "medical cookbook," or clinical guidelines and practice policies, which have become more widespread in recent years. Sidestepping the issue of clinical "freedom of decision making," guidelines and policies may offer an evidence-based approach to help the physicians make treatment decisions. Most guidelines have been derived through a systematic methodology, using the best available current information; if they are relevant to the present situation, they may be very useful. However, in the process of

creating clinical guidelines, authors have sometimes discovered significant gaps in current knowledge, where there is no definitive evidence to answer the current problem. Guidelines or practice policies that are consensus-based frequently suffer from validity issues. They are often written by special interests and may reflect significant biases. Too often guidelines and policies are long, are not written by or for primary care physicians, and present little of immediate relevance. Nevertheless, given that they form the basis of much of the quality assurance process to which physicians are increasingly exposed, it is important to be aware of their content and to incorporate relevant components into practice. The ability to access guidelines and policies via the Internet is an exciting new development and is addressed in a subsequent section.

Formal CME Programs

"Formal" CME offerings range from journal clubs and other educational meetings at the local hospital (some bringing in outside experts) through local/regional teleconferences to the out-of-town, "traditional" CME meeting. They use a variety of formats from lectures to group discussions to highly interactive and skill-building workshops. For certain areas of knowledge acquisition or skill building, there are formal traineeships, ranging from day-long workshops to extended fellowships. All formal CME courses are required to meet certain standards in order for the participants to receive credit. These include goals and objectives and an evaluation component, but in general they are not particularly rigorous. The literature indicates that the lower the level of physician interaction and the more generalized the information, the less the impact on physician behavior or patient outcomes. The problem with most CME meetings is that the relevance of the information offered does not always address specific needs with regards to patient care. Another problem with all formal CME conferences is assessing the validity of the information presented. Overall, the cost (work) factor of most formal CME is very high if one considers lost clinical revenue, registration and travel, and, in many cases, the limited relevance. Since many clinicians combine CME with nonprofessional activities, there are other variables to consider. Nevertheless, with proper planning and conference selection to meet specific goals, the usefulness of CME meetings can be high.

Opinion Leaders

All clinicians rely to a significant extent on their consultants, or "local experts," for guidance in patient care and treatment decisions. If the experts use POEMs and DOEs in combination with their own clinical experience, they increase their validity and become excellent sources of continuing education. They are available (low work), they are addressing specific patient problems (high relevance), and the literature has shown that they do affect physician behavior and patient outcomes. The down side of experts is their tendency to "near-sightedness." Thinking about issues from the perspective of their area of expertise can limit their ability to see the broader picture regarding the full range of patient needs. Since these sources of information are utilized regularly, they have great impact, but there must be a constant awareness of both the validity of the information and the potential biases of the "expert."

Outreach Visits

A special, more recently developed form of expert information is called "academic detailing."[1] Historically there has been significant experience with detailing by pharmaceutical representatives and CME lectures sponsored by pharmaceutical companies. These are often very convenient and have been clearly shown to change physician behavior. Pharmaceutical representatives can provide very relevant data for specific patients if asked, but physicians must remain aware of the issues of bias and must keep this in mind in determining the ways in which the information is used.

As managed care expands, a new form of "academic detailing" is emerging—educators whose purpose is to improve patient care. These individuals are often doctors of pharmacy whose major goal has been to help physicians understand and use drugs more effectively. But, increasingly, these academic detailers are branching into other areas of patient care and resource management. As in the case of the pharmaceutical representatives, it is important always to question the biases of educators and the validity of their information. Academic detailers are in a position to increase relevance and decrease work because they will come directly to the practitioner with the expressed purpose of improving specific patient care as well as controlling cost.

Patient-Linked Interventions

The literature has demonstrated that "patient-linked" interventions can affect physician behavior and patient outcomes.[1] The audit mechanism of chart review, coupled with feedback and focused educational efforts, can be a very effective means of CME. This is very specific, often requires little work, and, when utilizing EBM, can prove valid. Many rural group practices have used this approach to CME. A component of the American Board of Family Practice (ABFP) recertification process uses chart review for educational purposes. The audit process can incorporate local experts and peers in an interactive group learning process. Given that chart auditing is a component of the quality assurance process, it can be channeled into a positive means of continuing education to modify physician behavior and improve patient care and outcomes. Chart-based reminders for interventions (health maintenance) can also change behavior and outcomes. Materials designed for patient education, if used directly by the physician, can improve doctor-patient communication, resulting in better outcomes. The literature suggests that a combination of all the above patient-based methodologies improves outcomes.

Learning by Teaching

Learning by teaching is another form of CME. Many rural practitioners have had the opportunity, over the years, to serve as preceptors to students in their practices. Increasingly, academic medical centers are recognizing this rich resource. A learner constantly challenges the teacher and often brings new information that can be applied to patient care. The questions asked by the learner stimulate the preceptor to question current practices and will often direct both teacher and learner to access many of the means of continuing medical education mentioned above, particularly computer and Internet resources.

ELECTRONIC APPROACHES TO INFORMATION GATHERING

Chapter 15 addresses the broad topic of medical informatics and information access. With the increasing ease for both physicians and patients of accessing information via the Internet, it is important to examine this new resource for CME. As more rural providers and their patients begin to connect electronically to the information superhighway, a knowledge of these vast resources becomes a critical source of professional and patient care information for both parties. The ease of access and the nature of the information available make the Internet a significant tool in providing CME opportunities for the rural provider for whom isolation has been a major barrier. Literature searches can be done with a few strokes on the keyboard. Article abstracts are immediately printable and many popular journals are available on line in full text. Patient education materials are readily available, as is access to government-created clinical guidelines and documents. Actual CME and decision support for patient case management are available online. More and more patients will access the same information as their health care providers and will come to the office as educated consumers, willing and demanding to participate in management decision making. Although Internet access to vast amounts of information may decrease the work for rural providers in locating and securing these resources, the issues of relevance and validity remain as questions to be addressed.

It is clearly beyond the scope of this chapter to deal with the issues of accessing the Internet. Securing Internet access for rural providers may be easy or challenging, but this is largely a technical matter and access is becoming more readily available. Costs are variable depending on local access and provider networks. Most rural physicians who precept medical students should be able to access the Internet through their home teaching institutions. Generally all that is required is a bit of ingenuity and persistence.

This section addresses a variety of useful areas for continuing education on the Internet and how to access them. Hopefully this guide will help focus your Web travels, thereby increasing their usefulness. The referenced Web sites will be contained within carets (⟨ ⟩). Two cautions: (1) traveling on the Web can be addicting and time consuming and (2) your patient can generally visit the same sites you can and may already have done so.

Search Engines

Once you gain Internet access, the possibilities are literally limitless. Upon entering a Web address (<u>u</u>niform <u>r</u>esource <u>l</u>ocator, or URL), one can "travel" for days by simply clicking on "hot links" (as indicated by either different-colored print or the appearance of the little hand over an item), and moving from Web site to Web site. A mechanism to facilitate Web travel has been developed called a *search engine.* There are several dozen search engines, each with a slightly different method of searching. They all use key words or phrases to scan text. Web searching is a skill, like doing a literature search, which can be developed with tutorials (or the help of your friendly librarian or teenager). Alta Vista http://www.altavista.digital.com has been rated the best for finding scientific information on the Internet. Several resources are available on the Internet to help one choose and use a search engine:

- *Choose the Best Search Engine*: ⟨http://www. nueva.pvt.k12.ca.us./~debbie/library/ research/adviceengine.html⟩
- *Finding Information on the Internet: A Tutorial*: ⟨http//www.lib.berkeley.edu/ TeachingLib.Guides/Internet/FindInfo.html⟩
- *Search Engine Watch*: ⟨http://www.search enginewatch.com⟩
- *Tips on Popular Search Engines*: ⟨http://www. hamline.edu/library⟩

Medline

MEDLINE is the premier biomedical database produced by the National Library of Medicine (NLM). It contains citations that appear in the *Index Medicus* as well as the *International Nursing Index* and the *Index to Dental Literature*. It includes journal articles, reviews, letters, and editorials from over 3900 journals from 1966 to the present. Abstracts are available for many entries. Citations can be retrieved by author name, medical subject headings (MeSH), and text words from titles or abstracts. Free MEDLINE access is available through NLM's *Internet Grateful Med* ⟨http://igm.nlm.nih. gov/⟩ and *PubMed* ⟨http://www.ncbi.nlm.nih. gov/PubMed⟩. An excellent discussion of the use of MeSH in MEDLINE searching may be found in an article by Lowe.[9] Skills developed in MEDLINE searching are transferable to other databases as well and can be helpful in utilizing Internet search engines.

Evidence-Based Medicine

There is a wealth of information available on the Internet for health care practitioners who want to learn more about the principles of EBM and how to search for evidence-based informa-

tion to support clinical decision making. The following resources provide an excellent introduction to this topic:

- *Evidence Based Medicine: Finding the Best Clinical Literature*: ⟨http://www.uic.edu/depts/ lib/health/ebm.html⟩. This site provides a brief introduction to EBM, references to key publications about EBM, links to Internet resources on the topic, and advice to the novice on constructing and executing a search of MEDLINE using clinical filters to retrieve evidence-based information.
- *When and How to Use Original Medical Literature: An Introduction to Evidence Based Medicine*: ⟨http://www.urmc.rochester.edu/SMD/ Medicine/imclerk/literature.htm⟩. This site was prepared for third-year medical students at the University of Rochester and serves as a good tutorial for those starting to search the literature.
- *Evidence Based Medicine Tutorial*: ⟨http:// courses.hscbklyn.edu/ebm/chapters.htm⟩. This site provides an excellent introduction to EBM.

There are evidence-based medicine journals actually on line, such as the following:

- The ACP Journal Club includes structured abstracts and commentaries relevant to internal medicine: ⟨http://www.acponline.org/journals/acpjc/jcmenu.htm⟩.
- *Evidence-Based Medicine* uses the same format but includes studies relevant to pediatrics, obstetrics, surgery, psychiatry, general and family practice, as well as internal medicine: ⟨http://www.acponline.org/journals/ebm/ ebmmenu.htm⟩.
- The McMaster site is most widely known for its users' guides. These are a set of guides, originally published in the *Journal of the American Medical Association*, that aim to help clinicians keep up to date. It critically appraises different types of literature. ⟨http://hiru. mcmaster.ca/ebm/⟩.
- The *Journal of Family Practice* regularly features POEMs to support evidence-based practice. 80

journals are reviewed each month to identify 8 articles with patient-oriented outcomes that have the greatest potential to change clinical practice: ⟨http://www.infopoems.com⟩.

- The *Cochrane Database of Systematic Reviews* (COCH) includes the full text of regularly updated systematic reviews of the effects of healthcare interventions: ⟨http://www.cochrane.org/default.html⟩.
- *Primary Care Clinical Practice Guidelines* provides guidelines for clinicians, including MEDLINE plus health topics and clinical reviews; as well as cross-cultural health, teaching, and more: ⟨http://medicine.ucsf.edu/resources/guidelines/⟩.

Many of these sites have links to other useful information.

Continuing Medical Education

On-line continuing medical education is an important direction for future development. There are several places to search for CME conferences, listed by topic, specialty, and location, or a general search engine can be used to locate a variety of options. For example, the AMA home page can direct readers to a searchable CME listing for Category I credit, similar to the biyearly listing which has been in JAMA for many years: ⟨http://www.ama-assn.org/⟩. Two other good sites are:

- The *Doctor's Guide to Medical Conferences*: ⟨http://www.pslgroup.com/MEDCONF.HTM⟩;
- *Medical Conferences*: ⟨http://www.medicalconferences.com/⟩.

  Actual CME on line is rapidly changing and also of variable quality. There are "courses" that can be taken and CME credit received free as well as for modest fees. These are easily accessible (little work), may or may not be relevant, and suffer from the same validity problems of any CME course. Courses are often involve articles to read and questions to answer. Nevertheless, with the advent of "streaming" video (like

regular video, yet on-line), it may soon become possible to attend CME meetings on line. Eventually this technology may bring CME into the home or office and can be accessed at one's convenience. Again, one can use a general search engine and enter the phrase "continuing medical education," with desired modifiers, and see where it leads. Several focused URLs which may be of interest are:

- *Medical Matrix,* which has a section which has an editor and ratings of CME courses: ⟨http://www.medmatrix.org/⟩
- A site maintained by Bernard Sklar, MD, a graduate fellow at the University of California, San Francisco, which is on the *Medical Computing Today* Web site: ⟨http://medicalcomputingtoday.com/0listcme.html⟩
- *Information Today,* which reviews some of the better online CME resources: ⟨http://www.medscape.com/Medscape/featur...1999.it1601.01.smit/it1601.01.smit.html⟩
- The American Academy of Family Physicians' Web site also includes CME for AAFP members: ⟨http://www.aafp.org/⟩

A note of caution, however, is that the bottom line for on-line CME at this time is: "Let the buyer beware."

Health Related Web Sites

Finally, the following is a potpourri of informative Web sites,[10] which were chosen primarily because they were prepared by reputable organizations and are evaluated and regularly updated. These include information on sites for both physicians and consumers (patient education).

- *American Medical Association Home Page:* http://www.ama-assn.org/
  The *JAMA* information center includes peer-reviewed resources produced by *JAMA* on select subjects (e.g., women's health) and includes top news stories and the latest from the literature.

- *American Academy of Family Physicians:* http://www.aafp.org/
  This Web site provides patient with information from family physicians, members of the AAFP, on a broad range of medical problems that family physicians are trained to treat. This site also includes on-line CME for AAFP members.
- *HealthWeb:* http://www.healthweb.org/
  HealthWeb is a cooperative project of academic health sciences libraries and the Committee on Institutional Cooperation (CIC). The CIC produces a subject index of health-related topics, including consumer health, nursing and allied health, rural health, public health, and reference resources.
- *Healthfinder:* http://www.healthfinder.gov/
  Healthfinder is a consumer health information Web site prepared by the U.S. government. This site offers reliable health information for the public and leads to additional Web sites and support groups.
- *MayoHealth:* http://www.mayohealth.org/
  The Mayo Clinic web site features reliable health information. The interactive format allows you to find information specifically tailored to your personal health concerns or interests.
- *Medical Matrix:* http://www.medmatrix.org/
  Medical Matrix provides a ranked, peer-reviewed list of clinical medical resources, including a list of sites for patient education and support.
- *Virtual Hospital:* http://vh.radiology.uiowa.edu/
  Virtual Hospital, developed by the University of Iowa, contains information from over 350 peer-reviewed books and pamphlets. The sections are *Peer Reviewed Web Sources on Common Medical Problems* and *Peer Reviewed Web Resources on Primary Care Problems.*
- *Doctor's Guide to the Internet:* http://www.pslgroup.com/docguide.htm
  This site features medical news and alerts, new medical sites of the week, new drugs recently approved, and a listing of medical conferences and CME events.
- *Medical Tribune: the Physicians's News Source:* http://www.medtrib.com/
  The *Medical Tribune* Web page highlights top news stories and presents the MD Cyber Guide, which ranks medical sites on the Internet.
- *Alternative Medicine Home Page:* http://www.pitt.edu/~cbw/refe.html
  This site represents a "jumping off point'" for sources of information on unconventional, unorthodox, unproven, alternative, complementary, or integrative therapies. It links to references of studies describing experiences with some of these therapies.
- *National Cancer Institute:* http://www.nci.nih.gov/
  This site presents treatment statements for the patient or the health care professional, including patients, the public, and the mass media. There is valuable information for consumers, including prevention and early detection tips as well as detailed statements by cancer site or type.
- *Agency for Health Care Policy and Research:* http://www.ahcpr.gov
  Through the clinical information page, clinicians can access AHCPR-supported practice guidelines as well as updates on treatment effectiveness and outcomes research.
- *Chronic Illness Resources:* http://www.clearinghouse.net/
  This site accesses a variety of support groups for chronic illnesses.
- *Rural Family Doc Home page:* http://www.ruralfamilymedicine.org
  This site, created by the Group on Rural Health of the Society of Teachers of Family Medicine, accesses an enormous variety of rural health–related topics.

THE FUTURE OF CONTINUING MEDICAL EDUCATION

CME for rural practice will be an ongoing challenge for rural physicians. All health care providers face the problem of the exponential expansion of information and its implications for continuing competence. The additional issues of distance and access create more challenges for rural providers. The emergence of electronic linkages, enabling telemedicine and Internet access, should help shrink these distances and provide better access to information. Already these have had a significant impact on practice in more remote areas, opening a future that has limitless possibilities. Ultimately, real-time on-line consultations with distant experts may prove to be the most useful CME, providing relevance, validity, and timeliness.

In review, we have defined CME as a process that leads to changes in physician behavior that can lead to improved patient outcomes. The literature on CME is discouraging in that it suggests that traditional forms of CME have had limited effectiveness in these regards. What is hopeful is that the combination of different forms of CME does result in change. As all providers struggle to maintain competence, it is important to take an evidence-based approach to CME. As we attempt to "drink from the information firehose," we must look for POEMs—patient-oriented evidence that matters—the pearls that direct changes in practice behavior, resulting in better patient outcomes. This overview has looked at traditional forms of information gathering and CME and at newer, potentially more effective methods to change physician behavior and patient outcomes. It has defined an evidence-based methodology to assess new medical advancements in information and technology. Finally, it has but scratched the surface of the enormous universe of the Internet and its potential to provide information access and CME. Clearly, the discipline of CME must evolve to help practitioners maintain competence and achieve improved patient outcomes. With the electronic connectivity available on the Internet, access to new information will be vastly improved for rural physicians. Although this is only one part of CME, it holds great promise for those who have chosen to deliver care in rural areas.

ACKNOWLEDGMENTS

The author would like to acknowledge significant contributions and support for the section entitled "Electronic Approaches to Information Gathering" by Don Lanier and Sue Hollander from the Library of Health Sciences–Rockford, University of Illinois at Chicago. He also expresses thanks for professional advice and commentary on this chapter from members of the Rural Medical Education Program (RMED): Mike Glasser, Marge Stearns, Cheryl Carlson, and LaVerne Larson.

REFERENCES

1. Davis D: Does CME work? An analysis of the effect of educational activities on physician performance or health care outcomes. *Int J Psychiatry Med* 28:21, 1998.
2. Davis DA, Thomson MA, Oxman AD, et al: Changing physician performance: a systematic review of the effect of continuing medical education strategies. *JAMA* 274:700, 1995.
3. Davis D, Parboosingh J: "Academic" CME and the social contract. *Acad Med* 68:329, 1993.
4. Kwee JS: *Report on Oregon Rural Health Care Provider Continuing Education Survey.* Portland, OR: Oregon Geriatric Education Center Department of Veterans Affairs, 1992.
5. Evidence-Based Medicine Working Group: Evidence-based medicine a new approach to teaching the practice of medicine. *JAMA* 268:2420, 1992.
6. Slawson DC, Shaughnessy AF, Bennett JH: Becoming a medical information master: feeling good about not knowing everything. *J Fam Pract* 38:505, 1994.
7. Curley SP, Connelly DP, Rich EC: Physicians' use of medical knowledge resources: preliminary theoretical framework and findings. *Med Decision Making* 10:231–241, 1990.
8. Shaughnessy AF, Slawson DC, Bennett JH: Becoming an information master: a guidebook to the medical information jungle. *J Fam Pract* 39:489, 1994.
9. Lowe HJ: Understanding the medical subject heading vocabulary to perform literature searches. *JAMA* 271:1103–1108, 1994.

PART FIVE

Lessons from Abroad

P hysician shortages in rural areas are a worldwide problem, with other countries facing many of the same challenges described in earlier chapters for the United States. Although health care systems vary considerably from one country to another, the problems of education for rural practice are more similar than different across national boundaries. In each instance, selection, recruitment, and retention of clinicians in rural practice represent a universal challenge. With the exception of public health problems in the developing world, patterns of disease and the clinical needs of patients also tend to be more similar than different from one country to another. It therefore follows that curricula for a broad range of clinical competencies are needed for rural physicians to be prepared to practice anywhere in the world.

Five countries have been selected for Part V; these illustrate various and sometimes different approaches to the common problems of education for rural practice. In every case, each country has a sizable rural population and extensive experience in education for rural practice.

The overall goal here is to describe the various strategies that have been taken to meet the common needs of rural practitioners. Since many of the challenges are generic to rural practice without regard to national borders, physicians and educators have much to learn from the experience, successes, and failures from one country to another.

John P. Geyman

CHAPTER 25

Rural Practice in Canada

JAMES T. B. ROURKE

THE COUNTRY

Geography and People

Canada, at approximately 3.8 million square miles (approximately 10 million square kilometers) is the second largest country in the world (Russia is the largest) but has a population of only 28.8 million.[1] Three-quarters of Canadians live within 93 miles (150 kilometers) of the southern edge of the country that borders on the United States,[2] while northern Canada, with its harsh arctic and subarctic climate, is one of the most sparsely populated parts of the world. Three cities have populations of over 1 million—Toronto, Montreal, and Vancouver—and together they comprise one-third of the population.[3] At the other end of the spectrum, one-quarter to one-third of Canadians live in rural areas.

A commonly used definition of *rural* in Canada includes communities of up to 10,000 people. By this definition, 8,740,847 Canadians (30.3 percent) are rural.[4] Rural people can also be defined as those living outside census metropolitan areas and census agglomerations.* By this

counting method, 22.2 percent of Canadians (6,396,906) are rural people[5,6] (Table 25-1).

Canada has a very diverse population. Its exclusively Aboriginal First Nations people consist of 460,680 North American Indians, 36,215 Inuit, and 135,265 Metis. (These are the three Aboriginal groups recognized by the Constitution Act.) More than 1 million Canadians have some aboriginal ancestry. Aboriginal groups represent 4 percent of the total population; they are scattered from coast to coast. Nearly 300,000 live in isolated reserves.[7]

Fifty-six percent of Canada's Aboriginal people live in rural areas including reserves: 35.2 percent on reserves and 20.3 percent in nonreserve rural areas.[8] The Northwest Territories, with Canada's harshest environment, has the highest proportion of Aboriginal peoples—more than 60 percent.[7] In April 1999, the Northwest Territories divided into two when the new territory of Nunavut was created, encompassing the eastern Arctic.

The majority of Canada's people are of British and French descent. Both British and French settlement began in the 1600s. French-speaking people make up about 25 percent of Canada's population. Canada's rich cultural mix includes people of descent from almost every nation. In the 1991 census, the most common "single ethnic" origins reported after French and British were German, Canadian, Italian, Chinese, Aboriginal, Ukrainian, Dutch, and East Indian. The pattern of immigration to Canada is also chang-

---

* A Census Agglomerate (CA) is defined as "a large urban area (known as the urban core) together with adjacent urban and rural areas (known as urban and rural fringes) that have a high degree of social and economic integration with the urban core." A CA has an urban core population of at least 10,000, based on the previous census.[5]

TABLE 25-1   POPULATION COUNTS, SHOWING DISTRIBUTION OUTSIDE CENSUS METROPOLITAN AREAS AND CENSUS AGGLOMERATIONS FOR CANADA, PROVINCES AND TERRITORIES, 1996 CENSUS

	Rural Population	Percent	Total Population
Canada	6,396,906	22.2	28,846,761
Newfoundland	306,924	55.6	551,792
Prince Edward Island	61,332	45.6	134,557
Nova Scotia	351,668	38.7	909,282
New Brunswick	357,984	48.5	738,133
Quebec	1,595,735	22.4	7,138,795
Ontario	1,596,138	14.8	10,753,573
Manitoba	371,338	33.3	1,113,898
Saskatchewan	428,565	43.3	990,237
Alberta	694,474	25.8	2,696,826
British Columbia	576,663	15.5	3,724,500
Yukon Territory	8,958	29.1	30,766
Northwest Territories (includes Nunavut)	47,127	73.2	64,402

SOURCE: Statistics Canada.[6]

ing. In the past the vast majority of newcomers were European. Currently more immigrants come from Asia than from any other part of the world. The number of Chinese-speaking Canadians is increasing at such a fast rate that Chinese may soon overtake Italian as the third most widely spoken language in Canada.[9]

On average, Canada's rural people are older and have a lower income and educational status than their urban counterparts. Canada's economy still is heavily resource-based, with mining, fishing, farming, and forestry accounting for 7 percent of Canada's gross national product.[9] All of these industries pose a higher risk of accidental injuries for rural people, including not only rural workers but also their families. Farm families in particular have a much higher than average childhood risk of injury.

Tourism also abounds in Canada's wonderful wilderness areas. Tourists present to rural emergency facilities with a full range of illnesses from poison ivy dermatitis to myocardial infarctions as well as with injuries specifically related to activities such as skiing. A remarkable example was the worst bus accident in Canadian history.

Forty-seven senior citizens were out to see the autumn colours on October 13, 1997, when their bus crashed in Les Eboulements, Quebec, about 60 miles (100 kilometers) northeast of Quebec City. Seriously injured patients were taken to Baie-Saint-Paul, a community of nearly 4000 with a small hospital (under 50 beds) that served a large rural area. The administrator of the hospital was returning home to Quebec City when he saw the ambulances going in the other direction. He immediately returned to Baie-Saint-Paul. Family physician and medical director, Dr. Jacques Cloutier said, "By the time I arrived at the hospital there were 20 nurses, 8 family physicians, the surgeon, the anesthetist, as well as receptionists and secretaries already in place." The five survivors were stabilized and within about 5 hours of the accident had been transferred to the tertiary care trauma center in Quebec City. Past experience helped staff develop an emergency plan to guide them not only in dealing with the survivors, but also with the unexpectedly large number of dead. Having that plan in place was essential to the successful outcome for the survivors. This case illustrates how a small hospital can effectively deal with larger emergencies.[10]

Canada's diverse geography impacts directly on its people. Significant barriers include the enormous distances and geography such as the Rocky Mountains. Even in southern Ontario, where distances are small, winter can have a significant impact. The author's town of Goderich is only 60 miles (100 kilometers) from a major university/tertiary care center, the University of Western Ontario in London. Nevertheless, on the lee of Lake Huron, the winter blizzards during a recent year completely closed the roads for 8 days. This posed significant challenges, particularly on New Year's Day, when the roads were closed and a patient presented with premature labor and significant bleeding at one of the small area hospitals. Clearly she could be best cared for at a tertiary care center, but this required the coordination of police, ambulance, and snow removal teams to forge a pathway through the blocked roads for what was fortunately a successful outcome.

Health Care System

In Canada, most patients with primary care problems are seen by general practitioners/family physicians (GP/FPs), who refer patients to specialists for specialized investigations, surgery, or management of complex problems. Specialists mainly act as consultants and rarely see primary care nonreferred patients. There are approximately 28,983 general practitioners/family physicians and 26,836 specialists in Canada[11] (Table 25-2).

Medical care in Canada is funded directly by the provincial governments. The provinces, in turn, receive some funding for this from the federal government under a cost-sharing arrangement. Provincial medical associations negotiate fees directly with the provincial governments on behalf of their members. There is virtually no private pay or private insurance for medical services. Patients can, however, pay for upgraded accommodation to a private room in a hospital and at-home support services such as nursing care and physiotherapy. Chiropractic services are partially public and privately funded.

The Canada Health Act, passed in 1984, lists the five criteria that provincial governments must meet as part of their health insurance plans to qualify for federal contributions[12]:

- Universality—All residents in the province must have access to public health insurance and insured services on uniform terms and conditions.
- Accessibility—Insured persons must have reasonable and uniform access to insured health services, free of financial barriers.
- Comprehensiveness—The health insurance plan of each province must insure all services that are "medically necessary."
- Portability—Provinces are required to cover insured health services provided to their citizens while they are temporarily absent from their province of residence or from Canada.
- Public administration—Each provincial health insurance plan must be administered on a nonprofit basis by a public authority, which is accountable to the provincial government for its financial transactions.

RURAL PRACTICE IN CANADA

Rural Practice Settings

In Canada, a widely accepted definition of rural medical practice is "practice in nonurban areas, where most medical care is provided by a small number of general practitioners/family doctors with limited or distant access to specialist resources and high technology health care facilities."[13] The Rural Committee of the Canadian Association of Emergency Physicians (CAEP) defines "rural remote" as "rural communities about 130 to 645 miles (80 to 400 kilometers) or about 1 to 4 hours transport in good weather from a major regional hospital" and "rural isolated" as "rural communities greater than about 400 km or about four hours transport in good weather from a major regional hospital."[14]

Rural health care in Canada is provided in a wide range of diverse settings. Small, scattered, isolated communities in northern Canada may have a nursing station staffed by experienced registered nurses or nurse practitioners that are supported by periodic visiting family physicians. The following vignette, in the words of

TABLE 25-2 ACTIVE PHYSICIANS IN CANADA, JANUARY 1998, BY PROVINCE AND BROAD SPECIALTY CANADIAN MEDICAL ASSOCIATION MASTERFILE DATA

| | Broad Specialty | | | | |
	GP/FP	Medical Specialist	Surgical Specialist	Medical Scientist	Total
Canada	28,983	19,307	7,529	77	55,896
Newfoundland	579	262	97		938
Prince Edward Island	93	53	27		173
Nova Scotia	956	606	254	2	1,818
New Brunswick	692	291	192		1,175
Quebec	7,579	5,380	2,127	17	15,103
Ontario	10,215	7,588	2,798	37	20,638
Manitoba	1,064	722	276	7	2,069
Saskatchewan	872	392	197	2	1,463
Alberta	2,453	1,540	569	5	4,567
British Columbia	4,396	2,462	980	7	7,845
Yukon Territory	43	3	3		49
Northwest Territories (includes Nunavut)	41	8	9		58

an itinerant family doctor, captures the flavor of this support.*

The trip up this time was in the lumbering old Beaver. I had the honor of sitting beside the pilot, which was good because I could wear the earphones to help drown out the old Pratt and Whitney's merciless drone. En route, I noticed some searching in the engine, with slight variations in the revolutions per minute. I casually mentioned this to the pilot, who said, "Yeah, funny how it does that. . .but she's going in for service tomorrow." "Great," I said to myself. "That's really great."

The small clinic waiting room was full when we arrived, so there was no time to unpack and settle in. The community health representative (CHR) from nearby Fort Lonely* had borrowed a pickup truck to bring a young mother with her two babies to the clinic. The older child, age 20 months, was stuffed up and miserable with the ubiquitous problem of an infected, draining ear. The baby,

age 2 months, was a different story. It looked very ill, with a heart rate of more than 200, respirations of 80, and a sickening pale blue color. The CHR had started the baby on antibiotics after reporting its illness by radiophone 2 days ago. The young mother responded angrily to my questions about whether the baby was getting medication. "I've been away for 3 days. My sister Betty has been looking after her." Time to stop asking questions. Time for me to think of management options. The Beaver has already headed back south, and it is now dark. No flights until nearly noon tomorrow. Damn it.

The young couple lives in a log cabin with no electricity or running water. They do not have a telephone. Still, this young mother was determined not to surrender the baby to our care and definitely not to go to town with the baby. "All right, "I said with resignation, "you can take the baby home, but it is really important to give the medicine to the baby." The mother looked at me disparagingly as if I had rocks in my head, and I suddenly realized I probably did. She was more worried about the baby than I was and certainly planned to take good care of it. All bundled up, the Fort Lonely bunch loaded into the old pickup truck for the long trip home. I hoped the heater worked, as it was below freezing. . . .

* Certain details of this story have been altered to protect the identities of the individuals involved, but the essence of the tale is true. Its author, George Deagle, practices family medicine in Prince George, B.C.

I phoned my wife to tell her I wouldn't be home. This was not happy news. We were invited for dinner, and she had bought a new outfit and had her hair done especially for this holiday visit. It is not easy being a physician's spouse at times like these, and some damage is done even though events are out of our control. "No, the plane [to take us home] had to turn back. No one was able to get out of here today. I know we were. . .I'm sorry, why don't you go by yourself? Well, I am really disappointed, too, OK. . .OK. . .see you tomorrow. Love you."

I felt upset and saddened even though I had intellectually accepted the risk of being stranded. "Your wife mad at you?" the seasoned nurse asked when I got off the telephone. "Yeah, can't say I blame her," I replied. "Well," the nurse responded, "it's better to get home tomorrow than not to make it home today." That made sense to me, after I thought about it. . . .

The moon still illuminated the new fallen snow when I got up early the next morning. The nearby mountains had a fresh dusting of powder snow, right down to the level of the lake. The plane will make it in this morning. I'm sure.

I'm really looking forward to my next trip back in a month. I think it would be good to bring my wife with me, though. We really could use some more time together.[15]

A December plane crash in northern Manitoba, in which 4 people were killed and 13 injured, served to remind the province's fly-in physicians of the perils their work may entail. It left one of the physicians with the University of Manitoba's Northern Medical Unit in hospital for 4 months with a serious head injury.[16] Similar risks are faced by patients and their families flying out to receive medical care. Not only flying but also the long-distance highway travel associated with rural living and rural practice add to the risk of serious accident.

Small rural communities without a hospital may have a doctor's office or a clinic with one to three physicians. Most rural communities of 2500 or more have a small hospital staffed by FP/GPs providing primarily emergency and a few inpatient care services in addition to office/clinic-based primary care.

Larger rural communities (4000 to 10,000 people) have small active hospitals that provide a broader range of services. In this setting, family doctors—in addition to office/clinic-based family practice—have a major role doing emergency department shifts, attending births, providing anesthetics, and caring for a variety of in-hospital patients.[17,18] In some hospitals, GP/FPs do general surgery operations such as cesarean sections, appendectomies, and hernia repairs.[19] Some of the larger rural hospitals may have one or more specialists. The general surgeon is the dominant rural specialist, often providing common plastic, orthopedic, gynecologic (including cesarean section) procedures in addition to general surgery.[17,20,21] There is a scattering of other rural specialists—including general internists, radiologists, and psychiatrists—and most rural hospitals have a variety of visiting specialist clinics.

More recently, however, some highly specialized services such as dialysis units have been successfully decentralized to some larger rural hospitals. A small rural hospital in Clinton, Ontario (population 3183), provides weekly cataract surgery by visiting ophthalmologists from the University of Western Ontario, thereby reducing transportation difficulties for hundreds of elderly rural practice patients from a large surrounding area. Most highly specialized services, however, remain centralized in Canada. Only one community of less than 10,000 people in Canada has a computed tomography scanner. A number of telemedicine programs are being developed in Canada, but as yet this has had only limited impact on rural patient care. The potential, however, is enormous.

Rural Physician Distribution and Activities

As in many other countries, there is a maldistribution of physicians in Canada, with rural areas having a shortage of physicians compared with their urban counterparts. Using CMA (Census

Metropolitan Areas) and CA (Census Agglomerations) data analysis, 6,393,906 people (22 percent of Canada's population) can be considered "rural." Using the same definition of practice location, only 9.9 percent of Canada's doctors, or 4775 family doctors (16.5 percent of Canada's GP/FPs), and 756 specialists (2.8 percent of Canada's specialists) can be considered rural[11] [Canadian Medical Association Masterfile Database, January 1998] (Table 25-3). In other words, 1650 more rural family doctors/GPs would be needed to make the number of rural family doctors/GPs per population equal to the Canadian average.

The Canadian Institute for Health Information data analysis using the National Physician Data Base (NPDB) found 4866 rural physicians. This included 498 GP anesthetists and 123 FRCS specialty anesthetists; in 1995–96 they provided 6.4 percent of all anesthetic services in Canada. There were 121 GP surgeons and 151 FRCS general surgeons; in 1995–96 they performed 2605 appendectomies in rural Canada (9.5 percent of all appendectomies). Cesarean sections in rural Canada were provided by 200 GP obstetricians and 131 FRCS specialists (100 were FRCS general surgeons and 31 were FRCS obstetricians); together they performed 4292 cesarean sections, or 6.9 percent of all cesarean sections in Canada.[21]

The Janus Study by the College of Family Physicians of Canada established a broad profile of family physician/general practitioner activity in Canada.[22] The study used an overall denominator of 27,324 FP/GPs in Canada. Of these FP/GPs, 17.7 percent (4836) identified themselves as serving a rural or geographically isolated or remote population.[22] This number corresponds closely with the number identified by the Canadian Medical Association Masterfile Database.

Further analysis of the Janus data, excluding responses with confounding variables for population served (i.e. "other" or "urban and rural" or "urban and small town") provides a denominator of 25,956 Canadian FP/GPs with 4179 (16.1 percent) of physicians self-identified as primarily serving rural and/or remote populations. Using these data, family physicians/general practitioners serving a rural/remote population are 28 percent female, 32.6 percent provide on-call coverage for obstetric deliveries,

TABLE 25-3   *ACTIVE RURAL PHYSICIANS IN CANADA, JANUARY 1998, BY PROVINCE AND BROAD SPECIALTY CANADIAN MEDICAL ASSOCIATION MASTERFILE DATA*

	Broad Specialty			
	GP/FP	Medical Specialist	Surgical Specialist	Total
Canada	4,775	446	310	5,531
Newfoundland	254	12	8	274
Prince Edward Island	31	1	1	33
Nova Scotia	299	60	38	397
New Brunswick	243	17	24	284
Quebec	1,328	163	117	1,608
Ontario	1,022	82	61	1,165
Manitoba	306	18	7	331
Saskatchewan	230	6	7	243
Alberta	476	21	14	511
British Columbia	567	65	33	665
Yukon Territory	8			8
Northwest Territories (includes Nunavut)	11	1		12

TABLE 25-4   *FAMILY PHYSICIANS IN CANADA, JANUS DATA ANALYSIS*

	Rural, Number	Rural, Percent	Small Town, Number	Small Town, Percent	Urban, Number	Urban, Percent	Total, Number	Total, Percent
Total	4,179	16.10	4,630	17.84	17,147	66.06	25,956	100.0
Female	1,189	28.5	1,295	28.0	5,648	32.9	8,132	31.3
On-call OB	1,631	32.6	1,373	29.6	2,795	16.3	5,799	22.3
FP/GP anaesthetist	361	8.6	243	5.2	147	0.9	751	2.9
FP/GP surgeon	144	3.4	49	1.1	183	1.1	376	1.4

and 8.6 percent identified themselves as GP anesthetists (see Table 25-4 for rural/urban comparison).

Rural/remote family physicians in Canada provide a broad range of health care services (Table 25-5). Of note, 61 percent provide Aboriginal health care and 18 percent devote over 10 percent of their practice time to Aboriginal health care. Further analysis of rural-based family physician services and comparison with urban-based services will be published in *Canadian Family Physician.*

TABLE 25-5   *MEDICAL SERVICES PROVIDED BY RURAL PHYSICIANS IN CANADA, JANUS DATA ANALYSIS*

	Percent of Physicians Who Provide Service	Percent of Physicians Who Provide Service More Than 10 Percent of Their Time
Aboriginal health	61.7	18.0
Addiction medicine	63.7	10.1
Adolescent health	84.0	50.7
Adult health	92.5	89.2
Alternative/complementary	54.6	14.5
Anaesthesia	38.4	8.3
Care of elderly	92.5	76.4
Child health	91.2	69.9
Chronic disease	82.8	66.7
Emergency medicine	76.4	52.6
HIV/AIDS care	44.5	1.8
Immigrant health	39.1	1.7
Mental health/psychotherapy	83.0	53.5
Obstetric care	67.6	25.7
Occupational/industrial	52.1	9.1
Palliative care	77.4	16.2
Preventive medicine	78.3	53.3
Sports medicine	56.1	12.4
Surgery (minor)	78.2	14.2
Surgery (assisting)	52.1	6.2
Surgery (major)	31.5	3.0
Other	6.0	1.4

Challenges of Rural Practice

Rural health presents a major challenge in Canada. Canada's rural population of 6 to 8 million is spread over an enormous area. All of the provincial and territorial governments have identified rural health as an urgent and important problem. In 1998 the Canadian government established a Directorate of Rural Health to provide overall direction and development of rural health in Canada. Throughout Canada there is a growing concern regarding the need to maintain and indeed improve rural health care, as reflected in the Canadian Medical Association report published in 1992.[23] This report identified professional and personal isolation as major barriers to recruiting and retaining rural physicians. Recent graduates are reluctant to go into independent solo rural practice. Rural communities need to establish well-supported, sustainable group practice clinics to convert "needs" into attractive job opportunities with appropriate incentives to both recruiting and retaining rural doctors.

For many physicians, lack of spousal job opportunities in rural areas is a significant problem. Balancing doctor-patient-family relationships and boundaries is a challenge for all rural physicians. In areas of doctor shortages there can be inordinate demands on physicians' time resulting in "limit, leave, or be left" approaches.[24] Women rural physicians in particular have significant role strain when balancing the demands of medicine, marriage, and motherhood, especially as most rural communities are short of doctors to share the medical work and on-call load.

Access to rural emergency medical services is vital but difficult to provide to Canada's spread-out rural population. The need to manage high-acuity patient problems such as multiple traumas and myocardial infarctions with limited local resources makes this an exciting challenge for rural family physicians, who provide the vast majority of care for the patient visits to hospital emergency departments in Canada. The heavy night and weekend on-call burden can lead to burnout and/or midcareer transfer to urban practice. Many rural hospital emergency departments now pay a sessional salary for night shifts on-call to encourage doctors to take part of the next day off. In 1997 the Canadian Association of Emergency Physicians published a major report with recommendations for rural emergency care.[14]

The availability of obstetric birth services in rural Canada is in serious decline. Fewer small hospitals provide obstetric birth services and fewer rural family doctors attend births.[25] In addition, the local availability of cesarean section and epidural services is also declining. The provision of rural obstetric services was a major focus of attention in 1997 and 1998, culminating in the *Joint Position Paper on Rural Maternity Care* by the Society of Rural Physicians of Canada (SRPC), College of Family Physicians of Canada, and Society of Obstetricians and Gynaecologists of Canada.[26]

Aboriginal Health Care

Improving the health of Canada's Aboriginal people presents the greatest challenge, particularly in the vast rural and remote areas. This challenge is particularly well described in the Report of the Royal Commission on Aboriginal Peoples, published in 1996, from which the following discussion is derived.[27]*

Prior to the arrival of the Europeans most Aboriginals enjoyed an active rural lifestyle with a simple diet. They generally enjoyed good health, free of many of the illnesses common today. Today the state of Aboriginal health is poor by any measure and the gap separating Aboriginal from non-Aboriginal people, in terms of quality of life as defined by the World Health Organization, remains stubbornly wide:

* Original version, Report of the Royal Commission on Aboriginal Peoples, Gathering Strength, Privy Council Office. Adapted by Dr. James Rourke, Southwestern Ontario Rural Medicine, Education, Research and Development Unit, The University of Western Ontario. Reproduced with permission of the Minister of Public Works and Government Services Canada, 1999.

TABLE 25-6   ESTIMATED LIFE EXPECTANCY AT BIRTH, TOTAL AND ABORIGINAL POPULATIONS, 1991

Population	Male (years)	Female (years)
Total population	74.6	80.9
Total aboriginal population	67.9	75.0
Registered North American Indian	66.9	74.0
On reserve	62.0	69.6
Nonreserve, rural	68.5	75.0
Nonreserve, urban	72.5	79.0
Inuit	57.6	68.8

SOURCE: Adapted from Norris et al.[8]

- Life expectancy at birth is about 7 to 8 years less for registered Indians than for Canadians generally, with Indian males living on reserves having a life expectancy of only 62 years (Table 25-6).
- Part of this difference in life expectancy is explained by high rates of infant mortality among registered Indians. For infants, the death rate is about twice as high as the national average. Fetal alcohol syndrome is also a concern. There are also high rates of injury and accidental death among Aboriginal children and adolescents. Mortality in all age groups is higher for registered Indians than for Canadians generally.
- Infectious diseases of all kinds are more common among Aboriginal people than others. Otitis media is particularly common among Inuit children, with resultant high rates of deafness. Tuberculosis is 43 times more prevalent among registered Indians than among non-Aboriginals.
- The incidence of life-threatening degenerative conditions such as cancer and heart, liver, and lung disease—previously uncommon in the Aboriginal population—is rising. Diabetes in particular affects Aboriginal people disproportionately, with an incidence two to three times higher than among non-Aboriginals. This may be a result of an inherited tendency combined with modern day poor nutrition and little physical activity. The complications of diabetes are enormous.
- Suicide is a serious problem. The reported suicide rate for registered Indians is 3.3 times the national average and for Inuit, 3.9 times the national average. For registered Indian males aged 20 to 29, the highest-risk group, there are over 100 suicides per 100,000 per year.
- Overall rates of injury, violence, and self-destructive behavior are disturbingly high. Death by injury is twice as common among Aboriginal people as among Canadians generally. For young people aged 15 to 24, fully 85.5 percent of all deaths were the result of injury. Even among those aged 25 to 44, some 59 percent of all deaths resulted from injury. It is estimated that up to 25 percent of accidental deaths among Aboriginal people are really unreported suicides.
- Rates of overcrowding, educational failure, unemployment, welfare dependency, conflict with the law, and incarceration all point to major imbalances in the social conditions that shape the well-being of Aboriginal people.

Throughout much of Canada, isolated Aboriginal Indian, Metis, and Inuit settlements have health care provided by specially trained nurses/nurse practitioners with regular clinic visits by family doctors. Patients requiring investigations and treatment are transferred to regional centers that may be hundreds of miles away.

The author had the privilege of doing locums in Hazelton, northern British Columbia, serving an Aboriginal Indian population and in Iqualuit (Frobisher Bay) and surrounding settlements on Baffin Island, Northwest Territories (NWT, in the part now called Nunavut), serving an Inuit population. As a medical student doing a rural elective in Inuvik, NWT, the author was flown some 300 miles (500 kilometers) as part of a medical evacuation team to Fort Good Hope, a small Inuit community of 600 people in the remote Arctic. We had been called by the nursing station nurse to attend an Aboriginal Indian woman who, because of pneumonia, had gone into premature labor. Upon landing, the team immediately assisted this woman's delivery of a 28-week-gestation infant in the back of a station wagon beside the runway. Mother and baby were then flown back to Inuvik, where the baby was taken by jet more than 1250 miles (2000 kilometers) to Edmonton for advanced neonatal care. This case posed major challenges for the health care team and health delivery system. These challenges, however, pale by comparison with the perspective of the woman and her family, their difficulty accessing health care, and then interacting with the enormous social, cultural, and distance barriers of ongoing care for sick infants, children, or any family members requiring transfer to a strange and distant urban health care environment.

The Royal Commission concludes that the convergence between Aboriginal perspectives and health sciences research provide a powerful argument for adopting an Aboriginal health strategy based on:

- Equitable access to health services and equitable outcomes in health status
- Holistic approach to treatment and preventative services
- Aboriginal control of services
- Diversity of approaches that respond to cultural priorities and community needs

The start of good health care must begin with safe and adequate supplies of water and food, effective sanitation systems, and safe and adequate housing. The holistic approach to treatment and preventive services must be driven by and integrated with community needs and supported by appropriate resources to be effective. There is a major movement now for First Nations communities to assume administrative responsibility for health care services. In addition, there is a growing recognition that further steps need to be taken to ensure the successful application of more Aboriginal people into medical school.[23] Many Canadian family medicine programs give residents exposure to Aboriginal health issues but need more depth and expertise.[28] There is still a long way to go before the outcomes and the strategy are achieved.

EDUCATION FOR RURAL MEDICAL PRACTICE

Medical Education in Canada

In Canada, 14 of 16 medical schools have 4-year programs and two have 3-year programs. Most require 3 more years of undergraduate university education prior to entry into medical school.

Postgraduate training in Canada, for both family and specialist practice, is provided by the university medical school departments. The family medicine and specialist departments' involvement in and responsibility for both undergraduate and postgraduate medical education have led to strong vertically integrated family medicine and specialty departments within each university. All university programs must meet accreditation criteria set by either the College of Family Physicians of Canada (CFPC) or the Royal College of Physicians and Surgeons of Canada (RCPS). Residents take examinations set by one or the other of these bodies upon completion of their training programs. The autonomy of university departments in shaping medical education has led to a variety of postgraduate vocational training programs in response to regional needs and regional resources. Postgraduate family medicine residency training programs are 2 years long with an optional third year. Postgraduate specialty residency training programs are 4 to 5 years long. Residents' salaries in Canada are generally paid by the provincial governments through the universities. Resident training is coordinated by university department program directors. The residents have a strong union. These factors have led to educationally focused, compact, and intensive postgraduate training programs.

Rural Undergraduate Medical Education

Faced with the problem of educating and recruiting enough physicians for rural and remote areas, a number of educational initiatives are being taken in Canada. These are based on findings that rural-origin medical students and students who have positive rural clinical experiences at undergraduate and postgraduate levels are more likely to enter rural practice.[29]

Attempts are being made to encourage rural students to consider medicine as a career. These efforts include high school career-promotion days and the development and distribution of videos on rural medicine. Despite these attempts, students from rural backgrounds remain underrepresented in medical school.[23] This may reflect both a lack of quality secondary-level education and a paucity of opportunities available to talented rural students as well as medical school location and selection criteria that unintentionally favor urban-educated students. None of the medical schools in Canada have affirmative-action programs for increasing the number of students from rural areas.[23]

In Canada, all the medical schools provide the opportunity for a rural learning experience.[23] This is usually a 2- to 4-week experience during a senior medical year, which may be too little, too late. There are limited opportunities for early rural learning experiences.

Memorial University in Newfoundland, a very rural Canadian province, provides a rurally oriented, vertically integrated medical education. This begins prior to medical school with the opportunity for rural students to spend some time at the university medical school during their senior secondary school break time. The rural focus extends throughout medical

school, the postgraduate family medicine training program and to continuing medical education for rural doctors.[23]

This is an exciting time of change in rural undergraduate medical education. Many medical schools are expanding their rural undergraduate medicine components. The University of Western Ontario (UWO), for example, is located in the heart of a region of 1.4 million people, of which 40 percent live in communities of less than 10,000. In 1997, UWO radically revised its undergraduate medical curriculum to include an extensive integrated rural undergraduate medicine program that is needs-driven, community-focused, evidence-based, learner-centered, and outcome-measured. This curriculum provides core rural and regional components for all students with extensive "rural training track" opportunities for some students. All 96 first-year medical students now spend 1 week in groups of two to four in 33 communities in southwestern Ontario. This "rural week" rotation was the highest-rated learning experience of the first-year medical students. It is followed throughout medical school by extensive opportunities for rural undergraduate summer studentships, required clerkship rotations in rural and regional centers, and rural elective opportunities.

Medical school enrollment is being increased in several provinces. Several medical schools are considering developing rural medical streams. A northern Ontario rural medical school is being considered.

Postgraduate Medical Education for Rural Practice

In Canada, rural education initiatives at the postgraduate level have developed almost totally within provincial regions. The forces for education reform at this level have come from grassroots rural physicians' input, pressure from rural practice groups within some provincial medical associations, and educational leadership at some university medical school departments of family medicine, with some support from general medical organizations and governments.[23,30,31]

As a result, a variety of family medicine training programs have been developed in response to regional needs and resources available. In general these programs can be seen as educationally intense, learner-centered 2-year family medicine training programs with a varying rural focus. All family medicine programs offer the opportunity for residents to experience some training in the rural practice setting, and approximately 80 percent of all second-year family medicine residents in Canada participate (567 of 702 residents in 1993, for example).[32] This may be as short as 1 month or as long as 12 months of rural family medicine experiential training in a rural family practice setting. Of the 18 family medicine training programs, 12 have compulsory rural family medicine training blocks that vary from 1 to 6 months, depending on the program. In addition, residents may choose to do an optional third year for advanced skills in fields that may be helpful in rural practice, such as obstetrics, anesthesia, emergency medicine, and psychiatry, although the number of these positions is limited.[33] Government-supported, university-developed, advanced-skills-year training is being most successfully expanded and implemented in Alberta and British Columbia.

The advantage of the Canadian approach has been the development of a wide variety of postgraduate family medicine educational programs in response to regional needs and resources that offer family medicine residents a considerable choice of programs to suit their own needs. Outcomes of these programs in terms of the numbers of trainees who ultimately establish rural practice have not yet been fully determined.

There has, however, been no common curriculum for postgraduate education for rural family practice or for rural family medicine advanced skills. The College of Family Physicians of Canada in collaboration with the Society of Rural Physicians of Canada established a Working Group on Rural Family Medicine Education.

Their report, approved by The College of Family Physicians of Canada in May, 1999, recommends the following.[34,35]

1. Rural undergraduate exposure should be provided for all medical students.
2. Postgraduate rural family medicine education streams should be developed as appropriate training for rural family practice.
3. Postgraduate rural family medicine education stream positions should be provided in sufficient number in order to train more physicians for rural areas.
4. Postgraduate rural family medicine education streams should be identifiable upon entry, include at least 6 months of rural-based education, and be competency-based.

This extensive report outlines the knowledge, skills, and attitudes required for rural family practice and a curriculum for postgraduate rural family medicine education streams.

Advanced rural family medicine skills form an important part of rural practice, but until now such skills have generally been acquired in nonaccredited programs that have not necessarily been nationally recognized. The report's recommendations are for competency-based advanced rural family medicine skills training programs including GP anesthesia, advanced maternity care including cesarean section, and GP surgery, with psychiatry and other programs to be developed. Curriculums are being established by the College of Family Physicians of Canada, the Society of Rural Physicians of Canada, and appropriate specialist organizations. The advanced family medicine skills training programs will be accredited by the College of Family Physicians and will be competency-based. The length of training will usually be 6 to 12 months, depending on the preexisting abilities of the trainees. These may be accessed as a third year for residents after completing their 2-year postgraduate rural family medicine education streams or as reentry positions for physicians in rural practice who return with identified needs for further training.

Postgraduate Specialty Education for Rural/Regional Practice

General surgeons are the most dominant specialists in rural practice, followed by general internists, radiologists, obstetricians, pediatricians, psychiatrists, and others. Traditionally, residents interested in pursuing a rural or regional career have generally arranged their specific rotations in the hopes of developing the right knowledge and skills. Several universities have flexible informal rural or regional preceptor-based rotations for their specialty residents. Dalhousie University in Nova Scotia has had a successful rural and regional specialist training program for several years to coordinate community-based specialist training rotations.[36] The University of Western Ontario began its Multi-Specialty Community Training Network in 1997. The MSCTN develops and coordinates rural and regional training rotations for specialty residents in anesthesia, emergency medicine, obstetrics, pediatrics, psychiatry, general surgery, internal medicine, and pathology. Specific learning objectives and evaluations have been developed based on the Royal College of Physicians and Surgeons' CanMeds 2000 Project. Many residents have ranked this as their best learning experience.

Continuing Medical Education for Rural Physicians

Continuing medical education in Canada remains a challenge for rural doctors who require broad knowledge and skills to provide the many medical services needed in their communities. Barriers include time, distance, cost, and difficulties getting locum tenens coverage while the doctor is away. A variety of innovative programs are being developed to address these needs of rural doctors. The Society of Rural Physicians of Canada Annual National Conference provides an excellent rural focus on continuing medical education. The Society of Rural Physicians of Canada has also developed a traveling critical care course with built-in locum tenens support.[37] A wide variety of conferences and clinical traineeships are offered by medical schools and other organizations. In Ontario, rural physicians can receive $5000 per year to cover tuition, travel, accommodation, and other expenses for CME as part of the Ministry of Health/Ontario Medical Association funding agreement. Internet access to information and distance education are being used by more rural physicians. A master's level distance education rural medicine course is being developed at the University of Western Ontario by Dr. Leslie Rourke and Dr. James Rourke.

CONCLUSION

It is to be hoped that the increasing attention to rural health will result in responsive system development, with measurable improvements in rural health outcomes. The underlying social, cultural, and economic determinants of rural health care must be assessed and addressed. Providing better rural health care will require educating more doctors and other health care providers, giving the appropriate knowledge and skills for rural practice and interest in it. Improved clinical support, information technology, and funding for rural health care providers will also be necessary.

The goal is to provide excellent health care for the entire rural population by health care practitioners who are well supported by innovative programs seeking to minimize the disadvantages and who are thus able to enjoy the advantages of living and working in a rural area.

ACKNOWLEDGMENTS

I would like to thank Dr. Leslie Rourke, Mary Ann Kennard, and Diane Gauley for their help with this chapter. Thanks to Lynda Buske and the Canadian Medical Association (CMA) for the CMA Masterfile Data, to Dr. George Deagle for his vignette, and to Louisa Blair for her excerpt.

This chapter reports data from the 1997 College of Family Physicians of Canada's (CFPC) National Family Physician Workforce Survey. This database is part of the CFPC JANUS Project: Family Physicians Meeting the Needs of Tomorrow's Society. Principal investigators are Dr. Calvin Gutkin, MD, FCFP, and Dr. Raymond Pong, PhD. The JANUS Project Coordinating Committee is chaired by Dr. Nick Busing, MD, FCFP. The Centre for Rural and Northern Health Research was contracted to carry out the 1997 survey. The JANUS Project is supported by Associated Medical Services (AMS), the Canadian Medical Association (CMA), the Royal College of Physicians and Surgeons (RCPS), and Scotiabank.

REFERENCES

1. Statistics Canada: *A National Overview: 1996 Census of Canada.* Catalogue number 93-357XPB. Ottawa, Industry Canada, 1997.
2. Statistics Canada: *The Canada Year Book, 1994.* Ottawa, Statistics Canada, 1994.
3. Statistics Canada: *Focus on Canada* [an analysis of data collected by the 1991 Census of Population and Housing], Ottawa, Statistics Canada, 1994, table 1.2.
4. Statistics Canada: *A National Overview: 1996 Census of Canada.* Catalogue number 93-357XPB. Ottawa, Industry Canada, 1997, table 17.
5. Statistics Canada: *A National Overview: 1996 Census of Canada.* Catalogue number 93-357XPB. Ottawa, Industry Canada, 1997, p 353.
6. Statistics Canada: *A National Overview: 1996 Census of Canada.* Catalogue number 93-357XPB. Ottawa, Industry Canada, 1997. table 6.
7. Government of Canada: *Canada.* Ottawa, 1999, p 4. Online: http://Canada.gc.ca/canadiana/faitc/fal_e.html
8. Norris MJ, Kerr D, Nault F: *Projections of the Population with Aboriginal Identity, Canada, 1991–2016.* Research study prepared by Statistics Canada for the Royal Commission on Aboriginal Peoples. Ottawa, Canada Mortgage and Housing Corporation, 1996.
9. Statistics Canada: *The 1997 Canada Year Book.* Ottawa, Statistics Canada, 1996, p 33.
10. Blair L: Rural docs deal with Canada's worst bus crash. *Can J Rural Med* 4(1):111–112, 1999.
11. Canadian Medical Association: *CMA Masterfile.* January 1998.
12. Madore O: *The Canada Health Act: Overview and Options—Current Issue Review 94-4E.* Research Branch, Library of Parliament, Canada, 1995.
13. Rourke J: In search of a definition of "rural." *Can J Rural Med* 2(3):113–115, 1997.
14. Canadian Association of Emergency Physicians, Rural Committee (Thompson J, chair): *Recommendations for the Management of Rural, Remote and Isolated Emergency Health Care Facilities in Canada.* Ottawa: Canadian Association of Emergency Physicians, 1997, p 12.
15. Deagle G: Tales of a flown-in doctor. *Can Fam Physician* 45:277–279, 1999.
16. Square D: Manitoba crash a wake-up call for "fly-in" physicians. *Can Meal Assoc J* 158:1064–1065, 1998.
17. Rourke J: Trends in small hospital medical services in Ontario. *Can Fam Physician* 44:2107–2112, 1998.
18. Rourke J: Small hospital medical services in Ontario. part 1: overview. *Can Fam Physician* 37:1589–1594, 1991.
19. Iglesias S: The future of rural health: comprehensive care or triage? *Can J Rural Med* 4(1):32–33, 1999.
20. Rourke J: Small hospital medical services in Ontario. Part 5: General surgery services. *Can Fam Physician* 37:1897–1900, 1991.
21. Iglesias S, Strachan J, Ko G, Jones L: Advanced skills by Canada's rural family physicians. *Can J Rural Med* 4(4):227–231, 1999.
22. Kermode-Scott B: Gold mine of information: Researchers and CFPC are thrilled with Janus survey. *Can Fam Physician* 44:1581–1584, 1998.
23. Canadian Medical Association: Advisory *Panel on the Provision of Medical Services in Underserviced Regions.* Report of the Advisory Panel on the Provision of Medical Services in Underserviced Regions. Ottawa: The Canadian Medical Association, 1992.
24. Craig M: Limit, leave, or be left. Master's research project, department of family medicine, University of Western Ontario, London, Canada, 1994.
25. Rourke J: Trends in small hospital obstetric services in Ontario. *Can Fam Physician* 44:2117–2124, 1998.
26. Iglesias S, Grzybowski S, Klein M, et al: Rural

obstetrics: joint position paper on rural maternity care. *Can Fam Physician* 44:831–843, 1998.

27. Canada Royal Commission on Aboriginal Peoples: *Report of the Royal Commission on Aboriginal Peoples:* Vol 3. *Gathering Strength.* Ottawa, Minister of Supply and Services, 1996.

28. Redwood-Campbell L: Residents' exposure to aboriginal health issues: survey of family medicine programs in Canada. *Can Fam Physician* 45:325–330, 1999.

29. Rourke J: *Education for Rural Medical Practice: Goals and Opportunities: An Annotated Bibliography.* Moe, Victoria, Australia, Monash University, 1996.

30. Rourke, J: Politics of rural health care: recruitment and retention of physicians. *Can Med Assoc J* 148:1281–1284, 1993.

31. Barer ML, Stoddart GL: Toward integrated medical resource policies for Canada: Part 8. Geographic distribution of physicians. *Can Med Assoc J* 147:617–623, 1992.

32. Rourke J: Rural family medicine training in Canada. *Can Fam Physician* 41:993–1000, 1995.

33. Perkin RL: Rural practice. *Can Fam Physician* 40:632, 1994.

34. College of Family Physicians of Canada Working Group on Rural Family Medicine Education (Rourke J, Chair): *Postgraduate Education for Rural Family Practice: Vision and Recommendations for the New Millenium.* Mississauga, Ontario, approved by The College of Family Physicians of Canada in May 1999. www.cfp.ca/ruralpaperfull

35. College of Family Physicians of Canada. Working Group on Postgraduate Education for Rural Family Practice (Chair Dr. James Rourke): Postgraduate education for rural family practice: vision and recommendations for the new millennium. *Can Fam Phys* 45:2698–2704, 1999.

36. Gray JD, Steeves LC, Blackburn JW: The Dalhousie University experience of training residents in many small communities. *Acad Med* 69(10):847–851, 1994.

37. Kingsmill S: National Rural Critical Care Course: rural docs teaching rural docs. *Can J Rural Med* 2(3);143, 1997.

CHAPTER 26

Rural Practice in Australia

RICHARD B. HAYS

THE AUSTRALIAN HEALTH CARE SYSTEM

Geography

Australia is a geographically large nation whose population is concentrated in the southeastern corner, where approximately two-thirds of the her 18.5 million citizens live in cities with up to 4 million people.[1] With the exception of the southwestern corner, which is home to approximately 1.5 million urban Australians, the rest of the country is sparsely populated. The larger towns are scattered along the coastal fringe, so that Australia is essentially a coastal nation. Inland communities tend to be small and many are quite distant from major population centers. Because population growth is largely confined to urban areas, a nation once famed for its outback nature is each year becoming increasingly urbanized, even though most of the nation's wealth is derived from agricultural and mining industries in rural and remote areas.

As in other developed nations, defining rurality is a complex issue. The Australian approach is to combine several parameters, each of which contributes some understanding of what life is like in rural communities. The most relevant to health care is the Rural, Remote and Metropolitan Areas (RRMA) classification,[2] which considers population, population density, and distance from major urban centers to form seven categories. These are capital city; metropolitan; large rural center; small rural center; remote center; and other remote areas. As a rule, populations of communities in the first two categories are more than 100,000 people; large rural centers have 25,000 to 99,999 people, small rural centers have 10,000 to 24,999, and remote centers have more than 5000 people. The difference between the rural and remote categories is in the distance from capital cities or other metropolitan centers. This a simplified summary, as decision points about population levels and distances vary slightly between states, but it enables all Australian communities to be placed in a single national framework.

A weakness of the RRMA system, however, is that it does not necessarily define communities well.[3] The basic units for population estimates are statistical local authority (SLA) boundaries, but SLAs do not necessarily define communities, particularly in two situations. The first is where the SLA boundaries are geographically large, such that several small communities are regarded as being a single community when in fact they function independently. The second is where SLA boundaries are small, such that larger communities are regarded as several small communities when in fact they function as a single community. The latter is particularly relevant to urban fringe growth areas, where once-rural communities adopt urban characteristics as they merge. Another method of classifying rural populations is to use postal codes to define population boundaries. However, this is

TABLE 26-1   A FUNCTIONAL DEFINITION OF RURAL MEDICAL PRACTICE

Category	Characteristics
Large rural community	Population >18,000, 80–160 miles (50–100 km) or about 1 hour travel time from support services
Small rural community	Population <18,000, 160–480 miles (100–300 km) or 1–3 hours travel time from support services
Large remote community	Population >18,000, >480 miles (>300 km) from advanced facilities but usually with a reasonable range of local support services
Small remote community	Population <18,000, >480 miles (>300 km) or 3 hours travel time from support services

SOURCE: From Hays et al.,[4] with permission.

equally flawed, as postal delivery routes also do not necessarily define rural communities.

Hence, although the RRMA system is widely adopted in Australia to classify health care characteristics, it is not regarded as a good definer of rural medical practice. Instead, the system has been modified according to *what rural doctors do.*[4] This *functional* definition of rural practice is based on distance and travel time from health care support services; this is not always the same as the concept of the major center adopted by RRMA. Isolation from other health personnel, particularly procedural specialists, and major hospital facilities appears to predict more reliably the range of skills needed and performed by rural doctors. The most accurate method of measuring this isolation is surface travel time, as this allows for major geographic barriers (e.g., mountain ranges and flooding rivers) and poor transport systems. The functional classification system is illustrated in Table 26-1.

However, while this modified classification is a reasonable method of defining rural medical practice, it is not suited to the more complex task of allocating health care resources according to needs. Other models are being explored to develop a more equitable method of allocating resources, one of which combines an index of local economic resources with population and distance/travel time data in a method that has demonstrated validity for equity of access to educational resources.[5] Another recent approach produces an index of accessibility and

remoteness based on two scales—population of service centers and the distance from large service centers.[6] There are four population categories for the service centers: A (>250,000); B (48,000 to 249,999); C (18,000 to 47,999); and D (5000 to 17,999). The 12 categories of remoteness reflect increasing distances from service centers, using travel time by road as the main determinant. This approach combines traditional geographic data with a more functional understanding of how access to services is determined by travel time to service centers, not all of which are in large cities, and appears to better describe the variations between different rural and remote communities.

Organization of Health Care

An interesting feature of Australia that affects how health care is delivered is the structure of the government. When colonized and incorporated into the British Empire in the late eighteenth and early nineteenth centuries, each part of the country was established as an independent colony with autonomy over the management of local services, including health care. When Australia became an independent nation in 1901, this structure became a federation of states, each with an independent elected government that continued to manage health care for her own citizens. Hence Australia, with six states and two territories, has eight different health care systems, each with particular funding and management strategies. These differences have profound effects on how rural health care is organized and supported.

Like those of most developed nations, the Australian health care system provides comprehensive primary-, secondary-, and tertiary-level care that is regarded as being of a high standard, by international standards. The primary-care level is assigned substantial responsibility for providing illness prevention and for assessing patients who might need access to secondary- and tertiary-care levels. General practitioners are the most important group, as patients may not proceed to specialist care unless they are referred by a general practitioner or an emergency department. Nurse practitioners are not currently licensed to work independently or to prescribe drugs, although some states are planning to do this, particularly in rural areas. In some ways the Australian system could be seen as having elements of both the U.K. and the U.S. systems. As in the United Kingdom, the position of the general practitioner is central, with a "gatekeeper" role that could control flow-on costs in the secondary and tertiary sectors. However, there are as yet no formal controls on referrals—such as primary care budget-holding, where flow-on costs generated by primary care doctors are deducted from primary care budgets—nor are there U.S.-style health maintenance organizations (HMOs), which use protocols to define care pathways and restrain overall cost.

Funding of Health Care

The funding of health care reflects the shared responsibility borne by state and federal governments. Australia has two parallel health care systems: one called the "private" system and the other the "public" system. Both are heavily supported by the federal government from tax revenue. The federal government directly supports most aspects of primary health care and non-hospital-based ambulatory secondary care through a universal basic insurance scheme that underwrites a fee-for-service payment scheme.

Much of the funding for this scheme comes from an additional tax (the Medicare levy) on incomes. This is known as the "private" system, as patients may be billed directly in a direct contractual arrangement with a service provider.

State governments fund most hospital-based care, using a portion of a federal grant (derived from the Medicare levy), for which Australian residents are not charged a direct fee. This is known as the "public" hospital system. In addition, individuals may take out additional private health insurance, which provides greater choice of hospital, provider, and timing of health care, thus forming a "private" hospital system. However, although most government funding could be viewed as coming originally from the same source, management of hospital-based and ambulatory care is provided by different and at times conflicting organizational structures, and private hospitals are managed independently.

The inevitable barriers imposed by this complex organization are perhaps less obvious in rural communities. Although the models vary between states, most state governments directly fund some aspects of rural health care in response to local political concerns about communities with special needs. Examples of such special needs include remote locations with poor access to health care, Indigenous communities with poor health status, and small communities that might otherwise not support fee-for-service medical practitioners. Some states directly employ medical practitioners to serve such communities. Primary care medical practitioners are usually employed to reside in those communities, while secondary care services usually provide regional services from larger centers. Secondary services in key specialties (surgery, anesthesia, and obstetrics) are often provided by itinerant "flying specialist" services that visit both regular clinics and emergencies, while major trauma and other emergency patients are usually transported to regional hospitals by "retrieval" teams, often by air. The result is that rural initiatives sponsored by the federal and state governments often collaborate with and complement each other better than in urban settings to provide reasonable access to medical services, although the range of services is more restricted than in urban communities.

THE HEALTH OF RURAL AUSTRALIANS

Most comparisons of urban and rural health care status demonstrate that rural people are at a disadvantage.[7] Overall, there is a 40 percent higher rate of avoidable death.[8] There are higher rates of respiratory problems, asthma, allergies, and skin cancer and more frequent infectious diseases, such as leptospirosis and hydatid cyst disease.[9,10] Work-related injuries are more common, because farming and mining, the dominant industries, are relatively hazardous occupations.[11,12] Serious motor vehicle accidents are more common because of the long distances that must be traveled.[12,13] Rural people also consume more alcohol and tobacco and have poorer nutrition.[8] The effects of the recent rural recession have been severe, placing extreme pressure on rural communities. Counseling services, support groups, and other mental health services are either limited or unavailable.[14] Rural youth suicide rates are high, reflecting the high rates of youth unemployment and, perhaps, the availability of firearms.[15] Rural and remote Australia is also home to the majority of the Indigenous population, whose health status is significantly worse than that of the Australian population as a whole.[16]

Differences between urban and rural health status are due to more than rural occupational lifestyle and population subgroup differences. Rural people have restricted access to health care services. Those on farming or grazing properties might be more than an hour's drive from the nearest small town and often have to rely on the Royal Flying Doctor service for health care advice by radio. Health care for residents of small towns is provided by relatively few primary care nurses and medical practitioners, with little or no choice of provider possible.

Few specialist nursing, medical, or other health professionals (e.g., physiotherapists, psychologists, etc.) live outside of urban centers, so rural people may have to travel substantial distances to receive even basic hospital and procedural services that are taken for granted by urban people. The relative shortage of medical and other health care workers prevents rural people from receiving services equivalent to those available to urban people.[17]

The poor access is compounded by the continuing decline of rural communities through economic recession, international competition, and variations in commodity prices. Increasing farm mechanization and rationalization of government services exacerbate the continuing population drift to urban centers. As rural populations and economies decline, basic services—such as banks and post offices—close. Smaller and poorer communities with few services have even greater difficulty attracting and keeping health professionals. This spiral of decline affects the morale of many rural communities.[11]

Although the work-force issues remain significant barriers to equity of access, the way in which rural health care is delivered is changing. In some cases, information technology can overcome distance barriers, so that rural people have improved access to selected services. The widespread availability of videoconferencing technology in rural areas allows rural health professionals to obtain real-time consultations with urban specialists who may be several hundred miles away. Particularly in psychiatry, dermatology, and other disciplines that rely on visual cues, teleconferencing enables the patient and rural doctor to bring the specialist into the rural consulting room.[18] Early evaluations demonstrate a reduced need for travel for further opinions and more appropriate management of mental health problems. As technology develops further, the range and quality of telemedicine services will increase while their cost will fall.

The Health of Indigenous Peoples

Among the most disadvantaged populations in Australia are the Indigenous peoples, who were defeated in an undeclared war of invasion that was fought in early European colonial times, commencing with the first formal settlement in 1788. The key to understanding their health status lies in understanding Australian history. Aboriginal and Torres Strait Islander culture is rich with oral history and mythology of a long-standing civilization lasting perhaps 40,000 years. Documented contact occurred between Aboriginal communities and European explorers as early as the sixteenth century, but the history of European civilization in Australia is relatively short. Although there are no accurate data on Aboriginal and Torres Strait Islander peoples at the time of European settlement, the population was scattered in small clan groups, each of which cared for and lived off a particular geographic area. Their "hunter-gatherer" existence was well suited to the harsh climate and the natural vegetation and animals, and their social structure was strong. It is believed that infectious diseases were relatively uncommon and that their spread through the dispersed population would have been limited.[19]

However, the European settlers did not understand this different culture and lifestyle. Aboriginal culture was branded primitive and the absence of permanent settlement was interpreted as meaning that Aboriginal people did not "own" the land. Aboriginal people were not organized and equipped to fight one of the world's most powerful nations; therefore, with a few exceptions, they were easily beaten off to occupy parts of the country that Europeans did not want.[20] The decline in the population through warfare was exacerbated by the introduction of infectious diseases, to which the Indigenous peoples had little immunity. In one of the more remarkable legal decisions of the times, the continent that was named Australia was formally regarded as *terra nullius* or "empty land" by colonial governments, such that the dispossession became legal. This gave settlers the right to chase Aboriginal people off land that was needed for farming or grazing. Those who resisted were killed, while those that remained in contact with settler communities were used as cheap labor, and few attempts were made to educate or care for them. In a sense they were "chattels" that simply came with the land the settlers occupied.

The early years of European settlement were disastrous for Aboriginal people. Almost the entire Aboriginal population of some parts of the country was either killed or transported to remote locations as European settlement spread rapidly around the coastal fringe and to adjacent inland areas. The later years have hardly been better, as Aboriginal people developed into a permanent "underclass" of the dispossessed, poor, malnourished, and poorly educated.[16] The twentieth century brought a new challenge, when well-meaning groups forcibly removed children of mixed European and Aboriginal parentage to be brought up and partly educated, so that they would become part of mainstream Australian culture. However, many of these children, known as the "stolen generation," ended up in a twilight zone between cultures.[21,22]

Specific examples of the poor health status of Aboriginal and Torres Strait Islander peoples are listed in Table 26-2. Life expectancy is 15 to 20 years lower than for non-Indigenous Australians.[23] There are high rates of diabetes (up to 16 percent of some populations), renal disease, cardiovascular disease, respiratory disease, alcoholism, accidental and nonaccidental death, mental illness, and infectious diseases.[23] Infant mortality is high, although this has improved dramatically since the early 1970s, when up to 78 of every 1000 live births failed to survive. In some respects, the Aboriginal health status is closer to that of populations of developing nations rather than that of an apparently wealthy industrialized society. Indeed, the living conditions of some of the more remote communities are similar to those in the developing world, with poor basic community infrastructure (e.g., clean water, sanitation systems, and health care). Aside from the condition of the infrastructure (which is basic to health), direct spending on Indigenous peoples' health remains lower than that for other Australians.[24]

The key to improving the health of Indigenous Australians lies in a difficult process of acknowledging the past, reconciling differences,

TABLE 26-2   EXAMPLES OF HEALTH CARE STATUS COMPARISONS BETWEEN INDIGENOUS AND NON-INDIGENOUS AUSTRALIANS

	Indigenous	Non-Indigenous
Obesity (>13 years)	60%	
Smoking (>13 years)	50%	
Low birth weight (<2500 g)	7–16/100,000	6/100,000
Perinatal mortality	14–35/100,000	7–12/100,000
Meningococcal meningitis	13/100,000	2.2/100,000
Tuberculosis	12.5/100,000	5.7/100,000

SOURCE: From the Australian Bureau of Statistics.[23]

and empowering Indigenous peoples to work toward a common goal. This requires recognition that there are many different groups of Aboriginal and Torres Strait Islander peoples, with up to 700 languages or dialects. Each of these groups has a particular history and culture, such that Indigenous Australia is really a confederation of separate nations. The politics of reconciliation involve acknowledging land rights (different to the European view of land ownership), repairing self-esteem, and including all Australians in the healing process. Meanwhile, increased expenditure is required for basic community infrastructure needs and initiatives to improve the availability of an appropriately trained health care work force.

WORK-FORCE INITIATIVES

Rural Australians have always had to seek health care from the relatively few doctors and nurses who sought opportunities away form the comfort of an urban lifestyle—traditionally a mix of missionaries and misfits.[25] Initially, all medical graduates were trained in just two medical schools, one each in Sydney and Melbourne. This did not change until the 1930s, when moves began to establish schools in the other states. By the 1970s, each state had its own medical school. However, while the existence of a medical school in each state's capital city improved the national distribution of medical graduates, it did little to improve the distribution to smaller

communities. Even in the mid-1990s, students of rural background formed a disproportionately small proportion of entering cohorts, and the 30 percent of the Australian population that is rural was served by about 20 percent of the graduates—this is despite the fact that Australia has one of the highest doctor-population ratios in the world.[26]

With the exception of establishing medical schools in each state, Australian governments have relied on individuals wanting to work in rural areas and on market forces to drive excess urban doctors into rural and remote areas. The assumption has been that once the cities were full of doctors, the excess would overflow into rural areas. Schemes to place doctors in rural practice in exchange for undergraduate financial support have been moderately successful for over 40 years in the state of Queensland. However, this has relied on sending poorly trained recent graduates into difficult situations for short periods of time. Early burnout has been as frequent as a commitment to remain, so this has not been a successful long-term strategy.

By the late 1980s, it had become clear that the "overflow effect" was not occurring. The metropolitan areas had become overcrowded with general practitioners, with no significant change in rural work-force shortages. Major studies of rural medical practice in the late 1980s and early 1990s provided information about the personal and educational backgrounds of rural doctors, the nature of their practice, continuing education, attitudes toward practice, and issues in recruitment, training, and retention of rural general practitioners (GPs).[27–29] The findings from these studies were similar to those from research in other countries: rural doctors are busier, work longer hours, provide a wider range of services in relative professional isolation, and bear an increased professional indemnity responsibility than urban doctors. Rural practice offers professional rewards—such as greater clinical diversity, social cohesion, and professional autonomy[27–29]—but rural doctors do not stay long in small communities because of inadequate training, overwork, and poor opportunities for their spouses and children.[30] Publicity about the difficulties encountered in rural practice and the negative portrayal of rural practice and "learned helplessness" that is role-modeled in medical school combine to make rural practice appear to be more challenging than it really is. Is it surprising, therefore, that many students might not regard rural practice as their first choice?

A result of the many reviews of rural medical work force during the 1980s and 1990s has been a more coordinated, multilevel approach by governments to address the identified barriers to recruitment and retention. Financial incentives, improved continuing education programs (including replacement doctors), and improved medical school and postgraduate training initiatives have been developed.[31] Improved support must be provided for Indigenous students in health professional careers, as currently only 0.8 percent of health professionals are Indigenous Australians.[31]

EDUCATION AND TRAINING FOR RURAL PRACTICE

The nature of rural practice has implications for the training of an appropriately skilled medical work force. Rural doctors must be capable of dealing with a broader range of patient presentations, including emergencies, than urban general practitioners. The absence of other special-ists means that some rural doctors provide inpatient care and perform a range of procedures—such as general and regional anaesthesia, operative intrapartum care, and other urgent or semiurgent surgical procedures. The increased need for skills is not confined to procedures, as rural doctors must also function without close access to specialists in most other disciplines.

Medical school education and postgraduate training programs were once strongly city-oriented. Because this contributed to the urbanization of the medical work force, government policy now regards education strategies as work-force tools. Recent reforms to medical education have focused on both the content and context of curricula. Training is being decentralized to regional and rural areas and future rural doctors, in recognition of the emergence of rural medicine as a distinct discipline, receive training in the broader roles that will be required of them.[32]

Undergraduate

Australia has 10 medical schools whose curricula are accredited by the Australian Medical Council. Until recently, those curricula were similar in all except Newcastle University, which was one of the pioneers of problem-based learning (PBL). All took in students direct from secondary school at the age of 17 or 18, and all except Newcastle were 6-year courses (Newcastle was 5 years). However, during the 1990s, all medical schools have revised their curricula substantially. Three (Sydney, Flinders, and Queensland) have changed to 4-year, graduate-entry courses with "hybrid" curricula. That is, their curricula include a combination of PBL and traditional approaches. Students seek entry to these schools through a common, nationwide Graduate Australian Medical Schools Admission Test (GAMSAT), which includes tests of scientific reasoning, written expression, and aptitude and a structured interview. Most other medical schools have now adopted an alternate national admissions test called Undergraduate Medical Admissions Test (UMAT), which was developed by Newcastle University. These selection processes are usually not designed to achieve specific quotas for either rural background or Indigenous students, although some medical schools alter selection criteria to create small subquotas for students in these groups.

Coinciding with these curriculum changes, the federal government offered financial incentives for medical schools that introduce and achieve targets for selection of rural-background students, rural curriculum exposure, and decentralization of resources to rural and regional centers.[31] As a result, all medical students in Australia now experience substantially more rural teaching, in terms of both content and location, than previously.[32] All students receive at least 8 weeks of rural practice exposure, and some schools have developed programs that allow for up to 1 or 2 years in regional schools. Examples include the Flinders University Riverland Project and the Darwin Clinical School,[33] and the North Queensland Clinical School, which saw the relocation of a 40-student cohort school some 2100 miles (1300 kilometers) north into the tropics.[34] The latter initiative is evolving into Australia's 11th medical school, at James Cook University, where the whole program will reflect an emphasis on rural and remote, indigenous, and tropical health contexts.

Postgraduate

Rural doctors in Australia are regarded as a variant of general (family) practitioners, and their training is provided through the Royal Australian College of General Practitioners (RACGP) Training Program. There are two streams to this training program: a 3- to 4-year program for those intending to enter rural practice and a 3-year program for others. Both streams cover a similar core curriculum content and follow parallel learning paths, although learners in the Rural Training Stream (known as registrars) spend much of their training in regional and rural practices and have access to additional learning experiences.[35] These include opportunities for advanced rural skills training in surgery, anesthesiology, and obstetrics.[36] Other advanced-skills posts include Indigenous peoples' health, public health, mental health, child health, and emergency medicine.[37] The rural training program is shown diagrammatically in Table 26-3.

The curriculum is based on adult-learning principles and hence allows for substantial flexibility in the timing, location, and sequencing of training terms.[35] Increasingly, rural education programs rely on information technology.[38] Formative assessment is provided throughout training, and completion of training is certified by success in the college examination, the sole national entry route into general practice. The examination is common to both rural and nonrural streams, with additional rural components assessed separately either during training or at the end of discrete rural training units.

The rural training program has been the focus of debate, with many rural doctors believing that the RACGP was too urban-oriented and therefore failing to achieve the desired output of rural-trained doctors. A new Australian College of Rural and Remote Medicine was formed to remedy this,[39] and this now works in sometimes contentious collaboration with the RACGP Training Program to deliver an improved rural program. In an associated strategy,

TABLE 26-3   *RURAL TRAINING PROGRAM UNITS (TERMS) IN TYPICAL SEQUENCE: EACH UNIT IS 6 MONTHS IN DURATION*

Year 1		Year 2		Year 3		Year 4[a]	
Hospital	Hospital	Basic GP	Advanced GP	Mentor GP	Mentor GP	Advanced skills	Advanced skills

[a]Optional year-4 units may be done at any time after Basic GP terms in a rural community.

each state has established rural health training units in regional or rural centers; one of the more successful is in Western Australia.[40] These provide the regional and rural focus for the RACGP Training Program, including educational programs, mentoring by rural doctors, and other forms of rural-oriented support.

Continuing Professional Development

There have been substantial improvements in the availability and quality of continuing medical education (CME) since the Rural Incentives Program initiatives were introduced in 1995.[41] Each state now has federally funded organization that develops and implements CME programs, employing and coordinating replacement doctors to facilitate attendance by rural doctors. The programs adopt the principle of taking educational resources to rural doctors through extensive use of information technology, including telephone and videoconferencing (via ISDN, microwave and satellite technology) and the Internet and through taking more traditional face-to-face education programs to regional and rural locations.

FUTURE DIRECTIONS

Although the future cannot be predicted with certainty, it is unlikely that the urbanization of Australia will cease. Although much of the nation's wealth will continue to come from primary industries, mechanization, increasing use of "fly-in, fly-out" workers, and other efficiencies will limit the economic benefits received by rural communities. Communities along the coastal fringe will grow and coalesce further, and there will be a continuation of population migration from the south of the continent to the north and west—the "rust belt-to-sun belt" phenomenon. Inland communities will continue either to grow slowly or to decline. The likely result is that a minority of the population will continue to live in small communities that are distant from health care services. The extent to which nurse practitioners and other health care workers should replace or augment scarce medical graduates has yet to be resolved. The degree to which information technology will compensate for access problems is uncertain; meanwhile, rural information technology infrastructure will continue to develop.

In the short to medium term, governments will continue to apply financial incentives to encourage health care practitioners to commence and then remain in rural careers. Medical education initiatives will continue to develop in rural areas, particularly in northern Australia. Funding is also being directed toward addressing specific health problems. Examples include campaigns aimed at reducing tobacco consumption, youth suicide, and farm accidents and improving access to women's health services in rural communities. Although these have begun, it is too soon to measure their effectiveness. Improving the health care of the Indigenous population will remain a national priority. This will require continued allocation of substantial resources, both directly to health care and to improve housing, water supply, and sanitation services. It will also require resolution of the legal and moral dilemmas surrounding reconciliation of Aboriginal and European cultures.

REFERENCES

1. Australian Bureau of Statistics: *Regional Population Growth, 1996–97.* Canberra, Australian Government Publishing Service, 1997.
2. Commonwealth Department of Human Services and Health: *Rural, Remote and Metropolitan Areas Classification 1991 Census Edition.* Canberra, Australian Government Publishing Service, 1994.
3. Hays RB, Veitch PC, Franklin L, Crossland L: Methodological issues in medical workforce research: implications for regional Australia. *Aust J Rural Health* 6:32–35, 1998.
4. Hays RB, Craig M, Wise A, et al: A sampling framework for rural general practice. *Aust J Public Health* 18:273–276, 1994.
5. Griffith DA: A northern territory approach to quantifying access disadvantage to educational services in remote and rural Australia. In

McSwan D, McShane M (eds): *Proceedings of the International Conference on Issues Affecting Rural Communities.* Townsville, James Cook University, 1994.

6. Commonwealth of Australia: *Accessibility/Remoteness Index of Australia.* Occasional paper series no. 6. Canberra, Department of Health and Aged Care and University of Adelaide, 1999.

7. Trickett P, Titulaer I, Bhatia K: Rural, remote and metropolitan area health differentials: a summary of preliminary findings. *Aust Health Rev* 20:128–137, 1997.

8. Mathers C: *Health Differentials among Adult Australians Aged 25–65 Years.* Canberra, Australian Institute of Health and Welfare, 1994.

9. Humphreys J, Rolley F: *Health & Healthcare in Rural Australia.* Armidale, University of New England, 1991.

10. Clarke L: Analysis of the health status of rural people, in Cullin T, Dunne P, Lawrence G (eds): *Rural Health and Welfare in Australia.* Wagga, New South Wales, Centre for Rural Welfare Research, Charles Sturt University, 1990, pp 132–145.

11. Optimal Occupational Health and Safety Services: *Managing Change in the Face of Rural Sector Decline.* Melbourne, Sydney Myer Foundation, 1995.

12. Low JM, Griffith GR, Alston CL: Australian farm work injuries: incidence, diversity and personal risk factors. *Aust J Rural Health* 4:179–189, 1996.

13. Tolhurst HM, Dickinson JM, Ireland MC: Severe emergencies in rural general practice. *Aust J Rural Health* 3:25–33, 1995.

14. Human Rights and Equal Opportunities Commission: *Human Rights and Mental Health.* Canberra, Australian Government Publishing Services, 1993, pp 678–722, 936–939.

15. Dudley MJ, Kelk NJ, Florio TM, et al: Suicide among young Australians, 1964–1993: an interstate comparison of metropolitan and rural trends. *Med J Aust* 169:77–81, 1998.

16. Thomson N: A review of Aboriginal health status. In Reid J, Trompf P (eds): *The Health of Aboriginal Australia.* Sydney, Harcourt Brace Jovanovich, 1991, p 37.

17. Australian Health Ministers Conference: *National Rural Health Strategy.* Canberra, Australian Government Publishing Service, 1994.

18. Yellowlees P, Kavanagh S: The use of telemedicine in mental health service provision. *Australas Psychiatry* 2:268–270, 1994.

19. Saggers S, Gray D: *Aboriginal Health and Society.* Sydney, Allen and Unwin, 1991.

20. Reynolds H: *The Law of The Land,* 2nd ed. Melbourne, Penguin Books Australia, 1992.

21. Gray A, Trompf P, Houston S: The decline and rise of Aboriginal families, in Reid J, Trompf P (eds): *The Health of Aboriginal Australia.* Sydney, Harcourt Brace Jovanovich, 1991, p 80.

22. Human Rights and Equal Opportunity Commission: *Bringing Them Home: National Inquiry into the Separation of Aboriginal and Torres Strait Islander Children from Their Families.* Canberra, Sydney, Sterling Press, 1997.

23. Australian Bureau of Statistics: *The Health and Welfare of Australia's Aboriginal and Torres Strait Islander Peoples.* Canberra, Australian Government Publishing Service, 1997.

24. Australian Institute of Health and Welfare: *Australia's Health 1998.* Canberra, Australian Government Publishing Service, 1998, p 39.

25. Richards D: To minister to the sick: an historic socio-profile of the medical profession in northern Australia, in Pearn J (ed): *Outback Medicine.* Brisbane, Amphion Press, 1994, p 23.

26. Australian Medical Workforce Advisory Committee: *Australian Medical Workforce Benchmarks.* Canberra, Australian Institute of Health and Welfare, 1996.

27. Kamien M: *Ministerial Inquiry into the Recruitment and Retention of Country Doctors in Western Australia.* Perth, University of Western Australia, Department of Community Practice, 1987.

28. Strasser RP: Attitudes of Victorian rural general practitioners to country practice and training. *Aust Fam Physician* 21:808–812, 1992.

29. Wise A, Hays RB, Adkins P, et al: Training for rural general practice. *Med J Aust* 161:314–318, 1994.

30. Hays RB, Veitch PC, Cheers B, Crossland L: Why doctors leave rural practice. *Aust J Rural Health* 5:198–203, 1997.

31. Commonwealth Department of Human Services and Health: *Rural Doctors: Reforming Undergraduate Medical Education for Rural Practice.* Canberra, Australian Government Publishing Services, 1994.

32. Strasser R: Rural General Practice: Is it a Distinct Discipline? *Aust Fam Physician* 24(5):870–876, 1995.

33. Commonwealth Department of Health and Family Services: *The Current State of Undergraduate*

Medical Education for Rural Practice: Report of the Mid-term review of the General Practice Rural Incentives Program's Rural Undergraduate Component. Canberra, Australian Government Publishing Service, 1998.

34. Mudge P: A Clinical School for North Queensland. *Med J Aust* 158:501, 1993.

35. RACGP Training Program: *Training Program Handbook 1998,* Melbourne, Royal Australian College of General Practitioners, 1998.

36. Royal Australian College of General Practitioners (Faculty of Rural Medicine): *Training Curricula in Surgery, Anaesthetics and Obstetrics for Rural General Practice.* Sydney, RACGP, 1992.

37. Hays RB, Wallace DA, Sen Gupta TK: Training for rural practice in Australia. *Teaching Learning Med* 9:80–83, 1997.

38. Sen Gupta TK, Wallace DA, Clark SL, Bannon G: Teleconferencing: practical advice on implementation. *Aust J Rural Health* 6:2–4, 1998.

39. Hays RB, Strasser RP, Wallace DA: Development of a national training program for rural medicine in Australia. *Educ Health* 10:275–285, 1997.

40. Jackson WD, Jackson DJ: The West Australian Centre for Remote and Rural Medicine. *Med J Aust* 155:144–146, 1991.

41. Holub L, Williams B: The general practice rural incentives program, development and implementation: progress to date. *Aust J Rural Health* 4:117–127, 1996.

CHAPTER 27

Rural General Practice in the United Kingdom

IAIN J. MUNGALL   JOHN WYNN-JONES   JENNIFER DEAVILLE

WHAT IS RURAL PRACTICE?

Rural practice in Britain, like the countryside itself, is immensely diverse. Compare commuter villages in the Home Counties around London, the Cotswolds, and the West Country (swamped during the peak holiday season) with mining communities in the North of England, hill farms in mid-Wales, and the remote Scottish Highlands. Not only land use and culture but so also the economy varies widely between rural areas—which, in the United Kingdom, tend to have a wider spread of incomes than within urban areas. General practice, therefore, can be as varied within rural Britain as it is different from urban practice.

Currently, there is no universally accepted definition of rurality, but three factors are seen as relevant issues:

- A sparse population
- Distance from centers of population
- The perception of being rural

This chapter describes the current features of rural practice in the United Kingdom, including the health of rural populations, the organization of health care delivery, and recent developments in raising the profile of rural practice as a distinct discipline.

PATTERNS OF ILLNESS

Certain conditions commonly seen in the countryside are rarely seen elsewhere. Agriculture has its own risks—for example, trauma, poisoning with organophosphate insecticides, suffocation in silos, organic toxic dusts, and also the zoonoses to which those working closely with animals are exposed.

It is increasingly recognized that depression and indeed suicide are not uncommon in the countryside, possibly exacerbated by current pressures on the farming community. Mental health in the countryside is a rural health issue that has attracted increasing academic and policy attention in recent years. The Department of Health commissioned a program of research into suicide and stress among farmers in England and Wales because of concern over the increased risk of suicide in this group.[1]

It is very difficult to make valid comparisons of mortality and morbidity between rural and urban areas. Rural populations are dispersed and routine statistics gathered at a regional or county level fail to recognize small-scale differences. However, studies at a smaller geographical scale often suffer from having too few subjects to show any statistically significant difference between urban and rural areas. As a general rule, it would seem that country dwellers are healthier, being free of urban pollution and the risks of industrialization. This, however, is not universal, and the link between illness and deprivation is still more important than geography. Some northern rural areas have a worse mortality and morbidity than some southern urban areas.[2]

RURAL DEPRIVATION

Deprivation has long been understood to be associated with ill health, and efforts have been made to target additional resources at deprived populations. However, until the late 1990s, deprivation was seen to be largely an inner-city problem. Now it is more clearly understood that deprivation exists within rural areas but is more covert.[3]

A study in 1997 reported that around one-quarter of U.K. rural households live in or on the margins of poverty (defined as an income below 140 percent of Supplementary Benefit level).[4] Poverty is particularly associated with old age and low-wage employment. Large numbers of rural workers have part-time or seasonal employment.

In 1994 the average weekly earnings of agricultural workers was £217.18, compared with an average across England of £299.50.[5] In the late 1990s, agriculture is widely seen as under even greater financial strain.

EQUITABLE FUNDING

In the U.K., general practitioners (GPs) are funded for their National Health Service (NHS) work (typically under 10 percent is non-NHS) by a complicated formula that reflects the number of patients registered with them, the services provided, and whether certain targets for preventive health are achieved (see "Organization and Funding," below).

In recent years, additional payments have been made to GPs working in deprived areas in recognition of their additional workload. There is general agreement that standard deprivation indices are not sufficiently sensitive for use in rural areas. For example, car ownership is used in the formula as an indicator of wealth; but in the absence of public transport, it is a necessary expense, further compounding the problems of poverty. Furthermore, the relationship between self-reported morbidity and indices of deprivation has been shown to break down in nonmetropolitan areas.[6] An index of deprivation that is relevant and reliable is sorely needed if resources are to be distributed equitably in rural areas. The Rural Voice Health Group has listed many of the indicators of rural deprivation.[7]

In addition to the indices themselves being inappropriate for recognizing rural deprivation, the scale at which they are applied also discriminates against rural areas. Deprivation payments using the Jarman Index are currently calculated using a large (electoral registration) area. Studies have demonstrated, however, that were smaller geographical units like enumeration districts used, a considerable amount of extra deprivation money would flow into rural practices.[8]

ACCESS TO CARE

A big issue for the countryside is access to all services, not just health care. Public transport in rural areas has been increasingly run down in recent decades, and there is ongoing environmental pressure for the costs of private transport to increase. Patients may find that it is expensive (in money *and* time), difficult, or impossible to get to the nearest surgery or hospital. Studies have shown a clear "distance-decay" relationship in the United Kingdom with declining consultation rates and increasing distance from the point of health service provision. This has been shown for general practice and also for referrals to acute hospitals.[9] There is evidence that reduced access to care can have adverse effects on health; for example, Leese and colleagues in 1993 showed that diabetic retinopathy is likely to present in a more advanced state in rural areas.[10] Access problems particularly affect already disadvantaged groups, such as the handicapped and the elderly.

Mortality from roadside accidents is likely to be higher in rural areas because of the delay in accessing care. Home visiting may be more common where transport is difficult, though there is little evidence to show that this happens generally. Home visiting is likely to be arranged by geography as well as clinical urgency.

Solutions may lie in highly imaginative local transport initiatives, as well as national transport policies which are sympathetic to the needs of the countryside.

Two responses to the problems of access to care are branch surgeries and community hospitals.

Branch Surgeries

Branch surgeries are now much less common than they were a generation ago. They vary enormously in scope and size and may be identical to a main surgery or merely a room in a remote village hall. Equipment and staffing levels also vary widely. They tend to be popular with patients because of the easy access but unpopular with doctors who do the traveling and may offer a lower standard of care. It has been shown that branch surgeries can be closed down without increasing visiting rates in the main surgery,[11] yet no studies seem to have been done to measure the effect of closure on subsequent mortality and morbidity.

There would seem to be an inevitable conflict between access to care and quality of care. How this conflict is resolved depends on local circumstances.[12]

Community Hospitals

Community hospitals are generally run by local GPs, many of whom have or develop specialized skills to help to staff the hospitals with the aid of visiting consultants. There may be problems about the availability of these specialist skills—for example, as GPs move toward cooperatives for out-of-hours cover. There are similar problems for training of consultants, as general physicians and surgeons are threatened by increasing specialization.

A wide spectrum of services is provided by the hospitals. About 10 percent provide the majority of all care for the populations they service, including acute medicine, surgery, terminal care, and maternity care.[13–16] At the other end of the spectrum, another 10 percent of community hospitals provide extended nursing, long-term care, and respite care in much the same way as well-equipped nursing homes.[17] The remainder provide care that lies between these two extremes, usually including a minor casualty service, specialist outpatient clinics, x-ray facilities, and physiotherapy.

Good liaison with visiting consultants is an important issue for health care, and relationships with local GPs can be improved by close working. This is essential because of the need to seek advice when the consultant is at a distance from the community hospital. Innovative communication systems are vital to rural areas, and telemedicine is seen as a potentially invaluable resource for linking the community hospital with its local district general hospital (DGH) or distant specialist hospital.

Enthusiasm for local community hospitals has waxed and waned over the course of the century, but these hospitals are generally seen as an invaluable local resource. They are much appreciated by local people, helping to support the ideals of a local community.[18] By the end of the 1960s, only 300 remained, though recently they have increased in numbers. Costs per inpatient day have been shown to be lower than in the local DGH, though clearly such comparisons are invidious, since the clinical work is likely to be different.

Community hospitals are frequently seen as an easy source of revenue savings when local health authorities face financial crises. The tendency to centralize services within the NHS militates against community hospitals. However, arguments about better outcomes obtained in centers of excellence many miles from local communities need to be balanced by the costs, often unmeasured, of patients traveling long distances away from their communities and families. Baird, writing in *Rural Healthcare*, describes how patients often value being cared for in their own community, even at the expense of the high technology available at the remote center of excellence.[18] If community hospitals are phased out, then clearly an excellent transport infrastructure would be required.

ORGANIZATION AND FUNDING

Rural practices tend to be small and remote and may well provide dispensing services to their patients. They are likely to provide a wider range of services than more urban practices—for example, in casualty work, minor surgery, and immediate care at accidents. Similarly rural GPs carry a wider range of equipment than is usual—for example, a defibrillator and other resuscitation equipment.

Rural practices are funded in exactly the same way as urban practices, but extra funding is available through rural practice payments and dispensing payments to mitigate the effects of smaller-than-average list sizes, the lack of economies of scale, and traveling costs. Some very small practices may depend upon the inducement practitioner scheme whereby they are guaranteed a minimum income.

Rural practice payments are essentially a capitation mileage scheme, where doctors having more than 20 percent of patients living over 3 miles from their central surgery can claim money from the rural practice fund. The greater the distance of each patient from the center, the larger the sum payable. It is viewed by many as a very blunt instrument, with imprecise matching of resources with costs.[19]

Dispensing payments are made as a series of fees for providing a dispensing service to patients and are essentially similar to the system whereby community pharmacists are funded. The regulations concerning dispensing and which practices may dispense are complicated.[20] In essence, any GP in an area classified as rural may apply to dispense to any of his or her patients living over 1 mile from the local pharmacist as long as this would not render the pharmacist's business unviable. Many doctors feel that dispensing payments are needed to subsidize the provision of general medical services.

There is currently considerable unrest since this funding is not seen as secure in the long term. It is now clear that in Northern Ireland, for example, dispensing is being phased out throughout the province. The Royal College of General Practitioners (RGCP) Rural Doctors' Group has stated that general medical services in rural areas should be funded equitably without the need to rely on this extra source of income. This would mean that the question of who dispenses medicines could then be considered purely on its merits.

The Associate Practitioner Scheme

Established in 1990, this has been an undoubted success. Recognizing the particular difficulties of being single-handed with onerous on-call commitments, the scheme allows the deployment of an extra doctor between two single-handed remote GPs. It is funded at no cost to the practices concerned and allows the isolated doctors time away from the practice for study and relaxation. It has also given young doctors a taste of rural general practice without requiring an immediate commitment.

The Inducement Scheme

This has been in operation since the NHS's inception and follows a similar scheme that has been in operation in Scotland since 1912.[21] In effect, a minimum salary (currently around 81 percent of target net income)[22] is guaranteed for a GP in a rural area where the population is too small to make a practice viable under normal terms and conditions. Without this provision, many small (e.g., island) communities would not have any real access to medical services.

RECRUITMENT

During the 1990s, as recruitment to general practice became problematic, there have been particular anxieties about recruitment to remote rural practices. Studies in Scotland[23] have suggested that the number of vacant rural vocational training posts is significantly higher than the number of urban vacancies. Particular issues needing resolution include the following:

- Specific training needs for rural practice
- Out-of-hours work, especially in areas where cooperatives do not or cannot function*
- Difficulties of obtaining continuing education
- The particular needs of women doctors in isolated areas
- The lack of appropriate job opportunities for the doctor's family.

The World Organization of General Practitioners (WONCA) has made specific proposals to help address possible recruitment problems for rural doctors.[24] Many are applicable within the United Kingdom.

SOME RECENT DEVELOPMENTS IN RURAL PRACTICE

The Montgomeryshire Medical Society

The Montgomeryshire Medical Society (MMS) was founded by rural doctors in mid-Wales in the early 1980s. For the past 9 years the MMS has organized an annual conference at Gregynog Hall in Powys to provide locally based education for rural GPs. This has become an estab-

lished and successful annual event that has been highly influential in developing links both within the United Kingdom and internationally for health professionals interested in rural health issues.

The Institute of Rural Health

The Institute of Rural Health (IRH) was formed in 1996 as a U.K. organization. It is based at Gregynog Hall in Wales and is helping to establish a multidisciplinary academic foundation for rural practice. Current initiatives include:

- A program of research including Ph.D. research into developing computer-assisted learning for child asthmatics and research into adolescent substance abuse in rural Wales
- A community involvement project aimed at tackling rural stress in Powys
- A series of briefing papers on relevant topics such as zoonoses, farming accidents, and dermatology in rural areas
- The development of an academic course leading toward a diploma for rural practice
- Organization of an annual rural health forum
- Developing and evaluating the use of audio-conferencing to deliver an education program to rural primary care teams
- A rural health discussion board on the IRH Web site (www.rural-health.ac.uk) for use by health professionals, academics, and others with an interest in rural health issues
- Development and promotion of telehealth in rural health care

The Royal College of General Practitioners' Rural Practice Group

Formed in 1993 by Jim Cox, the RCGP group has worked to identify and address some of the issues relevant to rural practice.[25] There was general agreement that there was little research literature on rural health issues in the United Kingdom. Rural practice was then widely seen within the profession as the "rural idyll," and

---

* Out of Hours Cooperatives of General Practitioners have been in existence for many years but have increased in popularity enormously in the late 1990s with specific government funding. By 1999, some 80 percent of the U.K. population have their out-of-hours care from a cooperative doctor who is working a shift in a rotation. Rural areas present particular organizational difficulties, and additional funding is now available to allow even more remote areas to be served by cooperatives.

without significant problems. The aims of the group are as follows:

- To raise the profile of rural practice
- To stimulate research and education in rural general practice and to disseminate good practice
- To function as a "virtual faculty"

The RCGP group

- Has given evidence to government bodies
- Produces a regular newsletter, *Country Matters*, distributed free to all college members identifying themselves as rural
- Has produced an occasional paper, *Rural General Practice in the UK*[26]
- Has made an important contribution to *Rural Healthcare*, the first textbook of rural health care in the United Kingdom, published in 1998[27]

The RCGP Web site began hosting its first discussion group, for rural practice, in 1996 (www.rcgp.org.uk/special/rural/index.htm). The Scottish Council of the RCGP is in the process of forming, with others, a Scottish multidisciplinary rural health forum.

The Centre for Health Services Research

Based at the University of Newcastle Upon Tyne, the center completed important research on rural health issues in 1997, and this included a detailed literature review.[19] This work has been important in helping to develop the emerging research agenda into rural health in the United Kingdom.

The Scottish Office

In 1999 the Scottish Office established a resource center with £2 million annual funding to help address the issues of rural health. (It is interesting to note that, since the development of regional government in Scotland and Wales in 1999, we may anticipate some divergence in development in the NHS, especially since these two countries have a greater proportion of rural areas than does England.)

Euripa

EURIPA, the European Rural and Isolated Practitioners Association, was formed in 1997. It aims to help address the health needs of rural communities in Europe and the professional needs of those serving them. Current areas of interest include acting as a voice for rural health issues in Europe; setting up mechanisms for sharing information, skills, and knowledge using Internet technology; promoting recruitment and retention of rural health professionals; and initiating rural research and setting up links with other professional organizations (e.g., RCGP, WONCA).

At a recent meeting there were representatives from Wales, Scotland, England, Ireland, Denmark, Finland, Poland, Spain, Portugal, and Greece. The secretariat is currently based at the Institute for Rural Health in Wales. A Charter for Rural Practice has also been drafted. More details are available at the IRH Web site (for Web address, see above).

THE FUTURE

As the NHS increasingly looks to efficiency, there has been a tendency for services to be centralized, creating particular problems for some rural communities. The work over the last decade to raise the profile of rural health issues means that we now enter the new millennium confident that at last rural practice is becoming recognized as a distinct discipline. As the issues become more defined, so resources will be allocated equitably, ensuring high standards of care for the whole population irrespective of geography.

REFERENCES

1. Hawton K, Simkin S, Malmberg A, et al: *Suicide and Stress in Farmers.* Department of Health

funded research. London, Her Majesty's Stationery Office, 1998.

2. Phillimore P, Reading R: A rural advantage? Urban-rural health differences in northern England. *J Public Health Med* 14:290–299, 1992.

3. Cox J: Poverty in rural areas. *BMJ* 316:722, 1998.

4. University of Aberdeen: *Disadvantage in Rural Areas.* Rural research report no. 29. London, Rural Development Commission, 1997.

5. House of Commons: *Hansard.* London, HMSO, March 24, 1994.

6. Jessop EG: Individual morbidity and neighbourhood deprivation in a non-metropolitan area. *J Epidemiol Commun Health* 46:543–546, 1992.

7. Cox J: Rural general practice: a personal view of the current key issues. *Health Bull* 55(5):309–315, 1997.

8. O'Reilly D, Steele K: General practice deprivation payments: are rural practices disadvantaged? *J Epidemiol Commun Health* 52:530–531, 1998.

9. Haynes R, Bentham G: The effects of accessibility on GP consultations: out patients attendances and in patient admissions in Norfolk, England. *Soc Sci Med* 16:561–569, 1982.

10. Leese GP, Ahmed S, Newton RW: Use of mobile screening unit for diabetic retinopathy in rural and urban areas. *BMJ* 306:187–189, 1993.

11. McAvoy BR: Does closing branch surgeries affect home visiting? *BMJ* 290:120–122, 1985.

12. Mungall I: Rural diseases, in Cox J, Mungall I (eds): *Rural Healthcare.* Abingdon, Oxon, Radcliffe Medical Press, 1999.

13. Cavenagh AJM: How do community hospitals make economic sense? *BMJ* 2:392, 1974.

14. Williamson BCM: The work of a general practitioner surgeon. *Practitioner* 226:521–525, 1982.

15. Tucker H: *The Role and Function of Community Hospitals.* Project paper no, 70. London, King's Fund, 1987.

16. Thorne CP, Seamark DA, Lawrence C, et al: The influence of general practitioner community hospitals on the place of death of cancer patients. *Palliat Med* 8:122–128, 1994.

17. Whitehouse A, Pearce VR: The elderly in cottage-community hospital in Devon. *Concord* 24:17–21, 1983.

18. Baird AG: Community hospitals and maternity units, in Cox J, Mungall I (eds): *Rural Healthcare.* Abingdon, Oxon, Radcliffe Medical Press, 1999.

19. Rousseau N, McColl E, Eccles M: *Primary Health Care in Rural Areas. Issues of Equity and Resource Management—A Literature Review.* Report no. 66. Centre For Health Services Research; University of Newcastle-upon-Tyne, 1994.

20. National Health Service (Pharmaceutical Services): *Regulations, 1992.* London, Her Majesty's Stationery Office, 1992.

21. The Birsary Report CMND 3257 (June 1967) referring to The Dewar Committee (Dec 1912): *Report of Highlands & Islands Medical Services Committee.* Cd6559 and CdC920, Edinburgh, Her Majesty's Stationery Office.

22. Marshall L. Inducement practitioners, associates and the doctors' retainer scheme, in Cox J, Mungall I (eds): *Rural Healthcare.* Abingdon, Oxon, Radcliffe Medical Press, 1999.

23. Gillies JCM, Ross S: *Recruitment and Training for Rural Practice: Problems and Solutions.* Report for Scottish Council for Postgraduate Medical and Dental Education. University of Glasgow, 1996.

24. WONCA (Working Party for Training in Rural Practice): *Policy on Training for Rural Practice.* Hong Kong, WONCA. 1995.

25. Cox J. Rural general practice. *Br J Gen Pract* 44(386): 388–9, 1994.

26. Cox J: *Rural General Practice In the UK.* Occasional Paper no. 71. Exeter, Royal College of General Practitioners, 1995.

27. Cox J, Mungall I: *Rural Healthcare.* Abingdon, Oxon, Radcliffe Medical Press, 1999.

CHAPTER 28

Rural Medical Practice in South Africa

Stephen J. Reid   Ian D. Couper   Vanessa Noble

*A*t the brink of the new millenium, South Africa is poised at a fascinating point in history. Rural practice, like virtually every other activity in South Africa, has been deeply shaped and impacted by the political situation in the country over the past 50 years. The policies of apartheid had their most vicious effects on the health of the rural poor, in geographically designated "bantustans" separated by race. Rural health in South Africa, therefore, is synonymous with the health of the deliberately underdeveloped areas of the country, inhabited largely by black communities. As this chapter shows, this is a picture of disease that is similar to that of most developing countries throughout the world: a vast array of communicable diseases and other conditions of poverty such as malnutrition, and now the frightening and accelerating epidemic of heterosexually transmitted HIV.

However, with the first-ever democratic elections in the country in 1994, which were miraculously peaceful, a new hope infected the country. Plans and ideas conceived outside of the country while still in political exile formed the basis for the new national health plan of the African National Congress,[1] which came to power through a huge majority. This plan envisaged sweeping changes to the health care system, and a priority principle of the plan was that of equity. More than any other single issue, equity in South Africa is a driving force in the political arena, and this has direct impli-

cations for rural health care and practice. This ideal gave rise to the blueprint of the district health system, a system for the implementation of the principles of primary health care as articulated by the Alma Ata conference in 1978. It divides the country into manageable geographic health districts within which all health services are to be coordinated equitably. Many things are now possible in the country that were absolutely unthinkable less than 10 years ago.

In spite of this, the current harsh realities of the South African economy—resulting in tight health budgets, the rising HIV infection rate, the lack of middle-level management capacity and other professional skills in the public health service, and a raised public expectation of the health services—are some of the significant challenges that stand in the way of the broad health sector reform that was envisaged originally. The spirit in the country is still largely positive, riding the wave of optimism that resulted from the first democratic elections in 1994. As Nelson Mandela's era comes to an end and the country enters the new millenium, the quality of rural health services can be seen as a barometer of success of the broader social reforms undertaken by the government. With equity being the goal, the health of the country can be seen and measured in the children's ward of a rural hospital, where some of the most disadvantaged members of South African society end up as victims of the system.

A HISTORICAL VIEW OF RURAL PRACTICE IN SOUTH AFRICA

Current rural health care and practice in South Africa cannot be understood outside of the historical and political context of the country, which provides a rich and fascinating picture of the struggle for justice and equity. The history of health care provision in South Africa has been directly influenced by racist segregationist policies, through which a wide range of ideological forces, political considerations, and deep economic structural inequalities have combined to hinder the development of egalitarian health services.

At the turn of the century the regions or provinces that were to form the Union of South Africa (1910) were ill served outside of main urban centers by any organized form of health service. After the Union until the end of the 1920s and early 1930s, national and provincial responsibility for health care provision to black communities was not recognized: instead, it was passed from one department to another. The 1928 Public Health Act was supposed to have created a network of health clinics, hospitals, and services across the land, but the real result was that the provinces concentrated their efforts on providing hospital services in large urban centers for whites to the neglect of catering for blacks in rural areas.[2] A vastly ineffective district surgeon system resulted in doctor-to-population ratios in some rural areas as low as 1:200,000. Health services were based not on people's needs but on their ability to pay, and white doctors were not prepared to carry out their services in rural areas where the poor could not afford to pay. There was no training available for black doctors in South Africa at this stage. Provincial administrations also maintained that it was not their responsibility to provide hospital care for Africans in rural reserve areas, as it was legislated that they were the sole responsibility of the Union government, who alone could tax them. But at the same time, the Union government held firmly that hospital care was a provincial responsibility. They thus both evaded their

health responsibilities for rural black communities. The state therefore left health services for rural blacks to the work of small groups of missionary doctors and nurses scattered throughout remote rural areas. Christian medical missionaries have played an essential role in South Africa's rural health history, as they established and maintained an extensive health service for the black majority of the population for over 150 years, with external funds raised by their respective church denominations overseas.[3]

The Christian Medical Missionary Endeavor in Southern Africa

During the late eighteenth and ninteenth centuries, following closely on the establishment of the colonial power, Britain many churches set up missionary bodies in Southern Africa. Protestant denominations tended to establish themselves earlier (such as the London Missionary Society and the Anglican, Lutheran, Swiss, and American churches), followed later in the nineteenth century by the Roman Catholic and Dutch Reformed churches. They were numerous and established themselves as independent and uncoordinated bodies spread widely across the country. As "Christian soldiers," their aim was to bring the "light" of the Christian message to what they, the colonizers, perceived as "heathen," "uncivilized," and "backward" indigenous African societies.[4] Once settled, these missionaries recognized the vital need for trained medical doctors to help protect their own health but also to treat the indigenous black people suffering under the burden of disease. During the early years, medical practice was viewed as subservient to the main evangelistic work of the churches but increasingly became the "handmaiden" to religion. The colonizers viewed secular medicine as inferior to the rendering of combined spiritual and medical healing, which might also lead to religious conversions. However, delivery of health care by these doctors was frustrated by competing traditional medical practices among the indigenous black peoples. They viewed these traditions as "dangerous practices" of magic and witchcraft and felt that the only way to curb them was by providing effective biomedical cures as well as spreading the Christian faith.

It is important to note that the founding of these medical missionary institutions resulted in the establishment of the first western biomedical health services in numerous remote rural areas, where they would have started much later by the state if at all. During the first three decades of the twentieth century, secure foundations for rural medical services were laid: from small beginnings many missionary doctors almost single-handedly built successful hospital services through their own ingenuity, courage, and determination to help others.[5] Medicines had to be used sparingly, while equipment and instruments were restricted to the bare necessities. The missionary doctors recruited and trained local black nurses to assist them, and they increasingly shouldered the load of clinical care. There was little in the way of monetary reward and most of them passed unnoticed and unknown. As the years progressed, the character of the mission hospitals changed with advances in medical science as well as diagnostic and surgical procedures and medicines, especially leading up to and during World War II. With more patients and the need for skilled and trained staff to fill these growing modern hospitals, the greater expenditure requirements placed them well beyond most missions' financial capacities. Increasingly, subsidies from the national and provincial government health departments facilitated their progress from the late 1930s.

The Pholela Rural Health Center: A Successful Experiment

A unique strand of medicine that developed alongside mission medical endeavors from the 1940s was the more radical social, preventive, and community health center movement. This approach, inspired by such pioneer doctors as Sidney and Emily Kark at Pholela and Halley Stott at the Valley Trust, managed to combine the best of medical practice with new ideas of prevention at the family and community levels.

In the years leading up to the outbreak of World War II in 1939, the government proposed the establishment of three experimental health centers, each to serve a defined area, especially in black rural "betterment areas" that were simultaneously being planned by the agricultural section of the Department of Native Affairs.[6] However, the outbreak of the war hampered operations and only one such health center was established in Pholela, an African reserve area in southwestern Natal near Bulwer, a rural community typical of many others, laboring under the burden of communicable disease and poverty. The liberalism, euphoria, and optimism of social reform in the world at large, during and after the war, provided a rare window period of opportunity for innovative public health professionals to initiate and develop farsighted health reform policies.[7] In 1940, Sidney Kark took up his appointment as medical officer in charge of the center and became leader of a multiracial team of doctors, nurses, and health assistants who developed a progressive and integrated curative, promotive, and preventive extrahospital health service. Kark worked within the framework of "social medicine," which provided a more sophisticated and holistic understanding of social, political, and economic as well as biomedical causes of disease.[8] This approach challenged orthodox medical practice and clinical methods as it combined social science and medical research methods to develop a "socially oriented" form of epidemiology.[9] With this tool, the underlying social causes of disease were investigated at family and community levels. A unique aspect of Kark's approach was the establishment of an intensive "Family Welfare Service" with a 15- to 20-mile radius from the Health Center.[10] By training and using a new category of health worker—the "health assistant"—regular home visits could be conducted to survey and record health-relevant data while also disseminating information on health issues through group discussions. Practical demonstrations were undertaken to ensure low-cost, preventive, and pre-hospital recognition and hindrance of serious diseases. A general curative clinic and regular immunization programs were also established to address wider health needs and control infectious disease outbreaks. Pholela Health Centre was the first of its kind to embark on intensive research in a rural community and to demonstrate scientifically that a thorough family and community-based approach to the prevention of disease can be effective in this context. Kark's philosophy challenged the long-held tradition of centralized government policies and decision making, promoting instead the concepts of community participation and involvement in health.[11]

It is interesting to note that like the Christian medical missionary effort discussed earlier, this cadre of community health doctors was also marked by religious designation: an overwhelming proportion were of a progressive Jewish background who were against black oppression and saw medicine as a social service to the community. It is also important to note the ease with which these progressive socialist-inspired Jewish doctors connected with their Christian missionary counterparts on key issues of the day, but especially the provision of health services for rural, impoverished and disenfranchised black communities. This is especially evident with Kark's strong professional and personal links with the medical mission establishment of the McCord's Zulu Hospital in Durban. It was argued by one of Kark's community health doctor colleagues: "we were a closely knit group akin, I often thought, to secular missionaries. Many of the senior staff, particularly Sidney, were deadly serious and single-minded in their mission. They lived and breathed health centre ideology, leaving little room for the 'selfishness' of a private life. . . . In looking back, however, I know that many of us had personal problems that needed strong collegial support. 'Missionaries' however, are not encouraged to share their own dilemmas at work, and we were expected to be role models for new trainees."[12]

The National Health Services Commission and the Gluckman Report: 1942–1944

During the war years, in 1943, the community-based health center experiment in Pholela captured the imagination of the National Health Service Commission (NHSC), which was appointed by the state to develop a national policy of health reform.[13] The state's central Department of Public Health underwent a remarkable transformation in public health policy thinking during this time and, by incorporating Pholela's ideas, the radical social, preventive, and community health center movement became national government policy. Influenced by a far-sighted national minister and secretary for health, Drs. Henry Gluckman and George Gale, respectively, progressive plans were made for a comprehensive national health service. The Gluckman Report, as it became known, was based on a unified, nationally controlled and coordinated network of integrated preventive, promotive, and curative "health centers" countrywide, available to all sections of the population and linked to a national hospital system.[14] Because of their lack of coordination and the desire for uniformity in subsidy provision, the NHSC more than hinted that mission hospitals would be absorbed into the National Health Service. It was recommended that other health services—both curative but more importantly preventive—would be operated on a national basis, under one centralized authority responsible for their execution and financing. During this period, mission medical services in black "homeland" areas became more and more state-funded as the state recognized its health responsibilities, resulting in considerable growth as well as loss of church control.

The University of Natal and Durban Medical School: An Early Rural Health Orientation for Black Doctors

An important outcome of the NHSC was the recommendation to provide more extensive and diversified training facilities for the nationwide chain of health centers. As a result, the Institute of Family and Community Health (IFCH) was established in Durban, surrounded by seven practicing health centers, all under the direction of Sidney Kark. He left Pholela and took the techniques and skills learned in that rural community and adapted them to develop the first service, research, and training facility in community health work. While they were in positions of power, Gluckman and Gale also promoted Durban as the site of the first black medical school. They foresaw that the IFCH would provide facilities and contribute in concept and practice to the first black medical training institution with a new orientation toward preventive family and community health practice. It was envisaged that the majority of black doctors would enter health center services to be established among their own black communities and away from expensive curative-based hospitals. With the assistance of a 5-year grant from the Rockefeller Foundation, the IFCH was affiliated to Durban Medical School and brought into line with other research and educational institutions free from state control. However, the conservative, right-wing shift in government in 1948 brought the National party's conservative and racist policies to the fore, and subsequently a determined effort was made to undermine and replace what they viewed as a radical health movement at a national level.

State Control of Rural Health Services

During the late 1950s and 1960s rural health services were progressively constricted by the Nationalist government's tight control of all sectors during this period of "high apartheid." The grand scheme for the "separate development" of each of the country's racial groups led to the formal establishment of the "bantustans" or "homelands," which were largely rural areas for blacks. Health services were established in each of them, resulting in 14 separate government departments of health.

But they were each grossly underfunded relative to the provincial health services, which were for the exclusive use of whites. In many rural towns, as with all public service institutions, two hospitals served two completely different population groups: one for the whites and one for the blacks. Within the bantustans, the rural health services closely resembled the situation in many third world countries: mission hospitals struggling to cope with the effects of poverty and infectious disease as well as political and social disempowerment on a huge scale. Migrant labor, particularly for the mines in the Johannesburg area, contributed significantly to the disruption of rural families, with direct effects on their health. From 1973, the Department of Bantu Administration and Development (DBAD) progressively took control of all mission hospitals in the homelands prior to their being handed over to various bantustan governments fully supported by DBAD subsidies. Only a handful of mission hospitals remained independent, with provincial subsidies.

The New South Africa after Apartheid

The policies pursued by the new government and health department following the peaceful democratic elections in 1994 display a strong political will for equity and redistribution of resources in the public health sector of the new South Africa. The Truth and Reconciliation Commission, established by the government in 1995 specifically in order to examine the human rights abuses and injustices of the previous 35 years, heard a specific submission on human rights abuses in rural health. This described the systematic denial of access to reasonable health care services for the majority of rural people through the discriminatory policies of the previous government.[15] Social justice and equity are cornerstones of the policies of the new constitution, and the reelection of the ANC-led government in June 1999 means that these policies will be implemented over the next 5 years at least.

The broader policies of the national ministry aim at the implementation of a national health system based on the principles of primary health care and a decentralized district health system that is progressively able to take on autonomous functions of health service provision. Thus, one of the broad policies outlined in the 1997 White Paper for the Transformation of the Health Services aims to "distribute health personnel throughout the country in an equitable manner."[16] However, in a detailed quantitative analysis of the distribution of health personnel in South Africa, comparing the situation in 1994–95 with 1998, Makan found that there had been "very little, if any, shift towards the establishment of an equitable distribution of human resources in the South African public health sector."[17]

The sections that follow below outline the current situation in the country, including the efforts of all role players in rural health to overcome past injustices.

RURAL HEALTH IN SOUTH AFRICA TODAY

Demographics and Rural Health

Over half (52 percent) of the population of South Africa live in rural areas. However, enormous urban/rural differences between the provinces exist,[18] as shown in Fig. 28-1. Similarly, population density in each province varies greatly. The population is highly mobile, with large movements between rural and urban areas as the economically active members of rural communities migrate to urban areas to find employment and return to their rural homes when possible. Demographic surveillance of a rural area revealed that half of the males between the ages of 25 and 59 and 14 percent of the women of the same age were migrants, spending more than 6 months of the year living elsewhere.[19] This is the legacy of the forced removals of African people and the lack of landownership under the apartheid system. It means that rural areas

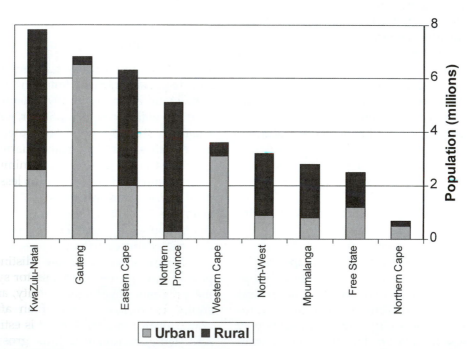

FIGURE 28-1 *Urban and nonurban population by province, 1994. (From CSS RSA Statistics in Brief, 1996,[37] with permission.)*

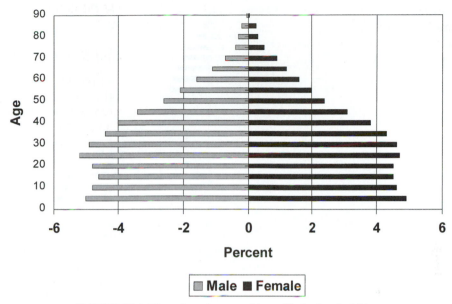

FIGURE 28-2 The urban demographic profile in South Africa.

in South Africa are populated largely by the very young and the elderly and that most employable men and women are absent, finding work in the cities. This has serious consequences for the health of rural families. Figures 28-2 and 28-3 display differences in demographics of urban and rural populations.

Another major factor influencing rural health is that of income and poverty.[20] The policy of racial capitalism under apartheid ensured a high level of privilege for white people and far lower standards of living for others. Although per capita incomes for whites in South Africa were estimated in 1991 as being 12.3 times higher than per capita incomes for black Africans, the 13 percent of the population who were white earned 62 percent of total income, while the 75 percent who were African earned 27.6 percent.

Certain groups are particularly vulnerable to disease and ill-health: the poor, the deprived, and the marginalized. In South African society, these groups are represented by the very young, women, and rural Africans. Broadly, more than one-third of all South African households, or half the population, can be classified as being poor. Some 75 percent of the poor live in rural areas, although only 53 percent of the population overall lives there: the rural poverty rate is thus much higher than the urban. The provincial distribution of poverty indicates the rural bias: the three most rural provinces (Eastern Cape, Northern Province, and KwaZulu-Natal) contain nearly two-thirds of the poor, whereas only 6 percent of the poor live in Gauteng province around Johannesburg. Three-quarters of rural households live below the minimum subsistence levels, as compared with less than one-third of urban households.[19]

Financing of Health Care

South Africa operates two distinct parallel health systems—the public sector system, providing care for the poor majority, and the private system, taking care of an affluent and largely employed minority. It is estimated that 8.5 percent of the country's gross domestic product is spent on health care. Out of this R42 billion total, the private health system consumes

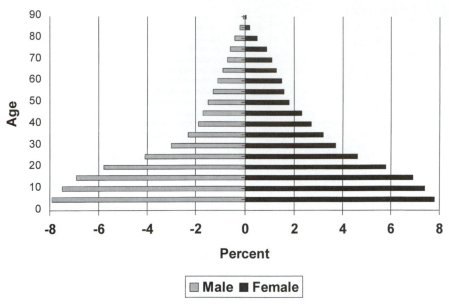

FIGURE 28-3 The rural demographic profile in South Africa.

over half of the total expenditure but caters to only 23 percent of the country's total population (Table 28-1). Only about one in five South Africans have health insurance. With the exception of nurses, a majority of health professionals (57 percent of doctors) practice in the private sector. The public health system, by contrast, caters to the majority of the population on an annual national budget of around R20 billion (US$ 3.4 billion).[21]

The historic maldistribution of public sector health care resources on a geographic basis has

TABLE 28-1   ESTIMATED HEALTH EXPENDITURE, 1995

	Rand (billion)	%
Public sector	19.2	45
Private sector	22.7	55
Medical schemes	14.9	35
Out of pocket payments	7.8	20
TOTAL	41.9	100

SOURCE: Palmer N, Wolvardt G: Chapter 4. In: Barron P (ed): *South African Health Review 1997.* Health Systems Trust, Durban, 1997.

been highlighted by a number of studies that have focused on the maldistribution of resources between the former homelands and the provinces.[22] The per capita budget for each province varies considerably, those provinces with a higher rural proportion of the population receiving considerably less than the more urban provinces. This issue is receiving specific attention from current government health planners, who are concerned with redressing the inequities of the past. Regarding the geographic distribution of private sector health care resources, most private hospital beds and practitioners are concentrated in the large metropolitan areas, where the majority of employed and therefore medically insured people reside.

A further challenge facing public health services is the relative concentration of resources within the hospital sector as compared with primary care. Some 76 percent of total public health care expenditures in 1992–93 were attributable to acute hospitals, with academic and other tertiary hospitals alone accounting for 44 percent.[20]

South Africa, therefore, devotes a relatively high proportion of its economic resources to the financing of health care. However, there is a maldistribution of these resources between the public and private sectors, between levels of care, and between urban and rural areas.

Health Status

South African society, like many other developing societies, is a society in transition, and this is reflected in its morbidity, mortality, and disability profiles. During the last century, both childhood and adult mortality have declined dramatically as a result of improved incomes, food and living conditions, and access to medical technology. However the effects of the HIV epidemic are expected to oppose this trend in the near future. There is a polarization of disease trends between the rich and the poor; however, the emergence of the diseases of affluence (hypertension, diabetes, coronary and cerebrovascular disease) in African people is an illustration of the transitional profile, as western diets become the norm for urbanized blacks.

By contrast, the health status of rural people in South Africa is similar to that of people in many developing nations around the world. The diseases of poverty are common, including a wide range of infectious disease, nutritional deficiencies, and chronic disability. HIV, tuberculosis, and diarrhea are the most common problems, with high rates in rural areas. KwaZulu-Natal, the most populous province, had a prevalence rate for HIV in the reproductive age group of over 30 percent in 1999.

The infant mortality rate (IMR) for the country as a whole is 40.2 per 1000 live births, but the variation between race groups and between urban and rural areas is large. The IMR for whites is 12.3 per 1000 births, while that for Africans is over 100. The national average IMR for urban areas is 33, while that of rural areas is 53. Access to health care for rural people is difficult: the high cost of transport and the large distances involved lead to late presentations of disease, particularly in rural areas. This is further complicated by traditional beliefs regarding illness: unregulated traditional healers of various levels of experience and skill make their services available to a somewhat fearful and tradition-bound public in rural areas. Although some beneficial diagnostic and treatment practices are rendered, the delayed presentations and dangerous side effects of herbal medication are frequently seen in the clinics and hospitals. This adds to the morbidity and mortality in rural areas.

Medical Practitioners and Rural Health Services

Health services in rural areas include both public and private systems. In the whole country there are approximately 12,000 general practitioners in the private sector and 9000 in the public sector. The doctor/population ratio for the country as a whole is 4.2 per 10,000, which compares well with the recommended international average of 4.9 per 10,000. However, these averages hide huge discrepancies between provinces and between urban and rural areas. In the Northern Province, which is largely rural, the doctor/population ratio is 0.9 per 10,000, and there are major shortages of medical staff in rural and remote hospitals. This contrasts with Gauteng province, which includes Johannesburg, with a ratio of 9.1 doctors per 10,000 population.[18]

Most of the private practitioners in rural areas are general practitioners offering primary care in small towns, where there are few private hospitals. However private practitioners are being increasingly squeezed by financial forces: increasing costs in the private sector and the policies of funders trying to insure low-risk individuals at the expense of the elderly and the sick have driven many patients away from health insurance and the private sector. Rural practitioners rely heavily on patients paying cash, and a number retain part-time government appointments as "district surgeons" or in government hospitals in order to provide a comprehensive service and bolster their income. The district surgeon system allowed indigent patients access to free health care, upon production of a magistrate's certificate approving this, for each consultation. The district surgeons were supplied with drugs and remunerated on a fee-for-service basis by the government health service and saw these patients in their practices. However, the system was open to abuse, and the new government has tried to amend it, amid great controversy. As a result, this arrangement has been partially withdrawn and replaced by sessional contracts for private practitioners within government health facilities.

The personal experiences of two rural practitioners in South Africa give an inside view of rural practice in the country.

Dr. Hoffie Conradie, a family physician in a small rural town, gives this account of his practice:

I am a South African–born doctor, qualified in 1973 at Stellenbosch University near Cape Town. I spent 2 more years at a teaching hospital before starting my rural career at Rietvlei Hospital as a missionary doctor. The hospital was soon taken over by the state and the hospital gradually lost its mission character. I spent the next 15 years in rural state hospitals in South Africa, followed by a 2-year stint in very rural Canada. I returned to South Africa and have since been in rural private practice. Presently I am in a two-man practice in Dordrecht in rural Eastern Cape, serving a farming community. There are few local job opportunities and able-bodied people go away to seek jobs in the larger cities and on the mines. The local people are often the young, the old, and the disabled. Dordrecht is also the centre for a large rural population of subsistence farmers.

Our day starts at the 50-bed state-aided hospital. We have sessional posts at the hospital where we do daily rounds, minor surgery, obstetrics, and provide 24-hour emergency care. We also admit our private patients at the hospital. At our office we see private patients as well as indigent patients referred by the local state clinics in our capacity as part-time district surgeons. We also do medico-legal work, which includes attending to rape victims, performing post-mortems, and assessing people for disability grants. We visit the state clinics once a week. Private patients are either on medical aid or pay an inclusive free for consultation and medicine. Twice a week we do a mobile

clinic route in the surrounding district. We carry all our medicines with us, and on the route of 140 km we have about 10 stops—at private houses, next to shops, or at schools—where patients wait for us. Patients in need of hospital admission come with us to the local hospital. I am also involved in the local state psychiatric clinic. Since the beginning of this year we also supervise a young doctor doing a year of compulsory community service. This has added new challenges to our practice.

A turning point in my rural career was when I enrolled for a postgraduate degree in family medicine. The emphasis was on the individual doctor-patient relationship and it opened a whole new world for me. It was difficult but challenging to apply the principles of family medicine in a third-world cross-cultural situation, communicating in a foreign language. My time in Canada allowed me to practice these principles in a first-world situation. Back in South Africa I chose to work in a rural setting where these two worlds meet. I can now communicate in the local black language, Xhosa, but also enjoy communicating with patients in my mother tongue, Afrikaans. Since completing my family medicine degree, I have had a part-time appointment with a university department of family medicine and have been involved in their postgraduate training program. This has been very stimulating for me as an isolated rural doctor.

For me the upside of rural practice is the continuity care I have with my patients, living in the same environment as my patients and the variety of medical problems we see and deal with. The downside is being on call every second day and every second weekend. I play squash regularly and whenever possible I take part in mountain-bike races.

Dr. Victor Fredlund, a British missionary doctor who has been working in South Africa for the past 18 years, gives this account of his work:

I came to Mseleni from London, U.K., in 1981 to join two other experienced practitioners. At the time Mseleni was a small hospital of 118 beds with a mobile clinic service and one residential clinic just opened at Mbazwana. Annual deliveries were around 350. I was sent by two U.K. churches through the African Evangelical Fellowship mission and had only completed house jobs and 6 months of obstetrics. However, within 1 week of arriving I had had to do an emergency hysterectomy for a ruptured uterus. The idea of learning from two other experienced doctors was a good one, but unfortunately one was already leaving by the time I came. As there had been three doctors for the previous year and now this was reduced to two, and one a novice, the work was unrelenting. Learning the Zulu language was a priority and an hour or two per day was spent on that. For the first 2 years, most Sundays I was on call while my colleague went out to one of the distant churches. In church there was a lot of time for listening to Zulu, as sermons were generally at least three-quarters of an hour long!

My work now as medical superintendent of a much busier 185-bed Mseleni—with nearly 2000 deliveries, eight clinics, and a mobile team plus other community groups and services and a team of nine doctors—is quite diverse. Planning, budgeting, fund raising, control, discipline, committees, and letter writing fill a lot of my days. I still have clinical duties with ward rounds and outpatients and do on call as well as provide an opinion to junior doctors and do most of the major surgery. My special interest in the Mseleni hip disease has led to my performing total hip replacements and to a number of research projects. It has also led to the area of community sanitation and water development and job-creation projects. In each of these activities as well as in the church, I have found many opportunities to share the greatest treasure I have with patients, colleagues, and community members.

The public health care system in rural areas has been rendered through a system of rural hospitals and clinics, many of which were built and operated as mission hospitals until the 1970s, when most of them were then taken over by the apartheid government in an effort to centralize planning. These same hospitals now form the infrastructure for the new National Health System, the aim of which is to decentralize to a district-based health system. The infrastructure and facilities available in rural hospitals are relatively good, although diagnostic services are limited. Most rural hospitals offer a comprehensive service and are staffed by generalist doctors who are largely foreign-qualified. A survey in 1997 found that 76 percent of rural doctors in the public sector in KwaZulu-Natal were foreign-qualified, and the figure rose to 89 percent in the Northern Province. A handful remain from the mission hospital era, but most arrived in the country from other parts of Africa and from Europe in the last decade. As foreign-qualified doctors are barred from working in the private sector and most urban posts in the public sector are filled, the majority ends up in rural hospitals. Private practitioners in rural areas, by contrast, are almost exclusively South African. Foreign-qualified doctors have made a very positive contribution to the health service, as they come with years of experience in third-world health problems and find that conditions in rural hospitals are similar to those in their countries of origin, especially other parts of Africa.

In an attempt to alleviate the difficulty in recruiting medical staff for rural hospitals, the South African government entered into a special agreement with the Cuban government in 1996, in terms of which 300 Cuban doctors were recruited to fill rural posts. This was a deliberate move by the Minister of Health, who was impressed by the Cuban health system, with its emphasis on prevention and population-based health planning. Subsequently a further group joined them, and they have shored up the staffing gaps in rural hospitals to a certain extent. However, they have been somewhat frustrated by the language gaps and the curative focus of the health system.

The most recent attempt by the government to address the issue of rural recruitment is the controversial introduction of compulsory community service for doctors in 1998. Initially proposed as "vocational training," the scheme generated stiff opposition from junior doctors, who stated that they were not opposed to community service in principle but that it needed to be fairly and honestly implemented. Other professional groups are therefore also being considered for national service. Before they can obtain full registration as independent practitioners, medical graduates are now obliged to spend a full year of community service after their internship in a government hospital. Many of these are in rural areas, and rural medical staffing in 1999 improved considerably as a result. However, the compulsory nature of the placements has caused resentment and a negative attitude on the part of some of these young graduates, and in a number of situations there is inadequate supervision by senior doctors to ensure a high standard of care. Most are intent on seeing through their year but feel no obligation to remain in rural practice after they have completed their time. Despite these problems, most community service doctors are tackling the challenge positively and are making a significant contribution in areas of need. The opportunities provided by the year of compulsory community service are enormous but are unlikely to be realized until a system of postgraduate vocational training is officially in place. The longer-term effects of this program on medical recruitment and retention in rural areas remain to be seen.

Financial incentives to retain doctors in rural areas include improved salaries and a rural allowance. Public sector salaries for medical doctors and nurses were substantially increased across the board in 1995 in an attempt to stem the tide of health professionals leaving the public service and the country. In addition, a special allowance is given to doctors working in areas designated as rural through a formula based on the "hospitability" of the situation. In the opinion of most practitioners, however, this is inadequate as a significant incentive for the recruitment of rural doctors relative to the lure of much higher incomes in the private sector, or outside of the country.

Rural Doctors' Initiatives

Despite these government attempts to address the issues, many problems and inequities with respect to rural practice persist: the urban drain of health professionals continues, in addition to the flow of doctors into the private sector and overseas, leaving public rural hospitals short of experienced professional staff. However, rural doctors themselves have been instrumental in initiating a number of programs aimed at overcoming the obstacles and the isolation of rural practice by forming collaborations and organizations in support of rural practice.

A significant factor in linking up rural professionals has been through the use of electronic mail. Healthlink, a project of the Health Systems Trust, a nongovernmental organization supported by grants, has established a nationwide system for electronic mail at low cost. Although subject to technical limitations of the telephone system in rural areas, the project has brought rural practitioners closer through more immediate communication and made discussion possible across the geographic barriers of distance. The electronic discussion group "mailadoc" makes it possible for rural doctors to obtain answers to clinical problems from specialists in urban centers as well as from rural colleagues.

The Rural Doctors Association of Southern Africa (RUDASA) was formed in 1995 and has grown to a membership of some 300 since then. The annual conference and a quarterly newsletter have been successful, and the association has addressed a number of issues of importance to rural doctors. Among these are the regulations governing continuing professional development (the equivalent of continuing medical education), which was introduced in the country in 1999. Before now, there was no formal obligation for practitioners to maintain their knowledge and skills. RUDASA has successfully lobbied for the inclusion of distance learning methods in the regulations.

The South African Academy of Family Practice and Primary Care, the largest single national organization of family doctors, has played a major supportive role for rural practitioners. A rural practice task team was formed in 1992 to address the particular issues affecting its rural members, and a number of vocational training programs around the country arose from this initiative. Through its links with the World Organization of National Colleges and Associations of Family Doctors (WONCA), an active part has been played by South African Academy in the establishment of an international rural practice task group. This led to the successful staging of the Second World Rural Health Congress in Durban in 1997, hosted jointly by the academy and WONCA. With the theme "The Rural Practitioner: A Model of Health Care for the 21st Century," the congress portrayed rural practice as an idea situation for the practice of holistic and cost-effective medicine.[23] Speakers from developed countries shared the platform with those from developing nations, in keeping with the spectrum of experience of the host, South Africa. It was striking that the areas of common concern far outweighed the differences in context and resources. The recruitment and retention of professional staff in rural areas is a global issue, as is the balance between personal and community care.

A certain amount of attention has been given to the issue of surgical skills of the rural generalist. The Pan-African Association of Surgeons devoted a 1996 symposium to the identification and training of medical practitioners to deal competently with surgery in the rural setting.[24,25] As most surgery in rural hospitals is performed by generalists rather than specialist surgeons, the scope of practice is often limited only by the level of skill of the generalist hospital doctor. A recent study found that the range of surgical procedures varied enormously between hospitals, depending on the experience of the practitioners.[26] The majority of anesthetics given in rural operating rooms are local and regional blocks, as there are insufficient doctors for routine general anesthetics. Nurse anesthetists and "clinical assistants" are not recognized in South Africa as they are elsewhere, and there has been no effort to train a midlevel cadre of health worker, as the trend toward increasing professionalism among health personnel precludes this. Ketamine is used extensively as a single agent, especially in children, and many operations are performed by one doctor acting as surgeon and anesthetist simultaneously. The tasks of establishing norms and standards for rural practice, both in procedural care as well as the

vast spectrum of other skills required by the rural practitioner, lie ahead.

EDUCATION FOR RURAL PRACTICE

Overview

Little specific training for rural practice exists in South Africa at present. There is a large procedural element in undergraduate training as well as during internship/postinternship positions because of the high patient numbers in South African teaching hospitals, such as the Chris Hani Baragwanath, Groote Schuur, and King Edward VIII hospitals. Thus the focus on skills that is often the driving force behind rural training for physicians in other countries is less marked. This, however, provides students, doctors, and their teachers with a false sense of security, because they do not realize how different their context is from the rural one and how separated they are from the communities they serve.

The reality remains that traditional training still focuses on the specialist, within specialist departments; for the most part, issues such as context, community, and culture, together with strategies in primary health care and public health are poorly addressed. Rural physicians are mostly seen as second-rate doctors who refer disasters to their hospital-based specialist colleagues, becoming the butt of their jokes. This is the pervasive attitude that small programs within most medical schools are working against, usually offering too little, too late.

One notable exception is the University of Transkei Medical School, which has adopted an integrated, problem-based curriculum and aims to do much of its teaching within the context of clinics, health centers, and hospitals outside of the urban zone.[27]

Student Selection

Selection of students should be the first step in making changes to training. Major changes are taking place in the country, as the traditionally "white" medical schools (Cape Town, Witwatersrand, Pretoria, Free State, and Stellenbosch) are steadily increasing the number of black students accepted for the course. At present, though, the focus is on racial composition rather than geographic origin. Schooling for black applicants in rural areas is by and large very inferior to that in most urban areas and is likely to remain so for some time to come, given the enormous disparities that exist. Therefore, unless specific programs are introduced to assist rural students, their representation in medical schools is likely to remain disproportionately low.

One attempt to address this is a new state-sponsored scheme whereby students from disadvantaged backgrounds, with poverty and rurality included as elements in the disadvantage, are being given the chance to study in Cuba. The wisdom of taking students totally out of their context and training them in a foreign country and a foreign language in order to equip them to serve in areas of need in South Africa must be questioned, but it is too early to see what impact this will have.

Undergraduate Programs

The extent of exposure to rural medicine in the 6-year undergraduate curriculum is very variable but generally limited. Usually it is the community health or family medicine department that takes the lead in organizing rural placements for students, as no departments of rural medicine or rural health yet exist in South African medical schools.

The University of the Witwatersrand has a 2-week rural block in the final year as part of its 6-week community-based medical practice program.[28] In contrast, the University of Natal offers 10 days in the final year. University of Cape Town offers a 2-week rural option in final year.[29] The University of Pretoria has established a department of community-based education under Professor Detlef Prozesky, a former rural doctor.[30] It has also established satellite campuses in Witbank and Nelspruit, which are smaller towns. Similarly, the Medical University of Southern Africa has established a satellite campus at Pietersburg in the Northern Province in addition to its main campus at Ga-Rankuwa outside Pretoria. From there, students are sent into surrounding health districts. As mentioned, the University of Transkei aims to integrate clinical attachments in a variety of contexts into the curriculum at an early stage and is pursuing an integrated, problem-oriented curriculum.

Postgraduate Training

No formalized postgraduate training currently exists for rural practice. Many rural doctors wishing to equip themselves better for their task look to formalized academic family medicine programs. Each medical school currently runs a master's in family medicine program, which can be completed on a part-time basis. Most of these, however, are urban-based and teach a traditional curriculum in family medicine. The University of Stellenbosch focuses on teaching specific skills required by rural doctors, with training posts in secondary and district hospitals.[31]

An exciting exception to the norm is the master's program of the Medunsa Department of Family Medicine, started in 1979 by Professor Sam Fehrsen, a former rural doctor from the Transkei territory. Particular features of this program are distance learning, student-centeredness, patient- and context-based learning, and a needs-driven approach,[32] making it very appropriate for rural doctors, among whom it has been very popular. More recently, Professor Khaya Mfenyana at the University of Transkei (a Medunsa graduate) has also begun to develop a similar program in the Eastern Province, an area of great medical need and minimal resources.

A number of vocational training schemes have also been running in an attempt to develop the skills required by rural doctors. Small schemes around East London in the Eastern Province and Pietermaritzburg in KwaZulu-

Natal were set up under the auspices of the South African Academy of Family Practice/Primary Care. During these 3-year programs, trainees spent 18 months in secondary and tertiary hospitals acquiring specific skills and then 18 months in rural hospitals. Both these schemes have since been disbanded for lack of support. In 1994, a 2-year vocational training program was launched at McCord Hospital, Durban, funded by the Christian Medical Fellowship of South Africa, with the stated aim of equipping doctors to serve the underserved.[33] One month in each year is spent in a rural hospital. The program continues and is a strong one, but its success in getting doctors into rural practice has been limited by resources and the urban context of most of the training.

Other rural doctors wishing to develop skills have either done so on an ad-hoc, personal basis, with the support of cooperative hospital superintendents or have elected to follow the route of acquiring one or more diplomas through the College of Medicine in South Africa, mainly in anesthesia, child health, or obstetrics and gynaecology. As each of these requires at least a 6-month rotation through a recognized secondary- or tertiary-level training institution, they cannot be obtained during actual rural practice.

The main relevant distance-education diplomas available are those in tropical medicine and hygiene, public health, and health services management, each requiring a year of part-time study. No specific rural health education of this type exists.

EDUCATION FOR RURAL MEDICINE: THE PRETORIA EXPERIENCE[34]

The University of Pretoria Medical School was previously an Afrikaans medium, conservative and racially exclusive institution. The curriculum was traditional, and the total exposure of students to rural medicine was 2 weeks in primary health care clinics in fourth year and 2 weeks in a district general hospital in sixth year. However, it has been undergoing rapid change over this last 10 years. The Department of Community-Based Education was established in 1995, with the aim of introducing students to medicine in the community in general and in rural communities in particular. An agreement was entered into with the Moretele District of North-West Province for training to be conducted in Jubilee District Hospital and its satellite clinics. In 1997 a new curriculum was launched, which is integrated and problem-orientated. Community Based Education is intended to be an integral part of all blocks in the new curriculum. In their first year students are introduced to doctors working in both urban and rural settings and are given small research projects to complete. In the second year they spend regular afternoons in rural communities near Pretoria, investigating environmental factors in health and disease. In the third year they spend 2 weeks focussing on Maternal and Child health in the primary health care and district hospital facilities. Fourth year will include a 2-week elective, and then there will be 2 weeks in fifth year and 6 weeks in sixth year with the Community Based Education Department. Further involvement in the course is envisaged in future. At the same time the composition of the student body is changing rapidly.

Synopsis

In spite of the high percentage of rural people in South Africa, undergraduate and postgraduate training has focused on urban and periurban centers. The lack of development often found here and the vast needs have led to a failure to look beyond these in most cases. Medical schools, by and large, have token rural programs for undergraduates. A few attempts are now being made to equip graduate doctors for rural practice, but there is still a long way to go.

THE FUTURE OF RURAL PRACTICE IN SOUTH AFRICA

The District Health System

The challenge facing the South African health system is to be part of a comprehensive programme to redress social and economic injustices, and to ensure that emphasis is placed on health and not just on medical care. The South Africa Government of National Unity, through its adoption of the Reconstruction and Development Programme in 1994, committed itself to the development of a District Health System based on the Primary Health Care approach, as enunciated at Alma Ata in 1978. A National Health System based on this approach is as concerned with keeping people healthy, as it is with caring for them when they become unwell. These concepts of "caring" and "wellness" are promoted most effectively and efficiently by creating small management units of the health system, adapted to cater for local needs. These units—the health districts—provide the framework for our health system, so that a single authority can take responsibility for the health of the population in its area.[35]

The country is divided into 160 geographic health districts, which are grouped into health regions within the nine provinces. A range of health services are offered within these districts, including private general practitioners, traditional healers, local and provincial government clinics, district hospitals, and environmental health services. In many of them, these various role players have never spoken to each other before, despite serving the same community for years.

In each of these districts, there are interim district health management teams in place, struggling to overcome the past fragmentation of health services and to establish rational and equitable systems for the deployment of resources and the delivery of health care. The challenge of the future is to build a whole new system that is more equitable and inclusive of all the providers. It will take years, but the vision is now there: possibilities now exist that were unthinkable under the old regime.

One specific aspect of the new health system concerns the role of the primary care doctor in the district. This is currently poorly defined and results in much insecurity on the part of private practitioners as well as government doctors. To a large extent, doctors in primary care have been marginalized in the DHS in favor of nurse practitioners. The national health plan has opted to place professional nurses in the primary clinical role, but they have not been given the training and support necessary to fulfil this role adequately. Nurse practitioners in government clinics around the country struggle to cope with basic diagnostic and prescription issues as well as activities outside of their clinics, again with notable exceptions. So, for example, drugs are often prescribed according to symptoms without a physical examination, and precious resources are wasted on meaningless clinic visits that add no value to patients' health. A major effort in education and training is needed here, and primary care doctors need to be involved in this training on a systematic basis.

With a few exceptions, doctors have stuck to the roles that were appropriate in the previous health system: namely, a hospital-based curative role, with little impact beyond this. General practitioners in private practice have also perpetuated this curative role and have similarly been largely excluded in the process of setting up the DHS. The pivotal role of the generalist physician in South Africa has not been recognized, as it has in the National Health System of the United Kingdom and many other countries. Unfortunately and erroneously, the skills and principles of family medicine have been perceived as appropriate only for private general practice in South Africa, with little application in the public sector and of no relevance to primary health care and the DHS.[36] This situation needs to be rectified, and the principles of family medicine incorporated into primary care practice in the public sector as well as the private sector.

The District Medical Officer

The concept of a district medical officer in support of primary health care in each health district is currently receiving attention. This individual needs to be a part of but not necessarily the leader of the district health management team, bringing a medical perspective to the evaluation and management of health services at a local level.

There is a need for doctors who see their districts as a population at risk and who use every consultation as an opportunity for education and prevention, who are part of a network of health resources, and who help to manage those resources. At the same time there is a need for a human and caring health system in which doctors are committed to people rather than to financial reward or to a particular group of diseases or technical skills. Generalists are needed for the public health service who understand the context of their patients: their families, their communities, their cultural or traditional belief systems, their language, their aspirations, and their sources of stress. They also need to be effective teachers and should be actively involved in post–basic nurse education for the primary care role.

CONCLUSION

The underlying assumption of the idea of "social medicine"—that health and illness has more to do with the social, economic, and political determinants of society than with the health care system itself—significantly informed the current national health policy. As Kark noted in 1942: "Clinical services must be brought within the sphere of a broader social health scheme." South Africa has witnessed the results of ignoring this advice for half a century, as political events impacted on the health and well-being of millions of rural citizens.

So we have now come full circle, returning to a model of health care conceived in rural South Africa, taken up and developed in other countries, but suppressed in its place of origin by the apartheid era for 50 years. South Africa has now set new standards for a peaceful transition to democracy; as Mandela retires, the focus turns to the equitable delivery of services to all South Africans. The new policy of decentralization of health services and the political will in favor of equity mean that rural health care is likely to receive appropriate attention and resources in the future.

REFERENCES

1. African National Congress: *A National Health Plan for South Africa.* Johannesburg, 1994.
2. Gilliland J: Health legislation—a historical review. *South Afr Med J* 61:133–139, 1979.
3. Gelfand M: *Christian Doctor and Nurse: The History of Medical Missions in South Africa.* Sandton, RSA, Mariannhill Mission Press, 1984.
4. McCord JB: *My Patients Were Zulus.* New York and Toronto, Rinehart, 1951.
5. McCord M: *The Calling of Katie Makanya.* Cape Town and Johannesburg, David Philip Publishers, 1995.
6. Kark SL: *Promoting Community Health: From Pholela to Jerusalem.* Johannesburg, Witwatersrand University Press, 1999
7. Marks S: South Africa's early experiment in social medicine: its pioneers and politics. *Am J Public Health* 87(3):452–459, 1997.
8. Jeeves A: Public Health and Rural Poverty in South Africa: "Social Medicine" in the 1940s and 1950s. Seminar paper presented at the University of the Witwatersrand Institute for Advanced Social Research, March 30, 1998, p 2.
9. Kark SL: *Epidemiology and Community Medicine.* New York, Appleton-Century-Crofts, 1974.
10. Trostle J: Anthropology and epidemiology in the 20th century: a selective history of collaborative projects and theoretical affinities, 1920–1970, in Jones CR et al (eds): *Anthropology and Epidemiology.* Dordrecht, The Netherlands, D Reidel, 1986, pp 72–80.
11. Kark SL: *The Practice of Community Oriented Primary Health Care.* New York: Appleton-Century-Crofts, a Publishing Division of Prentice-Hall, Inc., 1981.
12. Salber EJ: *The Mind is Not the Heart: Recollections of a Woman Physician.* Durham and London: Duke University Press, 1989, p 103.
13. Gluckman H: *Abiding Values: Speeches and Addresses.* Johannesburg, Caxton, 1970, p 504.
14. Harrison D: The National Health Services Commission, 1942–1944—its origins and outcomes. *S Afr Med J* 83:142–146, 1993.
15. Reid S, Giddy J: Rural health and human rights—summary of a submission to the Truth and Reconciliation Commission Health Sector Hearings, 17 June 1997. *S Afr Med J* 88(8):980–982, 1998.
16. *White Paper for the Transformation of the Health Services.* Pretoria, SA Government Printer, 1997.

17. Makan B: Health personnel distribution, in *South African Health Review 1998*. Durban, Health Systems Trust, 1998.

18. Barron P (ed): *South African Health Review 1997*. Durban, Health Systems Trust, 1997.

19. Harrison D, Barron P, Edwards J (eds): *South African Health Review 1996*. Durban, Health Systems Trust, 1996.

20. Southern Africa Labour and Development Research Unit: *Key Indicators of Poverty in South Africa*. Capetown, Office of the Reconstruction and Development Programme, 1995.

21. Harrison D (ed): *South African Health Review 1995*. Durban, Health Systems Trust, 1995.

22. Botha JL, Bradshaw D, Gonin R, Yach D: The distribution of health needs and services in South Africa. *Soc Sci Med* 26(8):845–851, 1988.

23. Rourke J, Reid S, Naidoo N, et al: Report from the Second World Rural Health Congress, Durban, South Africa. *J Rural Health* 14(2):87–90, 1998.

24. Mazwai EL: Training surgically competent doctors for South African rural settings. *S Afr J Surg* 35:147–148, 1997.

25. Damp MH: A rural surgeon's thoughts on surgery in South African rural areas. *S Afr J Surg* 35:145–146, 1997.

26. Reid S, Chabikuli N, Jaques P, Fehrsen GS: The procedural skills of rural hospital doctors. *S Afr Med J* 89:769–774, 1999.

27. Mfenyana K: Holistic Care in the context of South Africa. Plenary address, 11th General Practitioners Congress, Sun City, South Africa, 1998.

28. Sparks B, personal communication.

29. Schweitzer B, personal communication.

30. Gibson R, personal communication.

31. de Villiers M, personal communication.

32. Couper ID, Fehrsen GS, Hugo SFM: The development of a distance learning programme for a Masters in Family Medicine for Rural Practitioners. Paper presented at the 3rd World Conference on Rural Health, Kuching, Malaysia, 1999.

33. Reid S. The McCord-Christian Medical Fellowship Vocational Training Programme. *S Afr Med J* 89:765–769, 1999.

34. Gibson R, personal communication.

35. Extract from A Policy for the Development of a District Health System for South Africa. Health Policy Coordinating Unit, National Department of Health, Pretoria, 1995.

36. Williams RL, Reid S: Family practice in the New South Africa. *Fam Med* 30(8):574–578, 1998.

37. Central Statistical Services, Republic of South Africa. *Statistics in Brief 1996*. Pretoria, 1996.

CHAPTER 29

Rural Practice in China

M. Roy Schwarz   Katherine Hill Chavigny
Zhoada Zhang   Huiman Ren

THE HEALTH CARE SYSTEM IN CHINA

China has a population of 1.2 billion people, or almost 25 percent of the total population of the world. It is a large, agricultural, developing country covering an area of about 3.7 million square miles (9.6 million square kilometers). About 80 percent of China's population lives in rural communities, according to the 1990 national census.[1] China's agricultural sector constitutes the main element of the national economy and health care concerns. In China, the size of the country, the large number of people, and the nature of the agrarian economy present a special challenge for the practice of rural health care. Just as the United States has problems providing health care in rural areas, so does China—only on a larger scale.

Rural health care practice in China must be viewed in the context of the total Chinese health system—a system that is different in many aspects from that of the United States and those of western countries in general. The existing health care system of China was founded in 1949; its organization remains highly centralized and multisectorial. Since the end of the Cultural Revolution and the ensuing opening up of China to the outside world in the 1970s, the health care system has been undergoing important social and political changes. These changes are especially significant given that China still describes itself as a socialist country with a proletarian dictatorship.[2]

In 1982 the Constitution of the People's Republic of China was adopted at the Fifth National Peoples Congress. Article 21 of the Constitution stipulates that "the state develop(s) medical and health services, promotes modern medicine and traditional Chinese medicine, encourage(s) and supports the setting up of various medical and health facilities by the rural economic collectives, state enterprises, and institutions and neighborhood organizations, and promotes health and sanitation activities of a mass character, all for the protection of the people's health."[3]

In 1977 the World Health Organization put forward a global strategy of health care for everyone by the year 2000. In 1979 the United Nations held a summit meeting on children's health, which produced the world declaration entitled *Existence, Protection and Development for Children*. The Chinese participated actively in these international activities and continue to support global strategies for health. Subsequently, targets were set in China for attaining health care for everyone by the year 2000, which, in an agrarian economy, called for special attention to rural areas. The "ninth five-year plan of national economic and social development" from 1994 contains "long-term objectives for the year 2010" that strive to accomplish health targets in the next century for the entire Chinese population. In this context, rural practice in China and the health of the farmers and their families are critical to the realization of the country's well-being and social aims.

Organization of the Health System

China has a specific system of government administration under which the health system operates. The State Council is the top executive body of the central government. In China the word *state* refers to the country's entire population. The State Council is the governing committee of China and is more accurately described for westerners as the "National Governing Council for the country of China." The governments of the 31 provinces, municipalities, and autonomous regions (PMARs) are directly subordinate to the State Council. Several ministries are organized and supervised by the council, such as the Ministry of Education, the Ministry of Industries, and the Ministry of Health.

The designation *Ministry of Health* in China is synonymous with *Ministry of Public Health.* The Ministry of Health functions at the discretion of the State Council and is responsible for the professional guidance of organizational units at all levels of government. These organizational levels are (1) the provincial and municipal levels, (2) the city government, and (3) the county and township—a level that includes villages' residential committees. Health institutions are organized under the auspices of the Ministry of Health and include many different activities for health care, such as hospitals and clinics, research and pharmaceutical institutions, health publications, universities and colleges for health professionals, and antiepidemic stations, among others.

Each administrative organization, such as the PMAR health bureau or the country health department, sets up several institutions in accordance with its service objectives, including the "department of policy and legislation and hygiene monitoring" and "maternal and child health." The organizations manage various offices and incorporate professional guidance and/or directives from higher organizations[4] (Fig. 29-1).

The system is therefore designed to be a hierarchical structure that promotes institutional coordination at the lateral levels of government administration. The overriding authority of the central government is established and maintained through units of organization that are social and economic institutions.[5] The main duties of health administrative institutions are to develop health policies, to design and execute regional health strategies and plans, and to monitor, manage, coordinate, and guide the work of health establishments. The overall aim is to promote the development of health-related enterprises and promote the health of the people.

Looking at the country as a whole, administration of health care in China can be divided into four separate parts: (1) those institutions organized and responsible to the Ministry of Health for administration, education and service; (2) health organizations responsible for industrial and other ministries; (3) military health institutions; and (4) public or nongovernment voluntary organizations.

HEALTH PROFESSION INSTITUTIONS OF THE MINISTRY OF HEALTH

Health institutions not only provide health services but also conduct research. There are eight types of health profession institutions in China under the Ministry of Health whose functions are explained by the focus of their service, as follows: medical services, preventive medicine, maternal and child health, traditional Chinese medicine, pharmaceuticals, medical education, medical research, health education, and publications.

MEDICAL SERVICES INSTITUTIONS   Medical services institutions are among the most important components of the health care delivery system. These institutions are grouped into a pyramidal structure, most often described as a "three-tier system" consisting of primary, secondary, and tertiary institutions, according to the level of care delivered to patients. The primary level consists of township or street-level organizations and neighborhood hospitals and village clinics. The secondary institutions include prefecture, county, and district hospitals. The ter-

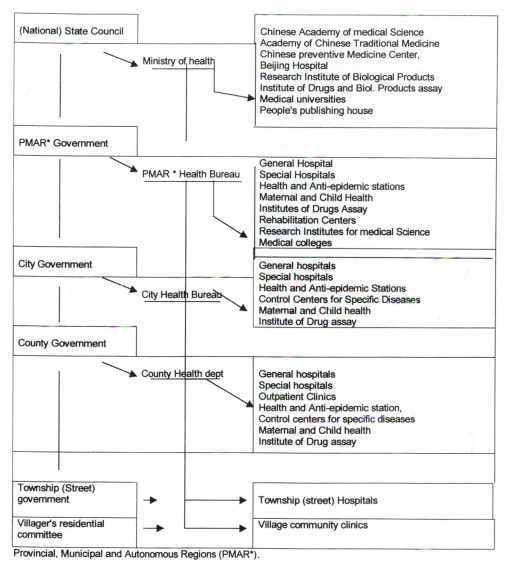

FIGURE 29-1 Organizational structure of the health system in China. (From He TW, Dai ZC: Organizational structure of the health system in China, in He TW, Dai ZC, Kang G (eds): Introduction to Health Administration. Chengdu, Sichuan, Scientific and Technologic Publishing House, 1986, p 32.)

tiary level consists of hospitals at the provincial and municipal levels as well as special institutions such as ophthalmic and oncology hospitals. As in the United States, tertiary-level institutions deliver the most complex, highly technical care through modern intensive care units and well-equipped operating rooms in large facilities. Tertiary institutions are responsible for comprehensive outpatient clinics; they offer enhanced preventive services and community-based health care as well as in-hospital services.

Primary, secondary, and tertiary institutions all have large geographic population bases to whom they deliver services. Rural care has few if any tertiary facilities; these are found almost exclusively in China's largest cities.

Medical education also follows the three-tiered system correlating with complexity of care. In general, higher medical education is taught in tertiary facilities and secondary medical education in secondary facilities; primary medical education correlates with less complex care taught in primary facilities[6] (Fig. 29-2).

PREVENTIVE MEDICAL INSTITUTIONS Usually, treatment (curative) and preventive care services are offered separately and generally in different locations in China. Preventive services are offered in the health and anti-epidemic stations, health quarantine institutions, special control centers for endemic and parasitic diseases, and other centers reserved for each type of infectious disease, such as tuberculosis, dermatologic problems, and sexually transmitted diseases. These preventive service centers are called Health and Anti-epidemic Stations and Centers for the Control of Communicable Diseases. The preventive medical institutions utilize practitioners who have different educational backgrounds from those practicing in the curative and diagnostic facilities.

Preventive services apply the theory and techniques of public health rather than accentuating the integrated principles of medical care and public health, as in America. In China, preventive services include the monitoring, supervision, and investigation of public health problems using epidemiology to study and monitor communicable and noncommunicable diseases and to collect morbidity and mortality statistics.

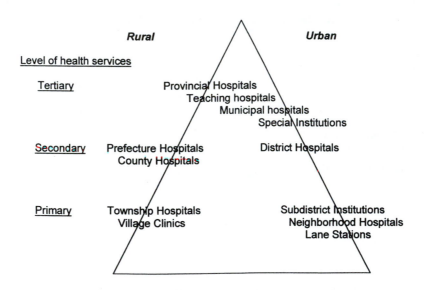

Note: The tertiary level of health services for rural and urban areas are provided by the same institutions.

FIGURE 29-2 *The three-tiered system of medical institutions in China. The tertiary level of health services for rural and urban areas is provided by the same institutions. (From Liu CJ: Three Tiered System of Medical Institutions in China. Department of Social Medicine, West China University of Medical Sciences, People's Republic of China. Chengdu, Sichuan, Scientific and Technologic Publishing House, 1998.)*

In the less urban areas, preventive care is also offered separately through medical institutions specifically dedicated to prevention and traditional public health services. They offer very few clinical services and are assigned to monitoring and surveillance of the community. They differ from the majority of public health clinics in the United States, which offer primary and secondary care with treatment capabilities. In 1996, there were 4919 health and anti-epidemic stations and 365 other preventive medical institutions within the public health system in China. This system had a total of 213,828 staff members.

MATERNAL AND CHILD HEALTH INSTITUTIONS   Maternal and child health institutions are preventive facilities that integrate clinical treatment and preventive services—the rare exception to the separation philosophy of preventive and clinical services. Maternal and child health institutions or clinics employ both physicians and (public health) primary care workers who provide both types of services for women and children. The services include family planning, premarital examinations, perinatal care, home visiting after delivery, developmental monitoring for children, and clinical management. Care is offered in either maternal and child health stations or in gynecologic and pediatric hospitals and clinics. In 1996 there were 2598 maternal and child health station within the public health system in China, with 23,000 beds and 82,400 health providers.

TRADITIONAL MEDICAL INSTITUTIONS   Traditional Chinese medicine remains popular despite the strong competition of western medicine, which is known in China as nontraditional medicine. The Chinese government continues to place emphasis on the growth of traditional medicine. Since 1949, the government has developed an important policy, namely "Combining traditional Chinese medicine and western medicine," and has established many research institutes, medical colleges, and hospital and pharmaceutical factories and plants for the

study and delivery of traditional medicine and medical care.

The main task of these institutions is to preserve traditional Chinese medicine and to investigate and develop traditional methods of practice. Their responsibilities include the training of modern personnel at advanced and intermediate levels and to integrate western and traditional methods of practice. In 1996 there were 2592 traditional Chinese medical institutions in China, with 237,488 beds and 347,846 physicians practicing traditional Chinese medicine.

PHARMACEUTICAL INSTITUTIONS   The pharmaceutical institutions prepare medications, conduct biological assays and research of biological products and related activities, and provide pharmaceutical plants for the pharmaceutical industry. They develop, produce, supply, and supervise drugs and biologicals and guarantee their effectiveness, their safety, and the rational use of therapeutic agents according to relevant legislation. They function at the national or state level as well as the city and county levels of organization.

WESTERN MEDICAL EDUCATIONAL INSTITUTIONS China has developed a stand-alone educational system in mainly western medicine that trains physicians for different levels of practice. The medical schools conduct medical research and their affiliated hospitals and pharmaceutical plants serve patients and produce drugs. These institutions also educate other health professionals and administrators of various ranks and carry out adult education for physicians, nurses, and medical technicians. They educate health workers in schools of nursing, schools of health administration, health worker colleges, and adult education schools. These latter organizations train health professionals and administrators of various ranks and carry out adult education for physicians, nurses, and medical technicians.

There are 10 key national medical universities that conduct medical education and function directly under the jurisdiction of the Ministry of Health. In 1996 there were a total of 123 medical universities and colleges in China, with 262,665 undergraduate students, and 550 middle health professional schools, which had 43,216 undergraduates.

MEDICAL RESEARCH INSTITUTIONS The Chinese Academy of Medical Sciences and the Chinese Academy of Preventive Medical Science are the leading research organizations. They conduct basic and applied research in medicine and collaborate with research centers in medical universities and colleges; they also interact with provincial or city medical schools. These organizations also identify, cultivate, and promote the distribution of scientific findings and are involved in international exchange of scientists and scientific information. In 1996 there were 401 medical research institutions, with 12,012 faculty members.

HEALTH EDUCATION AND PUBLISHING INSTITUTIONS Health education and publishing institutions include health education centers, health newspapers, and the people's health publishing organizations. The institutions act as information centers and clearinghouses for health knowledge. They study and transmit health information, seeking to correct health risk behaviors. The institutions report governmental health policy and principles, disseminate data on the status of health services, and publish medical books.

HEALTH INSTITUTIONS FOR INDUSTRIAL AND OTHER MINISTRIES
The ministries of industry, railway, and communications, etc., provide health institutions for their employees somewhat comparable to the occupational health clinics in large western industrial enterprises. These organizations in China are not administered by the Ministry of Health but by the ministry to which they are responsible. Their professional activities are supervised by their direct superior ministries and the local administrative organizations. These institutions deliver medical and public health care to staffs employed by their own system but may

also extend their services to parts of the local populations. They offer in-hospital services and medical and nursing care as well as other services for public health. In 1996 there were 10,239 health institutions of this type, with 750,201 beds and 1,337,637 staff members.[7]

MILITARY HEALTH INSTITUTIONS
The departments of health in the ministry of "rear guard services" of the People's Liberation Army—the PLA, direct these institutions. They include administrative organizations, the publishing house Medicine of the PLA, and the medical library of the PLA. All retired and current enlisted men of the PLA receive care in these facilities. The military institutions include military medical universities, the Academy of Military Medical Sciences, military hospitals, and local Ministry of Health Services centers. The military health organizations include medical education and research institutions

PUBLIC AND NONGOVERNMENTAL HEALTH ORGANIZATIONS
THE RED CROSS SOCIETY OF CHINA   The public and nongovernmental health organizations in China are similar to the voluntary organizations in western countries. The Chinese Red Cross Society was organized in 1904 and was recognized by the International Red Cross committee in 1912. It is a countrywide organization, which works in coordination with the government to encourage and coordinate people who are participating in patriotic health campaigns and medical and social services. Like the medical academies in China, the Red Cross fosters international friendships and exchanges. The Red Cross Society of China plays a very important role in providing assistance when disasters occur. For example, it set up an organ-donor coordinating association to facilitate organ transplantation. At present, it is one of the agencies that communicate with Taiwan for the delivery of medical services. In 1996, the Red Cross society had a membership of 22.8 million, of whom 1 million were trained as medical rescue workers.

VOLUNTARY HEALTH ASSOCIATIONS The China Medical Association, the China Nurses' Association, and the China Pharmaceutical Association were established in 1907, 1914, and 1915, respectively. Other associations, such as the China Association for Integration of Western and Traditional Medicine and the China Rural Health Association, were formed after 1949. Most associations have three levels of organization, national, provincial, and municipal, similar to the government organizational levels. In 1996 there were 57 voluntary health associations. The goals of voluntary associations are to organize scientific exchanges, complete and publish medical journals, popularize medical sciences, and make international contacts, and share information.

PRIVATE PRACTICE OF MEDICINE IN CHINA There is a small but growing sector of Chinese medicine in the major population centers that delivers privately paid care through the medical institutions. In some clinical facilities attached to the key universities, a floor may be dedicated to private patients. Private care was reported to make up almost 9 percent of physician practice in 1998, although this figure is not officially recognized (personal communication, 1998). It seems certain that private practice will probably continue to develop, especially when voluntary insurance becomes more feasible within China. This type of care is not yet available in rural communities.

Health Manpower and Health Education

Various disciplines are trained to provide appropriate health services in accordance with people's needs. For instance, when the hospitals identify a need for health technicians, they inform the universities and colleges, which activate their programs and recruit students to fill the need. The central government retains control of the work force. Work and employment rights are considered to be in the public domain. The government controls work units, such as medical institutions and pharmaceutical institutions. The government guarantees employment,

housing, and health benefits to all employees. According to Nan Lin and Gina Lai, the binding relationships between employees and the work units are firm.

Health manpower resources include professionals in clinical medicine, public health, rehabilitation, pharmacy and pharmaceuticals, nursing, health administration, and rearguard services for the military. In China, the average overall ratio between physicians and nurses is 1:0.73, according to a survey performed in 1995. In hospitals at the county level and above, the ratio is about 1:1. Rural hospitals and clinics use primary health care workers as well as nurses; a comparison of physicians to nurses in the rural areas is misleading, as it does not take the primary health work force into consideration. The education and training of health personnel, however, varies considerably from the cities to the rural areas. Professionals in urban county hospitals are better educated than those in less populated areas[8] (Table 29-1).

MEDICAL EDUCATION OF HEALTH PERSONNEL

EDUCATION OF PHYSICIANS The Ministry of Education and the Ministry of Health coordinate the organization and management of the medical education system. This system has three levels of health-worker training, which correlate with the levels of complexity of care. The first is higher medical education for tertiary care (5-, 7-, and 8-year curricula); the next is secondary medical education (usually a 3-year program); and the last is primary medical education (a 3- to 12-month certificate program).

For medicine, training programs vary in length. Some are 3 years long, others 5 years long, while others are 7 years long. One university has an 8-year program. The kind of recognition for successful completion of the training also varies, as follows: 3-year certificate, 5-year baccalaureate, 7-year master's degree, and 8-year medical doctor's degree. However, a great deal of experimentation is occurring at the present time, both as to length of training and curriculum content. This reflects, in part, a shift from a Russian type of model to a western model.

TABLE 29-1   HEALTH PROFESSIONALS IN VARIOUS INSTITUTIONS IN 1992

Level of Training	County Institutions		Township Hospitals
	Urban	Rural	
Bachelor's degree	20.8%	11.2%	1.74%
Higher education certificate	10.9%	14.2%	6.66%
Middle education certificate	48.4%	61.9%	38.95%
High school	11.0%	20.3%	19.75%
Middle school or below	8.9%	18.2%	32.90%

SOURCE: From *Education of Health Professionals in Various Institutions in 1992: China Health Annual Survey.* Ministry of Health, People's Republic of China. Beijing, People's Health Publishing House, 1997, p 407.

The 10 national key universities and research institutions identified and nominated by the (national) State Council also offer higher-level degree programs to train medical teachers and scientific researchers. They have programs of education for master's degrees, doctoral degrees, and postdoctoral programs for health scientists. The key universities are the most comparable to universities in the West.

Secondary medical education prepares health personnel in the secondary medical schools and colleges/universities that are operated by the local government, in contrast to the national oversight of the key universities. The education programs in secondary medical schools usually follow a 3- or 4-year curriculum. The objective of preparing physicians at this level is to fill any needs that are not met by the other programs. The candidates for the secondary medical education schools are those who have finished 9 years of general basic education. The work of these diploma physicians is limited mostly to outpatient clinics and rural areas.

Primary medical education occurs mostly at the local level and prepares the "barefoot physicians" through apprenticeship programs. The training used to be only 3 months in duration and now is usually about 12 months. The medical practice of certified doctors is limited to the villages and local clinics. Currently many programs encourage the village doctors to further their education.

The different levels of education define and rank "nontraditional" western-trained physicians as "high" and "midlevel" professionals. There are over 12 high-rank western-trained physicians per thousand population in institutions in China and 3 middle-rank western-trained physicians per thousand. All health professionals in China learn some traditional Chinese medicine even when they are enrolled in nontraditional programs.

Since 1949 both the absolute and relative numbers of health personnel have increased considerably. The total numbers of all employees in health institutions in China shows an almost exponential increase from 54.12 per 10,000 population in 1949 to 541.90 per 10,000 in 1996. In addition, there are physicians who specialize in traditional Chinese medicine, called "traditional professionals," who also work in hospitals and deliver patient care. These traditional physicians practicing Chinese medicine increased from 27.60 per 10,000 populations to 34.78 between 1949 and 1996[9] (Table 29-2).

The difference between physicians who work in urban areas and those who work in remote rural practice is not merely a matter of education, although this, of course, is important, as are the differences engendered by 5 years of training (baccalaureate) versus 3 years of education (diploma) and the certificate received by rural doctors, which can vary between 3 months and 1 year. The difference also occurs as a result

TABLE 29-2   THE NUMBER OF STAFF IN HEALTH INSTITUTIONS IN CHINA PER TEN THOUSAND POPULATION

Year	1949	1957	1965	1975	1985	1990	1995	1996
Total staff including nonprofessionals	54.12	125.44	187.23	259.35	431.30	490.62	537.34	541.90
Total health professional staff	50.50	103.92	153.16	205.71	341.09	389.79	425.69	431.18
Traditional Chinese Health Professionals								
Physicians	27.60	33.70	32.14	22.86	33.62	36.85	35.86	34.78
Traditional pharmacists	—	5.35	7.18	8.62	15.12	16.97	16.72	16.72
Subtotals	27.60	39.05	39.32	31.48	48.74	53.82	52.58	51.50
Nontraditional (Western) "High-Rank" Professionals								
Physicians	3.80	7.36	18.87	29.30	60.22	105.85	118.60	120.73
Nurses	—	—	—	—	6.83	43.15	63.38	67.43
Pharmacists	0.05	0.24	0.83	1.28	3.30	10.38	13.32	14.11
Other	0.04	0.19	1.25	1.27	5.67	15.37	21.09	22.48
Subtotals	3.89	7.89	20.34	31.85	75.02	174.75	216.39	224.75
Nontraditional (Western) "Middle-Rank" Professionals								
Physicians	4.94	13.57	25.27	35.61	47.28	33.12	36.48	37.45
Nurses	3.28	12.82	23.45	37.95	56.87	54.30	49.18	48.84
Midwives	1.39	3.58	4.56	6.49	7.56	5.84	4.90	4.90
Pharmacists	0.29	1.84	3.72	5.72	8.97	9.05	7.80	7.92
Other	0.33	2.35	4.99	7.07	13.27	12.91	10.39	11.20
Subtotals	10.33	34.16	61.99	93.84	133.95	115.30	109.75	110.31
Primary Care Givers								
Primary health care workers	8.69	22.82	31.5	48.54	83.38	45.93	46.93	44.61

SOURCE: *The Number of Staff in Health Institutions in China per Ten Thousand Population: China Health Annual Survey.* Ministry of Health, People's Republic of China. Beijing, People's Health Publishing House, 1997, p 409.

of limitations on practice through government regulation of all health personnel. These regulations compel less qualified physicians to restrict their practice in the cities to the outpatient clinics in hospital settings or to more rural areas. Most rural physicians receive training of this kind and replace, to a large extent, the need for nonphysician professional personnel, such as nurse practitioners and physicians' assistants. Diploma physicians and certified rural doctors are ineligible to practice in the cities; as a consequence, the retention of physicians in rural areas is less of a problem in China than in western countries.

All of these reasons do not account, however, for the differences in the numbers of available health personnel between urban and city areas. In 1996 the average number of physicians per 1000 persons in rural practice was 2.34 in the city compared with 1.08 in the county hospitals. Also the number of nurses in the city hospitals was greater than in county hospitals: 1.60 compared with 0.50 in the county. The same phenomenon of fewer resources for the less urban facilities is evidenced in the number of hospital beds per 1000 population, which is 3.49 in the city facilities but only 1.57 in the county hospitals.[10]

In Table 29-3, the county level is representative of rural practice. Initially, counties formed

**TABLE 29-3   AVERAGE HOSPITAL BEDS AND HEALTH PROFESSIONALS IN RURAL
PRACTICE PER 1000 POPULATION**

Year	1949	1957	1965	1975	1985	1990	1995	1996
Hospital beds								
Total	0.15	0.46	1.06	1.74	2.14	2.32	2.39	2.40
City	0.63	2.08	3.78	4.61	4.54	4.18	3.50	3.49
County	0.05	0.14	0.51	1.23	1.53	1.55	1.59	1.57
Health professionals	0.93	1.61	2.11	2.24	3.28	3.45	3.59	3.61
City	1.87	3.60	5.37	6.92	7.92	6.59	5.36	5.30
County	0.73	1.22	1.46	1.41	2.09	2.15	2.32	2.33
Physicians								
Total	0.67	0.84	1.05	0.95	1.36	1.56	1.62	1.62
City	0.70	1.30	2.22	2.66	3.35	2.95	2.39	2.34
County	0.66	0.76	0.82	0.65	0.85	0.98	1.07	1.08
Nurses								
Total	0.06	0.20	0.32	0.41	0.61	0.86	0.95	0.97
City	0.25	0.94	1.45	1.74	1.85	1.91	1.59	1.60
County	0.02	0.05	0.10	0.18	0.30	0.43	0.49	0.50

SOURCE: From *Average Hospital Beds and Health Professionals per 1000 Population: China Health Annual Survey.* Ministry of Health, People's Republic of China. Beijing, People's Health Publishing House, 1997, p 423.

"health units" established through the linkage of village, township, and county facilities. These health units were administrative and financial and established a referral procedure for rural populations. The health units constituted a vertical, three-level system attached to the collectives and were supported by government and local funds. When the reform of collectives to a market based economy occurred, this structure was reorganized mainly by shifting township hospitals from the county administration and promotion by the government of fee-for-service enterprises. However, county-level information still refers to rural practice conditions.[11]

NONPHYSICIAN PERSONNEL AND EDUCATION   In China the education for nonphysician personnel is not directly comparable to that of western workers. For instance, nurses are awarded diplomas after 3 years of education. Then, after an apprenticeship of 1 year in the teaching hospitals, the graduates sit for national registration. Candidates are eligible for entry into the diploma education programs after 9 years of basic education. National registration for nurses was

instituted in 1984 and is required by law for diploma graduates. Nurses seeking a 5-year baccalaureate degree must take demanding university entrance examinations and are trained with medical students for the first 3 years. Five-year-degree nurses, however, are exempt from the registration requirement.

Some student nurses, after 3 years studying with medical students, may opt to qualify as physicians with diplomas and work in clinics and rural areas. Most nurses work in hospitals and clinics run by the Ministry of Health. All nurses are responsible for patient health education in hospitals, but very few work as public health nurses in roles comparable to those of community health nurses in the United States.

The curricula in all medical school include general western medicine plus traditional Chinese medicine (TCM) and preventive medicine (more accurately, public health), medical administration, nursing, and short-term specialty training, especially in stomatology (dentistry).

In China the government retains control of health personnel. In recent years there has been a growing recognition of the compelling need to strengthen adult education and upgrade all health professional and technical education. Under consideration are continuing education programs—programs for graduates from medical schools at the tertiary, secondary, and primary levels. Adult or night school education is usually directed by various medical training centers, such as medical universities or colleges, adult medical schools, health workers colleges, health administrator training schools, and so on. Surveys in America have shown that retention in rural areas is better when the individual has resided in or has been trained in rural practice areas. The Chinese educational structure is organized to allow students to receive their training in local institutions, which increases the probability of retention of health workers in rural areas.

Financing Systems for Health Services

The money for health services comes mainly from national funds. The general financial policy is for every health institution to obtain its financial support from the government unit responsible for its administration. The National Health Service Fund is the national budget item that is routinely used for funding health services sectors by the government at different levels. There is another funding source for health care called a "construction fund" that is used for social security, medical education, and other targeted health costs. This construction fund is not included in the National Health Service fund.

The national funds for health care in China come from the government, from social enterprises (which take many forms of joint endeavors that integrate market-driven options with health care plans), and from individuals. Approximately 80% of the total health costs are financed through the government and group enterprises. The government funds for health care are gained through financial investments, charges to the public for medical care, investments through the basic construction fund, and some from charges for military medical care. Social enterprises include labor insurance, med-

ical care from the welfare funds in industrial enterprises, cooperative medical welfare funds in rural areas, medical insurance plans, and social medical aid.

Remaining health funds are garnered from individuals. These resources include out-of-pocket expenditures from patients and copayments for medical insurance. The cost of medical care is increasing and is expected to keep on rising in the future. In 1996, the average costs per patient per time spent in general hospitals were 52.5 yuan (US$6.50) and 2189.6 yuan (US$271) for outpatient and in-hospital services, respectively. These were 1.32 times and 1.31 times higher than those of 1995 and 4.8 times higher than those of 1990.

RURAL HEALTH CARE IN CHINA

The liberation of China in 1949 heralded considerable advancements in health care. Radical changes directly affected the whole of the Chinese population, including the many farmers and their families who live and work in the rural areas. National health policy called for the prevention of disease as well as early diagnosis and treatment. As a result, infectious disease rates fell dramatically and the overall mortality rates dropped from 20.0 per 1000 population in 1949 to 6.5 per 1000 in 1967. The infant mortality rate in 1949 rate was 200 per 1000. In 1973–1975, the rate was 47 per 1000 live births overall. The health status of farmers and development of rural health care delivery had improved considerably as part of the overall alterations in health policy by the new Chinese government.

After 1978 policy for health reform, the economic status of many agricultural areas changed for the better. In spite of these advances, the health status of rural dwellers continues to lag behind the health of those in the cities. The average life expectancy of the rural populations remains 2.85 years less than that in urban communities. In 1992 the infant mortality rate in rural China was twice as high as in urban areas. Liu and Hsiao report that in the very poor, remote counties, such as Yunnan near Burma, the infant mortality rate is three times the rate of average rural community. Unfortunately, the discrepancy between the health of rural and urban populations in China is real.[12]

The Development of the Rural Health System in China

Rural health care was organized into health units at the levels of the county, town or township, and village. In the 1960s and 1970s, wide health networks for rural practice were built on the basis of a cooperative health care system in rural China. Health centers and health stations were built at the county and town levels; the collectives utilized the production teams in villages and drew funds from public money for the building of cooperative health care clinics. The system educated village doctors, also referred to as "barefoot doctors," by selecting a farmer who would then be given at least 3 months of training to provide basic health services. Later this program developed into a 12-month training program, usually granting a certificate. The village doctor was paid through the award of a certain number of work points for the days spent in health care.

A collective economy was established through a Cooperative Medical Scheme (CMS), somewhat similar to a health plan. The CMS was a prepaid system that operated through its collectives and was organized into health units consisting of the three levels of county, township, and village. The communes and work brigades supervised the collection of welfare funds and the operation of the CMS. At its zenith, the free medical system and rural cooperative medical system covered 130 million people and more than 85% of the farming communes.[13]

In the late 1970s China began to overhaul the rural health care system following the Communist party plenum session of December 1978. The two main edicts were the decollectivization of the Chinese agricultural production system and the encouragement of a free market, with its accompanying pricing and production of ag-

ricultural commodities. The CMS, team-based, collective economy was converted to a household contract system, where families were responsible for their own contracts, which linked them to the production system.

The impact of health care reform was felt most keenly in the rural areas. Most of the collectives were weakened and many health units collapsed; the cooperative medical schemes deteriorated because they lost the financial support of the collective economy. Doctors in townships who opened offices and clinics had to live on their own earnings as the welfare fund supported by the collectives disappeared. Gradually, some cooperative clinics became enterprises consisting of individual businesses or joint clinics. In 1982, only 5% of village health posts were privately owned practices; however, by the 1990s, this proportion had increased to 48%.

Also by the 1990s, some 80% of all agricultural commodities were bought and sold in competitive markets. Multiple methods of economic development were promoted; the reforms were successful enough to increase the farmers' income, and in most rural areas income per capita rose. Nutrition, housing, and a healthier environment through cleaner water became available for many of the farmers, offsetting, it is claimed, some of the effects on health through the dismantling of the collectives. Many of the village "barefoot doctors" left health care for the more financially rewarding farm industries. Improved income for the farmers caused them to seek quality care at the county level, often bypassing the village and township facilities. In spite of the improvement in economic conditions, the difference between urban and rural health care remained, since the urban areas also benefited from economic improvements. This difference is particularly notable in very distant and very poor provinces.

As the compensation and management mechanisms of health centers changed, the percentage of the health centers' subsidies from the government decreased. Regular funding, including staff salaries of the state health centers, came mainly from the income received from health services and profits from prescription medications. As curative practice became more remunerative than preventive practice, many public health activities deteriorated. In these circumstances, the health centers were more likely to prescribe extra medications and to order unnecessary tests, as well as more profitable services, so as to ensure income.

As a result of the changes in delivery and financing, preventive health services were influenced negatively, including immunizations and maternal and child health programs. The system reverted to one where those who could pay received medical care but those who could not pay were largely without health services. Even cooperative health care systems, mainly financed by the agricultural community funds, now require all farmers to pay at least a nominal fee for their health care expenses.

In contrast, some rural areas, like Shandong and Jiangsu provinces, have retained some comparatively well-developed township industries with stronger collective economies that support their cooperative health care system. The old health units have survived by reorganizing their management systems and refocusing their goals. In these provinces, village-run clinics and village doctors are still actively working as part of the collective team. These successful cooperatives are relatively small in comparison to the size of the nation.

The change in the compensation and management mechanisms of health centers caused rapid increases in expenses for care. The average health care costs for a visit to a county hospital increased from 8.1 yuan (US$1) in 1990 to 18.1 yuan (US$2.24) in 1994, according to a survey conducted by the Chinese Ministry of Health. It increased 1.23 times in a period of 4 years, an annual growth rate of 22.3%. Individual health care payments grew fourfold from 1990 to 1995, which overtook the cost-of-living index by a large margin.[14]

As the collective system disintegrated in rural China, illness became one of the main reasons for impoverishment. The mushrooming medical expenses not only limited the farmer's basic services for health care but also became a big financial burden to seriously ill members. According to a survey conducted in 45 counties, 23% of farmers who became sick did not receive health services, and 25% of farmers who should have been hospitalized could not afford the high cost of health care expenses without assistance. Previous surveys had shown that 9.6% of the rural population use the cooperatives, in which health care is either free or has small deductibles; however, the survey also showed that 81% of the rural population had to pay their own medical expenses.

The State (National) Council of the Chinese Communist party has always considered that the countryside and its people are the focal point of government policy. To a large extent the collective system had provided the local farmers with free health services and ensured hundreds of millions of Chinese farmers the fundamentals of health care while optimizing limited health resources. The administrative organization of counties, towns, and villages, in conjunction with the cooperative system and the team of barefoot doctors, are still considered to be philosophically the foundation for the development of adequate health care practice in rural China. In the early 1990s, the National Council of the Chinese Communist Party and the State (National) Council called for the restoration of the cooperative health care units.[15] The national ninth 5-year plan included the important goal of "Primary Health for All by the year 2000." The key part of the program was aimed at the rural areas especially those areas that are impoverished. Currently the health care program in rural China is still precarious.

ORGANIZATION AND INFRASTRUCTURE FOR RURAL HEALTH CARE

China has hospital clinics and health stations in the counties, towns, and villages. There are also health and anti-epidemic stations and centers for the control of communicable diseases, health schools, and special preventive organizations, as described previously. County-level health institutions also function as preventive and treatment centers and are responsible for guiding health services, building up comprehensive township clinics for immunizations and child care, and launching public awareness programs for health and for family planning. Generally the village doctor and one or two health workers who are on the payroll in the clinic deliver care. In each village it is the clinic that is responsible for preventing and treating common and recurrent diseases.

To date, China has built its county, town, and village preventive and treatment health care organizational networks, in which traditional Chinese medicine as well as western care are delivered. In 1996 the number of China's county hospitals reached 2038. On an average, a county hospital had 67 doctors and 173 beds. There were 34,800 township clinics equipped with inpatient beds and 6967 township clinics without in-ward beds. The township clinic beds stabilized at 0.81 beds per 1000 people; the number of health workers reached 1.19 employees per 1000 people at that time. There are also 740,000 administrative villages or health units in China and almost 90% of them have health care clinics. The statistics indicate that the urban facilities have more resources and health workers than the rural areas. But, on the average, the latter appear to be within acceptable limits. Even so, availability of facilities and health personnel between rural and urban populations remains significantly unequal.[16]

OWNERSHIP OF HEALTH FACILITIES

The central government provides the national health institutions with funds for diagnostic and treatment services, for which China has adopted a low charge policy. The provinces organize rural health centers for preventive care, at the county and town levels, that is free of charge. The county hospitals are owned and run by the state. Township clinics are of two types, noncollective and collective. Some 58% of all township clinics are collective clinics, supervised by the town government, that receive subsidies from the state. Of other health facilities,

42% are affiliated with the county health bureaus and are state-run. More than half of the village health care clinics have adopted collective ownership or a combination of collective and individual joint ownership. Since the opening of China to the West and the reform of the health care system, self-owned, licensed village clinics are growing. A survey conducted in 1993 indicated that about 44% of the existing village clinics are privately owned.

HEALTH CARE FUNDING

THE PUBLIC SERVICE MEDICAL SCHEME   In China, the Public Service Medical Scheme (PSMS) refers to the provision of health care for public employees associated with government, partisan groups, government enterprises, and universities, including faculty and students. Rural health care is provided to partisan groups, handicapped veterans, and employees of the government at the levels of the county and the town. According to the 1993 national health services investigation, using a sample survey of 65 counties, 160,914 persons are covered by this system, which is only 1.6% of the total rural population and 14.5% of the nonagricultural population.

The average health care budget for each county rose 147% in the 7-year period between 1986 and 1992. The actual expenses in 1986 were cited as 599,000 yuan (US$74,134), increasing to 1,546,000 yuan (US$191,337) in 1992—a 158% increase. Overspending was identified as 15.6% in 1986 and 20% in 1992.

LABOR INSURANCE SCHEME   The national health care survey showed that nonagricultural populations who are employed by collective enterprises are included in the labor insurance scheme. They account for 1.13% of rural communities and 20% of the nonagricultural populations. People who enjoy semi–labor insurance schemes are protected in this category, which covers 0.27% of the rural population. Under labor schemes, the average health care budget for each county reached 1,120,000 yuan (US$138,600) in 1986 and 2,138,000 yuan

(US$264,600) in 1992—a 90% growth in this 7-year period. The actual expenses in 1986 were 1,580,000 yuan (US$195,550) and 3,580,000 yuan (US$443,000) in 1992. Again, overspending was a problem, increasing from 40 to 67%. Most of the people in this labor insurance scheme generally go for care to the clinics attached to their enterprises or to the county hospitals. A small number are referred to the hospitals above the county level.

OTHER HEALTH CARE FUNDING SYSTEMS   The Cooperative Medical Care Scheme (CMS) was widely developed in rural China in the decades of the 1960s and 1970s. In the early 1990s, when the central council of the Chinese Communist party and the National State Council called for the restoration of the cooperative health care units, another national health services survey was conducted. The 1992 survey showed little change from the previous investigation in 1988 (i.e., only 9.5% of the rural population use the cooperatives).

According to the Chinese Health Economics Society, health care has three basic types of organization: (1) health care for employees with the township enterprises, (2) countryside care, and (3) agricultural industry and commercial overall health care. They are funded as part of the work system to which they belong. As the economics of China have changed, township enterprises have grown rapidly. A fairly large number of local farmers have become employees of the townships. As a result, where township industries have developed, diversified forms of general health care have been established.

Health insurance pilot programs were launched in a few rural areas to experiment with the provision of western methods of funding health care. These insurance programs were based on cooperative health care and overall health care plans. Some of them were conducted by joint efforts from the insurance companies and the employers. Others were initiated through insurance companies alone. Only 0.33% of the rural population bought health insurance,

according to the Chinese Health Economics Society.

SELF-SUPPORT HEALTH CARE   There is a final category of health care funding called "self-support health care." Currently most of the rural populations have to pay their health care expenses—the average being 60 yuan (US$7.40) in 1992. Unfortunately, the funding systems for hospitals is also inadequate, and so unpredictable that it has caused between 40.6 to 60% of hospitals to have financial shortfalls. In addition, the national survey showed that 84.1% of rural populations must pay for their own health care as best they can.

Medical Needs and Utilization of Rural Health Care Services

Statistics collected in 1988 from a targeted population of 62,564 farmers in more than 20 counties and cities of 16 provinces revealed that the morbidity of diseases within 2 weeks before the study was 11%. Less than 13% of these patients had been to see a doctor, and the annual rate of hospitalization was about 3%. The survey showed that 20% of farmers could not visit a doctor because of inability to pay and 595 seriously ill farmers could not be hospitalized owing to economic difficulties. These statistics show that about one-fifth of the farmers did not benefit from available health care services. Stratification of the information from the survey by wealth of county as an index of socioeconomic status indicated that farmers in poverty-stricken regions are more likely to be deprived of medical care than those in more affluent regions.[17]

According to information from another survey completed by the Ministry of Health in 1993 showed that the medical needs of patients and utilization of health care services had both increased since 1988. The gap between the patient needs and utilization of care had become wider and wider, especially in the poverty-stricken counties. In 1993 the main problem occurred in hospitalization of patients. The average proportion of patients in China who had a need but did not receive hospitalization was 41% while the proportion in those areas designated as "poor" or poverty stricken was as high as 48% compared with 29% in the more wealthy counties (Table 29-4).[18]

Clearly, increased costs of care are widening the gap between medical needs and utilization of services. The cost of drugs and hospitalization, especially in rural areas, is rising at an alarming rate. For example, in the county hospitals, the cost of a clinic visit was 8.1 yuan (US$1) in 1990; it increased four times to 32.6 yuan (US$4) in 1996, with an annual 32% growth rate. The average cost of hospitalizations was 310 yuan (US$38.40) in 1990; it increased 3.8 times to 1182 yuan (US$146.30) in 1996, an average annual growth rate of 31%. According to this investigation, the per capita medical expenses of farmers was 60 yuan (US$2.45) in 1993, which was 9% of the per capita net income of 665 yuan (US$82.30). In one of the worst poverty stricken counties, 41% of patients could not visit a doctor merely because of unaffordable medical expenses, while 79 percent of the seriously ill could not be hospitalized for treatment owing to economic difficulties.

Effective use of physicians in practice for preventive and curative care is also declining. A national survey of general hospitals showed that in 1989, one physician served an average of 6.1 outpatient visits per day. This was lowered to 4.3 visits in 1993 and 3.89 in 1996. Furthermore, a national survey revealed that 32% of the patients who were admitted to hospitals in China had not followed physician's instructions, again decreasing the effectiveness of physician care.

It is not surprising that the gap between health levels of nonrural citizens and the farmers is growing, according to government statistics for 1996. Examples of this may be found in infant and maternal mortality. In the city, infant mortality averages 21 per 1000 live births, but it is 41 per 1000 overall in rural areas and 72 in those counties that are designated as poverty counties. Maternal mortality is 39 per 100,000 in the city and 80 per 100,000 in rural regions; it is as high as 503 per 100,000 in poverty-level rural counties. In addition, maternal health care in these counties is much lower in quality than that in the city. Only 29% of mothers receive prenatal care in rural areas (which drops to 18% in the poorest counties), compared with 96% in the cities. Another index, known as the ratio of deliveries in hospitals, is 87% among the city dwellers and 22% in the countryside, but it is 7% in poverty regions and as low as 3% in the impoverished counties.

TABLE 29-4   *NEEDS AND UTILIZATION OF HEALTH CARE FOR URBAN AND RURAL INHABITANTS, 1993*

	City	Rural Region	Wealthy Counties	Poor Counties
Incidence of medical complaints within previous 2-week time period (%)	17.7	12.8	12.4	12.7
Proportion of hospital visits 2-week time period (%)	19.9	16.0	15.3	15.7
Proportion of patients without hospital visits though needed (%)	42.0	34.0	33.0	37.0
Annual rate of hospitalization (%)	5.0	3.1	3.3	3.3
Proportion of patients without hospitalization though needed (%)	26.0	41.0	29.0	48.0

SOURCE: From *Needs and Utilization of Health Care for Urban and Rural Inhabitants, 1994.* Research in National Health Services. Ministry of Health, People's Republic of China. Beijing, People's Health Publishing House, 1994.

TABLE 29-5   NUMBERS OF HEALTH WORKERS IN RURAL CHINA PER 10,000 RURAL POPULATION, 1985–1990

	1985	1986	1987	1988	1989	1990
Total population of village doctors and health workers	129.3	128.0	127.8	124.7	124.1	123.2
Population of village doctors	64.3	69.5	72.4	73.2	75.4	77.7
Population of primary health care workers	65.0	58.5	55.5	51.5	48.8	45.5
Population of female workers	34.2	34.2	43.3	31.0	32.2	32.1
Population of midwives	51.4	50.8	48.2	46.7	44.5	47.1

SOURCE: From Huang YC: *Numbers of Health Workers in Rural China in Ten Thousand per Agricultural Population, 1985–1990: National Health Conditions in China.* People's Republic of China, Shanghai, Shanghai Medical University Publishing House, 1994, p 142.

Health Care Education and Personnel in Rural China

EDUCATION AND TRAINING OF RURAL HEALTH CARE WORKERS

Health workers in rural China can be divided into county physicians and village doctors, medical technicians, administrative officers, and primary health care workers. There are a total of 1,316,000 village health personnel, of whom 72.5% are village doctors and 27.5% are primary health care workers. A total of 1.45 providers per 1000 population were available in 1996 for delivery of services in rural populations.[19]

Rural medical education schools prepare primary health care workers. They offer a 3- to 12-month program depending on the focus of the worker. Primary health care workers are specifically trained for preventive services. These health workers are somewhat akin to "community health representatives" in the United States, who assist in the delivery of health care in underserved populations, as on Indian reservations. Primary health workers usually have 12 months of preparation.

PERSONNEL FOR RURAL HEALTH CARE

Even though there are fewer health personnel and health resources in rural areas in China than in the city, the total population of health workers in rural China seems to have remained relatively stable (Table 29-5). Some scholars attribute the decline in primary health care workers to the migration of these workers for education at a higher level. Other experts state that since the growth of the market economy, these workers have sought alternative employment in the farming industry. Nonetheless, most Chinese sources agree that there is an adequate number of primary care health personnel and physicians in rural areas at the present time.[20]

The numbers of all graduates from medical schools has steadily increased from 1949 through 1990. Within this group, the education levels of graduates also improved in the higher medical schools from 6.05 per 10,000 population to 36.86 per 10,000. The numbers of graduates from secondary medical schools have always been higher than the graduates from higher medical schools, and they, too, have increased from 23.84 per 10,000 to 80.62 per 10,000 in the 1985–1990 period. Presently, there are a total of 1334 health training schools being set up in over 2200 counties in China, which will become the bases for training primary health workers in the twenty-first century.[21]

THE FUTURE OF RURAL PRACTICE IN CHINA

Discussion of Problems in Rural Health Care

China is a country in transition. It is moving from a socialist society toward the incorporation of western ideas and customs that address its particular concerns. Nowhere is this truer than in the health care system; but the problems in rural practice are unique because they have the distinct imprint of the Chinese culture and its history. The familiar yardsticks for costs of care and access to care are applied somewhat differently. For example, transportation as a deterrent to accessing care—a familiar need in other parts of the world—is never mentioned in regard to rural practice in China. With these caveats in mind, it appears that the most salient problems in delivery of medical care in China are the following: (1) the need for financial reform, (2) the need for infrastructure and medical personnel, (3) the need for preventive services, (4) the need for telecommunications, and (5) the need for administrative innovation.

THE NEED FOR FINANCIAL REFORM

Costs of care are the most often quoted reason for problems in medical practice in China. Costs affect the rural and urban communities differently, as the poor are affected to a greater degree than the affluent, and the poor are to be found in greater numbers in rural areas. It follows that the increasing costs of health care prevent access to medical services more in rural China than in urban areas. What this means in practice is that patients in the rural areas are more often deprived of fundamental medical care than those in urban settings. In one instance a 12-year-old patient with miliary tuberculosis attended a clinic for diagnosis. The family allegedly told the medical staff that they could not afford the "expensive" medications. According to the clinical staff, he was therefore sent home with the expectation that he would die if untreated within 1 or 2 years.

Most countries are concerned about the costs of health care, and China views the control of costs as its prime concern, particularly for rural practice. The difference in China is that a collective system of health delivery had been in place since the 1950s. It is claimed that this cooperative system provided free care to the majority of the rural communities and at the same time applied judicious use of resources. This system is now being changed to a market economy through the incorporation of western approaches, such as health insurance and fees for services. China is struggling to hold onto its cardinal principles of socialism while incorporating western operations to help solve its economic problems. This mixing of philosophies is causing a considerable amount of uncertainty.

The rise in the costs of health care is prohibitive for patients with very low incomes. Investigation shows that the reason that many Chinese farmers, especially the poor, do not receive basic medical care is mainly due to lack of ability to pay. In addition, the burden of expensive medications is much heavier for poorer patients. Although the consumption of goods in poverty-stricken counties is lower than in the more affluent counties, the proportion of health care costs per net income is much higher.

THE NEED FOR INFRASTRUCTURE AND MEDICAL PERSONNEL

A lack of infrastructure and a lack of health personnel are *not* major problems in rural China. The long-standing difficulty of "seeing a doctor" has almost been resolved. Also, the total population of professionals in the field of health care is increasing year by year. Farmers in rural China often do not receive primary medical care not because of lack of infrastructure or physicians but because many rural residents, especially the very poor, cannot pay the for their care.

Resources for practice in facilities, clinics, and public health stations are available and are underutilized. Very few patients are not hospitalized because of lack of beds or medical resources or lack of access to a physician. The supply of physicians is adequate and retention of physicians in rural areas is better than in the United States and other developed countries. Again, not enough funds are allocated for these services. This is compounded by inadequate planning and inefficient operations.

THE NEED FOR PREVENTIVE SERVICES

It is important to emphasize that the main factor underlying inadequate preventive health services in rural areas is not lack of access to care. Access to public health services is facilitated through the infrastructure in China at all levels of government. In rural areas the "health units" consist of links between the county, township, and villages, constituting a reliable referral system. The health units may also be partly responsible for the deemphasis of transportation problems within rural areas. Also, in each county of China, there is an epidemic-prevention station in charge of preventive health care, and health centers are responsible for maternal and child health. This infrastructure remains intact administratively.

Many Chinese scholars believe that the deterioration of preventive care is due to the fact that most of the limited medical financial resources are spent on clinical medicine rather than preventive medicine and public health. As a result, the proportion of investments of time and money in rural health services is further reduced. It is significant that clinical and preventive services are mostly independent from each other, which hampers the distribution of community-based comprehensive health services within the changing system.

In order to solve these administrative problems, three methods are used by some preventive service organizations. One is to cut down expenses by reducing the services, another is to charge for preventive health care instead of delivering the care free of charge, and the third is to set up clinics to earn money through drugs sales. Fee-for-service preventive care clearly reduces the provision of these services to the rural poor. Some argue that only the improvement of environmental conditions through economic agricultural reforms can offset the rise in infant mortality and general health status.

THE NEED FOR TELECOMMUNICATIONS AND COMPUTER NETWORKS

Owing to the vastness of China's rural areas, the large numbers of people, and the poverty of many provinces, the development of telecommunications and computer networks holds great promise for the future. Government supervision of the rural areas is very difficult, especially in the villages. The government is acutely aware of the need to supply high-tech equipment, particularly computers, to health stations and village clinics. This would enable the gathering of reliable statistics and improve the accuracy of monitoring the delivery of health care; it would also facilitate assessment of the distribution and utilization of available resources in health administration.

THE NEED FOR ADMINISTRATIVE INNOVATION

The administration of health resources requires innovation. Finances remain limited for health care. In 1994, the health expenditure made up 3.81% of the GNP. This low level of expenditure means that many health care needs must go unattended. Excluding the cost of living, the average rate of increase for medical costs is 15% per annum. This is higher than the 6 to 8% increase in the GNP and higher than the increase in the personal income rate of 6%.[22]

Medical innovation in the financial, workforce, and material sectors have increased; however, some would assert that these improvements have been matched by a concomitant rise in the ineffective use of these innovations.[23] The social health insurance system is incomplete, leaving only a small percentage of the population with adequate coverage. In the past, the free medical system, specifically the public welfare medical plan for government employees and labor insurance for workers in large state-owned factories, as well as the Cooperative Medical Schemes, played a very important role in ensuring people's health. In recent years, medical insurance plans with individual contributions to the cost of premiums have been introduced in both urban and rural areas. In the rural areas only 20% of the rural population are covered by such insurance plans. The difficulties in adapting to the new concept of insurance and mastering the operational techniques necessary to be successful remain to be resolved.

Suggestions for Improving Rural Health Care in China

REORGANIZING AND STREAMLINING THE MANAGEMENT OF THE HEALTH SYSTEM

Some Chinese scholars regard the commune system of health care through the Cooperative Medical Scheme (CMS) as a more desirable method of delivery of care in rural China. The government is beginning to recommend some return to this cooperative system. The government has introduced policies of "civilian-run programs with governmental assistance, self-propelled within the resources available and a willingness to adjust measures to local conditions." What this exactly means is not clear.

Undoubtedly, in its time, the CMS improved rural health care delivery. What tends to be overlooked, however, is that the economy of China was already in trouble when the CMS was put in place; therefore a reversal in kind would not necessarily solve the cost problems of health care in China, especially if it is to be achieved at any high level of service. Perhaps of equal importance is that the "judicious use of resources" claimed by the cooperatives was and is overstated. The old CMS, despite its advantages, had serious administrative problems, including poor management and the lack of quality assurance and cost-control mechanisms. Also, corruption and self-interest were identified as the major problem of the CMS even before reform.

Health reform in rural China, therefore, does not necessarily require returning to "older" methods of delivery. The current era provides an opportunity to build new systems of delivery of rural care. For instance, the Chinese may consider building rural health maintenance organizations, which could be a model for rural care for the rest of the world. By combining the funding structure of health maintenance organizations with the infrastructure of the health units, a union between the collectives and western ideas might be accomplished.

This and other solutions would still require government and private regulatory mechanisms for cost containment. The Chinese government should also construct regulatory guidelines to ensure minimum standards of care. It is inevitable that the resources for rural and urban care will not be equally distributed—not in China or anywhere else, for that matter. In a country as vast as China, rural care will be associated with less sophisticated medical services. Nonetheless, regulatory strategies for controlling the use of resources and encouraging administrative reform would go far in assuring an acceptable level of care and should also help to contain the costs of care.

Changes in legislation should also facilitate controls on the market system and the government should enforce them. It is important to manage and supervise health services consistently and allocate resources according to local priorities. The health care system must be a dynamic force that responds to the needs and demands of the Chinese people.

ESTABLISHING FINANCIAL REFORMS

The application of western models of finance without consideration of the economic and cultural background of the health care system will exacerbate the problems in China. The core experiences from western countries—such as private health insurance, fee for service, and health maintenance organizations—must be adapted to the uniqueness of China itself. They are not transferable in western form. Experiments in China have demonstrated that health insurance for low-income groups is feasible, but a coordinated system is needed to operate such an insurance scheme.

The acquisition of money to invest in the health system is not a solution in and of itself, as the West has learned all too well. Without thoughtful planning and focused goals, no amount of fiscal resources will be sufficient. Targeted goals for their system within the fiscal constraints of the Chinese people must be developed. The goals may target selected groups of people, diseases, or regions, but it will have to take into account the unique needs of the rural areas if it is to be a success. That no other country has been able to accomplish this is scarcely a sufficient reason not to try.[24]

COMPUTERIZING MEDICAL PRACTICE IN THE HEALTH CARE SYSTEM

The use of computers and other technical advances is already being established in the provinces and urban areas of affluence in China. It is already known that the increased use of computers through local and wide-area networks improves the monitoring of emerging health problems and assists in the appropriate allocation of resources. Priority should be given to these technical advancements so that the Chinese people in both rural and urban areas can benefit from improved communications and medical practices. The monitoring of health indices should be a key strategy to enhance planning of care and economic development. If rural care is to be improved, it will have to be based on access to reliable information. Only through the availability of relevant current data can the impact of services in poverty-stricken areas be estimated.

Telemedicine can be a powerful method of improving care in rural areas through making the consultation services of specialists available to all and to make distance learning available to rural physicians. Although this is expensive, with careful planning it could be a method of bringing medical care to many farmers who have little or no access to modern medicine. Sophisticated telemedical centers are already available in the ten key Universities.

DEVELOPING COMPREHENSIVE COMMUNITY-BASED HEALTH SERVICES

Preventive medicine in China is confined to public health management, and preventive care is, for the most part, split from medical care. In China, public health and medical practice are parallel systems in terms of both application and education.

In contrast, preventive care is closely integrated into family practice and preventive medicine in the United States. The role of physicians emphasizes treatment and secondary prevention. Early diagnosis of preventable conditions necessitates the use of public health skills such as epidemiology and environmental health. These skills combined with those of curative medicine contribute to comprehensive care in any setting. Comprehensive care by definition must include the simultaneous delivery of curative and preventive care.

Chinese scholars point with pride to their successes in reducing rates of infant and maternal mortality and morbidity, even though rural rates are still higher than urban rates. They assign their success to effective prenatal and child care. In China, curative and preventive care were combined *only* in the maternal and child care clinics. It is not a coincidence that many of the most significant accomplishments of the Chinese health care system have come through the combined practice of medical and public health skills in those areas where they have been applied.

Nowhere is the combination of curative and preventive skills more needed than in rural China. This represents a major frontier for the future. The existing infrastructure sets the stage for an unprecedented marriage of these two tracks of medicine. However, for this future to be realized, a major modification must be made in the education of all levels of physicians.

CONCLUSIONS

The reforms currently taking place in China present the opportunity for rebuilding a unique system of health care. With change, it will be possible for physicians and primary health care workers together to deliver services for the good of the Chinese rural communities and for the improvement of the health of all the Chinese people. When comprehensive care is linked with other initiatives of financial reform and administrative change that are supported by effective technical communication networks, the Chinese system of health care will be able to meet most of the needs of the people. Not only can these changes benefit rural medical practice in China, but they can also provide models that could be adaptable to all the countries in the world.

ACKNOWLEDGMENTS

The invaluable help, consultation, and assistance of the following professors in preparing this manuscript are gratefully acknowledged. Their unfailing courtesy and good humor made their contributions to this work an invaluable experience in international cooperation and scholarship.

- Dr. Gao Jianmin, Dean and Professor of Health Administration, Xi'an Medical University Xi'an, Shaanxi, People's Republic of China
- Dr. Li Bing-Yu, Professor. Department of Social Medicine, School of Public Health, West China University of Medical Sciences, Chengdu, Sichuan, Peoples Republic of China
- Dr. Liu Chao-jie, Associate Professor Department of Social Medicine School of Public Health, West China University of Medical Sciences, Chengdu, Sichuan, People's Republic of China

REFERENCES

1. *China Population Statistical Yearbook 1990.* State Statistical Bureau, People's Republic of China. Beijing, Science and Technology Publishing House, 1991.
2. Liang HC: Health care in China; lecture delivered at Yale University, 1986; and personal communication, 1998.
3. *Constitution of the People's Republic of China.* Beijing, Foreign Language Press, 1982.
4. He TW, Dai ZC: Organizational structure of the health system in China, in He TW, Dai ZC, Kang G (eds): *Introduction to Health Administration.* Chengdu, Sichuan, Scientific and Technologic Publishing House, 1986, p 32.
5. Lin N, Lai G: Urban stress in China. *Soc Sci Med* 41(8):1131–1145, 1995.
6. Liu CJ: *Three Tiered System of Medical Institutions in China.* Department of Social Medicine, West China University of Medical Sciences, People's Republic of China. Chengdu, Sichuan, Scientific and Technologic Publishing House, 1998.
7. China Health Annual Survey: Ministry of Health. People's Republic of China. Beijing People's Health Publishing House, 1997, p 413.
8. *Education of Health Professionals in Various Institutions in 1992: China Health Annual Survey.* Ministry of Health, People's Republic of China. Beijing, People's Health Publishing House, 1997, p 407.
9. *The Number of Staff in Health Institutions in China per Ten Thousand Population: China Health Annual Survey.* Ministry of Health, People's Republic of China. Beijing, People's Health Publishing House, 1997, p 409.
10. *Average Hospital Beds and Health Professionals per 1000 Population: China Health Annual Survey.* Ministry of Health, People's Republic of China. Beijing, People's Health Publishing House, 1997, p 423.
11. Xiang Z, Hillier S: The reform of the Chinese health care system—county level changes: the Jiangxi Study. *Soc Sci Med* 41(8):1057–1064, 1995.
12. Liu YL, Hsiao CL, et al: Transformation of China's rural health care financing. *Soc Sci Med* 41(8): 1085–1093, 1995.
13. *Research on Rural Health Care System in China.* Ministry of Health, People's Republic of China. Shanghai, Shanghai Scientific & Technologic Publishing House, 1991.
14. *China Flagship Course on Health Sector Reform and Sustainable Financing.* China network for training and research in health economics and financing, unit three. CNEF. People's Republic of China. 1998, p 159.
15. *Survey Materials on Number of Health Services.* Ministry of Health: People's Republic of China. 1986.
16. *National Health Statistics Yearbook.* Ministry of Health, People's Republic of China. Beijing, People's Publishing House, 1997.
17. Gu XY: *Research on the Health Care System in Rural China.* People's Republic of China. Shanghai Science and Technology Publishing House. 1991.

18. *Needs and Utilization of Health Care for Urban and Rural Inhabitants, 1994*. Research in National Health Services. Ministry of Health, People's Republic of China. Beijing, People's Health Publishing House, 1994.

19. Huang YC: *National Health Conditions in China*. People's Republic of China. Shanghai Medical University Publishing House, 1994.

20. Huang YC: *Numbers of Health Workers in Rural China in Ten Thousand per Agricultural Population, 1985–1990: National Health Conditions in China*. People's Republic of China. Shanghai, Shanghai Medical University Publishing House, 1994, p 142.

21. Huang YC: *National Health Conditions in China*. People's Republic of China. Shanghai Medical University Publishing House, 1994, p 139.

22. *China Health Annual Survey*. Ministry of Health, Beijing, People's Health Publishing, 1997, p 140.

23. *National Health Survey*. Beijing, Ministry of Health, 1997, p 150.

24. *China Health Care Finance Study: Health Care Financing Reform 1990–2001*. China and Mongolia Department of Human Development. Washington DC, World Bank, September 1995.

Epilogue

For centuries rural life has been idealized as a pastoral, peaceful, and extremely desirable state of being. From Virgil's ancient exclamation of "Happy are those who worship the rural gods" to Garrison Keeler's recent assertions that Lake Woebegone is a place "where all the children are above average, the women are strong, and the men are good-looking," authors have told their readers that the "good life" is to be found in rural places.

As we enter the new millennium, it is an inescapable truth that good health care is an essential underpinning of the "good life." Yet the presence of good rural health care is by no means a certainty. As our world shrinks into a global village, there is no doubt that the challenges of providing optimal health care for rural people transcend national borders. The universal nature of the underlying "givens" of distance, population density, and scarcity of resources ensure that both problems and solutions will not be limited by place or country.

In spite of many challenges, there are numerous reasons to be optimistic. As detailed in the pages of this book, many factors are now present that *may* imbue the future of rural health care with positive attributes. Research providing evidence-based answers to important rural health questions, the absence of effects of distance on the travel of electrons or photons, systems management, clinical advances, educational progress, and social advances all provide us with strong reasons to be hopeful about the future. It is our hope that this book will be useful to those who face these challenges.

Editors

Index

ISBN 0-07-134540-X

90000

9 780071 345408

GEYMAN/RURAL MEDICINE